REDUCING RISKS FOR

Mental Disorders

FRONTIERS FOR PREVENTIVE INTERVENTION RESEARCH

Patricia J. Mrazek and Robert J. Haggerty
Editors

Committee on Prevention of Mental Disorders

Division of Biobehavioral Sciences and Mental Disorders

INSTITUTE OF MEDICINE

NATIONAL ACADEMY PRESS
Washington, D.C.   1994

NATIONAL ACADEMY PRESS • 2101 Constitution Avenue, NW • Washington, D.C. 20418

NOTICE: The project that is the subject of this report was approved by the Governing Board of the National Research Council, whose members are drawn from the councils of the National Academy of Sciences, the National Academy of Engineering, and the Institute of Medicine. The members of the committee responsible for this report were chosen for their special competences and with regard for the appropriate balance.

This report has been reviewed by a group other than the authors according to procedures approved by a Report Review Committee consisting of members of the National Academy of Sciences, the National Academy of Engineering, and the Institute of Medicine.

The Institute of Medicine was chartered in 1970 by the National Academy of Sciences to enlist distinguished members of the appropriate professions in the examination of policy matters pertaining to the health of the public. In this, the Institute acts under both the Academy's 1863 congressional charter responsibility to be an advisor to the federal government and its own initiative in identifying issues of medical care, research, and education. Dr. Kenneth I. Shine is the president of the Institute of Medicine.

The work on which this project is based was performed pursuant to Contract No. NIMH-OD-91–0014 with the National Institute of Mental Health.

Committee on Prevention of Mental Disorders

ROBERT J. HAGGERTY* *(Chair)*, Professor of Pediatrics Emeritus, University of Rochester School of Medicine and Dentistry, Rochester, New York

BEATRIX A. HAMBURG* *(Vice-Chair)*, President, William T. Grant Foundation, New York, New York

WILLIAM R. BEARDSLEE, Associate Professor of Psychiatry, Harvard Medical School, Boston, Massachusetts

ROLAND D. CIARANELLO, Professor of Psychiatry and Behavioral Sciences, Stanford University Medical Center, Stanford, California

JOSEPH T. COYLE,* Eben S. Draper Professor of Psychiatry and of Neuroscience, Chair of the Consolidated Department of Psychiatry, Harvard Medical School, Belmont, Massachusetts

WILLIAM W. EATON, Professor, Department of Mental Hygiene, School of Hygiene and Public Health, The Johns Hopkins University Hospital, Baltimore, Maryland

J. DAVID HAWKINS, Professor and Director, Social Development Research Group, School of Social Work, University of Washington, Seattle, Washington

FRITZ A. HENN, Professor and Chairman, Department of Psychiatry and Behavioral Medicine, State University of New York at Stony Brook, Stony Brook, New York

ROBERT P. LIBERMAN, Professor of Psychiatry, UCLA School of Medicine; Director, Clinical Research Center for Schizophrenia, Los Angeles, California

BEVERLY B. LONG, Chair, International Committee on Primary Prevention, and President-Elect, World Federation for Mental Health, Atlanta, Georgia

SPERO M. MANSON, Professor and Director, National Center for American Indian and Alaska Native Mental Health Research, University of Colorado Health Sciences Center, Denver, Colorado

DAVID MECHANIC,*† Director, Institute for Health, Health Care Policy, and Aging Research, Rutgers University, New Brunswick, New Jersey

RICARDO F. MUÑOZ, Professor of Psychology, University of California, San Francisco, San Francisco General Hospital, San Francisco, California

HERBERT W. NICKENS, Vice-President of Minority Health, Education, and Prevention, Association of American Medical Colleges, Washington, D.C.

RICHARD H. PRICE, Professor of Psychology and Research Scientist, Institute for Social Research, University of Michigan, Ann Arbor, Michigan

NAOMI RAE GRANT, Professor and Head, Division of Child Psychiatry, Department of Psychiatry, The University of Western Ontario, London, Ontario, Canada

---

*IOM Member
†NAS Member

Preface

Mental disorders cause an enormous burden on affected individuals, their families, and society. While impressive advances have been made in the past two decades in defining, diagnosing, and treating many of the major mental illnesses once they become full blown, many of these disorders are characterized by a chronic or relapsing course that has high personal and economic costs to all concerned. Cures are rare. Therefore, the logic of trying to prevent the occurrence of mental disorders is clear. Yet, in sharp contrast to the situation in the physical diseases, efforts to prevent mental disorders have had low priority. Many voices have been raised to correct this gap, including Congress, who charged the Institute of Medicine to prepare an integrated report of current research with policy-oriented and detailed long-term recommendations for a prevention research agenda for mental disorders.

The committee appointed by the IOM to carry out this task provided the diversity, the wide view, and the expert knowledge that this field demands. It included a range of disciplines, including adult and child psychiatry, psychology, pediatrics, epidemiology, sociology, anthropology, and public advocacy (see Appendix B).

The committee's process was a multipronged effort. It involved extensive review of a literature that is large in volume but limited in rigorous evaluation of interventions. Conferences were convened with experts who had conducted large-scale interventions to prevent physical diseases, and with experts in the fields of ethics and cultural diversity; and there were spirited committee meetings, in which the form and substance of the report were debated with an eye towards forging consensus in the final report. The committee examined some agency budget figures, but it was difficult to get firm data. In addition, several background papers were commissioned (see Appendix D). Committee members themselves contributed to many of the technical sections of the report. The conclusions and recommendations the committee makes in this report are based on its best judgment of the information and data that were available for review.

The committee concludes that the federal government should take several actions. For some mental disorders there have now been sufficient advances in knowledge to warrant the prompt mounting of intensive interventions designed to prevent mental disorders, so long as these programs are rigorously evaluated. For other conditions there is still the need for development of an adequate knowledge base before sound theoretically-based interventions are warranted. For the field in general there needs to be support for training of a cadre of investigators and for coordination of the currently fragmented efforts in prevention of mental disorders across the many departments of government and the private sector.

The committee recognized early that disparate definitions of the field of prevention were causing confusion in preventing mental disorders. The committee, therefore, developed a set of definitions to provide common terminology and to help achieve a common understanding of what is being done in the field. To date, the definitions have been so broad and flexible that almost everything has been labeled prevention at one time or another. The committee's more restrictive definition excludes interventions aimed at reducing recurrences among patients with diagnosed illnesses. Instead, we have labeled such programs as a part of good treatment. While there are honorable differences of opinion as to whether this should be called prevention, the committee recommends that for purposes of monitoring federal research and demonstration efforts, prevention research be limited to processes that occur before there is a diagnosable mental illness. When the new definition of prevention is used, we will be able to understand better what is being done in prevention per se. Our estimate is that the field of research on true prevention of mental illness, by our definition, is very small.

The committee recognizes the considerable barriers to progress in the prevention field. Currently there is little evidence from research that any specific mental disorder can be prevented. There is, however, considerable evidence that certain risk factors (some of which are causal of and some only markers of mental disorders) have been clearly identified. Using the model found effective in the prevention of physical disorders, it seems quite appropriate to initiate interventions designed to reduce these identified risk factors (and also to enhance known protective factors) with rigorous evaluations of outcomes. One advantage of targeting interventions on risk factors is that certain clusters of them are common to several disorders, and the potential for reducing more than one disorder by comprehensive intervention is appealing and is likely to be more cost effective.

For other disorders the knowledge base is yet too small and must be further developed before theoretically sound interventions can be tested. Promising areas of research are delineated. For many mental disorders, there is now convincing evidence for a genetic predisposition, but in practically all disorders there is also evidence that the genetic factors do not act alone, and that environmental factors can precipitate, or delay, onset. Therefore, research on understanding the causes of mental disorders must integrate biologic and behavioral sciences. In addition, there is considerable evidence that many mental disorders are brought on by physical diseases and that behavioral factors initiate or delay onset of physical disease. The committee urges more research in the interactions between physical and mental disorders.

The quality of the Institute of Medicine staff was crucial to the development of this report. Dr. Patricia J. Mrazek, the study director, brought a background in both service experience and research expertise, together with her organizational skills and uncompromising attention to scientific evidence, to all aspects of the committee's work. She did most of the writing of the report, ably assisted by Carolyn Peters and Carol Hospenthal. We are very grateful for their skills and dedication.

We believe that the U.S. Congress was wise to initiate this timely review of the field of prevention of mental disorders. The field is so important that the nation must invest the relatively small amounts recommended in this report to capitalize on the advances already made and to develop the knowledge base necessary for future advances. The one-third of our nation who today face the threat of mental disorder during their lifetime will be immediate beneficiaries when effective prevention programs are implemented, and the nation as a whole will ultimately benefit from the lifting of the burden mental disorders placed upon it. The time is right to move ahead with a national agenda to prevent mental disorders.

ROBERT J. HAGGERTY, M.D., *Chair*
BEATRIX A. HAMBURG, M.D., *Vice-Chair*

Acknowledgments

The Committee on Prevention of Mental Disorders expresses its appreciation to the agencies within the Department of Health and Human Services that co-funded this 24-month study: the National Institute of Mental Health (NIMH); the Administration on Children, Youth, and Families; the Maternal and Child Health Bureau; the Center for Substance Abuse Prevention; the Office of the Assistant Secretary for Planning and Evaluation; the Office of the Assistant Secretary for Health; and the Office of Disease Prevention and Health Promotion.

Many people outside of the committee contributed to this study in various ways. The committee gratefully acknowledges the enthusiastic support of Dr. Juan Ramos, Deputy Director of Prevention at NIMH and project officer for this study; the excellent assistance of Roseanne Price, who collaborated in the editing and writing of the report; and all of those who contributed by writing commissioned background papers, providing technical reviews of drafts of chapters, and making presentations to the committee. Many others contributed by providing preventive intervention research or service program materials, technical and funding information, and moral support. To all of you, the committee offers its sincere gratitude. The names and affiliations of contributors are listed in Appendix B; additionally, authors of commissioned papers are acknowledged in the relevant chapters. To anyone who was overlooked, please accept the committee's apologies and appreciation.

Abstract

Hardly a family in America has been untouched by mental illness. As many as one third of American adults will suffer a diagnosable mental disorder sometime in their life, and 20 percent have a mental disorder at any given time. Although research on the causes and treatment of mental disorders remains vitally important—and indeed major advances are leading to better lives for increasing numbers of people— much greater effort than ever before needs to be directed to prevention.

The Senate Appropriations Committee of the U.S. Congress believed that a strategic approach to the prevention of mental disorders was warranted. The Congress mandated the National Institute of Mental Health to enter into an agreement with the Institute of Medicine (IOM) to prepare an integrated report of current research with policy-oriented and detailed long-term recommendations for a prevention research agenda.

The specific tasks of the IOM committee, as negotiated with NIMH and the co-funding agencies, were as follows:

- Review the status of current research on the prevention of mental illness and problem behaviors and on the promotion of mental health throughout the life span. This should include an understanding of available research knowledge, research priorities, and research opportunities in the prevention research area.
- Review the existing federal presence in the prevention of mental disorders and the promotion of mental health, spanning the continuum from research to policy and services.
- Provide recommendations on federal policies and programs of

research support leading to a prevention research agenda as well as on opportunities for maximization of involvement and improvement of coordination among federal agencies.

• Render a "capacity-building" plan for the development of personnel and resources necessary to ensure a cadre of prevention researchers.

• Provide an estimate of resources (funding, manpower, training opportunities) necessary to make effective scientific progress in prevention research.

• Prepare a final report that will encourage universities, colleges, hospitals, and federal agencies to foster prevention research.

The committee concludes that a critical mass of knowledge relevant to the prevention of mental disorders has accumulated and that opportunities now exist to effectively use this knowledge to launch a research agenda. Therefore the committee strongly recommends that an enhanced research agenda to prevent mental disorders be initiated and supported across all relevant federal agencies, including, but not limited to, the Departments of Health and Human Services, Education, Justice, Labor, Defense, and Housing and Urban Development, as well as state governments, universities, and private foundations. This agenda should facilitate development in three major areas:

• Building the infrastructure to coordinate research and service programs and to train and support new investigators.
• Expanding the knowledge base for preventive interventions.
• Conducting well-evaluated preventive interventions.

The three major areas to be developed are recommended in conjunction with use of the definitions of interventions for mental disorders and of prevention research developed in this report. The term *prevention* is reserved for only those interventions that occur before the initial onset of a disorder. These preventive interventions can be further classified into universal, selective, and indicated types, depending on the targeted population group. The term *prevention research*, as used in this report, refers only to preventive intervention research and is distinct from research that builds a broad scientific base for preventive interventions. This latter research is prevention-related, but it is not prevention research per se.

BUILDING THE INFRASTRUCTURE

Preventive intervention research for mental disorders cannot thrive without providing for its infrastructure. Two areas are particularly important for moving ahead—coordination and research training.

- Coordination among federal agencies is needed for four reasons: (1) variation in the application of definitions has made it virtually impossible to assess the current activities and expenditures in preventive intervention research; (2) duplication of research activities and the lack of piggybacking of smaller projects onto larger ones contribute to waste of dollars and time, and, at the same time, gaps in research go undetected; (3) agencies conduct research or provide interventions for mental disorders (including addictions), educational disabilities, criminal behavior, and physical disorders as though these were separate conditions, whereas more often than not, coexisting disorders or problems occur; and (4) agencies have different strengths; for example, some are better at applying rigorous research methodologies to intervention programs, whereas others are better at reaching out into communities and forging alliances.

Therefore the committee strongly recommends that a mechanism be created to coordinate research and services on prevention of mental disorders across the federal departments. One model for accomplishing this would be the establishment of a national scientific council on the prevention of mental disorders by Congress and/or the President. Such an overarching federal council could be operated out of the White House Office of Science and Technology Policy or another coordinating office within the Executive Office of the President.

- The committee also strongly recommends that Congress encourage the establishment of offices for prevention of mental disorders at the state level.

- Agencies must be required to identify their funded programs for the prevention of mental disorders, separately accounting for universal, selective, and indicated preventive interventions, using the definitions developed in this report.

- The National Institute of Mental Health (NIMH), the National Institute on Alcohol Abuse and Alcoholism (NIAAA), and the National Institute on Drug Abuse (NIDA) should consider including prevention researchers with broad mental health perspectives on their national advisory councils.

- Mental health reimbursement from existing health insurance should be provided for preventive interventions that have proved effective under rigorous research standards such as those described in this report.

- Dissemination activities should receive much higher priority than they have in the past.

- Congress and federal agencies should take steps immediately to develop and support the training of additional researchers who can develop new preventive intervention research trials as well as evaluate the effectiveness of current service projects.

• Research training should be focused on two groups—mid-career scientists and postdoctoral students.

• The number of institutional training programs focusing on preventive intervention research should be increased from 5 to 12 over the next five years, including one at every specialized prevention research center, known at NIMH as Preventive Intervention Research Centers (PIRCs), that is productive.

• Support for faculty within institutional training programs should be increased.

• A major effort should be made to encourage the prevention research training of minorities.

• The proposed national scientific council on the prevention of mental disorders should reevaluate the training needs for preventive intervention research after the first five years.

EXPANDING THE KNOWLEDGE BASE

The committee believes that a viable research agenda for prevention of mental disorders rests on a firm stratum of health research in other fields. This knowledge base includes basic and applied research in the core sciences that is aimed at the causes and prevention of mental disorders. Included in this knowledge base are neurosciences, genetics, epidemiology, psychiatry, behavioral sciences (including developmental psychopathology), and risk research. It also includes evidence and lessons from other fields of research, such as prevention of physical illness and treatment of mental disorders. Therefore,

• Research to expand the knowledge base for preventive interventions should be continued.

• Support for research on potentially modifiable biological and psychosocial risk and protective factors for the onset of mental disorders should be increased. Priority should be given to research that illuminates the interaction of potentially modifiable biological and psychosocial risk and protective factors, rather than restricting the research to either biological or psychosocial factors alone.

• NIMH should support a series of prospective studies on well-defined general populations under the age of 18 to provide initial benchmark estimates of the prevalence and incidence of mental disorders and problem behaviors in this age group.

• A population laboratory should be established with the capacity for conducting longitudinal studies over the entire life span in order to generate understanding as to how risk factors and developmental transitions combine to influence the development of psychopathology.

• Whenever possible, research proposals relevant to the knowledge base for preventive interventions should explicitly state this connection, such as identification of potentially modifiable risk factors and possible avenues for preventive interventions.

• Treatment intervention research conducted under rigorous methodological standards that is directly relevant to preventive intervention research should continue to be supported—but not from the prevention research budget.

• Research should continue to be supported to determine which risk and protective factors are similar and which ones are different for treatment and prevention of a variety of mental disorders.

• Research should be supported to study the effects of social environments, such as families, peers, neighborhoods, and communities, on the individual and the effects of context on the onset of various mental disorders.

• Researchers working on relevant research in the core sciences should be encouraged to participate in activities such as forums and colloquia with preventive intervention researchers.

• A comprehensive, descriptive inventory of the activities in which the public engages to promote psychological well-being and mental health should be developed and supported.

CONDUCTING WELL-EVALUATED INTERVENTIONS

The knowledge base for some mental disorders is now advanced enough that preventive intervention research programs, targeted at risk factors for these disorders, can rest on sound conceptual and empirical foundations. Therefore,

• Increased methodological rigor in all research trials, demonstration projects, and service program evaluations should be required.

• The concept of risk reduction, including the strengthening of protective factors, should be used as the best available theoretical model for guiding interventions to prevent the onset of mental disorders.

• Universal preventive interventions should continue to be supported in the areas of prenatal care, immunization, safety standards such as the use of seat belts and helmets, and control of the availability of alcohol.

- Research on selective and indicated interventions targeting high-risk groups and individuals should be given high priority.
- Priority should be given to preventive intervention research proposals that address well-validated clusters of biological and psychosocial risk and protective factors within a developmental life-span framework.
- Increased attention should be given to preventive intervention research that addresses the overlap between physical and mental illness.
- Research support should be developed in two waves over the next decade, initially focusing primarily on increasing research grant support for individual investigators and later on increasing support for preventive intervention research centers.
- Research on sequential preventive interventions aimed at multiple risks in infancy, early childhood, and elementary school age to prevent onset of multiple behavioral problems and mental disorders should be increased immediately and substantially.
- Research on preventive interventions aimed at major depressive disorder should be increased immediately and substantially.
- Research on preventive interventions aimed at alcohol abuse should be increased immediately.
- Support for pilot and confirmatory preventive intervention trials should be increased for conduct disorder.
- Research should be supported on alternative forms of intervention for the caregivers and family members of individuals with mental disorders, especially Alzheimer's disease and schizophrenia, to prevent the onset of stress-induced disorders among these caregivers.
- Over the next decade, as new specialized prevention research centers are initiated across the federal government, priority should be given to those that are sponsored through interagency agreement.
- Knowledge base research at the specialized prevention research centers should be supported by new research grants (RO1s) that do not use preventive intervention research dollars.
- Dissemination mechanisms, including publication in peer-reviewed journals, and knowledge exchange opportunities with other researchers and with representatives from the community should be mandated as part of the mission of each specialized prevention research center.
- The preventive intervention research cycle as described in this report should be used as a conceptual model for designing, conducting, and analyzing research programs.
- Increased attention to cultural diversity, ethical considerations, and benefit-cost and cost-effectiveness analyses should be an essential component of preventive intervention research.
- Community involvement should be increased to help identify

disorders and problems that merit research and to support preventive intervention research programs.

There could be no wiser investment in our country than a commitment to foster the prevention of mental disorders and the promotion of mental health through rigorous research with the highest of methodological standards. Such a commitment would yield the potential for healthier lives for countless individuals and the general advancement of the nation's well-being. The committee recommends increased support for a research agenda, beginning with an increase of $50.5 million in fiscal year 1995. But even with the support of the federal government, the effort will not be easy. Overall, what is required is a national commitment to rigorous research and cooperation among federal, state, and local agencies, as well as universities, foundations, researchers, and communities.

Contents

APPENDIXES

List of Boxes, Figures, and Tables

REDUCING RISKS FOR

Mental Disorders

OVERVIEW

1

Introduction

In his 1963 message to Congress, President John F. Kennedy drew the nation's attention to the critical problem of mental illness and championed prevention as a promising approach. He contended that prevention could proceed along two fronts: "Prevention will require both selected specific programs directed especially at known causes, and the general strengthening of our fundamental community, social welfare, and educational programs which can do much to eliminate or correct the harsh environmental conditions which often are associated with mental retardation and mental illness" (Kennedy, 1963). These prevention activities were designated to take place in part within the newly created, federally mandated system of community mental health centers. However, other agendas took precedence within the centers, and little prevention work was actually done (Torrey, 1988; Klein and Goldston, 1977).

Thirty years after Kennedy's message, the problems of mental illness are still immense. In this country, it is estimated that 20 percent of adults suffer from an active mental disorder in a given year, and 32 percent can be expected to have such an illness sometime during their life (Robins and Regier, 1991). These estimates, which come from the National Institute of Mental Health's Epidemiologic Catchment Area (ECA) study, are the most current statistics based on government-supported research. The estimates are considerably higher than the 10 to 15 percent estimated as the annual prevalence of mental disorder by the President's Commission on Mental Health (1978) and reflect the growth of knowledge in this area. The ECA figures are larger—and probably more accurate—because of improvements in methodology and instrumentation. However, differences in diagnostic criteria may also account for some of the difference in the estimates. The ECA study defined active disorder as a disorder for which criteria (codified in the third edition of the *Diagnostic and Statistical Manual of Mental Disorders* [American Psychiatric Association, 1980]) had been met at some time in the person's life and at least one symptom (or one episode) had been present in the year prior to interview.

Mental disorders can occur throughout the life span, but the type and nature of the illnesses vary with age. At least 12 percent (or about 7.5 million) of our nation's 63 million children and adolescents suffer from one or more mental disorders—including autism, attention deficit hyperactivity disorder, severe conduct disorder, depression, and alcohol and psychoactive substance abuse and dependence (DHHS, 1991; IOM, 1989; OTA, 1986). Based on a review of seven epidemiological studies, the Office of Technology Assessment (OTA, 1991) reported that the prevalence of diagnosable mental disorders among individuals under age 20 may be closer to 20 percent. In 1990, suicide ranked as the third leading cause of death among 15- to 24-year-olds (National Center for Health Statistics, 1993). The American Academy of Child and Adolescent Psychiatry (1990) reported that growing numbers of children and adolescents are at exceptionally high risk for developing a mental disorder: for example, 1.5 million children and adolescents are reported abused or neglected each year, 300,000 are in the foster care system, and 7 million live with an alcoholic parent. In addition, more than 18,500 children and adolescents have been left motherless by the HIV/AIDS epidemic, and that number will more than double by 1995 (Michaels and Levine, 1992). Toward the other end of the life span are the 4 million older Americans who, according to a National Institute on Aging estimate, are likely to be suffering from Alzheimer's disease (Evans, Scherr, Cook, Albert, Funkenstein, Smith et al., 1990) and the 15 to 25 percent of the elderly in nursing homes who are clinically depressed (NIH Consensus Development Panel on Depression in Late Life, 1992).

Mental illness of this magnitude places an extraordinary burden on the financial and social resources of this country. Current expenditures in this area include not only core costs such as direct costs for treatment and indirect costs for lost worker productivity, but also related costs such as those resulting from investment of time while caring for mentally ill family members. One estimate put our annual total economic cost of drug abuse, alcohol abuse, and mental illness at just over $218 billion in 1985, of which $44 billion was for drug abuse, $70 billion for alcohol abuse, and $103 billion for other mental illness (Rice, Kelman, Miller, and Dunmeyer, 1990). Based on this study, using socioeconomic indexes, Rice and colleagues have estimated that for 1990 the totals were over $66 billion for drug abuse, $98 billion for alcohol abuse, and $147 billion for other mental illness (D. Rice, personal communication, April 1993). The concomitant cost in human suffering and lost opportunity is incalculable.

Mental and physical health are closely linked, and beyond the costs just described, the contribution of mental health to physical well-being has to be considered. Physical disorders can cause serious mental disorders, and physical disorders can have their origin in psychosocial processes (IOM, 1982). Studies estimate that 60 percent of visits to physicians for medical symptoms are due in part or whole to psychosocial problems (Regier, Goldberg, and Taube, 1978), and the frequency of diagnosable mental disorder found in studies of general practice ranges from 11 to 36 percent (Eisenberg, 1992; Barrett, Barrett, Oxman, and Gerber, 1988). In a comparison of the functioning of patients with depression and patients with chronic medical conditions, only chronic heart disease produced more disability than depressive symptoms (Wells, Stewart, Hays, Burnam, Rogers, Daniels et al., 1989). Contrary to the current rigid arbitrary separation of research on mental and physical disorders, the human condition is one in which the mental and physical processes inexorably intertwine.

Despite enormous expenditures attempting to contain the problem of mental illness, it is estimated that only 10 to 30 percent of those in need receive appropriate treatment (DHHS, 1991; IOM, 1989; NMHA, 1986). Thus it is time to take a fresh look at prevention to see if it can be made to function as a full partner with new treatment approaches in addressing our nation's mental health care crisis.

A NEW EMPHASIS ON PREVENTION: OPPORTUNITIES AND STRENGTHS

Several forces are coming together to enhance the timeliness of a new emphasis on research to prevent mental disorders. As is detailed in the chapters to come, the knowledge base for preventive interventions, which had been scanty in the 1960s, has undergone a remarkable expansion, fueled by a considerable research effort within the past decade. Fundamental advances in our understanding of the biological substrates and genetics underlying numerous mental disorders and of the role of environmental factors in the onset of specific disorders have been made. There is also a promising variety of new interventions that offer a much more optimistic view for the future of prevention of some specific mental disorders.

The concept of risk reduction is at the heart of prevention research. Risk factors are those characteristics, variables, or hazards that, if present for a given individual, make it more likely that this individual, rather than someone selected from the general population, will develop a disorder (Werner and Smith, 1992; Garmezy, 1983). In this report a broad definition of risk factors is used, encompassing biological (including genetic), psychological, and social factors in the individual, family, and environment. Recent research has demonstrated that many at-risk individuals also have variables in their background or life that serve as protective factors. A well-documented description of the interplay between risk and protective factors is a critical scientific first step in establishing successful preventive intervention programs. Such a description is now available for some disorders, and research is under way to identify such factors for a number of others. The next step is to identify causal risk factors that may be malleable, that is, that can be altered through interventions. Then the effects of these interventions are tested in systematic, empirical, and rigorous ways, most often in preventive intervention trials. This step also contributes to the fundamental knowledge base through the determination of causality and malleability. One way to determine causality and malleability of risk factors for specific disorders is through examination of preventive interventions aimed at a single factor or a cluster of factors. If risk factors can be decreased or in some way altered, and/or if protective factors can be enhanced, the likelihood that at-risk individuals would eventually develop the mental disorder would decrease.

This risk reduction model is widely used for prevention of physical illness. As described in Chapter 3 of this report, to prevent physical disorders due to complex multiple causes, such as cardiovascular disease, the strategy is to determine risk factors and then to target interventions to such risk factors or to people with these risk factors. As with any disorder with multiple causes, it is difficult to document that any specific physical illness can be prevented in a given individual by risk reduction. However, indirect evidence from matching trends of risk reduction across populations with decreases in mortality or morbidity in groups that have changed behaviors is highly consistent with this theory, and results are encouraging. For example, through behavioral changes in diet and smoking, declines in the risks of morbidity have been achieved.

The study of mental disorders is at the stage where the knowledge base is comparable to the knowledge base prior to the large trials in the prevention of physical illnesses. Because of the power of the risk reduction model, this report is entitled *Reducing Risks for Mental Disor-*

ders: Frontiers for Preventive Intervention Research. A large body of knowledge exists today about the risk factors associated with many major mental disorders, the preventive interventions directed at reducing these risk factors and improving protective factors, and the research methods to assess the effectiveness of these interventions. This body of knowledge reflects the major advances that have been made in the field of mental disorder prevention.

OBSTACLES TO PROGRESS

Despite these recent advances in the prevention field and the fact that the history of mental health efforts related to prevention dates back many decades (see Table 1.1), progress has been limited because the efforts have been sporadic and have often lacked focus. Why hasn't the field received more concentrated attention? In response to a request from Congress and the National Institute of Mental Health (NIMH), the Institute of Medicine's Committee on Prevention of Mental Disorders examined this question as part of a broad review of the status of prevention research.

The committee found several apparent reasons for this inattention, some of which reflect problems that are shared with the larger field of treatment of mental disorders. One of the most important is that mental disorders have long carried a stigma. Because many people consider such illnesses to arise from a defect in character or will, patients and their families still try to hide the disorder and thus never seek or receive needed attention. Even some federal agencies heavily involved in the prevention and treatment of mental disorders (e.g., agencies supporting interventions aimed at alcohol and substance abuse and dependence) do not use the term *mental disorder.* Another difficulty is that even though research has shown that a number of effective treatment interventions are available—such as those for depression and anxiety disorders—this information is not generally known by the public. Also, many believe that unless treatment for a particular disorder is highly effective, nothing can be done in regard to prevention. In fact, for some disorders, such as conduct disorder, prevention may have a particularly important role because treatment has been so ineffective.

Another problem has been the lack of an organizing theoretical framework in the prevention of mental disorders. Only recently has the concept of risk reduction begun to take hold. Also, current understanding of the mechanisms that link risk and protective factors with proximal and distal outcomes is not well established for mental disorders. A great deal more is known about how to prevent some physical diseases (e.g.,

TABLE 1.1 Time Line of Events Related to Prevention of Mental Disorders

1909 The Mental Health Association was founded; subsequently it became the National Association for Mental Health and then the National Mental Health Association (NMHA). Since its inception, it has advocated for prevention of mental illness and promotion of mental health.

1910 Public meeting on "Prevention of Insanity" organized by the New York Committee on Mental Hygiene. Topics included alcoholism, syphilis, drug addiction, head injuries, infectious diseases such as meningitis, and influences of fatigue and stress.

1915 *The Proceedings of the National Conference of Charities and Correction* contained papers on prevention of mental illness and mental retardation. The ideas included sterilization, reduced immigration, and more institutions to lower the numbers of "feeble-minded" in the community.

1920s The child guidance movement and the mental hygiene movement (fostered by the National Committee for Mental Hygiene that was organized by Clifford Beers) were begun. Both movements were committed to prevention as well as treatment of mental illness and highly valued the role of local communities in solving problems, including prevention of juvenile delinquency.

1930 The White House Conference on Child Health and Protection issued a report with an expanded focus that included social and environmental factors that affect the physical and mental health of children.

1930s The national commitment to prevention decreased, and the treatment-oriented approach began to dominate. Insurance plans created at this time reinforced the illness/treatment approach.

1946 Passage of the National Mental Health Act (P.L. 487) authorized the creation of the National Institute of Mental Health (NIMH).

1948 The World Federation for Mental Health, an independent organization with close ties to the United Nations, was created and included prevention within its purview.

1948 The Mental Health Study Center, a small NIMH community laboratory, was established in Prince Georges County, Maryland, to apply public health principles to the practice of mental health at the community level. For the next 34 years, research was done and treatment and prevention services were provided.

1954 The first organized training program in mental health consultation, which included a prevention component, began at the Harvard School of Public Health, Laboratory of Community Psychiatry.

1955 The Mental Health Study Act directed the Joint Commission on Mental Illness and Health to analyze and evaluate the needs and resources of the mentally ill and make recommendations for a national mental health program.

1961 The Joint Commission on Mental Illness and Health released *Action for Mental Health* to the Senate and House of Representatives.

1963 President John F. Kennedy, in a message to Congress, championed prevention as an approach to the problem of mental illness.

TABLE 1.1   (*Continued*)

1963   The Community Mental Health Centers Act listed mental health consultation and education, which included prevention, as one of the five essential services necessary for such centers to qualify for federal funds. This was the first time in any federal health statute that a preventive service was declared mandatory.

1969   The Joint Commission on Mental Health of Children produced a report saying that millions of children were in need of services, and millions were at risk.

1973   NMHA formed a Prevention Task Force.

1975   The first Vermont Conference on the Primary Prevention of Psychopathology was sponsored by the World Federation for Mental Health, NIMH, and the John D. and Catherine T. MacArthur Foundation.

1976   The Conference on Primary Prevention sponsored by NIMH resulted in *Primary Prevention: An Idea Whose Time Has Come.*

1978   The President's Commission on Mental Health reported that (1) efforts to prevent mental illness and promote mental health were unstructured, unfocused, and uncoordinated and (2) preventive efforts received insufficient attention at the federal, state, and local levels. The commission recommended establishing a Center for Prevention in NIMH.

1978   The position of Coordinator for Disease Prevention and Health Promotion was established at the National Institutes of Health (NIH).

1979   The first annual Alcohol, Drug Abuse, and Mental Health Administration (ADAMHA) Conference on Prevention was held.

1980   The NIH Prevention Coordinating Committee was formed, with the NIH Coordinator for Disease Prevention and Health Promotion as the designated prevention coordinator.

1980   The Public Health Service Act (in response to the presidential endorsement of the 1978 President's Commission on Mental Health) was amended to give special attention to efforts to prevent mental disability. Among other requirements, this act and a 1983 amendment (1) established the Office of the Deputy Director for Prevention and Special Projects in NIMH, and (2) designated an Associate Administrator for Prevention within ADAMHA to promote and coordinate prevention programs, including those run by NIMH, the National Institute on Drug Abuse (NIDA), and the National Institute on Alcohol Abuse and Alcoholism (NIAAA). The Associate Administrator was made responsible for an annual report to Congress describing the prevention activities undertaken by ADAMHA and its agencies.

1980   NIDA established its Prevention Research Branch.

1981   The Select Panel for Promotion of Child Health (established by Public Law 95–626) presented its findings to the U.S. Congress and the Secretary of Health and Human Services. The panel reported a need for better coordination of mental health and health services due to the frequent concomitance of health and mental health problems in children.

1981   The Omnibus Budget Reconciliation Act folded the community mental health centers into alcohol, drug abuse, and mental health block grants to the states and introduced large cuts in all human service appropriations.

(continued)

TABLE 1.1 *(Continued)*

1982 The Center for Prevention Research (CPR) was established at NIMH. This was a step toward consolidation of preventive intervention research throughout NIMH into one unit.

1983 NIMH Center for Prevention Research established its first Prevention Intervention Research Center (PIRC).

1983 ADAMHA Associate Administrator for Prevention was appointed, as mandated by an amendment to the Public Health Service Act, to promote and coordinate the research programs of its component agencies—NIAAA, NIDA, and NIMH.

1984 NMHA established the Commission on the Prevention of Mental-Emotional Disabilities.

1985 NIMH appointed its first Deputy Director for Prevention, mandated by the 1980 Public Health Service Act.

1985 The Office of Substance Abuse Prevention (OSAP) was established.

1985 NIDA published the first of several monographs dealing with preventing drug abuse.

1985 The Center for Prevention Research reorganized into the Prevention Research Branch within the newly created Division of Clinical Research in NIMH.

1986 A prevention initiative was undertaken by the American Academy of Child and Adolescent Psychiatry, and a Project Prevention Steering Committee was formed. The initiative resulted in a series of prevention monographs published by OSAP.

1986 NIAAA established the Prevention Research Branch within the Clinical and Prevention Research Division, created at the same time.

1986 The position of Assistant Director for Disease Prevention at the Office of Director level was established within NIH.

1986 The Office of Technology Assessment (OTA) issued a report entitled *Children's Mental Health: Problems and Services*. The report concluded that there was a substantial theoretical and research base to show that mental health interventions were effective for children.

1986 NMHA released a report by the Commission on the Prevention of Mental-Emotional Disabilities, *The Prevention of Mental-Emotional Disabilities*.

1987 NIMH published *Preventing Mental Disorders: A Research Perspective*.

1987 The National Prevention Coalition was established within NMHA.

1989 The U.S. General Accounting Office issued a report to Senator Inouye, *Mental Health: Prevention of Mental Disorders and Research on Stress-Related Disorders*, a critique of the implementation of prior recommendations in the prevention field.

1989 The Institute of Medicine (IOM) issued *Research on Children and Adolescents with Mental, Behavioral, and Developmental Disorders: Mobilizing a National Initiative*. Prevention was not emphasized.

1990 Because of a congressional mandate, NIMH entered into an agreement with IOM so that IOM could prepare an integrated report of current prevention research, with policy-oriented and detailed long-term recommendations for a prevention research agenda.

TABLE 1.1   (*Continued*)

1990   The American Psychiatric Association published a report prepared by the Task Force on Prevention Research of the Council on Research with a review of research on the prevention of psychiatric disorders.

1990   The American Academy of Child and Adolescent Psychiatry published *Prevention in Child and Adolescent Psychiatry: The Reduction of Risk for Mental Disorders.*

1990   *A National Plan for Research on Child and Adolescent Mental Disorders* (National Advisory Mental Health Council) emphasized scientific research concerning biomedical risk factors and capacity building for scientific researchers.

1990   NIMH held its first National Conference on Prevention Research, and a NIMH Steering Committee on Prevention was established to write a report on the current status of prevention research within NIMH.

1992   The ADAMHA Reorganization Act abolished ADAMHA, organized the three research institutes (NIAAA, NIDA, and NIMH) under NIH, and provided for an Associate Director for Prevention in each research institute. The service components from ADAMHA were reorganized into the Substance Abuse and Mental Health Services Administration (SAMHSA) as the Center for Substance Abuse Treatment, the Center for Substance Abuse Prevention, and the Center for Mental Health Services.

1992   The IOM Committee on Prevention of Mental Disorders was formed in accordance with the NIMH agreement.

1993   NIMH Steering Committee on Prevention released *The Prevention of Mental Disorders: A National Research Agenda* at the third NIMH National Conference on Prevention Research.

through immunizations for specific infections). The lack of clarity regarding risk mechanisms for mental disorders has contributed to a reluctance to launch preventive interventions without additional research (Sameroff, 1990). However, it is not generally realized that at the beginning of many large intervention programs to prevent physical diseases, such as heart disease, the part of the knowledge base regarding risk mechanisms was also small. Large-scale prevention efforts were instituted with clear concepts but a modest knowledge base with regard to mechanisms, and the resulting research has yielded important information about the etiology of these diseases, the malleability of identified risk factors, and the risk mechanisms in multiple causal chains.

Difficulties in identifying, defining, and classifying mental disorders also present barriers to successful prevention. A culture of the bacteria establishes the diagnosis of a streptococcal sore throat. In contrast, mental disorders rarely have a single cause and do not have such a "gold standard" confirmatory diagnostic test. Mental disorders are currently defined by a description of a cluster of symptoms associated with clinical dysfunction. These have been codified in an evolving classification system called the *Diagnostic and Statistical Manual of Mental Disorders* (DSM), published by the American Psychiatric Association. The first edition was published in 1952, the current edition is the third revised (DSM-III-R), and a fourth edition is expected imminently. This system conceptualizes each mental disorder as "a clinically significant behavioral or psychological syndrome or pattern that occurs in a person and that is associated with present distress or disability or with a significantly increased risk of suffering death, pain, disability, or an important loss of freedom" (American Psychiatric Association, 1987).

Valid and reliable classification of disorders is a prerequisite for advances in the scientific understanding of mental disorders across the life span. The goal is for the nosologic system to be reliable enough to ensure that different investigators assign diagnoses according to the same criteria so that cross-study comparisons can be made with confidence. At the same time, diagnostic categories aim to be as discrete as possible so that when an individual is diagnosed, a standardized treatment is available. These systems of classification are of course empirically derived and somewhat arbitrary, and they do not necessarily improve the process of making a diagnosis for a particular individual.

Major and continuing advances have been made in the validity and reliability of psychiatric classification over the past 30 years, especially for adult disorders. Despite these advances, many problems with the classification of mental disorders remain, all of which will increasingly affect the prevention field as it more specifically focuses not only on the reduction of risk factors but also on the reduction of initial onset of disorders:

• Not all scientists whose work is relevant to preventive interventions agree on which diseases to include in the category of mental disorders, and, for a few diagnoses, what constitutes a mental disorder. For example, despite general consensus on their psychiatric status and the fact that they are officially codified in DSM-III-R, alcohol and psychoactive substance abuse and dependence and Alzheimer's disease are sometimes classified as addictive and neurological disorders, respectively, rather than as mental disorders. In addition, conduct disorder as a diagnosis continues to raise controversy. Some clinicians and researchers say that it should be examined as a "social diagnosis" rather than as a mental disorder.

It should be noted that there are behavioral, psychological, and social problems that may merit intervention that, nonetheless, are not mental disorders themselves, nor are they necessarily attributable to mental disorders. For example, mild, transient depressive or anxiety symptoms, which are common throughout the life span, are not mental disorders. Likewise, teenage pregnancy is not a mental disorder, although mental disorders such as bipolar disorder or substance abuse are sometimes associated with it.

● Classification of children's mental disorders poses particular problems. Far too often, children's unique expression of complicated behaviors and feelings has not been appreciated, and children have been saddled with adult diagnostic criteria. To address this issue, a national epidemiological study of the status of children's mental health is needed. Methodological issues related to the design of such a study are currently being addressed prior to its full implementation.

● Another problematic area in diagnosis is the considerable co-occurrence of two or more different mental disorders in an individual and the ambiguity of classification in such instances. DSM-III-R recognizes this and makes no claim that each mental disorder as described is a discrete entity.

● In addition to DSM, there is another classification system, *The International Classification of Diseases* (ICD, 1992). Whereas DSM has been widely accepted in the United States, ICD is well established throughout Europe. Having two systems that had many differences has made comparison of international data more difficult. However, much progress has been made in increasing the compatibility of these two systems, and DSM-IV and ICD-11 promise to be quite similar for most diagnoses.

● The DSM and ICD classification systems for mental disorders have changed frequently, and they will continue to evolve as more is learned about these illnesses. Essentially, the disorders are "moving targets" as diagnostic power advances. Long-term follow-up studies that use diagnostic codes become more complicated as a result of these changes.

Confusion about terminology extends to the terms *prevention* and *prevention research*, which mean different things to different federal agencies, advocacy groups, and professionals (see Chapter 2). Even scientists within federal research institutes are unlikely to agree as to what constitutes prevention of mental disorders. Although this problem has been recognized for many years, it has remained intractable.

Because of this semantic confusion, it is difficult to compare data derived from different sources or to estimate the nature and scope of prevention services and research regarding mental disorders. Accordingly, it is also challenging, if not impossible, to obtain reasonably accurate estimates of the level of support of these activities. The lack of clarity has contributed to a manipulation of terminology to secure funds earmarked for prevention. This, in turn, has culminated in an intense, and at times antagonistic, competition for funds among agencies, research institutes, and advocacy groups.

LOOKING FORWARD

Despite the obstacles, there has been an expansion in the knowledge base for prevention of mental disorders, an increase in methodology, and the development of some promising preventive interventions. Circumstances have combined to present an extraordinary opportunity to investigate the prevention of mental disorders much more seriously. It is time for a new emphasis on a sophisticated prevention research agenda and a new stature for such research. To achieve this, the field will need to attract good people from a broad range of disciplines and be able to support their research endeavors.

Currently, society at large is placing greater emphasis on personal health and disease prevention. Many people are striving to improve their physical and mental well-being, not just to avoid illness but to achieve what they consider greater personal rewards, including a more active life and a generally more positive disposition (Breslow, 1990). People are beginning to recognize that their physical health and mental health are intertwined. Some government and business organizations are advocating prevention programs, not only to improve health, but also with the hope of reducing the nation's health care bill, now approximately 14 percent of the gross domestic product (Burner, Waldo, and McKusick, 1992). Three federal agencies have recently recognized the increasing importance of prevention. The U.S. Department of Health and Human Services issued national objectives for health promotion and disease prevention, including mental and physical health, in its report *Healthy People 2000* (DHHS, 1991). The U.S. Centers for Disease Control, one of the primary federal health agencies, officially changed its name in late 1992 to the Centers for Disease Control and Prevention, and the National Institute of Mental Health recently issued a report on a national research agenda for the prevention of mental disorders (NIMH, 1993). In this type of cultural climate, efforts to prevent mental disorders may well find fertile soil.

ORGANIZATION OF THIS REPORT

The committee began its work with a review of the definitions of prevention and prevention research. With a clearer definition of what constitutes preventive intervention, the committee undertook a review of the current state of research in and relevant to the prevention of mental disorders and the promotion of mental health throughout the life span.

The committee selected five illustrative disorders to outline what is currently known about opportunities for preventive intervention research: Alzheimer's disease, schizophrenia, depression, alcohol abuse and dependence, and conduct disorder. The disorders were selected to demonstrate a range of potential etiologies—from largely psychosocial (conduct disorder) to largely biological (Alzheimer's disease)—and a range of age of onset of disorder—from childhood to late adulthood. There are, of course, many other disorders that could be used as illustrations, but space precludes their inclusion in this report.

In its review of the field, the committee noticed a common inclination to view prevention research as implementation and evaluation of randomized controlled trials to assess the impact of a preventive intervention. In fact, however, these trials are only part of a multistage research cycle in which each of the steps is linked sequentially and logically to other steps. Ideally in this process, the results of earlier steps inform subsequent research steps in important ways. A brief explication of the preventive intervention research cycle is critical both to gain perspective on the knowledge base that provides the foundation for any preventive trial and to evaluate the actual contributions of subsequent research activities to the knowledge base. Figure 1.1 provides a schematized version of the various steps in this cycle and is explained more fully in a later chapter.

The committee found the framework of the preventive intervention research cycle useful as a loose guide to the structure of its review of the field. And with this framework in mind, the reader may be similarly guided through this report and experience conceptually the stages he or she would go through in designing a prevention program. Following the introduction and description of definitions in Chapters 1 and 2, the committee presents a series of chapters on lessons learned from prevention of physical illness (Chapter 3); from the core sciences that provide part of the knowledge base for preventive interventions (Chapter 4); from a description of illustrative mental disorders (Chapter 5); from research on risk and protective factors associated with the onset of mental disorders (Chapter 6); from a review of illustrative preventive interventions for mental disorders that serve as promising models for future interventions (Chapter 7); from treatment research (Chapter 8); and from a review of the field of mental health promotion (Chapter 9). Throughout this report, as throughout the preventive intervention research cycle itself, the critical issues of ethics, cultural diversity, and economics unfold and require our attention.

16

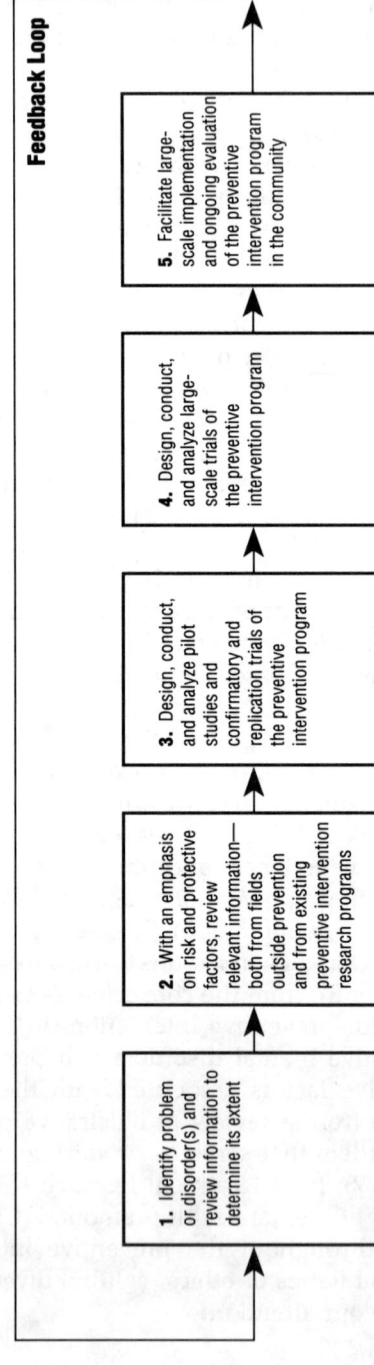

FIGURE 1.1   The preventive intervention research cycle. Preventive intervention research is represented in boxes three and four. Note that although information from many different fields in health research, represented in the first and second boxes, is necessary to the cycle depicted here, it is the review of this information, rather than the original studies, that is considered to be part of the preventive intervention research cycle. Likewise, for the fifth box, it is the facilitation by the investigator of the shift from research project to community service program with ongoing evaluation, rather than the service program itself, that is part of the preventive intervention research cycle. Although only one feedback loop is represented here, the exchange of knowledge among researchers and between researchers and community practitioners occurs throughout the cycle.

In the final section of the report the committee builds the agenda for the future: how to design, conduct, and analyze preventive interventions within the preventive intervention research cycle (Chapter 10) and how to exchange knowledge about preventive interventions and mental health promotion among researchers, practitioners, and communities (Chapter 11). The committee then assesses the infrastructure of the field, focusing on coordination, funding, and personnel (Chapter 12). In its major conclusions and recommendations (Chapter 13), the committee describes its vision for fulfilling the promise of the field of mental disorder prevention.

REFERENCES

American Academy of Child and Adolescent Psychiatry. (1990) Prevention in Child and Adolescent Psychiatry: The Reduction of Risk for Mental Disorders. Washington, DC: American Academy of Child and Adolescent Psychiatry.

American Psychiatric Association. (1987) Diagnostic and Statistical Manual of Mental Disorders (Third Edition—Revised). Washington, DC: American Psychiatric Association.

American Psychiatric Association. (1980) Diagnostic and Statistical Manual of Mental Disorders (Third Edition). Washington, DC: American Psychiatric Association.

Barrett, J. E.; Barrett, J. A.; Oxman, T. E.; Gerber, P. D. (1988) The prevalence of psychiatric disorders in a primary care practice. Archives of General Psychiatry; 45: 1100–1106.

Breslow, L. (1990) A health promotion primer for the 1990's. Health Affairs; 9: 6–21.

Burner, S. T.; Waldo, D. R.; McKusick, D. R. (1992) National health expenditures projections through 2030. Health Care Financing Review; 14(1): 14.

DHHS (Department of Health and Human Services). (1991) Healthy People 2000. Washington, DC: Government Printing Office; DHHS Pub. No. (PHS) 91–50212.

Eisenberg, L. (1992) Treating depression and anxiety in primary care: Closing the gap between knowledge and practice. The New England Journal of Medicine; 326(16): 1080–1084.

Evans, D. A.; Scherr, P. A.; Cook, N. R.; Albert, M. S.; Funkenstein, H. H.; Smith, L. A.; Hebert, L. E.; Wetle, T. T.; Branch, L. G.; Chown, M.; Hennekens, C. H.; Taylor, J. O. (1990) Estimated prevalence of Alzheimer's disease in the United States. Milbank Quarterly; 68: 267–289.

Garmezy, N. (1983) Stressors of childhood. In: N. Garmezy and M. Rutter, Eds. Stress, Coping and Development in Children. New York, NY: McGraw-Hill; 43–84.

ICD (The International Classification of Diseases [10th Revision]). (1992) Classification of Mental and Behavioral Disorders: Clinical Descriptions and Diagnostic Guidelines. Geneva, Switzerland: World Health Organization.

IOM (Institute of Medicine). (1989) Research on Children and Adolescents with Mental, Behavioral, and Developmental Disorders. Washington, DC: National Academy Press.

IOM (Institute of Medicine). (1982) Health and Behavior: Frontiers of Research in the Biobehavioral Sciences. Washington, DC: National Academy Press; Pub. No. 82–010.

Kennedy, J. F. (1963) Message from The President of the United States Relative to Mental

Illness and Mental Retardation; February 5, 1963; To the Congress of the United States. Washington, DC: Referred to the Committee on Interstate and Foreign Commerce and printed.

Klein, D. C.; Goldston, S. (1977) Primary Prevention: An Idea Whose Time Has Come. Washington, DC: Government Printing Office.

Michaels, D.; Levine, C. (1992) Estimates of the number of motherless youth orphaned by AIDS in the United States. Journal of the American Medical Association; 268(24): 3456–3461.

National Center for Health Statistics. (1993) Advance Report of Final Mortality Statistics, 1990. Monthly Vital Statistics Report; 41(7) Suppl.: 1–52.

NIH Consensus Development Panel on Depression in Late Life. (1992) NIH consensus conference: Diagnosis and treatment of depression in late life. Journal of the American Medical Association; 268(8): 1018–1024.

NIMH (National Institute of Mental Health). (1993) The Prevention of Mental Disorders: A National Research Agenda. Bethesda, MD: NIMH.

NMHA (National Mental Health Association). (1986) The Prevention of Mental-Emotional Disabilities. Alexandria, VA: NMHA.

OTA (Office of Technology Assessment), U.S. Congress. (1991) Adolescent Health. Volume II: Background and the Effectiveness of Selected Prevention and Treatment Services. Washington, DC: Government Printing Office.

OTA (Office of Technology Assessment), U.S. Congress. (1986) Children's Mental Health: Problems and Services—A Background Paper. Washington, DC: Government Printing Office.

President's Commission on Mental Health. (1978) Report to the President from the President's Commission on Mental Health. (Stock No. 040-000-00390-8, Vol. 1) Washington, DC: Government Printing Office.

Regier, D. A.; Goldberg, I. D.; Taube, C. A. (1978) The defacto U.S. mental health service system: A public health perspective. Archives of General Psychiatry; 35: 685–693.

Rice, D.; Kelman, S.; Miller, L. S.; Dunmeyer, S. (1990) Economic Costs of Alcohol and Drug Abuse and Mental Illness. Department of Health and Human Services: Washington, DC; DHHS (ADM)90–1694.

Robins, L. N.; Regier, D. A. (1991) Psychiatric Disorders in America: The Epidemiologic Catchment Area Study. New York, NY: The Free Press.

Sameroff, A. J. (1990) Prevention of developmental psychopathology using the transactional model: Perspectives on host, risk agent, and environmental interactions. Conference on The Present Status and Future Needs of Research on Prevention of Mental Disorders: Washington, DC.

Torrey, E. F. (1988) Nowhere To Go. New York, NY: Harper & Row; 142–150.

Wells, K. B.; Stewart, A.; Hays, R. D.; Burnam, A.; Rogers, W.; Daniels, M.; Berry, S.; Greenfield, S.; Ware, J. (1989) The functioning and well-being of depressed patients. Journal of the American Medical Association; 262(7): 914–919.

Werner, E. E.; Smith, R. S. (1992) Overcoming the Odds. High Risk Children from Birth to Adulthood. New York, NY: Cornell University Press; 185.

2

New Directions in Definitions

"To prevent" literally means "to keep something from happening." Different notions about what that something is—first incidence, relapse, disability associated with a disorder, or the risk condition itself—constitute a source of confusion in the field of mental health regarding the term *prevention*. An important first step in a renewed prevention effort is to arrive at commonly agreed upon definitions of the terms *prevention* and *prevention research*. Without this, prevention will continue to be a confused field with disagreement on its scope.

To begin the definitional process, it is necessary to look back over 100 years to the roots of public health concern with prevention. The original, and highly successful, prevention model addressed infectious disease. As a result of mass immunizations with specific vaccines and the introduction of hygienic measures, the infectious diseases that were the leading cause of death and disability in 1900 dramatically declined by 1970 (DHEW, 1979). Because of its record of success, this model was extended for use with a broad range of prevention efforts for noninfectious diseases and other chronic physical illnesses.

CLASSIFYING PREVENTIVE INTERVENTIONS FOR PHYSICAL ILLNESS

The original public health classification system of disease prevention was proposed by the Commission on Chronic Illness (1957). It consists of three types of prevention: primary, secondary, and tertiary. *Primary prevention* seeks to decrease the number of new cases of a disorder or illness (*incidence*). *Secondary prevention* seeks to lower the rate of established cases of the disorder or illness in the population (*prevalence*). *Tertiary prevention* seeks to decrease the amount of disability associated with an existing disorder or illness. Although the goals of these three types of prevention appear to be clear-cut, in practice there is considerable disagreement about their usage.

The classic example of primary prevention within a public health context was the history-making action in the nineteenth century of John Snow (Last, 1988), who removed the handle of the Broad Street water pump in London to halt the epidemic of cholera in the neighborhood. Despite very little understanding of cause and effect, the prevention effort was successful. Gradually, the knowledge base regarding infectious diseases expanded.

In the original classification system of primary, secondary, and tertiary prevention, there was an implied understanding of mechanisms linking the cause of the disease with the occurrence of the disease. Since the time this system was developed, research has advanced our understanding of the complexity of the association between risk factors and health outcomes. There is an increased appreciation for the importance of the interplay among the biological, psychological, and social, or biopsychosocial, factors in the expression of a physical illness. For the most part, knowledge of the intervening mechanisms is just beginning to be understood.

Recognition of this complex interaction regarding risk and protective factors and illness outcomes, and the lack of understanding about how risk factors lead to or are associated with the onset of illness, sometimes lead to a pessimistic view that prevention efforts are futile until etiology is better understood. Gordon (1987), however, was convinced that practically oriented disease prevention and health promotion programs could be based solely on empirical relationships, and this led him to propose an alternative classification system for physical disease prevention (Gordon, 1987, 1983). The system was based on a risk-benefit point of view; that is, the risk to an individual of getting a disease must be weighed against the cost, risk, and discomfort of the preventive intervention. Gordon's system consisted of three categories: universal, selective, and indicated. All three categories were meant to apply only "to persons not motivated by current suffering" (Gordon, 1983, p. 108). The three categories represented the population groups to whom the interventions were directed and for whom they were thought to be most optimal.

A *universal preventive measure* is a measure that is desirable for everybody in the eligible population. In this category fall all those measures that can be advocated confidently for the general public and for all members of specific eligible groups, such as pregnant women, children, or the elderly. In many cases, universal preventive measures can be applied without professional advice or assistance. The benefits outweigh the cost and risk for everyone. Examples include maintenance of an adequate diet, use of seat belts, prevention of smoking, many forms of immunization, and prenatal care.

A *selective preventive measure* is desirable only when the individual is a member of a subgroup of the population whose risk of becoming ill is above average. The subgroups may be distinguished by age, gender, occupation, family history, or other evident characteristics, but individuals within the subgroups upon personal examination are perfectly well. Because of the increased risk of illness, the balance of benefits against risk and cost can be justified. Examples include special immunizations, such as yellow fever, for individuals who travel to areas of the world where the disease is still prevalent, and annual mammograms for women with a positive family history of breast cancer.

An *indicated preventive measure* applies to persons who, on examination, are found to manifest a risk factor, condition, or abnormality that identifies them, individually, as being at high risk for the future development of a disease. The identification of persons for whom indicated preventive measures are advisable is the objective of screening programs. Gordon meant for the recipients of indicated preventive interventions to be asymptomatic regarding the disease but to have a "clinically demonstrable abnormality." Indicated preventive measures are usually not totally benign to the subject or minimal in cost. If they were, the balance in the benefit-cost analysis might favor their wider application, including segments of the population at lower risk of disease, and they would tend to move into the selective or universal classes. Examples of indicated measures include medical control of hypertension and frequent, careful examination of persons from whom a basal cell skin cancer has been removed (Gordon, 1983).

Unfortunately, over time there has been a simplistic blending of these two classification systems for the definition of prevention, that is, the original primary, secondary, and tertiary system and Gordon's universal, selective, and indicated system. At times, there even are attempts to use the three-tiered systems interchangeably. This sort of erroneous integration of terms has slipped into the prevention research field and added to the confusion regarding definitions.

Although universal prevention may at times be comparable to primary prevention, indicated measures have been compared to secondary prevention in a very narrow sense that Gordon thought was incorrect.

Further, even though the word *treatment* is often used in connection with indicated preventive measures, Gordon believed that there was a distinction between treatment and indicated prevention. Whereas the aim of treatment is to be immediately therapeutic, the aim of indicated prevention is to provide an intervention for an asymptomatic, clinically demonstrable abnormality that will result in the prevention of some later, anticipated symptoms or disability (Gordon, 1983). While others believed that this "asymptomatic, clinically demonstrable abnormality" was the first sign of illness, Gordon said that these signs were related to the biological origin of disease but were not the disease itself.

This distinction has compelling ethical ramifications. Treatment quickly provides benefits, including symptomatic relief, from an already existing diagnosable condition. On the other hand, indicated preventive interventions are based on probabilities. There is no sure way of knowing that the disease will occur, and potential benefits may be delayed for months or even years. When securing compliance from individuals for indicated interventions, these distinctions should be clarified.

CLASSIFYING INTERVENTIONS FOR MENTAL DISORDERS

Neither the original public health classification system of primary, secondary, and tertiary prevention nor Gordon's classification system of universal, selective, and indicated prevention was designed for use in the prevention of mental disorders. Rather, both focused on prevention of disorders traditionally identified as medical disorders. The application of these terms to a mental health framework is not straightforward. One of the main problems has been the notion of "caseness" that is used in public health. It is often more difficult to document that a "case" of mental disorder exists than it is to document a physical health problem. Agreement regarding the occurrence of a case of a mental disorder varies over time with the instruments and diagnostic systems employed and with the theoretical perspective of the evaluators. Also, symptoms and dysfunction may exist even though all criteria for a DSM-III-R diagnosis are not present. Finally, the outcomes in very young children (birth to age five) are often not diagnosable as "psychiatric caseness" but rather as impairments in cognition and psychosocial development.

The Mental Health Intervention Spectrum for Mental Disorders

Because of all the difficulties described above, the committee has chosen not to use the public health classification system of primary,

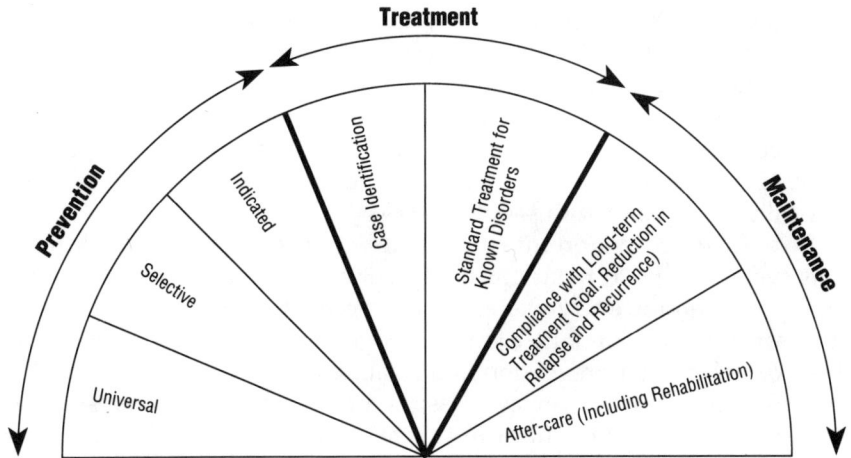

FIGURE 2.1   The mental health intervention spectrum for mental disorders.

secondary, and tertiary prevention. Rather, it presents an alternative system in which the term *prevention* is reserved for only those interventions that occur before the initial onset of a disorder. This system incorporates many of Gordon's ideas regarding prevention, including an adaptation of the concepts *selective* and *indicated*.

Although the committee's emphasis is on prevention, it realizes that a classification system is necessary that recognizes the importance of the whole spectrum of interventions for mental disorders—from prevention, through treatment, to maintenance (see Figure 2.1). Under this system, treatment interventions, which are therapeutic in nature (such as psychotherapy, support groups, medication, and hospitalization), are provided to individuals who meet or are close to meeting DSM-III-R diagnostic levels. There are two components in treatment intervention: (1) case identification and (2) standard treatment for the known disorder, which includes interventions to reduce the likelihood of future co-occurring disorders. The optimal treatment protocol aims to reduce the length of time the disorder exists, halt a progression of severity, and halt the recurrence of the original disorder, or if not possible, to increase the length of time between episodes. The clinician also aims to halt the occurrence of other disorders in the patient, a phenomenon known as co-morbidity. Some clinicians see this as a standard part of optimal treatment, whereas others view it as prevention within the original public health classification system. Maintenance interventions, which are supportive, educational, and/or pharmacological in nature, are provided on a long-term basis to individuals who have met DSM-III-R diagnostic levels and whose illness continues (especially the more severe disorders). The two components of maintenance intervention are (1) the patient's compliance with long-term treatment to reduce relapse and recurrence and (2) the provision of after-care services to the patient, including rehabilitation. The aim of both components is to decrease the disability associated with the disorder.

By setting prevention into a context within the mental health field, this system helps to point out the fallacy of the commonly voiced idea that prevention is everywhere, in all aspects of mental health research and service. The committee acknowledges that in clinical practice the boundary between prevention and treatment is not as clear-cut as this classification system conveys. Issues of co-morbidity, relapse, and recurrence can be thought of in several ways. For example, providing lithium medication to a patient with bipolar mood disorder is clearly treatment, but if the medication reduces the number and intensity of the depressive symptoms so that the patient is no longer at risk for becoming dependent on alcohol, the intervention may also be thought of as prevention, provided before the onset of a secondary problem, in this case alcohol dependence. Also, psychotherapy for an anxious mother of a healthy child can be conceptualized as treatment of the mother as well as prevention of later difficulties in the child. Finally, effective treatment of a physical illness may prevent a secondary mental disorder and vice versa.

While it is laudable for clinical practice to consider both treatment and prevention outcomes, this report focuses on prevention research as a separate entity. The change in terminology that is used throughout this report, although perhaps not particularly useful to clinicians, who may find themselves providing elements of prevention, treatment, and maintenance to the same patient, is critical to a review of prevention research. Without a system for classifying specific interventions, there is no way to obtain accurate information on the type or extent of current activities, either public or private, and no way to ensure that prevention researchers, practitioners, and policymakers are speaking the same language.

Preventive Interventions for Mental Disorders

In the mental health intervention spectrum, *universal preventive interventions* are targeted to the general public or a whole population group that has not been identified on the basis of individual risk. The intervention is desirable for everyone in that group. Prenatal care and childhood immunization, which have preventive effects not only for physical health but also for mental health, are examples, as is a program designed to prevent distress and divorce in couples who are married or planning marriage and are not currently experiencing difficulties in their relationship. All are described in Chapter 7 of this report. Universal interventions have advantages when their cost per individual is low, the intervention is effective and acceptable to the population, and there is a low risk from the intervention. However, it is crucial to be realistic about costs. An intervention provided to every prospective marital couple, although low in cost per couple, would be very expensive overall because of the size of the target group.

Selective preventive interventions for mental disorders are targeted to individuals or a subgroup of the population whose risk of developing mental disorders is significantly higher than average. The risk may be imminent or it may be a lifetime risk. Risk groups may be identified on the basis of biological, psychological, or social risk factors that are known to be associated with the onset of a mental disorder. Examples of selective preventive interventions include home visitation and infant day care for low-birthweight children, preschool programs for all children from poor neighborhoods, and support groups for elderly widows (see Chapter 7). Selective interventions are most appropriate if the interventions do not exceed a moderate level of cost and if negative effects are minimal or nonexistent.

Indicated preventive interventions for mental disorders are targeted to high-risk individuals who are identified as having minimal but detectable signs or symptoms foreshadowing mental disorder, or biological markers indicating predisposition for mental disorder, but who do not meet DSM-III-R diagnostic levels at the current time. The term *indicated* is used differently here from how Gordon originally meant for it to be applied. Whereas he meant it to apply only to asymptomatic individuals, within this mental health classification system it can be applied to asymptomatic individuals with markers as well as to symptomatic individuals whose symptoms are still early and are not sufficiently severe to merit a diagnosis of a mental disorder. An example of an indicated preventive intervention from this report is a parent-child interaction training program delivering an intervention for children who have been identified by their parents as having behavioral problems (see Chapter 7). Indicated interventions may be reasonable even if intervention costs are high and even if the intervention entails some risk.

Indicated preventive interventions are often referred to by clinicians as *early intervention* or an early form of treatment. One danger in this classification system is that individuals needing treatment interventions could be intentionally misclassified as needing indicated preventive interventions because of ethical concerns about labeling. Interveners are sometimes reluctant to apply diagnostic labels, especially to children, even when such diagnoses and their corresponding treatments are appropriate.

A critical component of universal and selective preventive interventions is that although some members of the group may have mental disorders when the intervention begins, this information is not relevant to the choice of the targeted groups. If individuals are chosen for a preventive intervention because of early psychological symptoms, by definition the intervention is an indicated one.

The overall aim of the three types of preventive intervention—universal, selective, and indicated—is the reduction of the occurrence of new cases. Usually, this is done through a risk reduction model, and even if outcomes are in the distant future and the goal of fewer cases has not yet been established, the decrease in risk and/or increase in protective factors can be documented. Another aim might be the delay of onset of illness and the short-term reduction of new cases in addition to the absolute prevention of new cases. Additionally, the aims of indicated preventive interventions might be to reduce the length of time the early symptoms continue and to halt a progression of severity so that the individuals do not meet, nor do they come close to meeting, DSM-III-R diagnostic levels. Even if the individual does eventually develop a DSM disorder, the prior preventive intervention may still have had an effect by reducing the duration and/or severity of the disorder.

Obviously, it is preferable to prevent a disorder throughout life, but the delay of onset of a disorder is also a worthwhile goal of prevention. Delay of onset has the potential for benefits not only to the individual but also to the family. For example, reducing the number of new cases of depressive disorder in mothers during their childrearing years may have a major effect on the incidence of depression in their children, even if, after the children leave home, the incidence of depressive disorders in these mothers returns to the usual level. Likewise, the delay of onset of Alzheimer's disease would result in a delay in the stress-induced problems experienced by family caregivers.

MENTAL HEALTH PROMOTION

The phrase *promotion of mental health* has definitional problems similar to those of *prevention*, meaning different things to different people. Norman Sartorius (1988, p. S3), director of the Division of Mental Health at the World Health Organization, noted that "For some, it means the treatment of mental illness; for others, it means preventing the occurrence of mental illness; and for others, promotion of mental health means increasing the ability to overcome frustration, stress, problems, enhancement of resilience and resourcefulness."

The committee has chosen not to include mental health promotion within the spectrum of interventions focused on mental disorders. Nevertheless, the committee recognizes that mental health promotion activities are important and widespread. The reason for not including it within the above spectrum is that health promotion is not driven by an emphasis on illness, but rather by a focus on the enhancement of well-being. It is provided to individuals, groups, or large populations to enhance competence, self-esteem, and a sense of well-being rather than to intervene to prevent psychological or social problems or mental disorders. This focus on health, rather than illness, is what distinguishes health promotion activities from the enhancement of protective factors within a risk reduction model for preventive interventions. (See Chapter 9 for a theoretical grounding in this perspective on health promotion.)

THE CLASSIFICATION SYSTEM IN PRACTICE

The committee's classification system can be applied to all research and service related to interventions for mental disorders. All three types of intervention—prevention, treatment, and maintenance—are fully compatible with empirical design and measurement and can yield important findings.

As mentioned above, the boundaries between prevention and treatment can be blurred in clinical practice. The same has been true in prevention research. The U.S. Public Health Service's 1984 definition of prevention research includes "only that research designed to yield results directly applicable to interventions to prevent occurrences of disease or disability, or the progression of detectable but asymptomatic disease." The lack of description of "occurrence," "disease," and "disability," as well as a breakdown of activities into "intervention," "preintervention," and "prevention-related research" (see Table 2.1), has led to a wide range of activities being labeled as prevention research. For example, a report to Congress from the Alcohol, Drug Abuse, and Mental Health Administration used this definition to justify the inclusion of everything from basic research to community support programs for the rehabilitation of the seriously mentally ill in its prevention research portfolio (ADAMHA, 1990). The committee recognizes that government officials value the flexibility and broader definition given

TABLE 2.1   U.S. Public Health Service Definition of Prevention Research

Prevention Research: Prevention research includes only that research designed to yield results directly applicable to interventions to prevent occurrences of disease or disability, or the progression of detectable but asymptomatic disease.

Pre-intervention
- Identification of risk factors for disease or disability
- Development of methods for identification of disease controllable in the asymptomatic state
- Refinement of methodological and statistical procedures for quantitatively assessing risk and measuring the effects of preventive interventions

Intervention
- Development of biologic interventions to prevent occurrence of disease or disability, or progression of asymptomatic disease
- Development of environmental interventions to prevent occurrence of disease or disability, or progression of asymptomatic disease
- Development of behavioral interventions to prevent occurrence of disease or disability, or progression of asymptomatic disease
- Conduct of clinical and community trials and demonstrations to assess preventive interventions and to encourage their adoption

Some interventions may be applicable to primary prevention as well as to disease treatment (e.g., diet and exercise as components of rehabilitation for coronary heart disease). Research into such interventions is considered prevention research.

Prevention-related research: More broadly defined, prevention research also includes that research which has a high probability of yielding results which will likely be applicable to disease prevention. Included are studies aimed at elucidating the chain of causation—the etiology and mechanisms—of acute and chronic diseases. Such basic research efforts generate the fundamental knowledge which contributes to the development of future preventive interventions.

them and that they are uneasy about targeted mandates from Congress. The committee also recognizes the importance of the whole continuum from basic sciences through treatment research and supports continued research in areas along the entire continuum. However, a too-inclusive definition of prevention research often underlies a neglect of interventions to reduce risks. Therefore the committee presents an alternative, using the term *prevention research* to refer only to preventive intervention research that can be further classified into universal, selective, and indicated types.

In service, these three general preventive intervention strategies can be integrated within an overall public health plan and are likely to occur in primary health care settings, schools, work sites, churches, and other community settings. For example, universal interventions can be applied when a program is believed to be beneficial for the general public and the benefits outweigh the costs and risks. Targeted campaigns can be mounted to implement selective preventive interventions for high-risk groups and for those individuals with high imminent or lifetime risk factors when the balance of benefits against risk and cost can be justified. Should individuals at risk begin to show early symptoms of the disorder, they would be candidates for an indicated preventive intervention program designed to avert the full-blown manifestation of the disorder through more intensive and focused preventive strategies. In a public health approach, each level of preventive intervention would be keyed to the nature of the target population's needs for reducing risk factors and strengthening protective factors.

Also within the public health care plan, adequate treatment and after-care interventions need to be readily available for those who have not had access to preventive interventions or for whom the interventions were not effective in preventing the onset of a mental disorder. Although the focus in this report is on prevention, the other components of the classification system outlined here deserve equal emphasis in a comprehensive and coordinated new approach to our nation's mental health.

REFERENCES

ADAMHA (Alcohol, Drug Abuse, and Mental Health Administration). (1990) Report on Programs and Plans in Prevention. Rockville, MD: Department of Health and Human Services.

Commission on Chronic Illness. (1957) Chronic Illness in the United States. Vol. 1. Published for the Commonwealth Fund. Cambridge, MA: Harvard University Press.

DHEW (Department of Health, Education, and Welfare). (1979) Healthy People: The Surgeon General's Report on Health Promotion and Disease Prevention. Office of the Assistant Secretary for Health and Surgeon General. Washington, DC: Public Health Service. DHEW (PHS) Pub. No. 79–55071.

Gordon, R. (1987) An operational classification of disease prevention. In: J. A. Steinberg and M. M. Silverman, Eds. Preventing Mental Disorders. Rockville, MD: Department of Health and Human Services; 20–26.

Gordon, R. (1983) An operational classification of disease prevention. Public Health Reports; 98: 107–109.

Last, J. M., Ed. (1988) A Dictionary of Epidemiology. New York, NY: Oxford University Press; 122.

Sartorius, N. (1988) Health Promotion Strategies: Keynote Address. Canadian Journal of Public Health; Suppl. 2; 79: S3–S5.

LESSONS FROM HEALTH RESEARCH

3

Prevention of Physical Illness

Major advances in the prevention of health-related problems have been made during recent decades in several areas of physical health (DHHS, 1991). Broad-based governmental actions as well as communitywide preventive intervention programs based on sound experimental research designs have produced significant changes in the health behaviors of many individuals, and declines in the risk of morbidity and premature mortality have been achieved. Progress has been notable in many areas, including the three used here as illustrations: cardiovascular disease risk reduction, smoking cessation and prevention, and injury prevention. The universal preventive strategies mounted in these areas have demonstrated that effective interventions are possible even when knowledge about the mechanisms causing illness is incomplete. Two experiments on cardiovascular disease risk reduction are reviewed, as is a series of experiments on smoking cessation. For injury prevention, a different approach is taken; rather than describing experiments, the effects of broad-based governmental action are reviewed.

The successful prevention campaigns in physical health can serve in several ways as a bridge in building effective mental health interventions. They provide powerful analogies and models for developing general strategic guidelines on approaches to prevention. In addition,

This chapter is based, in large part, on presentations at a workshop, convened by the Institute of Medicine, that focused on findings from prevention programs in physical health that might be applicable for mental health. (See Appendix C for participants and agenda of the meeting.)

the prevention programs in physical health can be directly useful by suggesting approaches and techniques—such as media presentations and strategies for community organization—that have proved their value in the physical health arena and may be readily modified and adapted to mental health.

CARDIOVASCULAR DISEASE

Cardiovascular disease, one of the leading causes of premature death and disability in the United States, is linked by extensive research to a variety of life-style components peculiar to the industrialized twentieth century. Smoking, little or no exercise, diets high in saturated fat and cholesterol, and chronic stress can lead to high blood pressure, high blood cholesterol, and obesity, all of which increase risk of cardiovascular disease.

Investigators at Stanford University have conducted two major studies designed to reduce the risk of cardiovascular disease. The prevention campaigns are based on the conviction that health risk factors associated with life-styles are most readily modified in the context of the community environment. It is important to note that although a connection between high fat intake, high cholesterol, and cardiovascular disease was reasonably well established by longitudinal data when the first of the Stanford studies began, the relative risk for cardiovascular disease (the ratio of the risk of disease or death among the exposed to the risk among the unexposed) had not been established experimentally, and the amount of change, or malleability, in the risk factors that was achievable from a community campaign was certainly not known.

The prevention programs—called the Stanford Three-Community Study and the Stanford Five-City Project—have demonstrated notable success in risk factor reduction through preventive interventions before the onset of illness. The results are promising because they suggest that it is possible to change the health habits of entire communities and to mobilize existing community resources to achieve those changes. The studies have become prototypes for comprehensive programs of planned social change to prevent many chronic diseases and other social problems (Flora, Maccoby, and Farquhar, 1989).

The goals of the Three-Community Study were to produce awareness of the probable causes of cardiovascular disease and of the specific measures that may reduce risk and to provide the knowledge and skills necessary to accomplish and maintain recommended behavior changes. The study encouraged reduction in body weight through caloric reduction and increased physical activity, and dietary changes to reduce intake of saturated fat, cholesterol, salt, sugar, and alcohol. Cigarette smokers were educated on the need and methods for ceasing or at least reducing their daily consumption.

Mindful of the powerful cultural forces that reinforce personal health habits, the investigators designed the study to combine an extensive mass media campaign with a considerable amount of face-to-face instruction. They also used three elements that had traditionally been ignored in health campaigns: (1) mass media materials devised to teach specific behavioral skills, as well as to offer general information to affect attitude and motivation; (2) the mass media approaches and, in particular, the face-to-face methods of instruction that were solidly grounded in theory and employed established social learning methods of achieving changes in behavior and principles of self-control training; and (3) an extensive analysis of the knowledge deficits and the media-consumption patterns of the intended audience, which was used to influence the campaign's ultimate design (Farquhar, Maccoby, Wood, Alexander, Breitrose, Brown et al., 1977).

The Three-Community Study was carried out from 1972 through 1975 in a trio of northern California towns: one received the intense media campaign and the face-to-face education, another just the media communications, and one served as a control. The media campaign consisted of about three hours of television programming, 50 television spots shown repeatedly, several hours of radio programming, weekly newspaper columns, newspaper advertisements and stories, billboards, posters, and printed material mailed to participants. The media materials incorporated elements of modeling and specific skill-building components designed to achieve participatory learning, which the investigators considered more effective than passive learning in promoting and maintaining behavior changes. For example, a televised hour-long "Heart Health Test" used self-scoring followed by instructions on how to reduce that particular risk, and another TV program modeled steps in preparation of healthful food alternatives. A specially tailored media campaign also was created for the sizeable populations of Spanish speakers in the communities. In the face-to-face component of the program, individuals identified as being at especially high risk received eight lessons (totaling 15 hours) of skills training, conducted in both group classes and at-home sessions and directed by expert counsellors trained in behavior modification techniques.

During its two-year period of active community education, the project achieved a statistically significant reduction in the composite risk score for cardiovascular disease, a result of significant declines in blood pressure, smoking, and cholesterol levels. The risk score decreased approximately 25 percent for the media-only community and 30 percent for the community receiving the combined campaign (Farquhar et al., 1977). Overall, the Three-Community Study demonstrated that (1) it is feasible to reach many individuals as opposed to targeting only high-risk individuals; (2) media-based strategies can be highly effective, but are even more so when supplemented with face-to-face communication; and (3) maintenance of the program requires mobilization of the community in addition to changes in individual behavior.

The Stanford Five-City Project extended the scope and objectives of the pioneering Three-Community Study, in particular by emphasizing community organization and including independent population surveys. It was a low-cost, comprehensive, communitywide program with the main goal of reducing risk of cardiovascular disease (Farquhar, Fortmann, Maccoby, Haskell, Williams, Flora et al., 1985). Other objectives included analysis of cost-effectiveness, development of educational and community organization methods, and gradual transfer of program control to community organizations.

Over a five-year period beginning in 1980, two medium-sized California cities received continual exposure to general education punctuated by four or five separate risk factor education campaigns per year (Farquhar, Fortmann, Flora, Taylor, Haskell, Williams et al., 1990). Three similar cities served as a control group, with the combined population of all sites reaching approximately 350,000. Education was carried out through the electronic and print media, and directly through classes, contests, and correspondence courses. Special programs were developed for Spanish-language radio, newspapers, and mass-distributed print materials.

In addition, school-based programs for grades 4, 5, 7, and 10 included special sessions on nutrition, exercise, and smoking, as well as multi-factor risk reduction classes for teachers and administrators and materials on exercise and nutrition for the students' parents. Work places were another major focus, and many large businesses participated by disseminating printed information, offering workshops and classes, sponsoring contests, and assessing environmental risks (such as smoking policy and exercise facilities). Heath care professionals participated in training programs, disseminated printed materials, and implemented risk reduction programs in their practices. There also were numerous point-of-purchase efforts. For example, many restaurants, cafeterias, and grocery stores participated in specially designed health food programs, such as a menu-labeling program that stressed the importance and versatility of low-fat foods.

The project's results proved quite encouraging. They definitively demonstrated the effectiveness of the intervention in reducing risk factors and suggested that similar programs could be tried. Although knowledge of risk factors increased in both the experimental and the control cities, the improvement in the experimental group was significantly greater in all follow-up surveys.

The knowledge apparently was put into practice, too. After 30 to 64 months, the experimental group registered an overall decrease in cardiovascular risk scores by 16 percent and a decrease in total risk score by 15 percent (Farquhar et al., 1990). On closer analysis, significant net reductions in community averages favoring the experimental group occurred in cholesterol level (about 2 percent) and blood pressure (4 percent). There also was a large decline in smoking level (13 percent) among the experimental group.

The decreases in cholesterol and blood pressure, although minor by clinical standards, may in fact have a potentially large public health significance (Farquhar et al., 1990). Because changes are greater in those at high risk and these changes apply to the entire population, a significant decline in the total number of cardiovascular disease events could be anticipated. The behavioral changes are also potentially sustainable and may even spread to other individuals as the changes are woven into the fabric of the community.

Not only effective, the campaign proved affordable. Over the project's span, each adult was exposed to an average of 527 educational episodes distributed fairly evenly over time—for a total exposure of about 26 hours per adult (Farquhar et al., 1990). Of these messages, about 70 percent were sent through television and radio, principally as 30-second spots. Annual radio and television exposure thus would be less than one hour per adult. The organizational and educational program was delivered at a per capita cost for adults of about $4 per year, excluding research costs.

Just as important as the specific details of the program are some broader issues that guided its development and implementation. For example, like its three-city predecessor the project was based on well-established models and theories. It effectively incorporated a communication-behavior change model, social learning theory, community organization principles, and social marketing methods. The program was designed to be comprehensive, encompassing multiple channels of communication, multiple objectives, and multiple targets of change (individuals, organizations, and larger community networks). It was also carefully evaluated at several stages, including pretesting the educational materials and conducting field assessments of whether the intended audience actually received the information.

SMOKING

Smoking kills approximately 434,000 Americans each year—more than the number who die from automobile crashes, fire, alcohol, homicide, suicide, drugs, and AIDS combined. In 1990, roughly 45.8 million persons age 18 or older, 25.5 percent of all adults, smoked cigarettes (CDC, 1992a). Young people smoke at about the same rate, which means we are replacing all the adults who either die or stop smoking with new smokers.

The picture would be even more grim were it not for major societal actions to discourage smoking. In the 1950s a series of epidemiological studies began to yield evidence that cigarette smoking could indeed cause lung cancer, as thoracic surgeons had been asserting for more than a decade (Breslow, 1982). Additional evidence accumulated, and in 1964 the Surgeon General of the U.S. Public Health Service issued *Smoking and Health*, which marked a watershed in alerting the public to the health hazards of tobacco (U.S. Public Health Service, 1964).

Since then, various organizations have conducted a large number of prevention programs, and there has been a series of public policy actions aimed at reducing smoking, such as restricting advertising, increasing public education, and requiring warning labels on tobacco products. These and other actions have produced a steady decline in smoking. From 1965 through 1985, smoking prevalence among adults dropped an average of 0.5 percentage points annually, and from 1987 through 1990 the decline averaged 1.1 percentage points annually (CDC, 1992a). Overall, the decline in smoking has been steady, with the exception of a minor increase of 0.3 percent between 1990 and 1991. This increase was not statistically significant, and the 1992 prevalence rate was below the prevalence rate of 1990 (SAMHSA, 1993). In 1989 the Surgeon General issued *Reducing the Health Consequences of Smoking: 25 Years of Progress* (DHHS, 1989). While reporting on dramatic changes in smoking behavior, he alerted the public to the need to focus increased efforts on preventing smoking initiation and encouraging smoking cessation among high-risk populations.

There have been some problems along the way, however, that are relevant for planning prevention efforts in mental health. Thomas Glynn of the National Cancer Institute's (NCI) Smoking, Tobacco, and Cancer Program has argued that, although there has certainly been success in reducing tobacco use, the early research and control activities did not provide the information necessary for even broader reductions (Glynn, 1991). That is, the series of intervention studies in the 1970s never were drawn together into a comprehensive plan of attack. Various reasons are cited for this, including competing or poorly coordinated funding agency priorities, inadequate research methodologies, lack of communication across disciplines, and an insufficiently coordinated data base. In addition, most investigators focused only on single causes of smoking (such as physical dependence on nicotine) or made use of single communication channels (such as mass media or physician office-based programs) for prevention.

Faced with this scattershot approach, NCI launched in 1982 the Smoking, Tobacco, and Cancer Program (STCP), a major planning and research effort to coordinate smoking prevention trials and develop large-scale comprehensive community interventions (Glynn, 1991). Lacking a consensus on how best to persuade people to quit or not begin smoking, the STCP mounted a well-planned, carefully phased three-phase campaign.

First, program administrators consulted with hundreds of experts to identify areas in which significant gains could be expected. They then called for and funded research to develop and evaluate prevention and cessation interventions that would be effective, cost efficient, durable, generalizable, and widely applicable. Between 1984 and 1987, NCI began 49 large trials, most of which were to last five years, at a total cost of $82 million.

Reflecting the multifactorial emphasis, these trials covered eight areas. First, there were school-based interventions with adolescents. These recognized that whatever can be done to prevent smoking by young people is doubly important, not only because it minimizes tissue damage during youth but also because it minimizes the hazard of addiction (few people start smoking after age 20, and those who do so may be less prone to addiction). There were self-help programs, based on the observation that 90 to 95 percent of all people who have stopped smoking claim they quit on their own. There were interventions conducted by physicians and dentists, who were considered a greatly underutilized resource. There were mass media interventions, which adopted many of the concepts developed in the Stanford cardiovascular risk programs. And there were interventions focused on four special populations: African-Americans, Hispanics, women, and smokeless tobacco users. At the time these trials began, the attributable risk of smoking (the rate of a disease or other outcome in exposed individuals that can be attributed to the exposure) had been fairly well established through epidemiological studies, although data were stronger for lung cancer than cardiovascular disease. There were few data, however, on the level of effect that the various types of interventions might have on smoking rates.

In order to assess as early as possible the effectiveness of these research efforts and their readiness to be applied on a larger scale, the STCP consulted on a regular basis with the various investigators to maximize cross-fertilization. As each trial area concluded, the STCP convened the principal investigators and their key staff. These meetings resulted in a series of consensus statements based on the empirical research, which have been used to select specific prevention and cessation activities to be further explored in the second and third phases of the program.

One example of the studies conducted during the first phase was school-based interventions, of which NCI funded 10 program trials. They covered both public and private schools, from elementary to high school levels. Some aimed at developing new curricula, some at revising existing curricula, and some at conducting long-term follow-up evaluations. When the investigators convened after the trials concluded, they agreed that school-based smoking prevention programs had had consistently positive effects, although the effects were modest and limited in scope.

The programs have been particularly effective in delaying the onset of tobacco use, but less successful in targeting use by high-risk and minority groups (Glynn, 1989). This should perhaps come as no surprise, given the barrage of advertising and media exposure that children steadily receive. For example, a recent study concluded that by the time U.S. children are six years old, they can just as easily identify "Old Joe the Camel," a cartoon character frequenting cigarette advertisements, as they can identify the logo for Mickey Mouse (Fischer, Schwartz, and Richards, 1991). Educational strategies to overcome such influences and boost success rates remain to be investigated, but may include earlier intervention and more frequent interventions throughout the junior high and high school years.

The second phase is a $45 million effort called the Community Intervention Trial for Smoking Cessation (COMMIT). Beginning in October 1988, a number of comprehensive community-based interventions (incorporating lessons from the first-phase studies) are being tested in 11 communities in North America, against the same number of control communities. The third phase, which will incorporate findings from the first two, will be the American Stop Smoking Intervention Trial for Cancer Prevention (ASSIST). This $150 million effort is set to begin in the fall of 1993. It will introduce large-scale interventions, emphasizing coalition development and policy change, in 17 states (reaching more than 50 million people), with work being carried out by state and local health departments. NCI believes that this sharply focused and coordinated strategy is the only means by which the nation will achieve further reductions in tobacco use (Glynn, 1991).

INJURIES

Injuries are the leading cause of death among Americans up to 44 years of age (IOM, 1985). Because they strike younger people disproportionally—children and teenagers are common victims—injuries also are the nation's leading cause of years of potential life lost through age 65. Of the approximately 150,000 persons who die from injuries each year, roughly one third are victims of intentional violence (homicide and suicide), one third die in motor vehicle crashes, and one third are killed by falls, burns, poisoning, drowning, and other unintentional injuries (CDC, 1992b). Many more persons are injured than killed. In 1987, a total of 62 million injuries caused Americans to restrict their activities for more than 600 million person-days and spend nearly 200 million person-days in bed (Brown, Foege, Bender, and Axnick, 1990).

When talking about preventing injuries, the first thing to note is that injuries are not "accidents." Too often, injuries are described as events that "just happen," unfortunate acts of fate beyond understanding and therefore beyond control. On the contrary, injuries are understandable, predictable, and potentially preventable. Indeed, given their importance in causing morbidity and mortality, injury prevention is increasingly becoming the focus of public health programs.

Among the most notable has been the effort to improve motor vehicle safety. The National Highway Traffic Safety Administration, led by its first administrator, William Haddon, launched a major initiative in the 1960s. When the program began, there was no consensus about the relative values of various intervention options. Would, for example, seat belts save more lives than vehicle modifications or driver education? Would seat belt use cause injuries? What was clear, however, was the very strong connection between driving a motor vehicle and sustaining motor-vehicle-related injuries.

The agency moved ahead with a variety of prevention programs— often in the face of considerable opposition from the automobile industry and other groups with vested economic interests. The efforts addressed the numerous factors that can play a role in causing injuries or contributing to their severity, and targeted a spectrum of audiences, including individuals, communities, businesses, regulatory agencies, and legislators. This comprehensive, well-coordinated campaign has yielded a range of safety-related advances, including increased use of seat belts; decreased drunk driving; better design and construction of highways and roadside structures; increased pedestrian, motorcycle, bicycle, and commercial vehicle safety; and engineering improvements in automobiles and trucks.

Promoting seat belt use, for example, was a particularly important component of the national safety program, and strategies to promote their use have included both mandatory-use state legislation and encouragement through public education campaigns. Investigators assessing these efforts have found that automobile fatalities have declined markedly as a consequence of increased seat belt use. They also have observed that enforcement of seat belt laws has proved necessary to ensure continued compliance with the laws (IOM, 1989; Campbell, 1988; Williams and Lund, 1988).

Overall, prevention campaigns have led to a decline in traffic fatalities by approximately 30 percent since the mid-1960s. Moreover, given the steadily increasing numbers of vehicles traveling many more miles, it is estimated that approximately 115,000 Americans would now be losing their lives in motor vehicle crashes each year if death rates common in the 1960s had not been reduced by the various safety interventions (U.S. National Highway Traffic Safety Administration, 1991).

From these years of experience, Haddon led other investigators in developing systematic ways to categorize prevention strategies that may extend well beyond injuries or highway safety. One result is called the Haddon Matrix (Haddon, 1972). This concept holds, among other things, that with any injury, there is a triad of factors at work: human factors, factors involving the vehicle and related equipment, and factors involving the physical and social environments. Each of these areas represents an opportunity to devise a prevention strategy. This challenges today's investigators not to become focused on any single option, but to think freely and fully about a range of possibilities. And it means fostering cooperation among a variety of scientific disciplines, because finding solutions to complex problems typically will require a wide range of experience and skills.

To break the chain of injury causation, investigators also have learned that it is best to aim at the weakest link first—that is, target the areas on which the greatest impact can be made for the smallest expenditure. In preventing injuries, this typically means modifying products or the environments in which they are used, rather than trying to modify human behaviors. For example, designing hot water heaters that do not circulate scalding water is more effective than mounting programs to remind millions of parents to be ever vigilant in not letting their children take unsupervised baths. This focus does not deny the success of behavior modification in other fields, but it does reflect an awareness that persistent behavioral changes are very hard to maintain.

Although all modes of injury need further investigation, one that is especially demanding—and perplexing—is violence, now recognized as a major national public health problem. Violence is linked with mental health in several ways. First, of course, violence begets mental health problems: victims of violence often experience severe emotional and psychological disturbances. Second, achieving a better understanding of mental disorders can help inform efforts to prevent such violent acts as homicide and suicide. Intertwined in this issue as well is the frequent association of alcohol and drugs with violent or abusive behavior.

Researchers have addressed the problem of violence in a number of studies. For example, there is evidence from studies conducted across societies and within societies that exposure, especially among some impressionable children and youths, to scenes of aggression and violence on television and in other media fosters our acceptance and expectation of violence in America and probably contributes to the frequency of aggressive acts themselves (Rosenberg, O'Carroll, and Powell, 1992). Studies also indicate that children who witness violence directly—an increasingly frequent situation in many urban areas—often develop symptoms associated with post-traumatic stress disorder, including diminished ability to concentrate in school, persistent sleep disturbances, disordered attachment behaviors with parents or significant caregivers, and changes in orientation toward the future that lead to increased risk-taking behaviors (Groves, Zuckerman, Marans, and Cohen, 1993). Children who witness domestic violence may be particularly vulnerable to emotional and developmental problems. Many aspects of the causes of violence and how violence can be prevented remain to be empirically tested, however, and the problem is presented here primarily to illustrate a broad-scale beginning in tackling one of the most destructive and powerful problems in society today, and one with important implications for prevention of mental disorders.

The Centers for Disease Control and Prevention (CDC) is now conducting a multifaceted community-based research effort devoted to youth violence prevention (Rosenberg et al., 1992). Multifaceted programs are needed because of the complex web of factors that cause violence and violence-related injuries, and community-based programs are needed to ensure community residents' involvement in, ownership of, and responsibility for the activities. Six key strategies have been identified, representing an orderly progression of research and implementation. The strategies are (1) developing prevention materials; (2) establishing community demonstration programs; (3) rigorously evaluating specific preventive interventions; (4) training public health workers, community members, and health professionals in violence prevention; (5) continuing surveillance, risk factor research, and evaluation; and (6) strengthening the capacity of state and local health departments.

The CDC investigators will first help local workers describe and define the problems of violence in their community and then select appropriate interventions. Toward these ends, specialized prevention materials are being developed, including a guidebook called *Prevention of Youth Violence: A Framework for Community Action* (CDC, 1993). This guidebook clearly spells out some relatively simple actions (though not all have been tested) that communities can adopt on their own to reduce violence. The next steps will be to help communities implement the interventions and then to evaluate the interventions and the overall program.

One facet of violence that has proved especially intractable involves firearms, particularly handguns. Firearm mortality dominates U.S. intentional injury statistics, accounting for 61 percent of all homicides and 59 percent of suicides, with the burden falling most heavily on minority and disadvantaged populations (Prevention of Violence and Injuries Due to Violence, 1991). For years, this issue had been approached strictly as a political or philosophical matter, with the debate polarized into those who favored some form of gun control and those who were against it. Beginning in the early 1980s, the CDC set about to change the nature of the debate by studying the problem scientifically, beginning with epidemiological studies, moving to analyses of risk factors and possible causes, and then developing an array of possible interventions and looking at their effectiveness.

Many of the studies are reviewed elsewhere (Taubes, 1992). For example, researchers learned that firearm attacks on family members and intimate acquaintances are at least 12 times more likely to result in death than are assaults using other weapons. When a woman is killed with a gun, the attacker is five times more likely to be her spouse, an intimate acquaintance, or a member of her family than to be a stranger. In another study, researchers compared overall rates of assaults, homicides, and suicides in two cities—Seattle and Vancouver—that were strikingly similar in all aspects but one: handguns were much easier to obtain in Seattle. The cities turned out to have similar levels of criminal activity, but homicide was 60 percent higher, and homicide by firearms was 500 percent higher, in Seattle than in Vancouver. Building on such studies, researchers are evaluating the effects of common approaches to preventing firearm injuries—including such interventions as prohibition of carrying guns in public, restrictive licensing, waiting periods for obtaining guns, and harsher sentences for crimes committed with guns.

Although conventional and innovative interventions remain to be more fully explored, some actions already have been proposed (Rosenberg et al., 1992). There is little controversy regarding children having unsupervised access to loaded guns—it is clear that controlling access to weapons can significantly limit accidental death among adolescents who may be suicidal or prone to impulsive acts. Alternatively, handguns themselves can be modified to reduce some of their lethal potential. For example, Smith & Wesson once manufactured a handgun advertised as being child-proof. Now discontinued, the gun could be fired only by depressing a special lever, which a child's hand would not be large enough or strong enough to accomplish. Such actions can begin to save countless lives as we develop and test effective and acceptable methods of reducing ready access to the most dangerous types of guns. Again, programs to break the chain of causation of injuries should be aimed at the weakest link, and modifying products and environments (for example, limiting access to guns) might yield the greatest impact.

FINDINGS AND LEADS

The underlying message from the prevention efforts in cardiovascular disease, smoking, and injuries reviewed here, of course, is that prevention can and does work—people have avoided injuries, reduced cardiovascular risk rates, and quit or never started smoking cigarettes. Some adults and youth have modified their life-styles as a result of multifaceted change strategies directed at individuals, groups, organizations, and communities. And people often have adopted such changes in the face of countervailing pressures, because the health habits altered are influenced heavily by social norms, peers, and environmental and economic factors. Paying close attention to the road signs these efforts have posted will help speed the journey that we must begin—immediately and together—toward preventing mental disorders and promoting mental health.

Other general lessons that, if carefully selected and applied, will contribute to success in developing mental health interventions include the following:

• **Preventive interventions for specific disorders are typically developed through a series of phases, each step building on its predecessor and supporting its successor.** The general stages are (1) recognizing and defining the problem; (2) delineating the risk factors involved; (3) conducting more detailed studies to describe the relative power of different risk factors, individually and in combination, and to describe protective factors; (4) developing and testing a variety of approaches to intervention to decrease risk and increase protection; (5) conducting large-scale confirmatory studies of the most promising interventions; (6) implementing and evaluating the interventions in large-scale demonstration projects at multiple sites; and (7) transferring the knowledge gained from the intervention programs into the public domain as widely and rapidly as resources allow.

Many areas of mental health are at the early stages of this development (that is, definition of risk factors), and longitudinal studies and other research efforts are only beginning to identify causal pathways. Some disorders, however, are ready (or nearly so) for various types of experimental preventive trials to begin. This report will identify where numerous disorders stand along this learning curve, which may help in planning the most appropriate next steps.

- **Preventive interventions need not always wait for complete scientific knowledge about etiology and treatment.** There is a distinction between knowing how to *treat* a disorder and knowing how to *prevent* it. Having effective treatment is not always necessary for effective prevention. For example, treatments for AIDS and fetal alcohol syndrome remain under active investigation, yet successful prevention is already possible. In addition, although there is no totally satisfactory treatment for lung cancer, smoking cessation interventions have proved effective.

Similarly, the fundamental biological mechanisms at work when a risk factor is associated with an adverse outcome may or may not be completely understood before undertaking prevention, or the relative importance of the risk factors may not be fully known. Indeed, preventive intervention trials—based on sound scientific theory and carefully conducted and evaluated—may themselves help to delineate mechanisms and to quantify the relative impact of various risk factors.

The Stanford group's program illustrates the value of this approach to prevention. Consider one risk factor: cholesterol. When the program began in 1970, scientists had established that there was a connection between high cholesterol levels in the body and increased risk of heart attack. They theorized that excessive dietary cholesterol might cause elevated levels in the body, which in turn might raise blood pressure, but they did not know precisely what effect reducing dietary cholesterol would have on cholesterol levels in the body, or what effect dietary change would ultimately have on rates of morbidity and mortality. Their solution was to target a constellation of related risk factors and employ a variety of intervention methods, and then determine the combined effect on health status. The immediate goal was achieved: promoting behavioral changes decreased risk of disease. The long-term goal of decreasing overall mortality requires further assessment. Over the years, researchers have delineated many of the mechanisms and relative risks involved—but had the Stanford group waited for fuller understanding of how and to what degree risk factors had an effect, their prevention insights might have been delayed by a decade or more.

In addition, in classic epidemiological terms, the amount of morbidity and mortality from vehicular injuries that could be affected by Haddon's proposed changes was certainly not known at the time intervention policies were adopted. But to wait until those studies had been done would not have been nearly as useful as what he did, which was to advocate and implement changes and to study carefully their effects—another example of the use of a prevention strategy both as an intervention and as an investigative tool.

• **Preventive interventions should be based on well-established theoretical frameworks.** A scientific theoretical orientation to the causation and mechanisms of a disorder is helpful in identifying "targets of opportunity" where intervention may best take place, and a developmental theoretical orientation helps in deciding when throughout an individual's development to direct intensive intervention.

Established theories also should guide how interventions are conducted. For example, many programs have used the principles of social learning theory. This model of self-directed behavior change assumes that people are able to regulate their own behavior and to participate actively in the learning and application of behavior change skills. The components of self-directed change include problem identification, goal setting, training in self-monitoring, and active training in the skills needed both to make changes and to avoid relapses. A cornerstone of the theory is that active practice of a new skill is more likely to achieve lasting change than is written or verbal persuasion or watching other people acting as models of a new behavior (Farquhar, Fortmann, Flora, and Maccoby, 1991). Social marketing principles then can help bridge the gap between theories and action. Among other things, social marketing calls for developing messages, products, or services from the perspective of the consumer, which allows the campaign designer to tailor messages to specific audiences.

• **Preventive interventions typically are most effective when they consider multiple domains of intervention.** This means using numerous communication channels to reach a variety of people repeatedly with a range of educational materials. The idea is that individuals are more likely to adopt new behavior if encouraged to do so in many ways and from many directions.

The Stanford program, for example, incorporates a wide range of communication channels—from electronic and print mass media to face-to-face personal counseling and mediated group sessions, from billboards and grocery store displays to the latest technologies of interactive personal computer systems and laser discs. Moreover, the components reinforce each other wherever possible; radio spots promote a contest that includes printed educational materials that in turn promote another radio program. This saturation can develop into what might be called environmental synergy, in which the sum of the messages becomes greater than their parts.

- **Preventive interventions should focus on the community, both in planning and in implementation.** Foremost, community involvement opens many doors for reaching people with educational materials. With local cooperation, materials can be routed through schools, work sites, recreation centers, churches, stores, and voluntary organizations. Community members also can be recruited as facilitators; for example, health care professionals can distribute materials and advice during patient visits. In general, as people come to feel that a program is "theirs," they are more likely to participate and to retain beneficial new behaviors.

Special attention may need to be given to critical subpopulations within a community. For example, in recognition of the disproportionate burden of violence that minority groups frequently bear, the Centers for Disease Control and Prevention has sought extensive input in developing its youth violence intervention guidelines from community minority leaders and others who already have implemented innovative prevention programs in urban centers. Also, as mentioned earlier, the Stanford program developed special programs for Spanish-speaking community members.

Developing community strength also may prove crucial for the long-term vitality of prevention efforts. The Stanford group, for example, believes that adoption of prevention programs by existing community organizations—including schools, hospitals, health agencies, and citizens groups—is generally necessary to supply ongoing reinforcement and reminders and to provide new knowledge and skills as they become needed (Farquhar, Fortmann, Flora, Taylor, Haskell, Williams et al., 1990). The form this process of "institutionalization" takes may vary considerably, but one possible model is to develop a council or consortium of local agencies that deal with health education and prevention programs. This not only will ensure an adequate base of expertise, but also may cut territorial wrangling and maximize interagency cooperation.

- **Preventive intervention programs should be rigorously designed, and the programs and their components evaluated extensively.** This should occur as the program is being developed (formative evaluation), while it is being conducted (process evaluation), and after it has been completed (summative evaluation).

In the Stanford programs, for example, investigators first analyzed the needs of the targeted audience to discover the interests, educational status, media use, and other characteristics of different subsections of the community, which helped determine the proper location and time for educational activities. They also developed prototypes of educational materials and programs and tested them among sample audiences to determine the appropriate content and method of delivery.

When the prevention campaign was under way, investigators carefully monitored the introduction of educational materials into the community to assess what was working and what needed to be revised. This process evaluation identified some of the factors that influenced participation in various aspects of the program, dictated how much was learned, and determined whether an event or program actually affected behavior.

During and after the intervention, investigators collected data on a number of health outcomes. They also evaluated specific risk reduction strategies (e.g., smoking cessation, dietary counseling) to determine their effects on individual knowledge, attitudes, and behavior. For example, the effects of a quit-smoking contest with 500 participants were evaluated through several measures: a mail survey of contest finishers, a telephone survey of selected nonrespondents, a carbon monoxide assessment of contestants who quit, and a one-year follow-up examination of those who tested positive for carbon monoxide—an indicator for smoking (King, Flora, Fortmann, and Taylor, 1987). Data from this study allowed investigators to see both the successes and the shortcomings of the contest. The findings showed that the quit rate for contestants was twice as high as the rate in the general population in the control communities, and the cost of the program—including its evaluation—was lower than that of traditional antismoking classes or groups. Program planners concluded that the contest could be strengthened by extending the program to add a relapse prevention element and by the use of incentives to maintain abstinence.

- **Prevention efforts must increasingly recognize the many areas of overlap between physical health and mental health.** To cite just one example, the causes and consequences of violence are not only physical but psychological. Traumatic brain injuries, frequently caused by gun shots or automobile and motorcycle crashes, induce severe mental disturbances in thousands of persons each year. Even victims of violence who recover from their physical injuries frequently bear long-lasting psychological scars. Indeed, entire communities can be destabilized by continuing outbreaks or threats of violence, reducing the quality of life and perhaps helping to perpetuate the cycle of violence. The integration of physical and mental aspects of health care in prevention will require a broad interdisciplinary approach.

• **Prevention efforts require a significant and sustained commitment on the part of the federal, state, and local governments and coordination across disciplines and agencies.** The prevention programs in physical health are complex and multifaceted, reflecting the nature of the health problems they are designed to address. Similarly, mental health interventions typically will be complex and multifaceted. There are likely to be multiple points in the causal chain where preventive interventions could be applied, which will require us to consider a wide range of prevention strategies. Outcomes will need to be assessed not only in the short term but also in the long term. Furthermore, as is true in the physical sciences, multidisciplinary approaches drawing on expertise from numerous scientific domains—ranging from the physical and mental health fields to the social sciences, education, political science, and communications—will prove most fruitful. It is therefore imperative that prevention efforts for mental disorders be carefully and systematically coordinated by the federal, state, and local governments across the gamut of agencies that will be involved. As the history of prevention programs in smoking and highway safety vividly illustrates, coordination within the government is crucial to success. While the federal government has a critical role in setting priorities and providing support for prevention services and research, state and local governments have important public health responsibilities, not only to set and enforce relevant laws and regulations, but also to generate their own hypothesis-driven prevention programs whose outcomes can be fully assessed.

An equally great challenge will be to muster the national political will—and corresponding financial support—required to move expeditiously ahead. Such an investment was necessary in order to move forward in cardiovascular disease, smoking, and injury prevention. The cost of prevention programs, based on the experience of some of the physical health care models, will not be small (Farquhar et al., 1990), and benefit-cost analyses are imperative as the prevention field moves ahead. However, the cost of *not* beginning to design and implement mental health intervention programs may be even greater. Given the successes in prevention of physical illness, the energies of citizens and communities can surely be harnessed to prevent mental disorders.

REFERENCES

Breslow, L. (1982) Control of cigarette smoking from a public policy perspective. Annual Review of Public Health; 129–151.

Brown, S. T.; Foege, W. H.; Bender, T. R.; Axnick, N. (1990) Injury prevention and control: Prospects for the 1990's. Annual Review of Public Health; 11: 251–266.

Campbell, B. J. (1988). Casualty reduction and belt use associated with occupant restraint. In: J. Graham, Ed. Preventing Automobile Injuries. Dover, MA: Auburn Publishing.

CDC (Centers for Disease Control and Prevention). (1993) National Center for Injury Prevention and Control. Prevention of Youth Violence: A Framework for Community Action. Atlanta, GA: CDC.

CDC (Centers for Disease Control and Prevention). (1992a) Cigarette smoking among adults—United States, 1990. Morbidity and Mortality Weekly Report; 41: 354–355 and 361–362.

CDC (Centers for Disease Control and Prevention). (1992b) Table 9. Provisional number of deaths and death rates for 72 selected causes: United States, 1990 and 1991. Monthly Vital Statistics Report; 40(13): 20.

CDC (Centers for Disease Control and Prevention). (1991) Injury Mortality Atlas of the United States, 1979–1987. Atlanta, GA: CDC.

DHHS (Department of Health and Human Services). (1991) Healthy People 2000. Washington, DC: Government Printing Office; DHHS Publication No. (PHS) 91–50212.

DHHS (Department of Health and Human Services). (1989) Reducing the Health Consequences of Smoking: 25 Years of Progress. A Report of the Surgeon General. Centers for Disease Control, Center for Chronic Disease Prevention and Health Promotion, Office on Smoking and Health: DHHS Publication No. (CDC) 89–8411; Prepublication version.

Farquhar, J. W.; Fortmann, S. P.; Flora, J. A.; Maccoby, N. (1991) Methods of communication to influence behavior. In: Oxford Textbook of Public Health. Volume 2. Methods of Public Health. New York, NY: Oxford University Press; 331–344.

Farquhar, J. W.; Fortmann, S. P.; Flora, J. A.; Taylor, C. B.; Haskell, W. L.; Williams, P. T.; Maccoby, N.; Wood, P. D. (1990) Effects of communitywide education on cardiovascular disease risk factors: The Stanford Five-City Project. Journal of the American Medical Association; 264: 359–365.

Farquhar, J. W.; Fortmann, S. P.; Maccoby, N.; Haskell, W. L.; Williams, P. T.; Flora, J. A.; Taylor, C. B.; Brown, B. W., Jr.; Solomon, D.; Hulley, S. B. (1985) The Stanford Five-City Project: Design and methods. American Journal of Epidemiology; 122: 323–334.

Farquhar, J. W.; Maccoby, N.; Wood, P. D.; Alexander, J. K.; Breitrose, H.; Brown, B. W., Jr.; Haskell, W. L.; McAlister, A. L.; Meyer, A. J.; Nash, J. D.; Stern, M. D. (1977) Community education for cardiovascular health. Lancet; 1(8023): 1192–1195.

Fischer, P. M.; Schwartz, M. P.; Richards, J. W., Jr. (1991) Mickey Mouse and Old Joe the Camel. Journal of the American Medical Association; 266: 3145–3148.

Flora, J. A.; Maccoby, N.; Farquhar, J. W. (1989) Communication campaigns to prevent cardiovascular disease: The Stanford Community Studies. In: R. Rice and C. Atkin, Eds. Public Communication Campaigns. Beverly Hills, CA: Sage Publications; 233–252.

Glynn, T. J. (1991) Comprehensive approaches to tobacco use control. British Journal of Addiction; 86: 631–635.

Glynn, T. J. (1989) Essential elements of school-based smoking prevention programs. Journal of School Health; 59(5): 181–188.

Groves, B. W.; Zuckerman, B.; Marans, S.; Cohen, D. J. (1993) Silent victims: Children who witness violence. Journal of the American Medical Association; 269: 262–264.

Haddon, W., Jr. (1972) A logical framework for categorizing highway safety phenomena and activity. The Journal of Trauma; 12: 193–207.

IOM (Institute of Medicine). (1989) Community approaches and perspectives from other health fields. In: Prevention and Treatment of Alcohol Problems: Research Opportunities. Washington, DC: National Academy Press; 109–127.

IOM (Institute of Medicine). (1985) Injury in America: A Continuing Public Health Problem. Washington, DC: National Academy Press.

King, A. C.; Flora, J. A.; Fortmann, S. P.; Taylor, C. B. (1987) Smokers' challenge: Immediate and long-term findings of a community smoking cessation contest. American Journal of Public Health; 77(10): 1340–1341.

Prevention of Violence and Injuries Due to Violence. (1991) In: Position Papers from the Third National Injury Control Conference. Setting the National Agenda for Injury Control in the 1990's. April 22–25, Denver, CO. Department of Health and Human Services; 161–241.

Rosenberg, M. L.; O'Carroll, P. W.; Powell, K. E. (1992) Let's be clear. Violence is a public health problem. Journal of the American Medical Association; 267(22): 3071–3072.

SAMHSA (Substance Abuse and Mental Health Services Administration). (1993) Office of Applied Sciences. Preliminary Estimates from the 1992 National Household Survey on Drug Abuse. Advance Report No. 3. Rockville, MD: DHHS.

Taubes, G. (1992) Violence epidemiologists test the hazards of gun ownership. Science; 258(5080): 213–215.

U.S. National Highway Traffic Safety Administration. (1991) Fatal Accident Reporting System: A Review of Information on Fatal Traffic Crashes in the United States in 1989. Washington, DC: U.S. Department of Transportation; Report No. DOT-HS 807–693.

U.S. Public Health Service. (1964) Smoking and Health. Report of the Advisory Committee to the Surgeon General of the Public Health Service. U.S. Department of Health, Education, and Welfare, Public Health Service, Centers for Disease Control; Atlanta, GA: PHS Pub. No. 1103.

Williams, A; Lund, A. (1988) Mandatory seat belt laws and occupant crash protection in the United States. In: J. Graham, Ed. Preventing Automobile Injuries. Dover, MA: Auburn Publishing.

4

The Core Sciences: Contributions and Frontiers

R esearch on the prevention of mental disorders, like all research, should be grounded in a rigorous scientific tradition. If prevention research can build on past contributions and integrate an immense amount of new knowledge from a wide range of core sciences, it will be able to expand its frontiers and open up new possibilities for intervention. Two broad areas of science provide the knowledge base for research on the prevention of mental disorders—the behavioral sciences, in which the study of mental disorders has its historical roots, and the biological sciences, which have begun to provide insights into these disorders more recently.

The boundaries between the behavioral and biological sciences should not be viewed as rigid and distinct. Interdisciplinary investigations that incorporate principles and findings from both the behavioral and the biological perspectives have vital implications for research on the prevention of mental disorders. The frontiers for the field of prevention can be moved forward through appropriate theoretical integration. In the sections that follow, this chapter presents four of these integrative core sciences as illustrations—neuroscience, genetics, epidemiology, and developmental psychopathology—to highlight how they have contributed and will continue to contribute to preventive intervention research.

NEUROSCIENCE

Neuroscience research encompasses the acquisition of knowledge about fundamental biological processes of the brain and nervous system and about the pathophysiology of neurological disease processes, including cellular mechanisms underlying etiology, course, and outcome. Knowledge about these biological processes can lead to the design of strategies aimed at treating specific symptoms and disorders and evaluating the efficacy and limitations of those treatments. Such understanding also can be important in framing and implementing a rational prevention strategy. The more that is known about etiology, the more possible it becomes to target preventive interventions to intervene in causal chains.

Neuroscience research varies in scope from highly theoretical to practical application, but, in general, the neuroscience research supported by the National Institutes of Health (NIH) takes a more disease-oriented focus, whereas the research supported by the National Science Foundation (NSF) focuses on acquiring basic knowledge about the functioning of the nervous system. The strategic value of having these complementary approaches is well recognized, but merits reaffirmation: knowledge from research in basic science is essential for applied investigations. Using worms or grasshoppers to study how nerve cells grow, differentiate, and reach their targets, and investigating the interaction between genetic and environmental factors in these processes, provides a simpler model system for understanding how more complex systems function.

Neuroscience research has provided important insights into how mental disorders arise. The discovery of chemical neurotransmission more than 70 years ago can be taken as the beginning of the modern neuroscience era. Prior to this discovery, understanding of the brain was limited to knowledge of its anatomy. Now, however, the functional relationship between certain classes of transmitters and specific neurons, the nature of transmitter receptors, and the consequences of receptor activation are being studied. Specific data are being gathered that define conditions in which channels will open or close, calcium will enter the cell or be excluded, and genes will be activated or silenced.

The basic function of nerve cells is to transmit information. Once chemical neurotransmitters are released, they act on neighboring cells to excite or inhibit them. There is a highly precise interaction between the neurotransmitter and a specific receptor protein on the target cell that regulates the latter's response, yet a single neurotransmitter can affect multiple receptors. For example, the neurotransmitter serotonin, which is important in both depression and schizophrenia, acts on at least 11 different specific serotonin receptors, and the neurotransmitter gamma-amino butyric acid (GABA) may act on as many as 100. These receptors differ slightly in their molecular structure and in the target functions they regulate, and are dispersed among cell clusters throughout the brain, thus providing great diversity in the cellular response to a single neurotransmitter. Serotonin released from a group of neurons may excite some neighboring cells and inhibit others, with gradations of activation and inhibition depending on the diversity of receptors it acts upon. There are also differences in where the receptors are found on a given cell, how avidly they respond to the transmitter, how long they respond, and what other cellular processes they regulate.

The production, liberation, and inactivation of neurotransmitters are highly regulated biological processes. Elucidating the mechanisms underlying these processes has contributed to the discovery of drugs used with varying degrees of success to treat schizophrenia, major depressive disorder, bipolar disorder, anxiety disorders, including obsessive compulsive disorder, and other conditions. Recent advances in molecular biology have led to an increase in our understanding of the scope and complexity of neuronal function. The practical outcome so far has been the discovery of new classes of drugs, such as the calcium channel blockers.

One goal of current research is to provide even greater effectiveness of drug therapy by increasing the number of cellular targets for drug action. These may include more receptor-subtype-specific agents, as well as drugs that act on ion channels (that regulate the influx and afflux of charged molecules) and protein kinases (that add phosphate groups to proteins), all of which are steps between the receptor and the cellular response to its activation. The potential implications of this research for indicated preventive interventions may be considerable if the medications are found to be safe enough to justify their use with high-risk individuals who have developed early signs and symptoms of a disorder.

GENETICS

Research into the genetic causes of disease is among the most active and exciting areas of biomedical investigation.* Within the next several years, genetic research promises to make substantial contributions to our understanding of mental disorders.

Genetic influences are quite relevant to prevention research. First, the accumulated results in genetic research have provided convincing evidence of the role of genetic factors both in normal variations in

---

*Portions of this section were based on a commissioned paper by M. Rutter, available as indicated in Appendix D.

psychological functioning and in psychopathology (Loehlin, 1992; Plomin, 1990, 1986; Rutter, Bolton, Harrington, Le Couteur, Macdonald, and Simonoff, 1990; Rutter, Macdonald, Le Couteur, Harrington, Bolton, and Bailey, 1990; Vandenberg, Singer, and Pauls, 1986). Heritability estimates for most mental disorders tend to be in the 30 to 60 percent range, so the genetic component, although not overwhelming, is by no means trivial. Second, interaction between environmental influences and genetic factors will be clearer as research gradually elucidates the specific impact of genes on mental functioning. Genetic studies have the power to be highly informative about developmental processes and psychopathological mechanisms (Rutter, Simonoff, and Silberg, in press; Rutter, Silberg, and Simonoff, 1993; Rutter, 1991). Because an understanding of such processes and mechanisms is crucial for the most effective planning of interventive measures, genetic research and genetic knowledge are potentially very valuable to prevention as well as treatment. Current and potential contributions to prevention center on the following topics:

- Nature of disorders. When planning preventive interventions, knowledge about the nature of the disorders to be prevented may often be helpful; genetic research findings can be useful in that connection. First, they may point to basic causal processes. Second, they can indicate which disorders are, and which are not, continuous with normally distributed characteristics. Third, disorders may come about through several rather different mechanisms, and genetics research may be helpful in determining which mechanism applies in each case.

In the future, research will seek to understand whether disease-specific genetic alleles controlling receptor-mediated processes lead to mental disorders. If this is found to be true, the initial application of this knowledge will be to screen individuals bearing the disease-specific allele so that earlier, and hopefully more effective, preventive strategies can be implemented. Some of these indicated preventive interventions may be pharmacological, but rich opportunities also exist for psychosocial interventions.

An example of such an opportunity may exist with infantile autism, a severe developmental disorder that strikes in infancy and leads to profound cognitive and social impairment. Autism represents a disturbance in the development of the brain centers that mediate language and information processing. One goal of research in autism is to identify a reliable marker for the disorder that will enable high-risk individuals to be identified in early infancy. Indicated prevention strategies, such as language and social skills training, could then be implemented to take advantage of the great plasticity of the brain in early childhood. One hypothesis of this research is that immature, still developing brain centers could be stimulated to acquire the function of the centers that are developmentally impaired, thus delaying or even eliminating the emergence of autism. This notion arises directly from the concept of sensitive periods, that is, periods in development during which relevant stimuli and transactions must occur or development is irreversibly altered, an important principle derived from basic research in developmental neurobiology.

• Mechanisms of genetic risk. In the past, much genetic research in the field of psychopathology has been concerned with quantifying the genetic contribution to overall population variance. In themselves, however, heritability estimates are not particularly useful because they carry no information about the mechanisms involved in genetic risk. Understanding genetic mechanisms is crucial for most effective interventions. Phenylketonuria constitutes an obvious example of a disorder in which such an understanding has led to an extremely effective environmental preventive intervention (low phenylalanine diet in childhood). Thus a disorder that is genetic nevertheless leads to disabilities that are environmentally preventable.

There is a rapidly growing body of evidence that major genes play a contributory role, as part of multifactorial inheritance, in a range of complex human diseases, including diabetes, heart disease, and hypertension (Weatherall, 1992). The value of these studies is that they are beginning to identify the mode of operation of genetic risk (Kurtz, 1992). Cambien and colleagues have reported that a deletion polymorphism in the gene encoding the angiotensin converting enzyme (ACE) may be a risk factor for myocardial infarction in a specific subgroup of individuals (Cambien, Poirer, Lecerf, Evans, Cambou, Arveiler et al., 1992). If confirmed, this particular finding could mean that genotyping could be used to identify people for whom administration of an ACE inhibitor might prevent recurrent myocardial infarction. The implication of this work, particularly for mental disorders, is that for most conditions we must move from thinking about a single cause of a disease (genetic or environmental) to thinking about how we may elucidate possible risk mechanisms. Examples relevant to mental disorders include the role genetic factors play in alcohol dependence, depressive disorders, physiological reactivity, temperamental characteristics, and emotional and conduct disturbances.

• Testing for environmental effects. Traditionally, studies examining differences between identical and fraternal twins have been classified as genetic research. However, when the phenotype being studied is a behavior, these studies provide the most satisfactory way of quantifying the strength of environmental effects. Other types of studies that have provided useful information include adoption studies; studies of various classes of relatives, using path models; and experimental studies, including experiments of nature, in which individuals are exposed to changing environments.

As Plomin and Bergman (1991) pointed out, the fact that a variable is labeled as "environmental" does not mean that its effects are environmentally mediated; many supposedly "environmental" measures actually index genetic, as well as environmental, influences. This point is best seen with the many risk factors that are based on someone's personal characteristics or behavior, such as low intelligence, aggressiveness, and behavioral inhibition. These involve a genetic component as well, and it is necessary to determine whether the psychiatric risk reflects genetic or environmental mediation.

● Individual differences in environmental effects. One of the most important recent findings from behavioral genetics research with twins has been the demonstration that, for many aspects of normal and abnormal psychosocial development, nonshared environmental effects tend to be substantially more important than shared ones in quantifying variability in outcomes (Plomin and Daniels, 1987). Shared risk factors that apply to the family as a whole, such as family discord or poverty, are indeed relevant, but they are likely to impinge on different children in the same family to varying degrees or in different ways, that is, to have nonshared effects. If we are to understand how such environmental risk factors operate, we must investigate the processes on a person-specific basis and not simply assume a uniform impact.

Relative differences between siblings in how they are treated in a home may be more important than the absolute level of this treatment in the home (Dunn and Plomin, 1990). That is, what appears to be a shared risk factor within the family may actually be an unshared risk factor, with its concomitant unshared effect, for, perhaps, only one child in the family. For example, it may be that it is less important whether parents respond to their children in a generally warm, or strict, or harsh fashion than whether one child in the family is consistently dealt with less warmly, or more strictly, or more harshly than his or her brothers and sisters. In other words, scapegoating or favoritism may be the operative risk factor (Boer and Dunn, 1992).

Attention needs to be paid to shared and unshared risk and protective factors and shared and unshared effects outside, as well as inside, the family. The body of evidence that school influences have effects on children's behavior and scholastic attainments (Maughan, in press;

Mortimore, in press) is particularly pertinent because it provides a setting for potential prevention that applies to all children. Peer group and community influences are also relevant (Quinton, in press; Reiss, in press).

• Individual differences in exposure to risk factors. During the last decade, behavioral geneticists have drawn attention to the various ways in which gene-environment interactions can arise. They have argued that, to a great extent, individuals shape and select their environments and that genetic factors play a part in this process (Scarr, 1992; Scarr and McCartney, 1983). Many nongeneticists have been reluctant to accept this possibility and have interpreted the suggestion as an argument against taking measures to improve environmental conditions. This suggests a point that may be vital to planning effective interventions, namely, that individuals vary greatly in their exposure to risk factors in their environments (Rutter and Rutter, 1993). Psychosocial stresses and adversities are not randomly distributed, and it is essential that we understand how those individual differences in risk exposure come about. This issue has not been addressed in any intensive and systematic manner, but we need to learn why some individuals suffer a host of environmental adversities, whereas others go through life with a string of generally positive experiences. Individual differences in environmental risk exposure should be treated as dependent, as well as independent, variables.

• Misleading environmental assumptions. Up until 10 or 20 years ago, there was a widespread assumption that birth trauma was an important environmental cause of brain damage and therefore a common cause of mental retardation and cerebral palsy (Hardy, 1965). More recent findings have forced a reassessment of this belief and now indicate that in most cases the causal factors operated at a much earlier stage in gestation (Nelson and Ellenberg, 1986). Nevertheless, there is still a tendency to treat obstetric complications as though they were only environmental risk factors. Recent evidence suggests that the process may also work the other way around: genetic or chromosomal abnormalities in the fetus may predispose to obstetric complications. For example, studies in children with Down's syndrome have indicated that the genetic abnormality is associated with a substantially increased risk of obstetric complications (Bolton and Holland, in press). This appreciation has also led to a reevaluation of the etiological role of obstetric complications in autism.

• Genetic counseling. Most medical genetic counseling has been based on the various patterns of risk associated with different types of genetic disorders: autosomal dominant, autosomal recessive, and so forth. But advances in molecular genetics now enable us to provide individualized risk information and not just actuarial probabilities. Genetic counseling is no longer confined to advising people about the risks involved if they have children or the risk involved in a particular pregnancy. It may now involve decisions on whether to take preventive action with people who are known to be at genetic risk through mechanisms involving susceptibility to environmental factors.

• Gene therapy. Gene therapy may become a possibility with some applications in the field of mental disorders. Some therapy is currently feasible in conditions caused by a single gene of major effect. Most mental disorders, however, involve multiple genes. It is now possible in tissue culture cells, and in limited cases in animals, to modify the expression of mutant genes and alter their pathologic outcome. This capability will only grow over the coming years, and the advent of gene therapy has led to a parallel realization of the ethical dilemmas it engenders. There is now growing agreement that somatic gene therapy to treat a disease, in which the genes of body (e.g., muscle) cells are modified, is ethical in certain circumstances. In contrast, there is currently an active debate over whether modification of genes in the germline cells (sperm and ova) can be considered ethical in any circumstances.

EPIDEMIOLOGY

Epidemiology also can take a developmental and integrative perspective on the etiology and course of psychopathology. Epidemiology is the study of the distribution of disorders in populations. Epidemiologists prefer to study well-defined populations, including community samples. The differential distribution of disorders is reported as incidence and prevalence of specified disorders. *Incidence* refers to the rate at which new cases of the disorder arise. *Prevalence* is the proportion of the population with the disorder. The prevalence of a disorder is a function not only of incidence but also of duration. Disorders can vary in duration from brief to lifelong. *Point prevalence* is the proportion in the population at a given point in time who have the disorder. Point prevalence is most useful for estimating need for services. *Lifetime prevalence* (sometimes called the proportion of survivors affected, or PSA) is the proportion of the population who, at some time during their lives up to the present, have had the disorder. Lifetime prevalence is most useful to those with interest in genetics. But because not everyone surveyed will have lived through the age of risk at the time of the interview, lifetime prevalence estimates are considered conservative.

Preventive interventions are directed toward reducing incidence, whereas treatment interventions seek to reduce prevalence by early detection and reduction of duration by effective intervention to reverse the symptoms and reduce the likelihood of relapse. Without effective treatment interventions, early case identification will have the paradoxical effect of increasing prevalence by increasing the count of a disorder that will then have lengthy duration because it is untreatable.

Epidemiological research has produced data on differential incidence and prevalence by demographic factors such as age, gender, educational level, employment status, ethnicity, and socioeconomic level; environmental factors such as hazardous conditions, toxic substances, stressful environments, availability of resources or supports, and ease of availability of drugs, alcohol, guns, and cars; personal attributes such as temperament, attractiveness, intelligence, and prior individual experience; and biological attributes such as genetics, health status, and other biological vulnerability.

Throughout epidemiological research, there is a common goal of identifying risk factors. There are two major research strategies for ascertaining the relation of risk factors to subsequent disorders. They are the *case-control* and the *cohort* designs. Case-control studies are often an initial and exploratory step in the identification of risk. An observed condition or disorder within an individual is called a "case." The cases are then compared with "controls," that is, similar individuals who do not have the disorder. On the basis of existing knowledge and reasonable hypotheses about antecedents, the cases and controls are compared retrospectively across a number of salient dimensions. This approach is often followed by a prospective cohort study, in which a group of persons who all have the antecedents of interest (that is, the risk factors) but do not have the condition or disorder of interest are compared with a group of persons who have neither the antecedents nor the disorder. These cohort studies yield actual estimates of the risk of disorder that follows a particular event or set of events.

Epidemiological studies of the occurrence of differential distribution of disorders across the population have yielded valuable data on both the origins and the life course of mental disorders. In studying the origins of a mental disorder, a prospective longitudinal design is particularly powerful. Epidemiological research designs that sample a range of populations and use repeated measurements permit inferences about causality. For some rare disorders and for disorders with onset in later life, case-control studies are the only practical method.

Two refinements of the concept of risk allow comparisons of various factors as they influence the development of disorder. One important refinement is *relative risk*. Relative risk is the ratio of incidence for a given disorder in an exposed population to the incidence in an unexposed population. For example, the risk of death by lung cancer might be 15 times higher among smokers than among nonsmokers—a relative risk of 15. Relative risk is obtained in a cohort study and can be approximated in a case-control study.

A second measure linked to risk is *attributable risk*. Attributable risk is the maximum proportion of cases that would be prevented if an intervention were 100 percent effective in eliminating the risk factor. Attributable risk combines information on relative risk with information on the prevalence of the exposure, in order to help judge which risk factor to target in trying to eliminate the disorder. The formula is $p(r - 1)/[p(r - 1) + 1]$, where p is prevalence of exposure and r is relative risk (Mausner and Kramer, 1985). If the relative risk of lung cancer for smokers versus nonsmokers is 15, as above, and the prevalence of smoking is about 50 percent, then the proportion of cases of lung cancer attributable to smoking, that is, the attributable risk, is approximately 88 percent.

Data on prevalence and on attributable risk are especially germane to research on the prevention of mental disorders. To acquire these data, diverse strategies of research are needed. The prevalence of the disorder is required in order to assess its impact on the population. Prevalence is obtained efficiently from a cross-sectional survey. The attributable risk for a range of risk factors is required in order to select interventions that will have the most powerful effect. Attributable risk probably is most efficiently obtained via the case-control strategy.

An even more recent frontier is the conceptualization of the age of onset for specific disorders. Determination of age of onset is required in order to time the intervention appropriately, that is, before the first incidence of a disorder or problem. Decisions as to when to target a high-risk population can be guided by epidemiological data regarding the range and mean age of onset in a population. Age of onset is best obtained from a longitudinal study of a cohort from the general population. Recognizing the importance of such data, the committee commissioned new analyses of data from the Epidemiologic Catchment Area study. The conceptualizations and methods used in these analyses, and the resulting fresh perspectives they permit, are presented in Chapter 5.

DEVELOPMENTAL PSYCHOPATHOLOGY

Many scientific areas of study with links to prevention research have their origin in the behavioral and social sciences. Developmental psychopathology is one of these areas. (See Box 4.1 for other illustrations.)

Box 4.1
Illustrations from the Behavioral and Social Sciences

Many theoretical concepts originating in the behavioral sciences have relevance to research on prevention of mental disorders. These include self-esteem, regulation of emotions, attribution, cultural and gender-based diversity, social networks, community context, and ecological perspectives. Other concepts are presented here as illustrations of specific areas of study that have had—and will continue to have—an impact on the conceptual design of prevention studies.

Psychological stress is associated with a variety of negative effects on health, although the specific mechanisms for this relationship are not well understood. Recent research in psychoneuroimmunology (Ader, Felten, and Cohen, 1991) has suggested that stress can directly affect interactions between the central nervous system and the immune system. Studies of the neuroendocrine correlates of stress, for example, may lead to a better understanding of the physiological pathways by which environmental stressors affect personal health (IOM, 1989, 1984, 1982b; CBASSE, 1988).

Social support mechanisms appear to perform an essential function in several areas, including increasing or decreasing an individual's sensitivity to certain stressors, increasing or decreasing an individual's likelihood of using or abstaining from drugs, and increasing compliance with therapeutic regimes. The quantity and quality of social support networks are also thought to have a role in the onset and course of mental disorders, including depression and schizophrenia. One line of inquiry has examined how perceptions of personal control mediate the effects of social networks on health outcomes, a factor that appears to be far more significant than has been recognized by health care providers (CBASSE, 1988; IOM, 1984, 1982a).

Analysis of the usage of health care delivery systems is also relevant to prevention. Research on the role of health maintenance organizations (HMOs), for example, has indicated that certain forms of public and private subsidies of diagnostic and preventive health care practices affect the use of such services by individuals and groups. Data from these studies strongly suggest that the delivery of health care services for the general population could be greatly improved by subsidizing expanded preventive interventions for people at risk for certain health disorders, although the economic and social consequences of such targeted practices have yet to be determined (CBASSE, 1988).

Interpersonal transaction research in recent years has defined a complex interplay among expectancies, self-concepts, and motives. For example, hostile acts are often stimulated and guided by expectations of aggression that may be influenced by early childhood experiences. If the individual has experienced aggressive behavior in the past, his or her perceptions may be negatively distorted, rather than assuming ambiguous acts to be benign or accidental (CBASSE, 1993, 1988; Dodge, Bates, and Pettit, 1990).

Attachment theory postulates that early relationships between infants and their caregivers, usually their mothers, have a critical role in the infants' later development, especially in social relationships. Infants show attachment behavior by seeking comfort and protection, and caregivers' responses demonstrate the quality of their sensitivity and responsivity. Mother-child pairs differ in their interactive styles, and there has been considerable research in the last 15 years, based on early work by Ainsworth and colleagues on the measurement and classification of these differences and their links to later behaviors (Ainsworth, Blehar, Waters, and Well, 1978). This theory has direct relevance to prevention and indeed has been applied in programs designed to enhance healthy parent-infant relationships. For example, a preventive intervention designed by Erickson, Korfmacher, and Egeland (1992) targeted prospective mothers in "a special window of opportunity" around the birth of their first child with the aim of having an impact on the mother's view of herself and her child as well as their relationship.

Self-efficacy theory is based on the premise that individuals who have a sense of control over their environment will live a more active and self-determined life. Perceived self-efficacy appears to be highly correlated with a wide range of health behaviors, affecting the onset, course, and sequelae of both mental and physical disorders (Schwarzer, 1992). For example, perceived self-efficacy is related to the appraisal and management of stressful experiences, to the onset of depressive symptoms, to problem-solving strategies that might influence decisions regarding use of cigarettes, to the alleviation of inappropriate fears of individuals recovering from heart attacks, and to the self-management capabilities of patients with chronic illnesses. A sense of self-efficacy is enhanced as individuals learn how to influence the risk factors and stressful experiences in their lives by setting attainable goals, enlisting incentives and social supports to sustain their efforts for behavior changes, and developing self-regulatory capabilities required for sustaining the new behavior over an extended period (Bandura, 1992).

Its developmental life span perspective reflects the impact of biological and psychological changes in the individual, and it provides the opportunity for an integrated empirical application of advances in other core sciences, including neuroscience, genetics, and epidemiology. In 1984, developmental psychopathology was defined by Sroufe and Rutter as "the study of the origins and course of individual patterns of behavioral maladaptation" (Sroufe and Rutter, 1984, p. 18). However, developmental psychopathologists are as interested in individuals who do not develop disorders despite severe adversity as in those who do succumb to illness. They also study children who appear emotionally healthy early in life, but develop mental disorders in adulthood. Prospective longitudinal risk research is at the heart of this new discipline; prospective designs help define etiologies and pathways for illness, illuminating changes in risk and protective factors for individuals over time. The task is complex. "Links between earlier adaptation and later pathology generally will not be simple or direct. It will be necessary to understand both individual patterns of adaptation with respect to salient issues of a given developmental period and the transaction between prior adaptation, maturational change, and subsequent environmental challenges" (Sroufe and Rutter, 1984, p. 17). Such a perspective provides a comfortable home for true integration of biological and behavioral influences.

Developmental psychopathology may indeed be the core integrative discipline for the knowledge base for preventive intervention research. Certainly its concepts, principles, and goals are similar to those in prevention. These concepts include risk and protective factors, precursors, sequelae, competence/incompetence, developmental antecedents of disorders, age-defined adaptation, resilience, and predictability. Sroufe and Rutter (1984) believed not only that the information gained from longitudinal risk research could yield valuable information for preventive interventions, but also that prevention was one of the central justifications for the existence of this special discipline. Developmentally based preventive interventions, moreover, have the potential to serve as tests of theory (Cicchetti and Toth, 1992).

Two examples highlight the research developments in developmental psychopathology. First, low birthweight and premature birth have long been thought to be risk factors associated with increased rates of behavioral and emotional symptoms. Early reports of these associations were largely retrospective and descriptive in nature, but with prospective longitudinal studies in many different disciplines the evidence is more sound. For example, Rose and colleagues reported that very low birthweight premature infants manifested more behavior problems than full-term infants at three and six years (Rose, Feldman, Rose, Wallace, and McCarton, 1992). Also, the overall prevalence of clinically significant problems in the low-birthweight premature infants increased with age: at age three, 30 percent had problems; by age six, 50 percent of them did. Studies such as this one add credence to the beliefs that some such infants are at risk not only for cognitive impairment but also for behavioral dysfunction and that the problems are not transient in nature. Other studies, however, have not shown such pessimistic outcomes, thereby raising research questions regarding degrees of risk and the role of protective factors.

Second, developmental approaches to depression—including epidemiology, risk and protective factors, precursor symptoms, onset, course, and sequelae—are needed across the life span. For example, during the transition to parenthood, depression can be a serious problem; about 10 percent of postpartum women develop a depressive disorder severe enough that it interferes with daily functioning (Campbell and Cohn, 1991; O'Hara, Zekoski, Phillips, and Wright, 1990).

Campbell and colleagues found that even though most postpartum depressions tend to be brief, they can last as long as two years; even those women whose depressive episode abates are likely to continue to experience more subtle difficulties (Campbell, Cohn, Flanagan, Popper, and Meyers, 1992). These problems eventually are reflected in the mother-infant relationship. In Campbell's study the infants of depressed mothers received less appropriate and less responsive care and more negative and rejecting care than the comparison group at two months. The impact of maternal depression on the infant's development can be seen quite early. Field (1992) found that these infants can develop a "depressed mood style" as early as three months and that this mood state persists over the first year of life if the mother's depression persists. By the end of the first year, this mood has affected both physical growth and scores on the Bayley Scales of Infant Development. There is also some evidence that by 11 to 17 months of age, infants of depressed mothers exhibit reduced activity in the right frontal area of the brain (Dawson, Klinger, Panagiotides, Spieker, and Frey, 1992). This finding raises the possibility that maternal behavior can influence not only an infant's developing psychosocial areas of functioning but also the development of the central nervous system.

Maternal depression is not the only, and perhaps not even the most frequent, risk factor for the development of depression during childhood. For example, other forms of parental psychopathology and child maltreatment, and especially the interactive effects when both risk factors are present, also significantly increase the likelihood that a child will become depressed in middle childhood (Downey and Walker, 1992; Toth, Manly, and Cicchetti, 1992).

The rate of depression rises overall between childhood and adolescence. In a sample of 3,519 8- to 16-year-old psychiatric patients, both boys and girls had increasing rates of depression across this age range, with no gender difference in rates before age 11 (Angold and Rutter, 1992). However, by age 16 girls were twice as likely as boys to have significant depressive symptomatology. When age was controlled for, pubertal status had no effect on depression scores. Depressed girls are at high risk for multiple problems, including early pregnancy. The babies of these girls can be, in turn, at risk for developing a similar affective style.

These two examples—low-birthweight premature births and depression—highlight new directions and frontiers for research in developmental psychopathology. First, there is value in understanding age variations in susceptibility to a wide range of phenomena, including low birthweight, parental psychopathology, brain injury, attachment problems, and hospital admissions. Second, it is essential to learn about continuities and discontinuities in development and about normal variation so that researchers can begin to clarify when preventive interventions are not warranted as well as when they are. Third, there is much more to understand about indirect causal chain processes, mechanisms, and biological and environmental interactions. Finally, there is a need to assess risk factors and the effects of intervention across multiple age periods in each individual and across generations, such as both mothers and their infants.

FINDINGS AND LEADS

• There is an increasing tendency within the biological and behavioral sciences to appreciate the complexity and interplay of genetic and environmental interactions. There has been some movement away from the traditional nature-nurture dichotomy toward a recognition that genetic inheritance (the genotype) provides a reaction range within which the environment can have some impact on the characteristic that is expressed (the phenotype).

• An understanding of etiology can contribute to the conceptualization and implementation of rational preventive interventions. Research in the core sciences to uncover the wide range of biopsychosocial etiological factors in mental illness is therefore critical to the long-term success of the prevention research initiative. Such basic scientific research endeavors have been the building blocks for the knowledge base on which prevention research has developed.

• Many of the interdisciplinary areas of investigation with relevance to prevention research have independently recognized the utility of a developmental focus. These areas include neuroscience, genetics, epidemiology, and developmental psychopathology. From this developmental focus has arisen the concept of sensitive periods.

• Eventually, it may become possible to determine the precise mechanisms by which environmental risk factors operate. In attempting to ascertain the relative contributions of the biological and environmental influences on expressed behavior or attributes, a number of paradigms have been useful, including twin, adoption, and experimental studies. In the absence of sound knowledge on risk mechanisms, there is some danger that prevention measures may be either wrongly targeted or so diffuse that they do not bring the expected benefits.

• There is considerable evidence that people act in ways that influence the level of risk in the environments they experience. What is less certain is the genetic influence in this process. Genetic influences on behavior may heighten or lower the likelihood of risk exposure. Investigations into genetic influences should lead to increased understanding as to how individual differences in environmental risk exposure come about.

• In the field of genetics, research findings are accumulating rapidly. Some of these are relevant to traditional genetic disorders that have psychiatric implications (e.g., mental retardations, Huntington's disease), but many have considerable value for the broader range of common, multifactorial mental disorders in which genetic factors play a variably prominent role, such as alcohol dependence and depressive disorder. To a limited extent, available genetic data have preventive implications in the area of genetic counseling, but, to a much greater extent, the findings identify the potential importance of environmental preventive interventions for individuals who are known to be at genetic risk through mechanisms involving vulnerability to environmental factors.

• Effective and efficient research on prevention of mental disorders requires that certain data on the epidemiology of the disorders be available—specifically, incidence, prevalence, relative risk, attributable risk, and age of onset. Such data are needed across the life span for an integrative, developmental understanding of mental disorders.

• Research studies on risk factors in the interdisciplinary area of developmental psychopathology have the potential for developing into preventive interventions targeting these risk factors with developmentally appropriate timing.

• Much can be learned from studies of individuals who do not develop mental disorders despite being at high risk as well as studies of individuals who appear emotionally healthy while young but develop mental disorders in adulthood.

• Contributions from areas of investigation rooted in the behavioral sciences offer substantial leads for research on the prevention of mental disorders. These include the impact of psychological stress on health; the role of social support mechanisms in decreasing risk factors and enhancing protective factors; usage of health care delivery systems; the relationship between theoretical concepts such as attachment, self-esteem, and self-efficacy and later social relationships and health behaviors; and the importance of social frames of reference, including race, culture, gender, and community context.

REFERENCES

Ader, R.; Felten, D. L.; Cohen, N., Eds. (1991) Psychoneuroimmunology. San Diego, CA: Academy Press.

Ainsworth, M. D. S.; Blehar, M. C.; Waters, E.; Well, S. (1978) Patterns of attachment: A psychological study of the strange situation. Hillsdale, NJ: Lawrence Erlbaum.

Angold, A.; Rutter, M. (1992) Effects of age and pubertal status on depression in a large clinical sample. Development and Psychopathology; 4: 5–28.

Bandura, A. (1992) Self-efficacy mechanism in psychobiologic functioning. In: R. Schwarzer, Ed. Self-efficacy: Thought Control of Action. Philadelphia, PA: Hemisphere Publishing.

Boer, F.; Dunn, J., Eds. (1992) Children's Sibling Relationships: Developmental and Clinical Issues. Hillsdale, NJ: Lawrence Erlbaum.

Bolton, P.; Holland, A. (in press) Chromosomal abnormalities. In: M. Rutter, E. Taylor, and L. Hersov, Eds. Child and Adolescent Psychiatry. 3rd ed. Oxford, England: Blackwell Scientific Publications.

Cambien, F.; Poirer, O.; Lecerf, L.; Evans, A.; Cambou, J. P.; Arveiler, D.; Luc, G.; Bard, J. M.; Bara, L.; Richards, S.; Tiret, L.; Amouyel, P.; Alhenc-Gelas, F.; Soubrier, F. (1992) Deletion polymorphism in the gene for angiotensin-converting enzyme is a potent risk factor for myocardial infarction. Nature; 359: 641–644.

Campbell, S. B.; Cohn, J. F. (1991) Prevalence and correlates of postpartum depression in first-time mothers. Journal of Abnormal Psychology; 100: 594–599.

Campbell, S. B.; Cohn, J. F.; Flanagan, C.; Popper, S.; Meyers, T. (1992) Course and correlates of postpartum depression during the transition to parenthood. Development and Psychopathology; 4: 29–47.

CBASSE (Commission on Behavioral and Social Sciences and Education). (1993) Understanding and Preventing Violence. National Research Council. Washington, DC: National Academy Press.

CBASSE (Commission on Behavioral and Social Sciences and Education). (1988) The Behavioral and Social Sciences: Achievements and Opportunities. National Research Council. Washington, DC: National Academy Press.

Cicchetti, D.; Toth, S. L. (1992) The role of developmental theory in prevention and intervention. Development and Psychopathology; 4: 489–493.

Dawson, G.; Klinger, L. G.; Panagiotides, H.; Spieker, S.; Frey, K. (1992) Infants of mothers with depressive symptoms: Electroencephalographic and behavioral findings related to attachment status. Development and Psychopathology; 4: 67–80.

Development and Psychopathology. (1992) Special issue: Developmental approaches to prevention and intervention; 4.

Dodge, K. A.; Bates, J. E.; Pettit, G. (1990) Mechanisms in the cycle of violence. Science; 250: 1678–1683.

Downey, G.; Walker, E. (1992) Distinguishing family-level and child influences on the development of depression and aggression in children at risk. Development and Psychopathology; 4: 81–95.

Dunn, J.; Plomin, R. (1990) Separate Lives: Why Siblings Are So Different. New York, NY: Basic Books.

Erickson, M. F.; Korfmacher, J.; Egeland, B. R. (1992) Attachments past and present: Implications for therapeutic intervention with mother-infant dyads. Development and Psychopathology; 4: 495–507.

Field, T. (1992) Infants of depressed mothers. Development and Psychopathology; 4: 49–66.

Hardy, J. B. (1965) Perinatal factors and intelligence. In: S. F. Osler and R. E. Cooke, Eds. The Biosocial Basis of Mental Retardation. Baltimore, MD: Johns Hopkins University Press.

IOM (Institute of Medicine). (1989) Behavioral Influences on the Endocrine and Immune Systems. Washington, DC: National Academy Press.

IOM (Institute of Medicine). (1984) Bereavement: Reactions, Consequences, and Care. Washington, DC: National Academy Press.

IOM (Institute of Medicine). (1982a) Health and Behavior: Frontiers of Research in the Biobehavioral Sciences. Washington, DC: National Academy Press; Pub. No. 82–010.

IOM (Institute of Medicine). (1982b) Stress and Human Health: Analysis and Implications of Research. New York, NY: Springer.

Kurtz, T. W. (1992) Myocardial infarction: The ACE of hearts. Nature; 359: 588–589.

Loehlin, J. C. (1992) Genes and Environment in Personality Development. Newbury Park, CA: Sage Publications.

Maughan, B. (in press) School influences. In: M. Rutter and D. Hay, Eds. Development Through Life: A Handbook for Clinicians. Oxford, England: Blackwell Scientific Publications.

Mausner, J.; Kramer, S. (1985) Mausner and Bahn Epidemiology: An Introductory Text. 2nd ed. Philadelphia, PA: W. B. Saunders & Company; 173.

Mortimore, P. (in press) The positive effects of schooling. In: M. Rutter, Ed. Psychosocial Disturbances in Young People: Challenges for Prevention. Cambridge, England: Cambridge University Press.

Nelson, K. B.; Ellenberg, J. H. (1986) Antecedents of cerebral palsy: Multivariate analysis of risk. New England Journal of Medicine; 315: 81–86.

O'Hara, M. W.; Zekoski, E. M.; Phillips, L. H.; Wright, E. J. (1990) Controlled prospective study of postpartum mood disorders: Comparison of childbearing and non-childbearing women. Journal of Abnormal Psychology; 99(1): 3–15.

Plomin, R. (1990) The role of inheritence in behavior. Science; 248(4952): 183–188.

Plomin, R. (1986) Development, Genetics and Psychology. Hillsdale, NJ: Lawrence Erlbaum.

Plomin, R.; Bergman, C. S. (1991) The nature of nurture: Genetic influence on "environmental" measures. Behavioural and Brain Sciences; 14(3): 373–427.

Plomin, R.; Daniels, D. (1987) Why are children in the same family so different from one another? Behavioural and Brain Sciences; 10(1): 1–16.

Quinton, D. (in press) Cultural and community influences. In: M. Rutter and D. Hay, Eds. Development Through Life: A Handbook for Clinicians. Oxford, England: Blackwell Scientific Publications.

Reiss, A., Jr. (in press) Community influences on adolescent behavior. In: M. Rutter, Ed. Psychosocial Disturbances in Young People: Challenges for Prevention. Cambridge, England: Cambridge University Press.

Rose, S. A.; Feldman, J. F.; Rose, S. L.; Wallace, I. F.; McCarton, C. (1992) Behavior problems at 3 and 6 years: Prevalence and continuity in full-terms and preterms. Development and Psychopathology; 4: 361–374.

Rutter, M. (1991) Nature, nurture and psychopathology: A new look at an old topic. Development and Psychopathology; 3(2): 125–136.

Rutter, M.; Bolton, P.; Harrington, R.; Le Couteur, A.; Macdonald, H.; Simonoff, E. (1990) Genetic factors in child psychiatric disorders: I. A review of research strategies. Journal of Child Psychology and Psychiatry; 31: 3–37.

Rutter, M.; Macdonald, H.; Le Couteur, A.; Harrington, R.; Bolton, P.; Bailey, A. (1990) Genetic factors in child psychiatric disorders. II. Empirical findings. Journal of Child Psychology and Psychiatry; 31(1): 39–83.

Rutter, M.; Rutter, M. (1993) Developing Minds: Challenge and Continuity Across the Lifespan. New York, NY: Basic Books.

Rutter, M.; Silberg, J.; Simonoff, E. (1993) Whither behaviour genetics? A developmental psychopathology perspective. In: R. Plomin and G. E. McClearn, Eds. Nature, Nurture and Psychology. Washington, DC: American Psychiatric Association.

Rutter, M.; Simonoff, E.; Silberg, J. (in press) How informative are twin studies of child psychopathology? In: T. J. Bouchard and P. Propping, Eds. Twins as a Tool of Behaviour Genetics. Chichester, England: John Wiley and Sons.

Scarr, S. (1992) Developmental theories for the 1990's: Development and individual differences. Child Development; 63(1): 1–19.

Scarr, S.; McCartney, K. (1983) How people make their own environments: A theory of genotype greater than environment effects. Child Development; 54(2): 424–435.

Schwarzer, R., Ed. (1992) Self-efficacy: Thought Control of Action. Philadelphia, PA: Hemisphere Publishing.

Sroufe, L. A.; Rutter, M. (1984) The domain of developmental psychopathology. Child Development; 55: 17–29.

Toth, S.; Manly, J. T.; Cicchetti, D. (1992) Child maltreatment and vulnerability to depression. Development and Psychopathology; 4: 97–112.

Vandenberg, S. G.; Singer, S. M.; Pauls, D. L. (1986) The Heredity of Behavior Disorders in Adults and Children. New York, NY: Plenum Medical.

Weatherall, D. (1992) The Harveian Oration. The Role of Nature and Nurture in Common Diseases: Garrod's Legacy. London, England: The Royal College of Physicians.

5

Description of Five Illustrative Mental Disorders

The diagnosis of mental disorders is made on the basis of signs and symptoms of aberrant thoughts, words, and behaviors. As yet there are no laboratory tests to diagnose these illnesses. Clinical research continues to refine our understanding of the symptomatology, natural course, co-morbidity, and treatment effectiveness for mental disorders. Continuing research on epidemiology provides needed data on incidence, prevalence, prodromal periods, and age of onset. In this chapter, the discussion of this knowledge is organized around five major mental disorders: conduct disorder, depressive disorders, alcohol abuse and dependence, schizophrenia, and Alzheimer's disease. In Chapter 6, the same disorders are examined for risk and protective factors that may eventually offer targets for intervention.

These five disorders were chosen as illustrations—for use in this chapter as well as in the rest of the report—because they are all serious disorders that have enormous emotional and financial costs associated with them. They demonstrate that specific disorders have their onset at varying stages in the life cycle, and that when they do occur, they often are disruptive to further stages of development. In addition, they represent the great diversity of mental illness and reflect a spectrum of causation, arising from clear genetic contributions in Alzheimer's disease to primarily psychosocial factors in conduct disorder. The choice of these five disorders is by no means meant to imply that these are the only disorders that should be targeted for preventive intervention research programs. Anxiety disorders, post-traumatic stress disorder, obsessive-compulsive disorder, and other adult and childhood mental disorders may also be appropriate for the introduction of preventive research strategies. These five disorders are simply illustrative of the range of factors and approaches that must be considered in designing preventive intervention research programs. The brief descriptions presented here, each highlighting slightly different points, are examples of how the information that is available for a particular disorder should be reviewed. The disorders are presented here in developmental sequence to emphasize the importance of a life course perspective.

DATA SOURCES, CONCEPTS, AND METHODOLOGIES USED IN THE DISORDER DESCRIPTIONS

Epidemiologic Catchment Area Study

The prevalence data for the five disorders are from several sources, including the National Institute of Mental Health's Epidemiologic Catchment Area (ECA) study, which has been discussed in more detail in other reports (various chapters of Robins and Regier, 1991, as cited below). Data on age of onset during the adult years are taken from the prospective one-year follow-up ECA study, designed, in part, to estimate the incidence of specific mental disorders (Eaton, Regier, Locke, and Taube, 1981). The onset data are not widely available elsewhere and so are highlighted here, along with their new application to delineation of prodromes, as well as explanations of the special utility of these concepts in preventive intervention research.

The ECA study consisted of community surveys carried out by five university-based research teams in different locations in the United States. The data presented below are from four sites: Baltimore, Maryland (Johns Hopkins University); St. Louis, Missouri (Washington University); Durham, North Carolina (Duke University); and Los Angeles, California (University of California). At each of these sites, both the prevalence survey and the one-year follow-up were done. For the fifth site, New Haven, Connecticut (Yale University), the longitudinal aspects of the design, and the questionnaire used, were sufficiently different to make pooling of data problematic.

The methods of the ECA study are described elsewhere (Eaton and Kessler, 1985). In brief, area probability samples of households were drawn, and household members 18 years of age or older were selected at random for interview. About 75 to 80 percent of those designated as respondents completed a 90-minute interview that included the Diagnostic Interview Schedule (DIS) (Robins, Helzer, Croughan, Williams, and Spitzer, 1981). At the one-year follow-up, a second interview was conducted with about 80 percent of those interviewed at the first wave. The DIS portion of the interview consisted of specified questions directly pertinent to diagnostic criteria from the third edition of the *Diagnostic and Statistical Manual* (DSM-III) of the American Psychiatric Association. The revised DSM-III-R is the best classification system available at the current time (DSM-IV is in press) and is the basis for the definitions used throughout the rest of this report. However, operational definitions of specific mental disorders as given in DSM-III, when major diagnostic criteria changes were made, were used in the ECA study and are used for determining onset in the analyses below. Onset is defined here as the first diagnosis of the disorder. Diagnoses were made from the DIS symptom data by means of computer algorithms that simulated the application of DSM-III criteria (Boyd, Burke, Gruenberg, Holzer, Rae, George et al., 1984). Because the ECA results depended on both the diagnostic criteria chosen and the method of ascertainment, the mental disorders as classified therein are referred to here as "DIS/DSM-III disorders."

Conceptualization of Onset

The absence of firm data on the validity of the DSM-III system for classifying mental disorders enjoins us to be careful about conceptualizing the process of disease onset. It is particularly difficult to establish the validity of a threshold for the presence versus the absence of disorder, because signs and symptoms of mental disorders are widespread in the population and do not always reflect the presence of a mental disorder. From the clinical standpoint, subtle differences in how behaviors are categorized may suggest quite varied thresholds for making diagnoses; from the epidemiological standpoint, subtle differences in threshold may produce widely varying prevalences.

A disorder that has a complex causal chain, where no particular cause is regarded as sufficient, may be preventable up to the point of onset, when the individual meets full criteria for diagnosis. The concept of attributable risk (see Chapter 4) allows quantitative comparison of risk factors in the population, which helps in selecting risk factors for intervention programs. Risk factors having high attributable risk for a specific disorder, or especially risk factors having high attributable risk for multiple disorders, would be prime targets for preventive interventions. But each risk factor may operate differently, and may be differentially malleable, that is, modifiable, at different times in life. Also, each risk factor may have a sensitive period in which an important contribution to the disorder may occur only at a particular phase of development, such as infancy, adolescence, or old age. Interventions should be planned before or during sensitive periods. Unfortunately, the sensitive periods of the risk factors are not well known, but they must occur before onset.

The *first incidence* of a disorder is the first onset of the disorder in the lifetime of the individual. It is usually simply called *incidence* in referring to age of onset in a population. The numerator for the *incidence rate* is composed of those individuals who have had an onset for the first time in their lives, and the denominator includes only persons who start the period of study with no history of the disorder. The incidence rate is the best quantitative expression of the force of morbidity in the population at a given age. Onset of first episode is a key concept for prevention because it is assumed that the causal structure producing morbidity changes after that point; that is, the risk factors that initiate the onset of a disorder may not be the same as the risk factors that prolong or exacerbate the disorder once it has occurred. Incidence rate is distinct from *attack rate* (also sometimes referred to as incidence, especially by those studying acute diseases such as respiratory infections), which is the rate at which episodes of disorder develop in a population not currently in an episode. The denominator for the attack rate is different from that for first incidence in that it may include persons who have had an episode of disorder earlier in their lives, but who do not currently meet the criteria for disorder; that is, it includes remitted cases.

For mental disorders and for many physical disorders, the force of morbidity may be expressed by the rate at which individuals cross a variety of thresholds, including onset, in the process of development of a disorder. These thresholds may be below the current diagnostic criteria or above them. The causal structure is not well understood for either initiation, prolongation, or exacerbation. Therefore the relative value of incidence versus attack rate is an empirical question that has not yet been resolved.

The *prodrome* is the period prior to onset of a disorder, when some early signs or symptoms are nevertheless present. Given the widespread prevalence of individual signs and symptoms of mental disorders in the general population, it is likely that many individuals with early signs and symptoms of disorder will not go on to develop the full criteria for diagnosis, perhaps because there is a dynamic flux of risk and protective factors over time. In this situation the signs and symptoms are not prodromal, in the strict sense of the word. For a particular individual a prodrome can be known only in retrospect, after he or she has developed the disorder. If he or she never develops it, the early signs were not part of a prodrome. Signs and symptoms from a diagnostic cluster that precede disorder, but do not predict the onset of disorder with certainty, are referred to here as *precursor signs and symptoms*. Signs and symptoms from a diagnostic cluster that do precede the development of a disorder in a particular individual are referred to as *prodromal signs and symptoms*. At the present state of our knowledge of the onset of mental disorders, there are few or no signs and symptoms that predict onset with certainty. Nevertheless, precursor signs and symptoms can be helpful in identifying groups at much higher risk for onset than the general population.

Methods for Analyzing Onset

An important problem in presenting data on age of onset is *censoring* (Lawless, 1982). In the context of age of onset, censoring occurs when the exact age of onset is known for only a portion of the sample; for the remainder, the age is known only to exceed some given age (right censoring) or to be below some given age (left censoring). Most presentations on age of onset arise from cross-sectional data and are right censored (e.g., Christie, Burke, Regier, Rae, Boyd, and Locke, 1988). In field surveys, the cross-sectional method is used to determine the presence or absence of disorder over the history of an individual, through retrospective recall, and then to determine age of onset for those with a positive history. In such surveys the vast majority of individuals do not report a history of disorder, and some of the individuals without disorder will develop a disorder after the survey is completed. Therefore the right-censored data from such a survey are inevitably biased in the direction of earlier age of onset. The degree of bias is difficult to know without knowledge of the age of onset, but it can be sizable. For example, imagine ascertaining age of onset for a disorder that typically has a very late onset, such as Huntington's disease, through a cross-sectional survey of the general population. Most persons in the sample would be too young to have had onset; only a handful would have lived through the age of risk for the disorder. Therefore the age of onset would appear younger than it really is. The prospective aspect of the data presented below avoids the problem of right censoring. But because the target population in the ECA surveys was defined as adults 18 years of age or older, onset for earlier years cannot be displayed. Data on psychopathology for population-based samples of children are discussed later in this chapter.

Age of onset is presented here in cumulative form because that form is, for reasons explained below, most relevant to prevention. However, cumulative presentation can obscure important relationships of the force

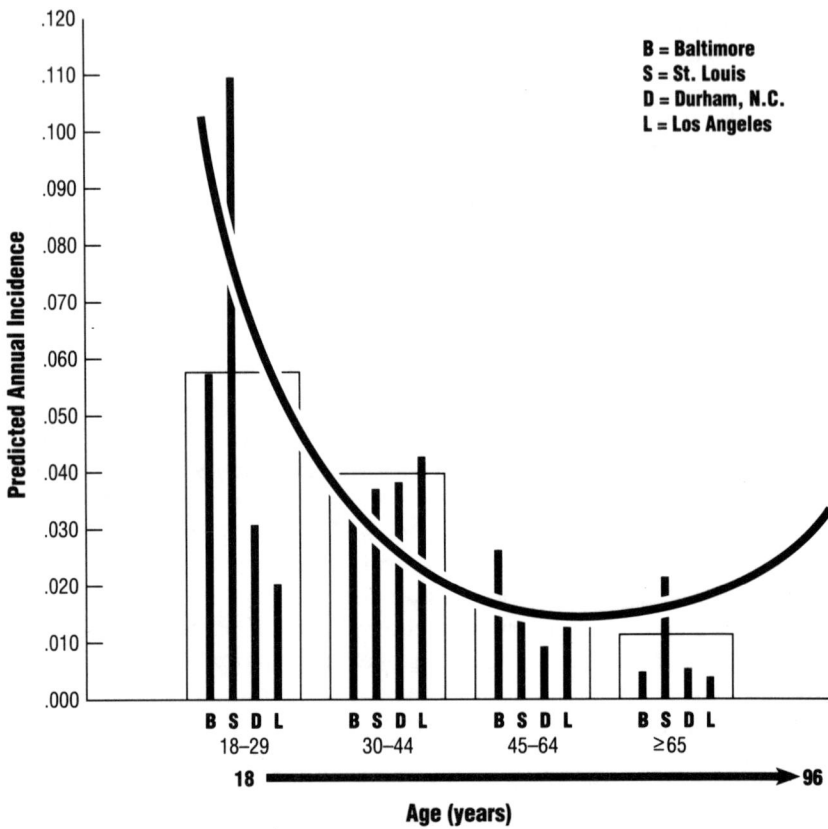

FIGURE 5.1   Annual incidence of DIS/DSM-III Alcohol Abuse/Dependence.

of morbidity to the life course, which may have etiological significance. For example, Figure 5.1 presents data on the incidence of DIS/DSM-III alcohol abuse or dependence among males at four sites of the ECA study (Eaton, Kramer, Anthony, Dryman, Shapiro, and Locke, 1989). The figure shows an upturn in incidence in the later years of life. The upturn is due to only a few individual onsets in a total sample of over 10,000, but a similar pattern in the only other comparable study (Hagnell, Lanke, Rorsman, and Ojesjo, 1982) suggests it is not a statistical artifact. The upturn in late life may indicate causal factors such as a decline in physical functioning or the effects of retirement. In the cumulative form presented in Figure 5.2, however, the upturn in later life is obscured.

Figure 5.1 illustrates other methodological issues. One issue is the considerable statistical volatility of the prospective data, which is based

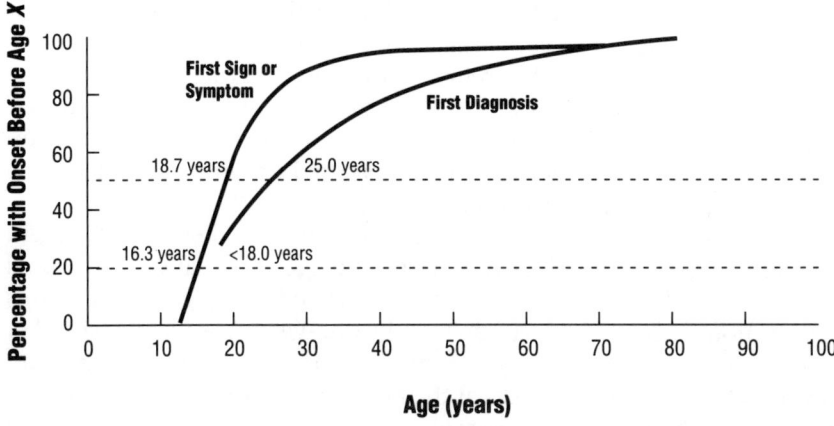

FIGURE 5.2   Age of onset of DIS/DSM-III Alcohol Abuse and Dependence. Population estimates are from 125 new cases (with 20th and 50th percentiles marked). Source: NIMH Epidemiologic Catchment Area Study, Four Sites, 1978 to 1983.

on the occurrence of a handful of new cases among many thousands of persons at risk for developing the disorder over the one-year follow-up. The volatility is best demonstrated by the thin black bars, which represent age-specific rates at each site. The open rectangle is the age-specific rate for all four sites collapsed, and it shows more stability due to pooling of data. The curve itself involves the maximal smoothing of the data, using only two degrees of freedom. The cumulative form of presentation obscures this statistical volatility. The cumulative distributions presented for the five disorders below are weighted statistically to represent a population with age, gender, and race characteristics identical to those of the U.S. population (as in Robins and Regier, 1991).

The cumulative form of presentation, along with the statistical weighting, links the data to the concept of attributable risk. The cumulative form allows one to estimate the proportion of cases in the United States that would be prevented if a 100 percent effective preventive intervention were applied at or before a given age. The *attributable risk proportion,* which is the percentage effectiveness of the intervention in eliminating the risk factor, and the cumulative percentage drawn from the figures below, can be chain multiplied to estimate the effectiveness of a given intervention program and to compare various intervention strategies. Data on the cost of modifying risk factors could also be incorporated in such calculations in designing a preventive intervention research program.

A variety of malleable risk factors may be available for intervention for any given disorder. Intervention should start as early in life as possible, other things being equal. But in many situations, an intervention later in life may still be effective, even if some will already have the disorder. Combining the cumulative distributions with the attributable risk and with cost and outcome factors can aid policymakers in making decisions on priorities in the use of resources.

Figures 5.2 through 5.5 present two cumulative distributions each. The distribution on the right focuses on the age at which the individual first meets full criteria for the given DIS/DSM-III diagnosis. For this distribution, onset must occur during the one-year prospective period of follow-up. The population being studied includes all those who had never met criteria for diagnosis at the beginning of the follow-up period. It includes those with no symptoms, as well as those with some symptoms of disorder, but not meeting full DSM-III criteria. The distribution on the left focuses on the age at which a prodromal sign or symptom related to that disorder first occurred, as reported by the individuals who had developed the disorder by the end of the follow-up period. Dotted lines mark the twentieth and fiftieth percentiles, and age values for these are recorded on the figure. The area between the two curves gives a rough outline of the prodromal period.

In the text and figures below, data are presented regarding prevalence and prodromal periods in individuals who have experienced the onset of disorder.* During these prodromal periods, precursor signs and symptoms were present, and ideally these individuals could have been identified as being at high risk. The data were, however, subject to the problems of retrospective recall by individuals with a current mental disorder.

ILLUSTRATIVE DISORDERS

Conduct Disorder

The essential feature of conduct disorder, according to DSM-III-R, is a persistent pattern of conduct in which the basic rights of others and major age-appropriate societal norms or rules are violated. This diagnosis is made among children and adolescents under age 18 when at least 3 of 13 possible criteria have been present for at least six months (see Table 5.1). The behavior pattern may be simultaneously present in

---

*These data were prepared in 1992 by William Eaton and Mohamed Badawi, both from The Johns Hopkins University, explicitly for this report.

TABLE 5.1 DSM-III-R Diagnostic Criteria for Conduct Disorder

A. A disturbance of conduct lasting at least six months, during which at least three of the following have been present:

 (1) has stolen without confrontation of a victim on more than one occasion (including forgery)
 (2) has run away from home overnight at least twice while living in parental or parental surrogate home (or once without returning)
 (3) often lies (other than to avoid physical or sexual abuse)
 (4) has deliberately engaged in fire-setting
 (5) is often truant from school (for older person, absent from work)
 (6) has broken into someone else's house, building, or car
 (7) has deliberately destroyed others' property (other than by fire-setting)
 (8) has been physically cruel to animals
 (9) has forced someone into sexual activity with him or her
 (10) has used a weapon in more than one fight
 (11) often initiates physical fights
 (12) has stolen with confrontation of a victim (e.g., mugging, purse-snatching, extortion, armed robbery)
 (13) has been physically cruel to people

Note: The above items are listed in descending order of discriminating power based on data from a national field trial of the DSM-III-R criteria for Disruptive Behavior Disorders.

B. If 18 or older, does not meet criteria for Antisocial Personality Disorder.

Criteria for severity of Conduct Disorder:

Mild: Few if any conduct problems in excess of those required to make the diagnosis, **and** conduct problems cause only minor harm to others.

Moderate: Number of conduct problems and effect on others intermediate between "mild" and "severe."

Severe: Many conduct problems in excess of those required to make the diagnosis, **or** conduct problems cause considerable harm to others, e.g., serious physical injury to victims, extensive vandalism or theft, prolonged absence from home.

SOURCE: American Psychiatric Association, 1987, p. 55.

several settings—home, school, with peers, and in the community—but often it is not. Reports by parents and teachers on a particular child's behavior have shown remarkably little agreement (Loeber, Green, Lahey, and Stouthamer-Loeber, 1989; Offord, Boyle, and Racine, 1989b; Rutter, Tizard, and Whitmore, 1970).

For many years, there has been considerable debate regarding the definition of conduct disorder. Robins (1991) has described the changes in both the ICD and the DSM classification systems and the differences between the systems. Indeed, there are those who question the validity of the disorder itself. For example, F. Earls (personal communication,

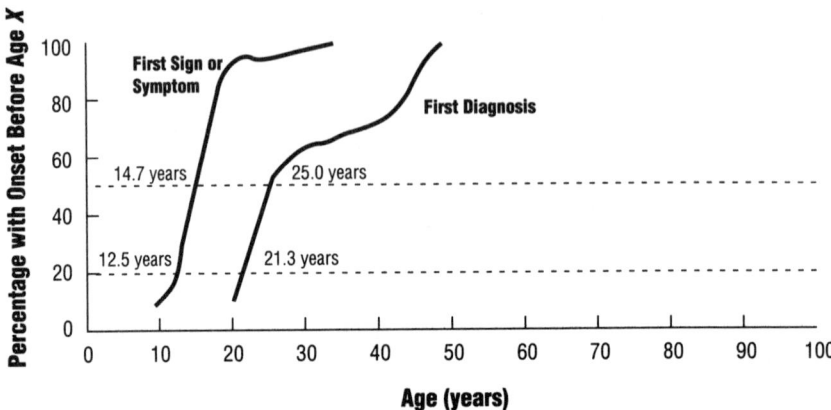

FIGURE 5.3 Age of onset of DIS/DSM-III Antisocial Personality Disorder. Population estimates are from 46 new cases (with 20th and 50th percentiles marked). Source: NIMH Epidemiologic Catchment Area Study, Four Sites, 1978 to 1983.

1992) has suggested that conduct disorder is not a condition, or even a series of conditions, but rather an emotional or behavioral symptom of disorder analogous to fever as a marker of infection. Robins (1991) has suggested, alternatively, that conduct disorder might better be viewed as the middle phase of a chronic mental disorder that typically begins early in life and continues into adulthood but which can abort at any time along the way. DSM recognizes the chronicity of the disorder but labels it differently at each stage. Taylor and colleagues found that children meeting the criteria for conduct disorder were quite heterogeneous in their symptoms (Taylor, Schachar, Thorley, and Wieselberg, 1986). This heterogeneity adds support to the increasingly held view that conduct disorder is really a cluster of disorders or subtypes. All of these variations in conceptualization, including definition and subtyping, affect apparent changes in prevalence, contribute to ethical dilemmas regarding labeling and deciding whom to treat, and complicate both treatment and prevention research.

Conduct disorder is the most common disorder seen in child mental health clinics in North America. Six-month and one-year prevalence rates obtained from general and health care clinic populations in the United States, Canada, and New Zealand range from 1.5 to 11.9 percent, depending on the gender and age range of subjects, but generally boys are diagnosed as having conduct disorder more often than girls and the rate for girls and boys increases with age (Costello, 1989; Offord, Boyle,

Fleming, Blum, and Grant, 1989a; Velez, Johnson, and Cohen, 1989; Bird, Canino, Rubio-Stipec, Gould, Ribera, Sesman et al., 1988; Anderson, Williams, McGee, and Silva, 1987; Offord, Boyle, Szatmari, Rae Grant, Links, Cadman et al., 1987). The costs to society of having such a high prevalence are not known, but obviously they are high, for they include the costs of damage to other people's property, the costs of educational, legal, and social service interventions, and the costs of loss of potential and eventual productivity of these individuals. Conduct disorder is not easily treated. Although many treatments are being applied and some, including problem-solving skills training, parent management training, and functional family therapy, have achieved positive short-term outcomes (Kazdin, 1993), the long-term success of these interventions is not known.

Symptoms of conduct disorder may arise from many different pathways. Loeber and colleagues (Loeber, Wung, Keenan, Giroux, Stouthamer-Loeber, Van Kammen, and Maughan, 1993) have postulated three routes: (1) an aggressive-versatile route with early onset, with symptoms that are already severe in preschool; (2) a nonaggressive, antisocial pathway with onset in late childhood to early adolescence, with conduct problems but no hyperactivity or aggression; and (3) an exclusive substance abuse pathway with onset in middle to late adolescence. There is a marked difference between the early-onset form of conduct disorder in a temperamentally difficult child who has accompanying attention deficit disorder and learning difficulties, and the late-onset form appearing in an adolescent who has previously functioned well but who in response to environmental stress suddenly changes patterns of behavior. Robins's (1980) work has suggested that late-onset conduct disorder is typically predated by early experimentation with sex, drugs, and alcohol. Adolescents who are most likely to be chronically antisocial are those who show early-onset, pervasive disorder, and co-occurrence of early hyperactivity (White, Moffitt, Earls, Robins, and Silva, 1990).

Within the DSM classification system, a majority of children with conduct disorder also have other concomitant psychiatric diagnoses. Conduct disorder often occurs in tandem with attention deficit disorder. Forty percent of children with attention deficit disorder go on to develop symptoms of conduct disorder (Offord, Boyle, Racine, Fleming, Cadman, Blum et al., 1992). The salient difference between those who remain attention deficit disordered but do not develop conduct disorder may lie in the level of family functioning. Families who provide a supportive, consistent environment with clearly defined limits presumably allow these children to develop enough social skills that they can function reasonably well in school and with their peers (Offord et al., 1992; Weiss and Hechtman, 1986).

Conduct disorder is important not only because of its relatively high frequency and occurrence with other disorders, but also because of its persistence into adolescence and adulthood. In one community study, 6 percent of boys and 1.6 percent of girls aged 6 to 11 and 10.4 percent of boys and 4.1 percent of girls aged 12 to 16 were diagnosed as having conduct disorder (Offord et al., 1989a). Forty percent of children with conduct disorder between ages 8 and 12 still had the disorder at follow-up four years later (Offord et al., 1992). Still other children who had conduct disorder at 8 to 12 years had substance abuse at follow-up four years later, although they did not show other features of conduct disorder. The pattern of conduct disorder symptoms most predictive of later drug abuse or delinquency is a combination of aggression and shyness (Moskowitz and Schwartzman, 1989; McCord, 1988; Kellam, Brown, Rubin, and Einsminger, 1983). Aggression accompanied by peer rejection, rather than aggression alone, predicts later delinquency. Furthermore, 50 percent of adolescents with conduct disorder go on to show persistent antisocial disorders in adult life (Rutter and Giller, 1983). Conduct disorder not only predicts later mental disorders in adulthood but also has wide-ranging poor prognosis in adult life with higher rates of school failure, joblessness, and poor interpersonal skills, especially marital difficulties (Robins, 1970). As adults, males have more externalizing disorders (such as antisocial personality disorders and alcohol and drug abuse) than females, and females have more internalizing disorders (such as mood and anxiety disorders) (Offord, 1989).

The antisocial behavior patterns that form the core of the conduct disorder diagnosis show considerable stability over the life course. When the patterns that had their onset in childhood or adolescence continue into adulthood, the name of the disorder changes, but the diagnostic criteria remain very similar. For the DSM-III-R diagnosis of antisocial personality disorder to be made, the individual must be at least 18 years of age, have a history of conduct disorder beginning before age 15, and demonstrate a pattern of irresponsible and antisocial behavior (meeting at least 4 of 10 diagnostic criteria) since age 15 (see Table 5.2). In adulthood the failure to conform to social norms often takes the form of impulsive and reckless behavior, poor work behavior, irritability and aggressiveness, and illegal activity that may result in incarceration and early death through various forms of violence. In the ECA study, about 0.5 percent of adults met the criteria for DIS/DSM-III antisocial personality disorder at a given point in time (conduct disorder was not studied because the focus in the ECA study was on adults), and

TABLE 5.2 DSM-III-R Diagnostic Criteria for Antisocial Personality Disorder

A. Current age at least 18.

B. Evidence of Conduct Disorder with onset before age 15, as indicated by a history of *three* or more of the following:

(1) was often truant
(2) ran away from home overnight at least twice while living in parental or parental surrogate home (or once without returning)
(3) often initiated physical fights
(4) used a weapon in more than one fight
(5) forced someone into sexual activity with him or her
(6) was physically cruel to animals
(7) was physically cruel to other people
(8) deliberately destroyed others' property (other than by fire-setting)
(9) deliberately engaged in fire-setting
(10) often lied (other than to avoid physical or sexual abuse)
(11) has stolen without confrontation of a victim on more than one occasion (including forgery)
(12) has stolen with confrontation of a victim (e.g., mugging, purse-snatching, extortion, armed robbery)

C. A pattern of irresponsible and antisocial behavior since the age of 15, as indicated by at least *four* of the following:

(1) is unable to sustain consistent work behavior, as indicated by any of the following (including similar behavior in academic settings if the person is a student):

(*a*) significant unemployment for six months or more within five years when expected to work and work was available
(*b*) repeated absences from work unexplained by illness in self or family
(*c*) abandonment of several jobs without realistic plans for others

(2) fails to conform to social norms with respect to lawful behavior, as indicated by repeatedly performing antisocial acts that are grounds for arrest (whether arrested or not), e.g., destroying property, harassing others, stealing, pursuing an illegal occupation
(3) is irritable and aggressive, as indicated by repeated physical fights or assaults (not required by one's job or to defend someone or oneself), including spouse- or child-beating
(4) repeatedly fails to honor financial obligations, as indicated by defaulting on debts or failing to provide child support or support for other dependents on a regular basis
(5) fails to plan ahead, or is impulsive, as indicated by one or both of the following:

(*a*) traveling from place to place without a prearranged job or clear goal for the period of travel or clear idea about when the travel will terminate
(*b*) lack of a fixed address for a month or more

(continued)

TABLE 5.2 *(Continued)*

(6) has no regard for the truth, as indicated by repeated lying, use of aliases, or "conning" others for personal profit or pleasure

(7) is reckless regarding his or her own or others' personal safety, as indicated by driving while intoxicated, or recurrent speeding

(8) if a parent or guardian, lacks ability to function as a responsible parent, as indicated by one or more of the following:

    (*a*) malnutrition of child
    (*b*) child's illness resulting from lack of minimal hygiene
    (*c*) failure to obtain medical care for a seriously ill child
    (*d*) child's dependence on neighbors or nonresident relatives for food or shelter
    (*e*) failure to arrange for a caretaker for young child when parent is away from home
    (*f*) repeated squandering, on personal items, of money required for household necessities

(9) has never sustained a totally monogamous relationship for more than one year

(10) lacks remorse (feels justified in having hurt, mistreated, or stolen from another)

D. Occurrence of antisocial behavior not exclusively during the course of Schizophrenia or Manic Episodes.

SOURCE: American Psychiatric Association, 1987, pp. 344–346.

it occurred in about 2.5 percent of the population over the life course up to the point of the interview (Robins and Regier, 1991). For antisocial personality disorder, the diagnostic requirement that some symptoms begin before age 15 ensures that the curve on the left of Figure 5.3 reaches nearly 100 percent prior to the age of 18. The accretion of signs and symptoms over the life course led to individuals at risk meeting the criteria for antisocial personality disorder for the first time over the year of follow-up. Twenty percent of cases first meeting criteria during adulthood had onsets before the age of 26, and 50 percent met criteria for diagnosis for the first time before age 40.

Depressive Disorders

Mood disorders, known as affective disorders in DSM-III, are disturbances of emotion that affect an individual's whole psychic life. There are two types of mood disorders, the first of which, bipolar disorder, is not the focus of this report. The second is depressive disorder, which has two subtypes: major depressive disorder (single episode or recurrent) and dysthymia (a chronic condition). Both types of depressive disorder are discussed below, with somewhat more detail given on major depressive disorder, which has greater severity. Frequently, they are referred to here jointly as depressive disorders. Both are diagnosed by inclusion and exclusion criteria based on severity of symptoms (see Tables 5.3 and 5.4). In general, the clinical picture involves a pervasive mood disturbance with feelings of sadness and loss of interest or pleasure in most activities in conjunction with disturbances in sleep, appetite, concentration, libido, and energy.

Depressive disorders are common and are associated with impairment at all levels of functioning. There have been remarkable scientific advances in the understanding of depressive disorders over the last three decades. These have included the development and application of reliable methods to diagnose depressive disorders, to describe their course, outcome, and associated impairments, and to elucidate the underlying biological changes that accompany them.

Some people have only a single major depressive episode in their entire lifetime; following it, they return to their previous level of functioning. However, about 50 percent of those in clinical samples who have one episode will go on to have another (American Psychiatric Association, 1987), thus meeting the criteria for recurrent major depression and underscoring the need to prevent the first episode. Also, women are much more likely than men to have major depressive disorder, with the lifetime prevalence being 8.7 percent for women and 3.6 percent for men (Robins and Regier, 1991). Dysthymia is a milder disorder, but the symptoms are chronic (two years in adults and one year in children).

Depressive disorders have a substantial cost to society. In terms of productivity, they are responsible for more missed days of work than any other health problem with the exception of cardiovascular disorders. They are the most common of all health problems encountered by primary care physicians in their offices. Estimates of the impact of effective interventions for depression can be approached by looking at the savings generated by the use of lithium to reduce recurrent episodes of bipolar mood disorder. Here the best estimate is that over $40 billion has been saved through the use of lithium since its widespread use began in 1970.

Depressive disorders have a high rate of co-morbidity; that is, they are associated with a number of other serious mental disorders, in particular substance abuse, anxiety disorders, and schizophrenia. They frequently accompany severe life stress such as divorce, job loss, or bereavement. They are strongly associated with suicide, one of the leading causes of death. In fact, more individuals in the United States die as a result of

TABLE 5.3 DSM-III-R Diagnostic Criteria for Major Depressive Episode and for Major Depression

Major Depressive Episode

Note: A "Major Depressive Syndrome" is defined as criterion A below.

A. At least five of the following symptoms have been present during the same two-week period and represent a change from previous functioning; at least one of the symptoms is either (1) depressed mood, or (2) loss of interest or pleasure. (Do not include symptoms that are clearly due to a physical condition, mood-incongruent delusions or hallucinations, incoherence, or marked loosening of associations.)

   (1) depressed mood (or can be irritable mood in children and adolescents) most of the day, nearly every day, as indicated either by subjective account or observation by others
   (2) markedly diminished interest or pleasure in all, or almost all, activities most of the day, nearly every day (as indicated either by subjective account or observation by others of apathy most of the time)
   (3) significant weight loss or weight gain when not dieting (e.g., more than 5% of body weight in a month), or decrease or increase in appetite nearly every day (in children, consider failure to make expected weight gains)
   (4) insomnia or hypersomnia nearly every day
   (5) psychomotor agitation or retardation nearly every day (observable by others, not merely subjective feelings of restlessness or being slowed down)
   (6) fatigue or loss of energy nearly every day
   (7) feelings of worthlessness or excessive or inappropriate guilt (which may be delusional) nearly every day (not merely self-reproach or guilt about being sick)
   (8) diminished ability to think or concentrate, or indecisiveness, nearly every day (either by subjective account or as observed by others)
   (9) recurrent thoughts of death (not just fear of dying), recurrent suicidal ideation without a specific plan, or a suicide attempt or a specific plan for committing suicide

B. (1) It cannot be established that an organic factor initiated and maintained the disturbance
   (2) The disturbance is not a normal reaction to the death of a loved one (Uncomplicated Bereavement)

   Note: Morbid preoccupation with worthlessness, suicidal ideation, marked functional impairment or psychomotor retardation, or prolonged duration suggest bereavement complicated by Major Depression.

C. At no time during the disturbance have there been delusions or hallucinations for as long as two weeks in the absence of prominent mood symptoms (i.e., before the mood symptoms developed or after they have remitted).

D. No superimposed on Schizophrenia, Schizophreniform Disorder, Delusional Disorder, or Psychotic Disorder NOS.

Major Depressive Episode codes: fifth-digit code numbers and criteria for severity of current state of Bipolar Disorder, Depressed, or Major Depression:

1-Mild: Few, if any, symptoms in excess of those required to make the diagnosis, **and** symptoms result in only minor impairment in occupational functioning or in usual social activities or relationships with others.

TABLE 5.3 *(Continued)*

2-Moderate: Symptoms or functional impairment between "mild" and "severe."

3-Severe, without Psychotic Features: Several symptoms in excess of those required to make the diagnosis, **and** symptoms markedly interfere with occupational functioning or with usual social activities or relationships with others.

4-With Psychotic Features: Delusions or hallucinations. If possible, **specify** whether the psychotic features are *mood-congruent* or *mood-incongruent*.

Mood-congruent psychotic features: Delusions or hallucinations whose content is entirely consistent with the typical depressive themes of personal inadequacy, guilt, disease, death, nihilism, or deserved punishment.

Mood-incongruent psychotic features: Delusions or hallucinations whose content does *not* involve typical depressive themes of personal inadequacy, guilt, disease, death, nihilism, or deserved punishment. Included here are such symptoms as persecutory delusions (not directly related to depressive themes), thought insertion, thought broadcasting, and delusions of control.

5-In Partial Remission: Intermediate between "In Full Remission" and "Mild," **and** no previous Dysthymia. (If Major Depressive Episode was superimposed on Dysthymia, the diagnosis of Dysthymia alone is given once the full criteria for a Major Depressive Episode are no longer met.)

6-In Full Remission: During the past six months no significant signs or symptoms of the disturbance.

0-Unspecified.

Specify chronic if current episode has lasted two consecutive years without a period of two months or longer during which there were no significant depressive symptoms.

Specify if current episode is **Melancholic Type.**

Major Depression

296.2x Major Depression, Single Episode

For fifth digit, use the Major Depressive Episode codes (p. 223) to describe current state.

A. A single Major Depressive Episode (p. 222).

B. Has never had a Manic Episode (p. 217) or an unequivocal Hypomanic Episode (see p. 217).

Specify if **seasonal pattern** (p. 224).

296.3x Major Depression, Recurrent

For fifth digit, use the Major Depressive Episode codes (p. 223) to describe current state.

A. Two or more Major Depressive Episodes (p. 222), each separated by at least two months of return to more or less usual functioning. (If there has been a previous Major Depressive Episode, the current episode of depression need not meet the full criteria for a Major Depressive Episode.)

B. Has never had a Manic Episode (p. 217) or an unequivocal Hypomanic Episode (see p. 217).

Specify if **seasonal pattern** (see p. 224).

SOURCE: American Psychiatric Association, 1987, pp. 222–224 and 229–230.

TABLE 5.4   DSM-III-R Diagnostic Criteria for Dysthymia

A. Depressed mood (or can be irritable mood in children and adolescents) for most of the day, more days than not, as indicated either by subjective account or observation by others, for at least two years (one year for children and adolescents).

B. Presence, while depressed, of at least two of the following:
   (1) poor appetite or overeating
   (2) insomnia or hypersomnia
   (3) low energy or fatigue
   (4) low self-esteem
   (5) poor concentration or difficulty making decisions
   (6) feelings of hopelessness

C. During a two-year period (one-year for children and adolescents) of the disturbance, never without the symptoms in A for more than two months at a time.

D. No evidence of an unequivocal Major Depressive Episode during the first two years (one year for children and adolescents) of the disturbance.

   Note: There may have been a previous Major Depressive Episode, provided there was a full remission (no significant signs or symptoms for six months) before development of the Dysthymia. In addition, after these two years (one year in children or adolescents) of Dysthymia, there may be superimposed episodes of Major Depression, in which case both diagnoses are given.

E. Has never had a Manic Episode (p. 217) or an unequivocal Hypomanic Episode (see p. 217).

F. Not superimposed on a chronic psychotic disorder, such as Schizophrenia or Delusional Disorder.

G. It cannot be established that an organic factor initiated and maintained the disturbance, e.g., prolonged administration of an antihypertensive medication.

Specify primary or **secondary type:**

   Primary type: the mood disturbance is not related to a preexisting, chronic, nonmood, Axis I or Axis III disorder, e.g., Anorexia Nervosa, Somatization Disorder, a Psychoactive Substance Dependence Disorder, an Anxiety Disorder, or rheumatoid arthritis.

   Secondary type: the mood disturbance is apparently related to a preexisting, chronic, nonmood Axis I or Axis III disorder.

Specify early onset or **late onset:**

   Early onset: onset of the disturbance before age 21.

   Late onset: onset of the disturbance at age 21 or later.

SOURCE: American Psychiatric Association, 1987, pp. 194–195.

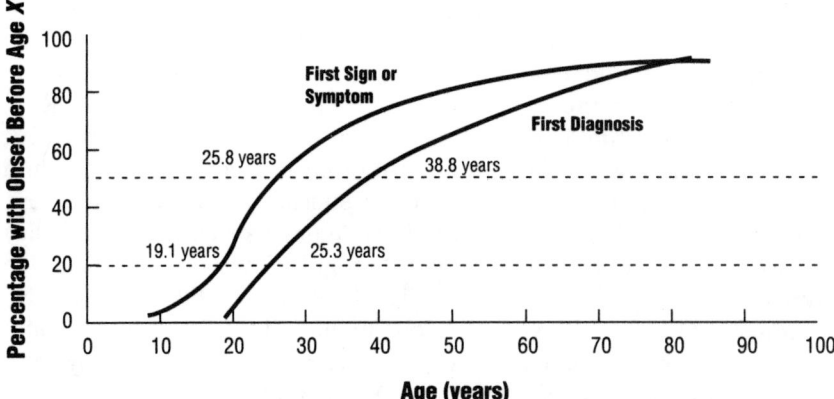

FIGURE 5.4   Age of onset of DIS/DSM-III Major Depressive Disorder. Population estimates are from 148 new cases (with 20th and 50th percentiles marked). Source: NIMH Epidemiologic Catchment Area Study, Four Sites, 1978 to 1983.

suicide than as a result of homicide (National Center for Health Statistics, 1993). Although the definitions of depression have varied, many studies link depression and suicide. More than half of suicides occur in adults suffering from depression (Barraclough, Bunch, Nelson, and Sainsbury, 1974). The lifetime risk of suicide in persons suffering from depression is 15 percent (IOM, 1990a). The risk of suicide among depressed persons of all ages is 30 times higher than in the general population (Guze and Robins, 1970). Twenty percent of all suicides occur in persons over 65 (Vital Statistics of the United States, 1975). Rates are strikingly higher for elderly white men than for other groups.

Both pharmacological and psychological treatment methods for depression have shown considerable success (Klerman, 1988; Weissman, 1988). There is also evidence that high-quality maintenance therapy substantially increases the likelihood of a good outcome for depressive disorders (Frank, Kupfer, Perel, Cornes, Jarrett, Mallinger et al., 1990). Thus clinical depression is unusual among the major mental illnesses in having good treatments available. It is therefore particularly important for clinicians to recognize the signs and symptoms of depressive disorders as well as note the existence of risk factors in susceptible patients' lives, because much suffering can be eliminated by the effective treatments available. Depressive disorders, especially if untreated, have profound effects on families, in particular on the children and spouses of those who are afflicted (Beardslee and Wheelock, in press; Keitner and Miller, 1991; Downey and Coyne, 1990).

However, there is strong evidence that clinical depression in adults is underrecognized and undertreated in medical practice (Pérez-Stable, Miranda, Muñoz, and Ying, 1990; Cleary, Goldberg, Kessler, and Nyez, 1982) and that treatment is often suboptimal (Keller, Lavori, Rice, Coryell, and Hirschfeld, 1986). It is evident that adults with depressive disorders, if they are treated at all, are often treated by internists and general practitioners, not mental health specialists (Regier, Goldberg, and Taube, 1978). This has prompted the Agency for Health Care Policy and Research to publish clinical practice guidelines on depression in primary care (Depression Guideline Panel, 1993a,b,c). Evidence has also accumulated that children with serious mental disorders in general and clinical depression in particular (Beardslee, Keller, Lavori, Staley, and Sacks, 1993; Keller, Lavori, Beardslee, Wunder, and Ryan, 1991) are also undertreated. In addition, Mexican-Americans and probably other minorities as well, significantly underutilize mental health services when in need of treatment for mental disorders in general. In the UCLA ECA study, utilization rates were low for the general population, at 22 percent, but for Mexican-Americans rates were only half that, or 11 percent (Hough, Landsverk, Karno, Burnam, Timbers, Escobar, and Regier, 1987).

A developmental perspective is necessary in the understanding of depressive disorders because the nature of clinical depression changes across the life span. Estimates of the rate of depressive disorders also vary depending on the instruments and diagnostic systems employed and on the samples studied. A useful technique is a structured interview scored according to standard diagnostic criteria, such as the DIS/DSM-III system used in the ECA study. ECA data suggest an overall lifetime disorder rate of 7.8 percent for all affective disorders (now classified as mood disorders in DSM-III-R), with major depression as the most common affective disorder, followed by dysthymia (with lifetime rates of 4.9 and 3.2, respectively) (Weissman, Bruce, Lief, Florio, and Holzer, 1991). Higher rates of depressive disorders have been reported when slightly broader diagnostic nomenclatures and semistructured interview schedules are used. For example, data collected from community samples using the Schedule of Affective Disorders and Schizophrenia suggest rates as high as 8 to 12 percent for men and 20 to 26 percent for women (Boyd and Weissman, 1981).

According to ECA data, the prevalence of major depression among the elderly living in the community is less than 3 percent. However, depressive symptoms occur in approximately 15 percent of community residents over 65 years of age. Thus clinical depression may have a different form in the elderly. The rates of major or minor depression among elderly people in nursing homes range from 15 to 25 percent (NIH Consensus Development Panel on Depression in Late Life, 1992). Major depressive disorder among children is rarer than among adults, as reviewed in more detail below.

There appears to be a cohort effect in the prevalence of depressive disorder. Birth cohorts born in successive decades in this century show higher prevalence of depression (Klerman, Lavori, Rice, Reich, Endicott, Andreason et al., 1985; Hagnell et al., 1982). The increase in depression, to some extent, parallels the increase in suicide. Recent evidence has shown that for the United States and several other nations, the more recent birth cohorts are at increased risk for major depression (Cross-National Collaborative Group, 1992).

In the ECA study, which included only persons age 18 and older and did not assess childhood or adolescent depression, major depressive disorder was shown to have its onset in young adulthood (Figure 5.4). Twenty percent of cases met criteria for diagnosis for the first time before the age of 25.3 years, and 50 percent before age 39. The prodromal period appeared to be about 6 years long for those with earlier onset, and more than 10 years long for those with later onset.

Alcohol Abuse and Dependence

Drinking problems generally are viewed as a continuum, ranging from occasional misuse by social drinkers to alcohol abuse and dependence. In DSM-III-R, alcohol is one of nine classes of psychoactive substances associated with abuse and dependence. Alcohol abuse is a maladaptive use pattern, demonstrated by either continued use despite knowledge of harmful effects or recurrent use in situations when use is physically hazardous, as well as symptoms that have persisted for at least one month or have occurred repeatedly over a longer period of time. Abuse of alcohol progresses to alcohol dependence, frequently referred to as "alcoholism," when three of nine possible diagnostic criteria related to quantity and length of use and effects are met (see Table 5.5).

According to the National Institute on Alcohol Abuse and Alcoholism (NIAAA), dependence is now recognized as a disease characterized by four main clinical features: craving, impaired control over drinking, physical dependence, and tolerance (NIAAA, 1991) (see Table 5.5). Whereas craving is a hunger for alcohol before drinking begins, impaired control over drinking refers to the difficulty that alcoholics experience in stopping once drinking has started. Unlike nonproblem drinkers, alcoholics may lack internal signals that would allow them to

TABLE 5.5   DSM-III-R Diagnostic Criteria for Psychoactive Substance Abuse and Psychoactive Substance Dependence

Psychoactive Substance Abuse

A. A maladaptive pattern of psychoactive substance use indicated by at least one of the following:
   (1) continued use despite knowledge of having a persistent or recurrent social, occupational, psychological, or physical problem that is caused or exacerbated by use of the psychoactive substance
   (2) recurrent use in situations in which use is physically hazardous (e.g., driving while intoxicated)

B. Some symptoms of the disturbance have persisted for at least one month, or have occurred repeatedly over a longer period of time.

C. Never met the criteria for Psychoactive Substance Dependence for this substance.

Psychoactive Substance Dependence

A. At least three of the following:
   (1) substance often taken in larger amounts or over a longer period than the person intended
   (2) persistent desire or one or more unsuccessful efforts to cut down or control substance use
   (3) a great deal of time spent in activities necessary to get the substance (e.g., theft), taking the substance (e.g., chain smoking), or recovering from its effects
   (4) frequent intoxication or withdrawal symptoms when expected to fulfill major role obligations at work, school, or home (e.g., does not go to work because hung over, goes to school or work "high," intoxicated while taking care of his or her children), or when substance use is physically hazardous (e.g., drives when intoxicated)
   (5) important social, occupational, or recreational activities given up or reduced because of substance use
   (6) continued substance use despite knowledge of having a persistent or recurrent social, psychological, or physical problem that is caused or exacerbated by the use of the substance (e.g., keeps using heroin despite family arguments about it, cocaine-induced depression, or having a ulcer made worse by drinking)
   (7) marked tolerance: need for markedly increased amounts of the substance (i.e., at least a 50% increase) in order to achieve intoxication or desired effect, or markedly diminished effect with continued use of the same amount

   Note: The following items may not apply to cannabis, hallucinogens, or phencyclidine (PCP):

   (8) characteristic withdrawal symptoms (see specific withdrawal syndromes under Psychoactive Substance-induced Organic Mental Disorders)
   (9) substance often taken to relieve or avoid withdrawal symptoms

B. Some symptoms of the disturbance have persisted for at least one month, or have occurred repeatedly over a longer period of time.

TABLE 5.5 *(Continued)*

Criteria for Severity of Psychoactive Substance Dependence:

Mild: Few, if any, symptoms in excess of those required to make the diagnosis, and the symptoms result in no more than mild impairment in occupational functioning or in usual social activities or relationships with others.

Moderate: Symptoms or functional impairment between "mild" and "severe."

Severe: Many symptoms in excess of those required to make the diagnosis, and the symptoms markedly interfere with occupational functioning or with usual social activities or relationships with others.[a]

In Partial Remission: During the past six months, either no use of the substance and some symptoms of dependence.

In Full Remission: During the past six months, either no use of the substance, or use of the substance and no symptoms of dependence.

[a]Because of the availability of cigarettes and other nicotine-containing substances and the absence of a clinically significant nicotine intoxication syndrome, impairment in occupational or social functioning is not necessary for a rating of severe Nicotine Dependence.

SOURCE: American Psychiatric Association, 1987, pp. 167–169.

regulate alcohol intake. Physical dependence is an adaptive state manifested by intense physical disturbances that occur when drinking is discontinued. Dependence results from the adaptation of central nervous system structures and functions (and probably those of other organs as well) to the presence of alcohol. Tolerance refers to the diminished effect of a given amount of alcohol that tends to develop with regular use. In spite of this diminished effect, however, many aspects of brain functioning are impaired, and vital organs may be damaged.

Alcohol is involved in over 100,000 deaths annually in the United States (from motor vehicle crashes, unintentional injuries, suicides, and the medical effects of alcohol dependence) and plays a major role in numerous medical and social problems (NIAAA, 1991; IOM, 1989a). Motor vehicle crashes are the nation's leading cause of injury deaths, and approximately half of all crash fatalities are alcohol related (DHHS, 1990; IOM, 1985). Such crashes, of course, leave many others with permanent disabilities, including head injuries. About half of all fire deaths are associated with alcohol use, 20 to 77 percent of fatal falls involve alcohol, and 25 to 50 percent of drowning deaths may be the result of drinking (IOM, 1989a). Alcohol is estimated to be involved in approximately 30 percent of all suicides and plays a particularly significant role in adolescent suicide and in suicide with the use of firearms, and it is also highly associated with homicides (NIAAA, 1991).

Because of the heterogeneity of age of onset and behaviors related to maladaptive use of alcohol, Cloninger and colleagues (Cloninger, Sigvardsson, Gilligan, von Knorring, Reich, and Bohman, 1989) have postulated two different forms of alcoholism: Type I and Type II (see Chapter 6).

Alcohol has effects on virtually every organ system in the body. The liver, the primary site of alcohol metabolism, is susceptible to injury of three major types: fatty liver, alcoholic hepatitis, and cirrhosis. Chronic alcohol abusers also may develop clinical signs of cardiac dysfunction. Heavy alcohol consumption is a well-documented cause of brain damage. Damage can result from alcohol's toxic effects; alcohol-related damage to other organs can impair proper brain functioning; and the poor dietary habits that frequently accompany chronic drinking can lead to nutritional imbalances that, in turn, can impair the nervous system. Neurological complications include dementia, blackouts, seizures, hallucinations, and peripheral neuropathy. Alcohol-related dementia accounts for nearly 20 percent of all admissions to state mental hospitals. Moreover, heavy drinking can seriously impair a person's ability to remember and to perform intellectual tasks. The recent development of imaging techniques has enabled researchers to identify certain structural abnormalities in the brain—possibly resulting from alcohol abuse—that may account for the impaired intellectual and memory functions. In addition, autopsy studies have shown that alcoholics have general brain atrophy as well as specific cell loss in at least two structures of the brain that control memory (DHHS, 1990). Alcohol also can affect the immune, endocrine, and reproductive systems and may be associated with increased risk of certain kinds of cancers, especially those of the liver, mouth, esophagus, and larynx.

Alcohol even reaches across generations by causing fetal alcohol syndrome (FAS), a cluster of permanent physical deformities and mental retardation in the newborn child that results from the mother's drinking heavily during pregnancy. There are approximately one to three FAS babies for every 1,000 live births in the United States; among known alcoholic mothers, this rate increases to a range of 23 to 29 for every 1,000 live births (IOM, 1989a). Alcohol abuse and dependence can cause various other psychiatric conditions or increase their severity, or the abuse of alcohol may be a response to other psychiatric problems. Data from the ECA study indicate that alcoholics are 21 times more likely than nonalcoholics to also have a diagnosis of antisocial personality disorder, 6.2 times more likely to have mania, 4 times more likely to have schizophrenia, and 1.7 times more likely to have a diagnosis of major depressive disorder. Other studies indicate that approximately 10 to 30 percent of alcoholics have panic disorder, and about 20 percent of persons with anxiety disorders abuse alcohol (DHHS, 1991). ECA data also indicate that persons dependent on alcohol are more likely to abuse drugs. The increased odds ratios are as follows: cocaine (35 times); sedatives (17 times); opioids (13 times); hallucinogens (12 times); stimulants (11 times); and marijuana or related drugs (6 times). Surveys of both clinical and nonclinical populations indicate that at least 90 percent of alcohol-dependent persons are also nicotine dependent (DHHS, 1991).

Despite the national downward trend in alcohol consumption, projections for 1995 suggest that 11.2 million adults will exhibit symptoms of alcohol dependence, while the number of alcohol abusers will remain at current levels (DHHS, 1990). More men than women are heavy drinkers. For both men and women, drinking problems are especially common among younger age groups. In a 1984 national survey, for example, the proportion of male drinkers reporting at least a moderate level of drinking problems was highest among those aged 18 to 29 for both dependence symptoms (14 percent) and drinking-related consequences (20 percent). The proportions dropped with increasing age, reaching respective lows of 5 and 7 percent among men aged 60 and older. Among female drinkers, the proportion reporting at least a moderate level of dependence symptoms remained stable at 5 to 6 percent from age 18 to age 49 and then dropped to 1 percent. For drinking-related consequences, the proportion reporting at least a moderate level of problems was relatively high in the 18-to-29 age group (12 percent), but dropped to 6 percent for women in their thirties and forties and was negligible for those aged 60 and older (Hilton, 1987).

There are characteristics other than gender and age that are related to patterns of alcohol consumption; one of these is homelessness. People who are homeless have higher levels of alcohol abuse and dependence than the general population, with prevalence estimates ranging from 20 to 45 percent and estimates of lifetime prevalence as high as 63 percent (DHHS, 1990). Unlike the pattern in the general population, the incidence of problem drinking among the homeless appears to be highest in the middle years, and is substantially lower among both the young and the old. This finding lends some support to the thesis that many homeless people continue to drink heavily as a means of coping with the physical and emotional stresses associated with homelessness, although it is probably also true that alcoholism itself puts middle-aged alcoholics at relatively high risk for becoming homeless.

Overall drinking levels are lower among African-Americans than among the majority white population, but there are notable differences within age-group categories and African-Americans suffer to a greater extent from alcohol-related problems. A survey conducted in 1984 found that while white males were at highest risk for alcohol use problems in the 18-to-29 age group, African-American males of similar age were at a much lower risk. For men in their thirties, however, problem rates increased sharply for African-Americans and decreased sharply for whites. Problem rates remained higher for African-Americans than for whites throughout middle and old age. African-American males also reported higher rates of drinking-related problems (medical, personal, and social) than white males (Herd, 1989). One possible explanation for the high level of health problems among African-Americans may be the later onset of heavy drinking. This late onset may be associated with more sustained patterns of high consumption, in contrast to patterns among whites, for whom heavy drinking is more likely to be a short-term phenomenon at a younger age.

Hispanics have a higher prevalence of drinking-related problems than other racial and ethnic groups, despite the fact that more Hispanics abstain from drinking. A representative national sample of Hispanics in 1984 revealed marked differences in alcohol consumption between men and women. Approximately 70 percent of Hispanic men reported drinking more than once a month, whereas almost the same percentage of Hispanic women drank either less than once a month or not at all (Caetano, 1989). Rates of heavier drinking increased sharply among Hispanic men in their thirties but declined thereafter. About 18 percent of the men experienced at least one alcohol-related problem during the year preceding the survey. Problem rates varied by national origin; much higher proportions of Mexican-American men reported problems than did Puerto Ricans or Cubans.

Native American and Native Alaskan groups vary widely in alcohol use, but as a whole they have very high mortality rates from alcohol-related causes. The 1985 age-adjusted rate for alcohol-related deaths among Native Americans and Native Alaskans was 26.1 deaths per 100,000 population, a significant decline from the 1973 high of 66.1 deaths, but still four times higher than the rate for the general population (Indian Health Service, 1988). Alcoholism death rates were twice as high for men as for women and, among age groups, ranged as high as 96.8 deaths per 100,000 for men between the ages of 45 and 54.

There have been significant efforts focused on treatment strategies, particularly to ameliorate alcohol abuse and dependence. Advances and research needs in treatment have been reviewed extensively elsewhere (IOM, 1990b; IOM, 1989a). Researchers have demonstrated that treatment can contribute to prolonged abstinence in some patients. During the past decade alone, several hundred new studies have been published reporting outcome data on various treatment methods. Some of the areas covered include pharmacotherapies, aversion therapies, psychotherapy and counseling, mutual-help groups such as Alcoholics Anonymous, behavioral self-control training, and relapse prevention procedures. Typically, alcohol treatment programs offer a combination of modalities, ranging from detoxification and health care to occupational therapy and after-care group meetings. Even though treatment can be effective, however, many alcohol-dependent individuals either do not seek help or resist treatment, and most patients experience at least one relapse to drinking following treatment.

To better understand the benefits of treatment and to improve the percentage of patients who experience those benefits, researchers are working to define the active ingredients of various treatment strategies and to determine which patient factors influence treatment outcome (NIAAA, 1991). Related efforts include refining diagnostic classifications; developing improved tools for screening, diagnosis, and assessment; and improving treatment outcome evaluation.

Researchers also are working to provide information that will help to ensure that treatment services reach the populations in need. It has been well established that general medical expenditures by alcoholics and their families are reduced substantially following treatment—and the benefits derived from treating alcoholics offset costs to the general health care system (IOM, 1990b; IOM, 1989a). In light of these findings, increasing efforts will focus on expanding information about the capacities, quality, availability, utilization, and costs of alcoholism treatment services in relation to the need and the demand for those services.

Alcohol abuse and dependence is present in about 3 percent of the adult population at any given time (point prevalence), and occurs in about 14 percent of the population over the life course (lifetime prevalence) (Helzer, Burnam, and McEvoy, 1991). It begins early in adolescence (Figure 5.2). The twentieth percentile for age of diagnosis occurred during the earliest age of respondents in the ECA sample (18 years old), and 50 percent of the cases had their onset before age 25. For those cases that began in adulthood, the prodromal period was short: the difference between the twentieth percentile for diagnosis versus the twentieth percentile for first problem was less than two years.

Schizophrenia

Schizophrenia in DSM-III-R is an illness defined by inclusion and exclusion criteria with regard to psychotic symptoms, deterioration in functioning, and duration (see Table 5.6). The criteria for diagnosis have

TABLE 5.6   DSM-III-R Diagnostic Criteria for Schizophrenia

A. Presence of characteristic psychotic symptoms in the active phase: either (1), (2), or (3) for at least one week (unless the symptoms are successfully treated):

    (1) two of the following:
        (*a*) delusions
        (*b*) prominent hallucinations (throughout the day for several days or several times a week for several weeks, each hallucinatory experience not being limited to a few brief moments)
        (*c*) incoherence or marked loosening of associations
        (*d*) catatonic behavior
        (*e*) flat or grossly inappropriate affect
    (2) bizarre delusions (i.e., involving a phenomenon that the person's culture would regard as totally implausible, e.g., thought broadcasting, being controlled by a dead person)
    (3) prominent hallucinations [as defined in (1)(*b*) above] of a voice with content having no apparent relation to depression or elation, or a voice keeping up a running commentary on the person's behavior or thoughts, or two or more voices conversing with each other.

B. During the course of the disturbance, functioning in such areas as work, social relations, and self-care is markedly below the highest level achieved before onset of the disturbance (or, when the onset is in childhood or adolescence, failure to achieve expected level of social development).

C. Schizoaffective Disorder and Mood Disorder with Psychotic Features have been ruled out, i.e., if a Major Depressive or Manic Syndrome has ever been present during an active phase of the disturbance, the total duration of all episodes of a mood syndrome has been brief relative to the total duration of the active and residual phases of the disturbance.

D. Continuous signs of the disturbance for at least six months. The six-month period must include an active phase (of at least one week, or less if symptoms have been successfully treated) during which there were psychotic symptoms characteristic of Schizophrenia (symptoms in A), with or without a prodromal or residual phase, as defined below.

Prodromal phase: A clear deterioration in functioning before the active phase of the disturbance that is not due to a disturbance in mood or to a Psychoactive Substance Use Disorder and that involves at least two of the symptoms listed below.

Residual phase: Following the active phase of the disturbance, persistence of at least two of the symptoms noted below, these not being due to a disturbance in mood or to a Psychoactive Substance Use Disorder.

Prodromal or Residual Symptoms:
(1) marked social isolation or withdrawal
(2) marked impairment in role functioning as wage-earner, student, or home-maker
(3) markedly peculiar behavior (e.g., collecting garbage, talking to self in public, hoarding food)

TABLE 5.6   (Continued)

(4) marked impairment in personal hygiene and grooming

(5) blunted or inappropriate affect

(6) digressive, vague, overelaborate, or circumstantial speech, or poverty of speech, or poverty of content of speech

(7) odd beliefs or magical thinking, influencing behavior and inconsistent with cultural norms, e.g., superstitiousness, belief in clairvoyance, telepathy, "sixth sense," "others can feel my feelings," overvalued ideas, ideas of reference

(8) unusual perceptual experiences, e.g., recurrent illusions, sensing the presence of a force or person not actually present

(9) marked lack of initiative, interests, or energy

Examples: Six months of prodromal symptoms with one week of symptoms from A; no prodromal symptoms with six months of symptoms from A; no prodromal symptoms with one week of symptoms from A and six months of residual symptoms.

E. It cannot be established that an organic factor initiated and maintained the disturbance.

F. If there is a history of Autistic Disorder, the additional diagnosis of Schizophrenia is made only if prominent delusions or hallucinations are also present.

Classification of course. The course of the disturbance is coded in the fifth digit:

1-Subchronic. The time from the beginning of the disturbance, when the person first began to show signs of the disturbance (including prodromal, active, and residual phases) more or less continuously, is less than two years, but at least six months.

2-Chronic. Same as above, but more than two years.

3-Subchronic with Acute Exacerbation. Reemergence of prominent psychotic symptoms in a person with a subchronic course who has been in the residual phase of the disturbance.

4-Chronic with Acute Exacerbation. Reemergence of prominent psychotic symptoms in a person with a chronic course who has been in the residual phase of the disturbance.

5-In Remission. When a person with a history of Schizophrenia is free of all signs of the disturbance (whether or not on medication), "in Remission" should be coded. Differentiating Schizophrenia in Remission from No Mental Disorder requires consideration of overall level of functioning, length of time since the last episode of disturbance, total duration of the disturbance, and whether prophylactic treatment is being given.

0-Unspecified.

SOURCE: American Psychiatric Association, 1987, pp. 194–195.

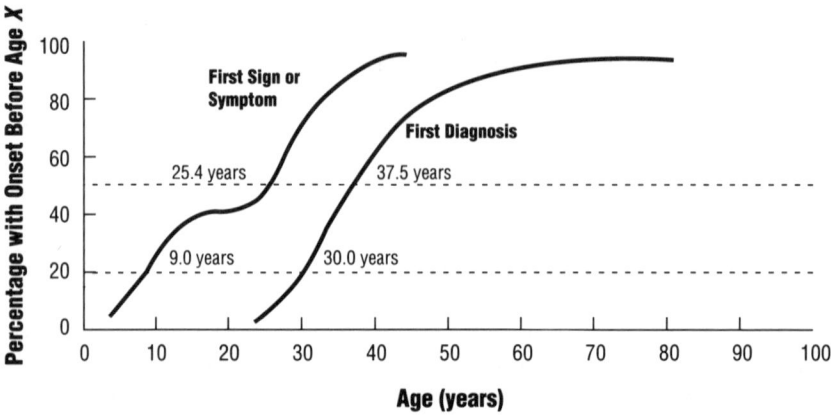

FIGURE 5.5 Age of onset of DIS/DSM-III Schizophrenia. Population estimates are from 35 new cases (with 20th and 50th percentiles marked). Source: NIMH Epidemiologic Catchment Area Study, Four Sites, 1978 to 1983.

changed somewhat from DSM-III and are likely to change again in DSM-IV. Also, the definition in the U.S. classification system differs somewhat from that in the diagnostic system used in Europe (ICD-10). The establishment of criteria has been complicated by the fact that schizophrenia has been considered by some to be a "group of schizophrenias" (Bleuler, 1950). From the time of Kraepelin, phenomenology and course have been used to group illnesses under the schizophrenic label, but valid subtyping of these illnesses has not yet been achieved because etiological factors are not yet clear. In general, schizophrenia is characterized by delusions and hallucinations, disorganized speech and behavior, deficits in social, emotional, expressive, and initiating behaviors, and a lack of motivation leading to decreased social and occupational functioning.

Schizophrenia is a major mental illness that drastically alters the life course of many individuals (Harding, 1988; Harding, Brooks, Ashikaga, Strauss, and Breier, 1987), causes enormous family suffering, and results in an immense economic burden to families and to the nation. The burden of the disease increases because it afflicts adolescents and young adults and lasts throughout the lifetime of most individuals. In follow-up studies, about one third of schizophrenic patients have a relatively unremitting course requiring constant or intermittent institutional care, one third function minimally in the community and require continuous support, and one third function semiautonomously in the community but rarely reach the level of functioning expected before the onset of schizophrenia. The course of the disorder is usually most malignant during its first 5 to 10 years; it then tends to stabilize and can even improve somewhat. The course also depends on the quality and quantity of available treatment and rehabilitation (Harding, 1988).

Keith, Regier, and Rae (1991, p. 34) have described these social and economic costs:

Patients with the disorder occupy over 30 percent of the nation's mental hospital beds—more than 100,000 beds on any given day (Manderscheid and Barrett, 1987). Treatment costs alone exceed $7 billion annually, and indirect costs—for example, of social services, loss of productivity, and premature mortality—account for at least double that figure, making the financial burden of schizo-phrenia in the United States approximately equal to that of all cancers combined (Hall, Goldstein, Andrews, Lapsley, Bartel, and Silove, 1985; Gunderson and Mosher, 1975). The demoralizing effects of this devastating illness are partly revealed by the exceptionally high suicide attempt and completion rate of its victims. Past clinical studies have estimated that one in four patients with schizophrenia will attempt suicide and one in ten will succeed in the first ten years of the illness (Roy, 1986; Winokur and Tsuang, 1975). Further, compared to the general population, persons with schizophrenia have a twofold increase in overall mortality, with excess mortality particularly likely to be caused by "unnatural death" (Allebeck and Wistedt, 1986). Schizophrenic patients at the greatest risk for premature death are those younger than 40 years (Black and Winokur, 1988).

The co-morbidity of schizophrenia with substance abuse is a major problem and can complicate the initial diagnosis. For patients with chronic schizophrenia who are in either state or Department of Veterans Affairs hospitals, alcohol and drug abuse appear to dominate as coex-isting conditions, with some 20 to 50 percent of such hospitalized patients having drug and alcohol problems (Shaner, Khalsa, Roberts, Wilkins, Anglin, and Hsieh, 1993). The lower rates are often biased by invalid reports given by the patients themselves. Shaner et al. (1993) found rates of higher than 50 percent when based on toxicological data. Substance abuse combined with schizophrenia can undermine the treat-ment of both disorders.

The widely reported data from the ECA study deserve special com-ment because this study reports on coexistence of symptoms, without invoking the hierarchy implicit in the DSM and ICD classification systems. When symptoms can be part of two disorders and a hierarchial system is used, the more severe disorder becomes the diagnosis. The ECA type of analysis, which relied on symptoms only, concluded that over 90 percent of schizophrenic patients have at least one concurrent mental disorder at some time. These data indicate that at some point the schizophrenic patient exhibits symptoms consistent with either affective disorders (60 percent) or anxiety disorders (60 percent) (Robins and Regier, 1991). However, a careful analysis of these results suggests that the symptoms that give rise to the second diagnosis may well be part of the original illness. In other words, depressive or anxiety symptoms may exist in the normal course of schizophrenia, not as separate diseases. Nevertheless, when such symptoms do coexist, they need to be identified and targeted for treatment.

Significant progress has been made in the reduction of the adverse outcomes of schizophrenia. Structural, educational, and behaviorally based treatments, such as skills training, and interventions that promote family coping and support, when combined with antipsychotic medication have substantially improved the course of psychosis and reduced the relapse rate (Falloon and Fadden, 1993; Liberman, 1992; Wyatt, 1991). The favorable impact of continuous and comprehensive treatment is readily observed in one- and two-year controlled clinical trials, but it has only begun to be established for longer periods. The efficacy of treatment for primary negative symptoms and for the subset of patients with persistent psychosis has improved with the use of new antipsychotic medications and social learning programs (Glynn and Mueser, 1992; Kuehnel, Liberman, Marshall, and Bowen, 1992; Meltzer, 1992; Brenner, Dencker, Goldstein, Hubbard, Keegan, Kruger et al., 1990).

The estimated annual incidence of schizophrenia across the world appears to range between 0.1 and 0.5 per 1,000 (Eaton, 1991). The lifetime prevalence of schizophrenia is roughly the same for men and women, although women have a later onset. The lifetime risk of schizophrenia in the general population in the United States is 1.0 percent. That is, 1 out of 100 people born today will develop schizophrenia by the time they are 55. But of course, not everyone's risk is equal because some have a strong family history of schizophrenia and other risk factors that can multiply the risk for onset of the disorder by tenfold or greater.

Schizophrenia usually appears after puberty, with the peak age of onset at about 20 to 24 years for males and 25 to 29 years for females (Lewine, 1988). These figures are somewhat misleading because onset is only the point in time that characteristic and florid psychotic symptoms bring the individual to psychiatric attention. A broader description of onset suggests a range of about 17 to 28 for males and about 20 to 40 for females. First-episode studies suggest that psychotic symptoms have been present for about two years (Mintz, Mintz, and Goldstein, 1987; Goldberg and Huxley, 1980) at the time of initial diagnostic and treatment services (Lieberman, Jody, Geisler, Alvir, Loeber, Szymanski et al., 1993). However, there are obvious problems in using mental health service contacts to determine age of onset. It seems likely that aspects of cognitive dysfunction and prodromal symptoms are present in many patients much earlier in life, and some features may be present from birth. About 10 percent of schizophrenics have their first hospital admission after age 45 (Gottesman, 1991); therefore a criterion in DSM-III that age of onset be before age 45 was dropped in DSM-III-R.

The prodrome for schizophrenia may be surprisingly long, according to ECA data. The first symptoms obtained by questions asking about the onset of hallucinations and delusions suggest that those patients with early onset may have had over-20-year histories of symptoms, whereas those with late onset may have had symptoms for about 12 years. The ECA data confirm that schizophrenia has its onset in young adulthood (Figure 5.5). The twentieth percentile is 30 years of age, and 50 percent of onsets occur prior to age 37.5.

Alzheimer's Disease

Alzheimer's disease (AD) is the most common cause of deteriorating cognitive function (dementia) in adults. AD accounts for 60 to 70 percent of dementia cases in most studies (Katzman, Lasker, and Bernstein, 1986), although one survey, the East Boston study, found a higher proportion; that is, 91 percent of those with moderate or severe dementia had AD (Evans, Funkenstein, Albert, Scherr, Cook, Chown et al., 1989). The onset of AD is typically heralded by a deterioration in recent memory with relative preservation of reference, or long-term, memory (see Figure 5.6 and Table 5.7 for DSM-III-R diagnostic criteria). The course is insidiously downward, with the progressive loss of the ability to read and write and increasing disability in speaking, learning, and planning of complex actions. The speed of cognitive deterioration varies markedly, and periods of decline are often punctuated by periods of slight recovery or plateaus during which symptoms remain stable for months. At end-stage, the affected person becomes mute, incontinent, and bedridden.

The annual costs of severe dementia have proved difficult to quantify precisely. Two studies of overall costs estimated $38 billion in 1983 dollars, and $24 billion to $48 billion in 1985 dollars (Huang and Hu, 1986; Battelle Memorial Institute, 1984). Diagnostic costs were estimated at between $500 million and $1 billion in 1987 (OTA, 1987), and direct costs of treatment at $10 billion in 1983 (Huang and Hu, 1986).

A recent study of costs, the most rigorous empirical study to date, was

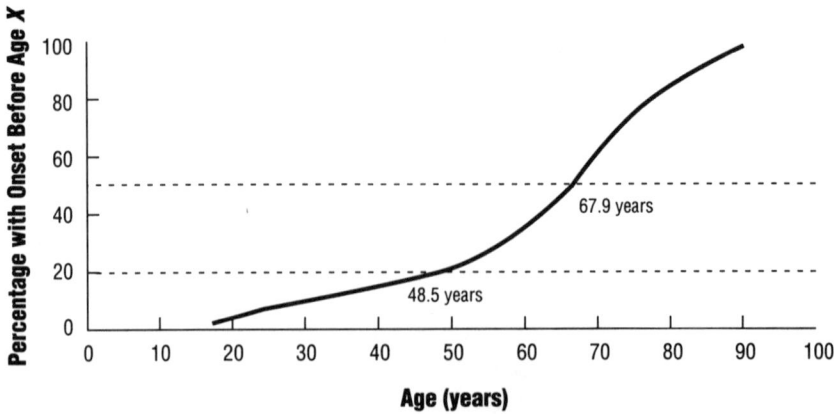

FIGURE 5.6   Age of onset of DIS/DSM-III Cognitive Impairment. Population estimates are from 187 new cases (with 20th and 50th percentiles marked). Source: NIMH Epidemiologic Catchment Area Study, Four Sites, 1978 to 1983.

reported by Rice and colleagues (Rice, Fox, Hanck, Max, Webber, Lindeman, and Segura, 1991). The study directly estimated costs for a cohort of dementia patients from the San Francisco Bay area, both institutionalized and residing in the community. This study suggested that previous cost estimates may well have been far too low. The study assessed the costs of formal care (including costs for nursing homes, physician services, hospitals, paid social services, and medications) and informal care (using cost estimates for services provided by family members or others based on the cost of the same services if performed by paid substitutes) for dementia patients. The costs per patient in a nursing home were remarkably similar to the costs per patient in the community, approximately $47,000 in 1990, but the fraction of costs due to formal services was predictably much higher for those in nursing homes. Three quarters of the costs among community-dwelling patients were for informal care. Among nursing home residents, 88 percent of the costs were for formal services, with 81 percent for nursing home charges alone. The $47,000 cost per patient cannot be generalized nationally, but it is more than double the per capita cost estimated in the previous studies.

The largest cost component is long-term care. Historical data on dementia prevalence in nursing homes are notoriously unreliable, but the data make clear that dementia is a serious problem among nursing home residents. National surveys show that at least half of those residing in nursing homes, and perhaps a much higher fraction, suffer

TABLE 5.7   DSM-III-R Diagnostic Criteria for Primary Degenerative Dementia of the Alzheimer Type and Dementia

Primary Degenerative Dementia of the Alzheimer Type

A. Dementia (see p. 107).

B. Insidious onset with a generally progressive deteriorating course.

C. Exclusion of all other specific causes of Dementia by history, physical examination, and laboratory tests.

Note: Code 331.00 Alzheimer's disease on Axis III.

Dementia

A. Demonstrable evidence of impairment in short- and long-term memory. Impairment in short-term memory (inability to learn new information) may be indicated by inability to remember three objects after five minutes. Long-term memory impairment (inability to remember information that was known in the past) may be indicated by inability to remember past personal information (e.g., what happened yesterday, birthplace, occupation) or facts of common knowledge (e.g., past Presidents, well-known dates).

B. At least one of the following:
   (1) impairment in abstract thinking, as indicated by inability to find similarities and differences between related words, difficulty in defining words and concepts, and other similar tasks
   (2) impaired judgment, as indicated by inability to make reasonable plans to deal with interpersonal, family, and job-related problems and issues
   (3) other disturbances of higher cortical function, such as aphasia (disorder of language), apraxia (inability to carry out motor activities despite intact comprehension and motor function), agnosia (failure to recognize or identify objects despite intact sensory function), and "constructional difficulty" (e.g., inability to copy three-dimensional figures, assemble blocks, or arrange sticks in specific designs)
   (4) personality change, i.e., alteration or accentuation of premorbid traits

C. The disturbance in A and B significantly interferes with work or usual social activities or relationships with others.

D. Not occurring exclusively during the course of Delirium.

E. Either (1) or (2):
   (1) there is evidence from the history, physical examination, or laboratory tests of a specific organic factor (or factors) judged to be etiologically related to the disturbance
   (2) in the absence of such evidence, an etiologic organic factor can be presumed if the disturbance cannot be accounted for by any nonorganic mental disorder, e.g., Major Depression accounting for cognitive impairment

Criteria for severity of Dementia:

Mild: Although work or social activities are significantly impaired, the capacity for independent living remains, with adequate personal hygiene and relatively intact judgment.

Moderate: Independent living is hazardous, and some degree of supervision is necessary.

Severe: Activities of daily living are so impaired that continual supervision is required, e.g., unable to maintain minimal personal hygiene; largely incoherent or mute.

SOURCE: American Psychiatric Association, 1987, pp. 107 and 121.

from a dementing disorder (OTA, 1992). The Office of Technology Assessment estimated that of the $53.1 billion paid for nursing home care in 1990, $11 billion was dementia-related government expenditure, roughly matched by dementia-related out-of-pocket payments from individuals and families or other private sources (OTA, 1992). The costs of respite care, day care, and informal care through relatives and friends are also significant and were estimated at $27 billion in 1983 (Hu, Huang, and Cartwright, 1986; Huang and Hu, 1986). Here again, the more recent study by Rice, although it did not project a national cost figure, suggests that this estimate is probably low by a factor of two or more (Rice et al., 1991).

Data on use and costs of day care, respite care, and other services increasingly available to assist families dealing with a dementing illness are extremely sparse. Many new services have been created over the past half decade, and most have been created for private payment, at times supplemented by contracts with local or state government, but with limited federal participation (and thus minimal national data reporting). The few studies that have been done to assess the use of community services have generally been in service-rich environments with access to case management, and so these studies do not represent the national norm. As uncertain as these cost estimates are, they are certain to escalate rapidly as the expected prevalence of AD triples over the next four decades, owing to the aging of the population.

The certain diagnosis of AD requires microscopic examination of brain tissue to look for the distinctive pathological stigmata: neurofibrillary tangles (accumulations of biochemically altered fibrous proteins inside nerve cells) and senile plaques (accumulations of fibrillar proteins between nerve cells, concentrated near points of cell-to-cell contact). Contrary to previous assumptions that AD represented a rather non-specific age-related deterioration of nerve cells throughout the brain, especially in the cerebral cortex, more recent studies have indicated a selective pattern of neuronal vulnerability among clusters of cells (Coyle, Price, and DeLong, 1983). Nerve cells in a cluster, called the nucleus basalis of Meynert, preferentially die off (Whitehouse, Price, Struble, Clark, Coyle, and DeLong, 1982; Whitehouse, Price, Clark, Coyle, and DeLong, 1981). These nerve cells communicate with those in the cortex by releasing the transmitter molecule acetylcholine, a phenomenon that has led to treatment attempts based on replacing the loss of this transmitter. Other neuronal cell clusters in different parts of the brain are also lost selectively, including neurons that use other transmitters, such as norepinephrine and several short protein molecules (peptides), somatostatin, and corticotropin releasing factor (CRF) (Coyle et al., 1983). Recent studies have suggested that a loss of synapses in specific brain regions, specifically the hippocampus and association cortex, may be associated with the loss of cognitive abilities in AD (R. Katzman, personal communication, 1993; Terry, Masliah, Salmon, Butters, DeTeresa, Hill et al., 1991; DeKosky and Scheff, 1990; Hamos, DeGennaro, and Drachman, 1989). The clinical and anatomic pattern of neuronal loss is thus more selective than once believed, but nonetheless involves multiple neuronal clusters and transmitter systems. Basic neuroscience as well as clinical studies suggest that the degeneration of these neuronal systems accounts for the cognitive and emotional symptoms of AD (Koo and Price, 1993).

Treatment of AD is confined currently to treating its behavioral and emotional symptoms. Only a small fraction, perhaps 3 to 5 percent, of all dementia cases are truly reversible (Katzman et al., 1986). Although the reversible cases of dementia are not AD, a careful diagnostic assessment is important to identify such cases, so they can be appropriately treated. Treatment of behavioral and emotional symptoms is nonetheless important, as is treatment of any other medical condition the patient may have, to keep the overall level of disability to a minimum (Katzman and Jackson, 1991). Because the overall level of disability, including the agitation, depressive symptoms, behavioral problems, and psychotic symptoms often associated with AD, contributes to family burden—and family burden is the strongest predictor of transfer to a nursing home or other formal care—antidepressants, antipsychotics, antianxiety agents, and other medications to diminish psychosis and behavioral problems are the most commonly used drugs with Alzheimer's patients.

Although the management of behavioral symptoms is important in the daily lives of those with dementia and those who care for them, the research literature on the effectiveness of these management techniques and on the frequency with which AD is co-morbid with other psychiatric symptoms and disorders is sparse (Deutsch and Rovner, 1991). A recent review of AD and depression, for example, found only a single controlled clinical trial (Teri and Wagner, 1992). Despite the weak research base, the use of medications intended to address psychiatric symptoms is common among those with AD. Various surveys suggest that one half to three fourths of those admitted to nursing homes with AD and other dementias are receiving psychotropic medications (OTA, 1992). Indeed, concern about the possible misuse of psychotropic medications has led to regulations in the Omnibus Budget and Reconciliation Act of 1987 intended to thwart misuse. This large gap in the clinical literature has obvious implications for the treatment of those with dementia, and direct relevance also to preventing sequelae among those who care for them, such as depression in caregivers.

Improved management of psychiatric symptoms associated with AD has strong implications for reducing the expression of some of the most troublesome aspects of AD. Improved care of AD patients—in homes, respite care centers, day care centers, clinics, nursing homes, hospitals, and special care units—offers the hope of reducing the load of excess disability, although research to validate this promise is only preliminary.

Research advances have been substantial, however, in the area of pathophysiology and genetics of AD. We now have reasonable evidence that several genetic forms of the illness exist with linkage to at least three different chromosomes. This finding suggests that there may be a collection of specific diseases with a single common pathway. One hope is that as we understand the nature of the final common pathway leading to cell death and discover a marker that will identify individuals at high risk for developing AD, ways can be found to inhibit a crucial step such as amyloid formation and prevent the emergence the illness. This might lead to indicated preventive interventions for high-risk individuals.

Conservative estimates suggest that severe dementia afflicts 5 to 7 percent of those over age 65 (Cross and Gurland, 1986), and such cases are expected to number 2.4 million by the year 2000. A community survey that included mild to moderate symptoms of AD found that 10.8 percent of those over age 65 had probable AD (Evans et al., 1989). In the ECA study, prevalence estimates for severe cognitive impairment were highly influenced by the age distribution of the population: in adults, the prevalence was less than 1 percent; in those over age 55, the prevalence was greater than 2 percent (George, Landerman, Blazer, and Anthony, 1991). The prevalence of AD escalates rapidly after age 65. The East Boston study showed that the prevalence of probable AD rose from 3 percent among those aged 65 to 74, to 18.7 percent among those 75 to 84, to 47.2 percent among those over 85 (Evans et al., 1989). As mentioned above, the prevalence of AD is expected to increase more than threefold during the next four decades, in large part because the oldest segments of the U.S. population, those most at risk for AD, are growing the most rapidly (Evans, Scherr, Cook, Albert, Funkenstein, Smith et al., 1990).

Projecting future AD prevalence hinges critically on assumptions about the growth of the over-85 population and the prevalence of AD in this group, both of which are well-known weak points in the epidemiological data. The projected prevalence among those aged 65 to 74 would increase only modestly from 1980 to 2050 in one recent projection, for example, but would increase sevenfold among those over 85 (Evans et al., 1990). Past census projections have been particularly inaccurate regarding expansion of the oldest age groups, and the anticipated rise of AD over the next four decades is especially sensitive to such uncertainty.

International epidemiological studies have shown relatively little variation among populations in the incidence or prevalence of dementia, when adjusted for late age of onset (Rocca, Hofman, Brayne, Breteler, Clarke, Copeland et al., 1991). Earlier reports had suggested a low incidence and prevalence of AD among Asian populations. More systematic recent studies have found prevalence among Asians within the range of Western surveys (Zhang, Katzman, Kashani, Salmon, Jin, Cai et al., 1990), although the ratio of AD to other causes of dementia may differ between predominantly Caucasian populations, in North America and Europe, and populations in Japan and China (Jorm, 1991). The consistency of findings suggests that AD is found among all geographic areas and population groups. Differences in prevalence from exposure to different risk factors, if they can ultimately be found, are too small to be detected consistently in population surveys.

The onset of severe cognitive impairment in the ECA study is shown in Figure 5.6. In the ECA study, AD was not separated out from other forms of severe cognitive impairment. The operational measure was the Mini-mental Status Exam. The Mini-mental Status Exam is used as a screening tool for dementia, but it also identifies those with cognitive impairments from other causes, such as delirium, substance-induced hallucinosis, and mental retardation. The at-risk population for onset consists of those with a Mini-mental score of 17 or more, and, among these, the new cases are those whose score at the second wave was 17 or less. The respondents' ability to recall the age of onset was limited because of their cognitive impairment. Hence it was not possible to inquire about the age of occurrence of the first prodromal sign or symptom, for those with cognitive impairment at the second wave, and therefore the figure shows only one distribution. Twenty percent of the onsets occurred before the age of 48, and 50 percent occurred before the age of 68.

GAPS IN OUR KNOWLEDGE

Age-Specific Prevalence in Children

The most important limitation of the ECA data presented above for the illustrative mental disorders is the truncation at age 18. Although the bias of censorship is avoided, there may be significant numbers of incident cases before the age of 18. If the cumulative age of onset were to include those under 18, that is, the total population, the curves would move to the left by an amount equal to the proportion of cases having incidence before the age of 18. Unfortunately, the data necessary to estimate age of onset correctly for the total population do not exist. Available data are either retrospective or do not use standard diagnostic nomenclature.

Lack of prospective data is less important at the level of diagnosis than for the occurrence of the first precursor sign or symptom, because diagnosis occurs later. Prospective data are less crucial for schizophrenia, alcohol abuse or dependence, and cognitive impairment, which begin later, than for depressive and conduct disorders, which arise earlier in life. Prevalence data on major depressive disorder from published sources are presented in Table 5.8 to give the reader some indication of how early in life prevention efforts might have to start. The standard assessment of depression in children and adolescents has involved the application of diagnostic interview schedules scored according to criteria for adults, with no modification for children. Using these techniques, the prevalence of depression in youngsters under six years of age is extremely low, as shown in Table 5.8 (Kashani and Carlson, 1987). The rate of depression increases by at least severalfold during adolescence. Major depressive disorder is present in less than 3 percent of children before the age of puberty, as shown in the first five rows of Table 5.8. The lower seven rows show the prevalence in adolescents to be 2 to 8 percent, with one low outlier estimate of 1 percent (McGee, Feehan, Williams, Partridge, Silva, and Kelly, 1990). Because the DSM-III diagnosis is required for entry into this table, these results are constrained to have been produced after the introduction of the DSM-III in 1980. But with the exception of one study (Kashani, McGee, Clarkson, Anderson, Walton, Williams et al., 1983), the findings in Table 5.8 have all been published within the past five years and represent a recent ballooning of information about psychopathology in children. For both prepubertal and postpubertal ages, the findings display a relatively large range, with the highest reported prevalence being about three times the lowest reported prevalence. The exact age distribution, the locale and culture, and methodological differences all presumably contribute to the range of rates shown in Table 5.8. At some time during late adolescence, the prevalence of major depressive disorder approaches that found in the adult population.

Table 5.8 presents point prevalence data, which are useful for estimation of need. But incidence data are required to estimate age of onset and to guide the timing of prevention efforts. Incidence data require a

TABLE 5.8   Prevalence Data on DSM-III Major Depressive Disorder in the General Population by Age: A Review of Selected Studies of Children and Adolescents

Age Range	Current Prevalence[a]	Reference
2–6	0.9	Kashani and Carlson, 1987
9	1.8	Kashani et al., 1983
6–11	2.7[b]	Fleming et al., 1989
11	0.5	Anderson et al., 1987
9–12	2.5	Velez et al., 1989
11–14	2.5	Velez et al., 1989
15	1.2	McGee et al., 1990
12–16	7.8[b]	Fleming et al., 1989
14–16	4.7	Kashani et al., 1987
13–18	3.7	Velez et al., 1989
14–18	2.6	Lewinsohn et al., 1993
15–20	3.1	Velez et al., 1989

[a]Current prevalence includes point prevalence and one-year or six-month prevalence.
[b]"DMS-III-like" major depressive syndrome; high and medium levels of diagnostic certainty.

NOTE: Studies selected had the following characteristics: they were published in English; they used DSM-III criteria for major depressive disorder; and the general population sample was larger than 100.

prospective design in which lifetime prevalence data are gathered at the baseline, so that an at-risk population can be defined. Only two of the point prevalence estimates in Table 5.8 were accompanied in the original studies by lifetime prevalence data or data that allowed for inference of estimation of lifetime prevalence (Lewinsohn, Hops, Roberts, Seeley, and Andrews, 1993; Kashani et al., 1983). Only one study estimated incidence (Lewinsohn et al., 1993).

The data presented in Table 5.8 display what is known about the epidemiology of major depressive disorder in childhood. Considerable good work has been done for this disorder in particular. The data nevertheless reveal many gaps in knowledge, which present opportunities for further study, discussed in more detail below. Data (not shown) on conduct disorder, would reveal a similarly wide range in estimates and similar gaps in definitive epidemiological knowledge.

Child Psychiatric Nosology

A series of studies have shown that between 12 and 20 percent of all children suffer from emotional and/or behavioral disorders at some point in their childhood and that the vast majority are untreated (Offord et al., 1989a,b; also see Chapter 1). There is compelling evidence of the need for much more systematic investigation of the course and natural history of these disorders as well as of preventive intervention studies, as was recommended in an IOM report (1989b).

The incidence figures given earlier in this chapter are for adult disorders. Large-scale epidemiological studies are needed to provide compatible data about disorders in children. But even more urgent is the recognition of the need for a developmental perspective. Even though signs and symptom patterns of serious disturbance vary over the age span of childhood, it is possible at each developmental stage to identify individuals who are seriously disturbed. The use of semistructured diagnostic interviews for mental disorders in children under 8 or 9 years has only limited value because the validity of applying standard diagnostic criteria is not well-established. Also, impairments in cognitive and social functioning are more important in children, both as outcomes and as targets for preventive interventions. Finally, the notion of what constitutes a case of mental disorder in childhood is less well established—hence the need for broad-based assessment of child functioning in addition to a diagnostic assessment.

Limited knowledge about the development of psychopathology in children constrains our ability to engage in preventive intervention efforts. More epidemiological research in the area of developmental psychopathology is needed (Rutter, 1989). The range of prevalence figures for major depressive disorder in children, presented in Table 5.8, is quite broad, and there is no consensus in these data on the age at which major depressive disorder can first manifest itself. Even though it is possible to operationally define major depression using the DSM-III criteria, it is not clear that the disorder is the same in children below the age of puberty, because important features of the disorder, such as the gender ratio, differ in prepubertal versus postpubertal depression. It is difficult to define a population "at risk" for onset of disorder and therefore difficult to estimate the age of onset, except in adults, as is done in Figures 5.2 through 5.6 above. Ideally, prevention efforts ought to be directed to specific age periods during which the causal events underlying the disorder are taking place: if the preventive intervention occurs too early, its positive effects may be washed out before onset; if it occurs too late, the disorder may already have begun. There is no consensus on exactly how signs and symptoms should be configured into disorders at various ages. Therefore epidemiological research on children should gather and retain data on a wide range of signs and symptoms, as well as disorders, to ensure that maturational changes or changes in the diagnostic classification system do not hamper the ability to study the development of psychopathology over time.

Empirical Search for Prodromes

The study of precursor signs and symptoms, and prodromal periods, might prove useful in prevention efforts, but there is little knowledge from prospective and population-based data. The precursor signs and symptoms that are most predictive of disorder should be identified in epidemiological surveys, because they might suggest particular indicated preventions. For example, using the same base of data as in Figure 5.4, it is estimated that persons at risk for the first incidence of major depressive disorder, who have in the prior year experienced two weeks or more of sad mood, are 5.5 times more likely to have a first onset of major depressive disorder during the next year as those who have not had this precursor symptom. Individuals who have had the two-week period and symptoms in two or more symptom groups in the diagnostic criterion level B in DSM-III (sometimes called "depression syndrome") have 5.7 times the risk of having a first onset. Estimated relative risks for the criterion B symptom groups are available elsewhere (Dryman and Eaton, 1991).

The formula for estimating attributable risk can be usefully applied to these relative risks if the prevalence of the precursor is known (Eaton, Badawi, and Melton, 1993). For example, the one-year prevalence of a two-week period of sad mood is about 5 percent, but the one-year prevalence of the depression syndrome is only about 0.5 percent. Applying the attributable risk formula to these data yields an estimate of 18.4 percent for sad mood and 2.4 percent for depression syndrome. Therefore, if an efficient screening device could be found, the two-week period of sad mood is a much more logical choice for locating a population for indicated preventive intervention than is the depression syndrome. The yield from application of the formula is not the same as for other risk factors, because precursors that prove to be prodromal are part of the disorder that eventually occurs. But the exercise is useful in quantifying precursors and searching for prodromes. Converting what is known about precursors into true prodromes is an important topic of research for epidemiologists interested in prevention.

Co-morbidity

The notion of precursor signs and symptoms can usefully be extended to co-morbidity (Kessler and Price, in press). Over the life span, the mental disorders overlap to a large degree (Regier, Farmer, Rae, Locke, Keith, Judd, and Goodwin, 1990; Boyd et al., 1984). The study of epidemiological data on age of onset for co-morbid disorders (to determine which of two disorders came first) has begun only recently (e.g., Merikangas, Eaton, Angst, Kraemer, Canino, Rubio-Stipec et al., 1993). The relative risks for symptoms of one disorder, or for the disorder itself, in predicting first onset of a second disorder, are probably not as high as for the precursor signs and symptoms that specifically belong within the diagnostic cluster of the second disorder; but these relative risks may be higher than other risk factors, and sufficiently high to warrant use in screening in some situations. For example, the relative risk for first onset of major depressive disorder for those with a panic attack is 3.4, as estimated in a time-dependent proportional hazards model (Andrade, Chilcoat, and Eaton, 1993). The prevalence of panic attack is about 10 percent (Eaton, Dryman, and Weissman, 1991). Applying the formula for attributable risk yields an estimate of 19 percent. The distinction between indicated preventive interventions and treatment interventions can be further clarified as the precursor symptoms of coexisting disorders become more understood.

Transition to Adulthood

The transition to adulthood is poorly understood, in spite of the fact that it is probably the age period when most adult disorders have their peak rates of incidence. There are prevalence surveys of mental disorders in adults, such as the ECA study, and in children, such as those reviewed in Table 5.8. The ECA study is the only one in the United States that estimates incidence of specific disorders in adults, and there is only one study estimating incidence rates for a DSM-III disorder in a population under age 18 (Lewinsohn et al., 1993). There are no studies that estimate incidence of specific disorders during the age period of the transition to adulthood, that is, from about age 15 to about age 25. Studies under way using synthetic cohort designs (in which the effects of aging can be studied by using a cross-sectional design that includes a range of ages but requires strong assumptions about the effects of birth cohort and historical period [Beltes, Cornelius, and Nesselroade, 1979]) have the capacity to yield estimates of incidence, and to study the effects of risk factors that are relatively close to the time of the beginning of the study. But synthetic cohort designs will not be able to study the effects of combinations of these risk factors and ones that occur later. Because these combinations may be very important in the transition to adulthood, this is a stark gap in our epidemiological knowledge relevant to the prevention of mental disorders.

FINDINGS AND LEADS

- A disorder may be preventable up to the point of onset of first episode. Although onset can rarely be accurately pinpointed, the time at which an individual meets full criteria for diagnosis can be used as an approximation. As more becomes known about precursors and pro-dromes, the age of onset will become more accurately known.
- Epidemiological research on children and adults should gather and retain data on a wide range of signs and symptoms, as well as disorders, to help ensure that maturational changes and changes in the diagnostic classification system do not interfere with the study of the development of psychopathology over time.
- Prospective epidemiological studies that estimate incidence of specific risk factors and disorders in childhood, adolescence, and during the transition to adulthood, from age 15 to 25, are greatly needed for prevention research. Such studies could help clarify the mechanisms linking risk factors to the first occurrence of disorders.
- For a particular disorder, a review of what is known about prodrome, age of onset, diagnostic criteria, course, co-morbidity, inci-dence and prevalence, effectiveness of treatment, and costs to society can help the investigator determine if the knowledge base is sufficient to consider designing a preventive intervention. For example, the inci-dence of a disorder will help determine the necessary size of the sample so that statistical analyses are meaningful (Muñoz and Ying, 1993); the demographics of a disorder will help determine who is at highest risk and what population groups should be targeted; and if a specific treatment is known to be effective, it could be considered for use before onset. Such a review could in turn help policymakers set priorities for preventive intervention programs.
- Many mental disorders, including conduct disorder, depressive disorders, alcohol abuse and dependence, schizophrenia, and Alzhei-mer's disease, are thought to be a cluster of several different illnesses or to have subtypes. Identification of these groups and clearer delineation of their etiologies may clarify which individuals may be most amenable to preventive interventions.
- Risk factors that have a role in the etiology of a mental disorder may be differentially malleable at different phases of the life course. More research regarding the sensitive periods of risk factors, that is, when they contribute most to etiology, could lead to more strategic

timing of preventive interventions, that is, before or during those sensitive periods.

● From a clinical perspective, the prodromal periods for some of the illustrative mental disorders may seem unusually lengthy. Because the prodromal data presented here were subject to retrospective recall by individuals who currently had a disorder, the time of the first sign or symptom may not be accurate. Also, the signs and symptoms may not have been sufficiently specific to differentiate them from a range of normal behavior. The only way of determining true prodromal periods is through prospective studies with cutoff points for carefully defined signs and symptoms. However, if through such studies prodromal periods are indeed found to be quite lengthy, the timing of preventive interventions may be adjusted accordingly.

● Prospective epidemiological studies could identify precursor signs and symptoms that are below the criterion level for the diagnosis of a mental disorder, as well as the age of the first occurrence of these precursor symptoms. Thus it may be possible to identify individuals at heightened risk for developing the full-blown disorder, who would then become candidates for indicated preventive interventions. For example, populations could be screened for precursors, such as a two-week period of sad mood.

● Research advances in understanding of the cause of Alzheimer's disease (AD) have been substantial. Genetic evidence suggests that AD may be a collection of specific diseases with a single common pathway. If this pathway can be clarified and a marker found to identify individuals at high risk for developing AD, an intervention may eventually be found that could inhibit a crucial step, such as amyloid formation, and prevent emergence of the disease or at least delay its onset.

REFERENCES

Alleback, P.; Wistedt, B. (1986) Mortality in schizophrenia. Archives of General Psychiatry; 43: 650–653.

American Psychiatric Association. (1987) Diagnostic and Statistical Manual of Mental Disorders (Third Edition—Revised). Washington, DC: American Psychiatric Association.

Anderson, J. C.; Williams, S.; McGee, R.; Silva, P. A. (1987) DSM-III Disorders in Preadolescent Children. Archives of General Psychiatry; 44: 69–76.

Andrade, L.; Chilcoat, H.; Eaton, W. W. (1993) Comorbidity of panic and depression: Age of onset. Unpublished manuscript.

Barraclough, B.; Bunch, J.; Nelson, B.; Sainsbury, P. (1974) A hundred cases of suicide: Clinical observations. British Journal of Psychiatry; 125: 355–373.

Battelle Memorial Institute. (1984) The Economics of Dementia. Contract report prepared for the Office of Technology Assessment. Washington, DC: U.S. Congress.

Beardslee, W. R.; Keller, M. B.; Lavori, P. W.; Staley, J.; Sacks, N. (1993) The impact of parental affective disorder on depression in offspring: A longitudinal follow-up in a non-referred sample. Journal of the American Academy of Child and Adolescent Psychiatry; 32(4): 723–730.

Beardslee, W. R.; Wheelock, I. (in press) Children of parents with affective disorders: Empirical findings and clinical implications. In: W. R. Reynolds and H. F. Johnston, Eds. Handbook of Depression in Children and Adolescents. New York, NY: Plenum Publishers.

Beltes, P. B.; Cornelius, S. W.; Nesselroade, J. R. (1979) Cohort effects in developmental psychology. In: J. R. Nesselroade and P. B. Beltes, Eds. Longitudinal Research in the Study of Behavior and Development. New York, NY: Academic Press; 61–84.

Bird, H. R.; Canino, G.; Rubio-Stipec, M.; Gould, M. S.; Ribera, J.; Sesman, M.; Woodbury, M.; Huertas-Goldman, S.; Pagan, A.; Sanchez-Lacay, A.; Moscoso, M. (1988) Estimates of the Prevalence of Childhood Maladjustment in a Community Survey in Puerto Rico. Archives of General Psychiatry; 45: 1120–1126.

Black, D. W.; Winokur, G. (1988) Age, mortality and chronic schizophrenia. Schizophrenia Research; 1:267–272.

Bleuler, E. (1950) Dementia praecox or the group of schizophrenias (J. Zinkin, Trans.). New York, NY: International Universities Press. (Original work published 1911.)

Boyd, J. H.; Burke, J. D.; Gruenberg, E. M.; Holzer, C. E., III; Rae, D. S.; George, L. K.; Karno, M.; Stoltzman, R.; McEvoy, L.; Hestadt, G. (1984) Exclusion criteria of DSM-III: A study of co-occurence of hierarchy-free syndromes. Archives of General Psychiatry; 41: 983–989.

Boyd, J. H.; Weissman, M. M. (1981) Epidemiology of affective disorders: A reexamination and future directions. Archives of General Psychiatry; 38(9): 1039–1046.

Brenner, H. D.; Dencker, S. J.; Goldstein, M. J.; Hubbard, J. W.; Keegan, D. L.; Kruger, G.; Kulhanek, F.; Liberman, R. P.; Malm, U.; Midha, K. K. (1990) Defining treatment refractoriness in schizophrenia. Schizophrenia Bulletin; 16: 551–561.

Caetano, R. (1989) Drinking patterns and alcohol problems in a national sample of U.S. Hispanics. The Epidemiology of Alcohol Use and Abuse among U.S. Minorities. NIAAA Monograph No. 18. Rockville, MD: DHHS Pub. No. (ADM) 89–1435.

Christie, K. A.; Burke, J. D., Jr.; Regier, D. A.; Rae, D. S.; Boyd, J. H.; Locke, B. Z. (1988) Epidemiologic evidence for early onset of mental disorders and higher risk of drug-use in young-adults. American Journal of Psychiatry; 145: 971–975.

Cleary, P. D.; Goldberg, I. D.; Kessler, L. G.; Nyez, G. R. (1982) Screening for mental disorders among primary care patients. Archives of General Psychiatry; 39: 837–840.

Cloninger, C. R.; Sigvardsson, S.; Gilligan, S. B.; von Knorring, A. F.; Reich, T.; Bohman, M. (1989) Genetic heterogeneity and the classifications of alcoholism. In: E. Gordis, B. Tabakoff, and M. Linnoila, Eds. Alcohol Research from Bench to Bedside. New York, NY: The Haworth Press; 3–16.

Costello, E. (1989) Child psychiatric disorders and their correlates: A primary care pediatric sample. Journal of the American Academy of Child and Adolescent Psychiatry; 28: 851–855.

Coyle, J. T.; Price, D. L.; DeLong, M. R. (1983) Alzheimer's disease: A disorder of cortical cholinergic innervation. Science; 219(4589): 1184–1190.

Cross, P. S.; Gurland, B. J. (1986) The epidemiology of dementing disorders. Contract report for the Office of Technology Assessment. Washington, DC: U.S. Congress.

Cross-National Collaborative Group. (1992) The changing rate of major depression. Journal of the American Medical Association; 268(21): 3098–3105.

DeKosky, S. T.; Scheff, S. W. (1990) Synapse loss in frontal cortex biopsies in Alzheimer's disease: correlation with cognitive severity. Annals of Neurology; 27: 457–464.

Depression Guideline Panel. (1993a) Depression in Primary Care: Vol. 1, Diagnosis and Detection. Clinical Practice Guideline, No. 5. Rockville, MD: Department of Health and Human Services, Public Health Service, Agency for Health Care Policy and Research. AHCPR Pub. No. 93–0550.

Depression Guideline Panel. (1993b) Depression in Primary Care: Vol. 2, Treatment of Major Depression. Clinical Practice Guideline, No. 5. Rockville, MD: Department of Health and Human Services, Public Health Service, Agency for Health Care Policy and Research. AHCPR Pub. No. 93–0551.

Depression Guideline Panel. (1993c) Depression in Primary Care: Detection, Diagnosis and Treatment. Quick Reference Guide for Clinicians, No. 5. Rockville, MD: Department of Health and Human Services, Public Health Service, Agency for Health Care Policy and Research. AHCPR Pub. No. 93–0552.

Deutsch, L. H.; Rovner, B. W. (1991) Agitation and other noncognitive abnormalities in Alzheimer's disease. The Psychiatric Clinics of North America; 14(2): 341–351.

DHHS (Department of Health and Human Services). (1991) Alcoholism and Co-occurring Disorders. Alcohol Alert. Rockville, MD: NIAAA; No. 14; PH 302.

DHHS (Department of Health and Human Services). (1990) Seventh Special Report to the U.S. Congress on Alcohol and Health. Rockville, MD: DHHS Pub. No. (ADM) 90–1656.

Downey, G.; Coyne, J. C. (1990) Children of depressed parents: An integrative review. Psychological Bulletin; 108: 50–76.

Dryman, A.; Eaton, W. W. (1991) Affective symptoms associated with the onset of major depression in the community: Findings from the U.S. National Institute of Mental Health Epidemiologic Catchment Area Program. Acta Psychiatrica Scandinavica; 84(1): 1–5.

Eaton, W. W. (1991) Update on the epidemiology of schizophrenia. Epidemiologic Reviews; 13: 320–328.

Eaton, W. W.; Badawi, M.; Melton, B. (1993) Prodromes and precursors for four DIS/DSM-III disorders: Epidemiologic data for prevention of disorders with slow onset. Unpublished manuscript.

Eaton, W. W.; Dryman, A.; Weissman, M. M. (1991) Panic and phobia. In: L. N. Robins and D. A. Regier, Eds. Psychiatric Disorders in America: The Epidemiologic Catchment Area Study. New York, NY: The Free Press; 155–179.

Eaton, W. W.; Kessler, L. G. (1985) Epidemiologic Field Methods in Psychiatry: The NIMH Epidemiologic Catchment Area Program. New York, NY: Academic Press.

Eaton, W. W.; Kramer, M.; Anthony, J. C.; Dryman, A.; Shapiro, S.; Locke, B. Z. (1989) The incidence of specific DIS/DSM-III mental disorders: Data from the NIMH Epidemiological Catchment Area program. Acta Psychiatrica Scandinavica; 79: 163–178.

Eaton, W. W.; Regier, D. A.; Locke, B. Z.; Taube, C. A. (1981) The Epidemiologic Catchment Area Program of the NIMH. Public Health Reports; 96: 319–325.

Evans, D. A.; Funkenstein, H. H.; Albert, M. S.; Scherr, P. A.; Cook, N. R.; Chown, M. J.; Hebert, L. E.; Hennekens, C. H.; Taylor, J. O. (1989) Prevalence of Alzheimer's disease in a community population of older persons. Journal of the American Medical Association; 262(18): 2551–2556.

Evans, D. A.; Scherr, P. A.; Cook, N. R.; Albert, M. S.; Funkenstein, H. H.; Smith, L. A.; Hebert, L. E.; Wetle, T. T.; Branch, L. G.; Chown, M.; Hennekens, C. H.; Taylor, J. O. (1990) Estimated prevalence of Alzheimer's disease in the United States. Milbank Quarterly; 68: 267–289.

Falloon, I. R. H.; Fadden, G. (1993) Integrated Mental Health Care. London, England: Cambridge University Press.

Fleming, J. E.; Offord, D. R.; Boyle, M. H. (1989) Prevalence of childhood and adolescent depression in the community: Ontario Child Health Study. British Journal of Psychiatry; 155: 647–654.

Frank, E.; Kupfer, D. J.; Perel, J. M.; Cornes, C.; Jarrett, D. B.; Mallinger, A. G.; Thase, M. E.; McEachran, A. B.; Grochocinski, V. J. (1990) Three year outcomes for maintenance therapies in recurrent depression. Archives of General Psychiatry; 47: 1093–1099.

George, L. K.; Landerman, R.; Blazer, D. G.; Anthony, J. C. (1991) Cognitive impairment. In: L. N. Robins and D. A. Regier, Eds. Psychiatric Disorders in America: The Epidemiologic Catchment Area Study. New York, NY: The Free Press; 291–327.

Glynn, S.; Mueser, K. T. (1992) Social learning programs. In: R. P. Liberman, Ed. Handbook of Psychiatric Rehabilitation. New York, NY: Academic Press.

Goldberg, D. P.; Huxley, P. (1980) Mental Illness in the Community: Pathway to Psychiatric Care. London, England: Tavistock.

Gottesman, I. I. (1991) Schizophrenia Genesis: The Origins of Madness. New York, NY: W. H. Freeman and Company.

Gunderson, J. G.; Mosher, L. R. (1975) The cost of schizophrenia. American Journal of Psychiatry; 132: 901–906.

Guze, S.; Robins, E. (1970) Suicide and primary affective disorders. British Journal of Psychiatry; 117: 437–438.

Hagnell, O.; Lanke, J.; Rorsman, B.; Ojesjo, L. (1982) Are we entering an age of melancholy? Depressive illnesses in a prospective epidemiological study over 25 years: The Lundby Study, Sweden. Psychological Medicine; 12: 279–289.

Hall, W.; Goldstein, G.; Andrews, G.; Lapsley, H.; Bartel, R.; Silove, D. (1985) Estimating the economic costs of schizophrenia. Schizophrenia Bulletin; 11: 598–611.

Hamos, J. E.; DeGennaro, L. J.; Drachman, D. A. (1989) Synaptic loss in Alzheimer's disease and other dementias. Neurology; 39: 355–361.

Harding, C. M. (1988) Course types in schizophrenia: An analysis of European and American studies. Schizophrenia Bulletin; 14(4): 633–643.

Harding, C. M.; Brooks, G. W.; Ashikaga, T.; Strauss, J. S.; Breier, A. (1987) The Vermont longitudinal study of persons with severe mental illness. American Journal of Psychiatry; 144: 718–735.

Helzer, J. E.; Burnam, A.; McEvoy, L. T. (1991) Alcohol abuse and dependence. In: L. N. Robins and D. A. Regier, Eds. Psychiatric Disorders in America: The Epidemiologic Catchment Area Study. New York, NY: The Free Press; 81–115.

Herd, D. (1989) The epidemiology of drinking patterns and alcohol-related problems among U.S. blacks. The Epidemiology of Alcohol Use and Abuse Among U.S. Minorities. NIAAA Monograph No. 18: DHHS Pub. No. (ADM) 89–1435.

Hilton, M. E. (1987) Drinking patterns and drinking problems in 1984: Results from a general population survey. Alcoholism; 11: 167–175.

Hough, R. L.; Landsverk, J. A.; Karno, M.; Burnam, M. A.; Timbers, D. M.; Escobar, J. I.; Regier, D. A. (1987) Utilization of health and mental health services by Los Angeles Mexican Americans and non-Hispanic whites. Archives of General Psychiatry; 44: 702–709.

Hu, T. W.; Huang, L. F.; Cartwright, W. S. (1986) Evaluation of the costs of caring for the senile demented elderly: A pilot study. The Gerontologist; 26: 158–163.

Huang, L. F.; Hu, T. W. (1986) The Economic Cost of Senile Dementia in the United States, 1983. Contract report prepared for the National Institute on Aging; No. 1-AG-3-2123.

Indian Health Service. (1988) Indian Health Service Chart Series Book. DHHS Pub. No. 0–218–547:QL3 ed.

IOM (Institute of Medicine). (1990a) Depression. In: The Second Fifty Years: Promoting Health and Preventing Disability. Washington, DC: National Academy Press; 202–223.

IOM (Institute of Medicine). (1990b) Broadening the Base of Treatment for Alcohol Problems. Washington, DC: National Academy Press.

IOM (Institute of Medicine). (1989a) Community approaches and perspectives from other health fields. In: Prevention and Treatment of Alcohol Problems: Research Opportunities. Washington, DC: National Academy Press; 109–127.

IOM (Institute of Medicine). (1989b) Research on Children and Adolescents with Mental, Behavioral, and Developmental Disorders. Washington, DC: National Academy Press.

IOM (Institute of Medicine). (1985) Injury in America: A Continuing Public Health Problem. Washington, DC: National Academy Press.

Jorm, A. F. (1991) Cross-national comparisons of the occurrence of Alzheimer's and vascular dementias. European Archives of Psychiatry and Clinical Neuroscience; 240: 218–222.

Kashani, J. H.; Carlson, G. A. (1987) Seriously depressed preschoolers. American Journal of Psychiatry; 144(3): 348–350.

Kashani, J. H.; Carlson, G. A.; Beck, N. C.; Hoeper, E. W.; Corcoran, C. M.; McAllister, J. A.; Fallahi, C.; Rosenberg, T. K.; Reid, J. C. (1987) Depression, depressive symptoms, and depressed mood among a community sample of adolescents. American Journal of Psychiatry; 144(7): 931–934.

Kashani, J. H.; McGee, R. O.; Clarkson, S. E.; Anderson, J. C.; Walton, L. A.; Williams, S.; Silva, P. A.; Robins, J.; Cytryn, L.; McKnew, D. H. (1983) Depression in a sample of 9-year-old children. Archives of General Psychiatry; 40: 1217–1223.

Katzman, R.; Jackson, J. E. (1991) Alzheimer disease: Basic and clinical advances. Journal of the American Geriatric Society; 39: 516–525.

Katzman, R.; Lasker, B.; Bernstein, N. (1986) Accuracy of diagnosis and consequences of misdiagnosis of disorders causing dementia. Contract report prepared for the Office of Technology Assessment. Washington, DC: U.S. Congress.

Kazdin, A. E. (1993) Treatment of conduct disorder: Progress and directions in psychotherapy research. Development and Psychopathology; 5: 277–310.

Keith, S. J.; Regier, D. A.; Rae, D. S. (1991) Schizophrenic disorders. In: L. N. Robins and D. A. Regier, Eds. Psychiatric Disorders in America: The Epidemiologic Catchment Area Study. New York, NY: The Free Press; 33–52.

Keitner, G. I.; Miller, I. W. (1991) Family functioning and major depression: An overview. American Journal of Psychiatry; 147: 1128–1137.

Kellam, S. G.; Brown, C. H.; Rubin, B. R.; Einsminger, M. E. (1983) Paths leading to teenage psychiatric symptoms and substance use: Developmental epidemiologic studies in Woodlawn. In: S. B. Guze, F. J. Earls, and J. E. Barratt, Eds. Childhood Psychopathology and Development. New York, NY: Raven Press; 17–51.

Keller, M. B.; Lavori, P. W.; Beardslee, W. R.; Wunder, J.; Ryan, N. (1991) Depression in children and adolescents: New data on "undertreatment" and a literature review on the efficacy of available treatments. Journal of Affective Disorders; 21(3): 163–171.

Keller, M. B.; Lavori, P. W.; Rice, J.; Coryell, W.; Hirschfeld, R. M. A. (1986) The persistent risk of chronicity in recurrent episodes of nonbipolar major depressive disorder: A prospective follow-up. American Journal of Psychiatry; 143: 24–28.

Kessler, R. C.; Price, R. H. (in press) Primary prevention of secondary disorders: A proposal and an agenda. American Journal of Community Psychology.

Klerman, G. L. (1988) Introduction. In: W. H. Reid, Ed. Treatment of Psychiatric Disorders: Revised for the DSM IIIR. New York, NY: Brunner-Mazel.

Klerman, G. L.; Lavori, P. W.; Rice, J.; Reich, T.; Endicott, J.; Andreason, N. C.; Keller, M. B.; Hirschfield, R. (1985) Birth-cohort trends in rates of major depressive disorder among relatives of patients with affective disorder. Archives of General Psychiatry; 42: 689–693.

Koo, E. H.; Price, D. L. (1993) The neurobiology of dementia. In: P. J. Whitehouse, Ed. Dementia. Philadelphia, PA: F. A. Davis; 55–91.

Kuehnel, T. G.; Liberman, R. P.; Marshall, B. D.; Bowen, L. (1992) Optimal drug and behavior therapy for treatment refractory, institutionalized schizophrenics. In: R. P. Liberman, Ed. Effective Psychiatric Rehabilitation: New Directions for Mental Health Services. No. 53. San Francisco, CA: Jossey-Bass Publications.

Lawless, J. F. (1982) Statistical models and methods for lifetime data. In: Wiley Series in Probability and Mathematical Statistics. New York, NY: John Wiley and Sons.

Lewine, R. (1988) Gender and schizophrenia. In: Handbook of Schizophrenia. New York, NY: Elsevier Science Publishers; 379–397.

Lewinsohn, P. M.; Hops, H.; Roberts, R. E.; Seeley, J. R.; Andrews, J. A. (1993) Adolescent psychopathology: I. Prevalence and incidence of depression and other DSM-III-R disorders in high school students. Journal of Abnormal Psychology; 1993; 102(1): 133–144.

Liberman, R. P. (1992) Handbook of Psychiatric Rehabilitation. New York, NY: Macmillan.

Lieberman, J.; Jody, D.; Geisler, S.; Alvir, J.; Loeber, A.; Szymanski, S.; Woerner, M.; Borenstein, M. (1993) Time course and biologic correlates of treatment response in first-episode schizophrenics. Archives of General Psychiatry; 50: 369–377.

Loeber, R.; Green, S. M.; Lahey, B. B.; Stouthamer-Loeber, M. (1989) Optimal informants on childhood disruptive behaviors. Development and Psychopathology; 1(4): 317–337.

Loeber, R.; Wung, P.; Keenan, K.; Giroux, B.; Stouthamer-Loeber, M.; Van Kammen, W. B.; Maughan, B. (1993) Developmental pathways in disruptive child behavior. Development and Psychopathology; 5: 103–133.

Manderscheid, R. W.; Barrett, S. A., Eds. (1987) Mental Health, United States. Washington, DC: Government Printing Office; DHHS Publication No. (ADM) 87–1518: 79.

McCord, J. (1988) Identifying developmental paradigms leading to alcoholism. Journal of Studies on Alcohol; 49(4): 357–362.

McGee, R.; Feehan, M.; Williams, S.; Partridge, F.; Silva, P. A.; Kelly, J. (1990) DSM-III disorders in a large sample of adolescents. Journal of the American Academy of Child and Adolescent Psychiatry; 29: 611–619.

Meltzer, H. Y. (1992) Treatment of the neuroleptic-nonresponsive schizophrenic patients. Schizophrenia Bulletin; 18: 515–542.

Merikangas, K. R.; Eaton, W. W.; Angst, J.; Kraemer, H. C.; Canino, G.; Rubio-Stipec, M.; Wittchen, H. U.; Wacker, H. C.; Helzer, J. E.; Andrade, L.; Kupfer, D. (1993) Comorbidity in the affective disorders: Results from an international task force. Unpublished manuscript.

Mintz, J.; Mintz, L.; Goldstein, M. G. (1987) Expressed emotion and relapse in first episodes of schizophrenia. British Journal of Psychiatry; 151: 314–320.

Moskowitz, D. S.; Schwartzman, A. E. (1989) Painting group portraits: Studying life outcomes for aggressive and withdrawn children. Journal of Personality; 57(4): 723–746.

Muñoz, R. F.; Ying, Y. W. (1993) The Prevention of Depression: Research and Practice. Baltimore, MD: Johns Hopkins University Press.

National Center for Health Statistics. (1993) Advance Report of Final Mortality Statistics, 1990: Monthly Vital Statistics Report; 41(7) Suppl.: 1–52.

NIAAA (National Institute on Alcohol Abuse and Alcoholism). (1991) Alcohol Research: Promise for the Decade: DHHS.

NIH Consensus Development Panel on Depression in Late Life. (1992) Diagnosis and treatment of depression in late life. Journal of the American Medical Association; 268(8): 1018–1024.

Offord, D. R. (1989) Conduct disorder: Risk factors and prevention. In: Prevention of Mental Disorders, Alcohol and other Drug Use in Children and Adolescents. OSAP Prevention Monograph—2.: DHHS Pub. No. (ADM) 89–1646: 273–307.

Offord, D. R.; Boyle, M. H.; Fleming, J. E.; Blum, H. M.; Grant, N. I. (1989a) Ontario Child Health Study. Summary of selected results. Canadian Journal of Psychiatry; 34(6): 483–491.

Offord, D. R.; Boyle, M. H.; Racine, Y. (1989b) Ontario Child Health Study: Correlates of disorder. Journal of the American Academy of Child and Adolescent Psychiatry; 28: 856–860.

Offord, D. R.; Boyle, M. H.; Racine, Y. A.; Fleming, J. E.; Cadman, D. T.; Blum, H. M.; Byrne, C.; Links, P. S.; Lipman, E. L.; Macmillan, H. L. (1992) Outcome, prognosis and risk in a longitudinal follow-up study. Journal of the American Academy of Child and Adolescent Psychiatry; 31(5): 916–923.

Offord, D. R.; Boyle, M. H.; Szatmari, P.; Rae Grant, N. I.; Links, P. S.; Cadman, D. T.; Byles, J. A.; Crawford, J. W.; Blum, H. M.; Byrne, C.; Thomas, H.; Woodward, C. A. (1987) Ontario Child Health Study: Six month prevalence of disorder and rates of service utilization. Archives of General Psychiatry; 44: 832–836.

OTA (Office of Technology Assessment). U.S. Congress. (1992) Special Care Units for People with Alzheimer's and Other Dementias: Consumer Education, Research, Regulatory, and Reimbursement Issues. Washington, DC: Government Printing Office; OTA-H-543.

OTA (Office of Technology Assessment). U.S. Congress. (1987) Losing a Million Minds: Confronting the Tragedy of Alzheimer's Disease and Other Dementias. Washington, DC: Government Printing Office; OTA-BA-323.

Pérez-Stable, E. J.; Miranda, J.; Muñoz, R. F.; Ying, Y. W. (1990) Depression in medical outpatients: Underrecognition and misdiagnosis. Archives of General Internal Medicine; 150: 1083–1088.

Regier, D. A.; Farmer, M. E.; Rae, D. S.; Locke, B. Z.; Keith, S. J.; Judd, L. L.; Goodwin, F. K. (1990) Comorbidity of mental disorders with alcohol and other drug abuse: Results from the Epidemiologic Catchment Area study. Journal of the American Medical Association; 264: 2511–2518.

Regier, D. A.; Goldberg, I. D.; Taube, C. A. (1978) The defacto U.S. mental health service system: A public health perspective. Archives of General Psychiatry; 35: 685–696.

Rice, D. P.; Fox, P. J.; Hanck, W. W.; Max, W.; Webber, P.; Lindeman, D. W.; Segura, T. (1991) The burden of caring for Alzheimer's disease patients. Paper presented at the NCHS Public Health Conference on Records and Statistics; July 15–17.

Robins, L. N. (1991) Conduct disorder. Journal of Child and Adolescent Psychiatry; 32(1): 193–212.

Robins, L. N. (1980) The natural history of drug abuse. Acta Psychiatrica Scandinavica; 62(Suppl. 284): 7–20.

Robins, L. N. (1970) Follow-up studies investigating childhood disorders. In: E. H. Hare and J. K. Wing, Eds. Psychiatric Epidemiology. London, England: Oxford University Press.

Robins, L. N.; Helzer, J. E.; Croughan, J.; Williams, J. B. W.; Spitzer, R. L. (1981) National Institute of Mental Health Diagnostic Interview Schedule: Version III. Rockville, MD: National Institute of Mental Health.

Robins, L. N.; Regier, D. A. (1991) Psychiatric Disorders in America: The Epidemiologic Catchment Area Study. New York, NY: The Free Press.

Rocca, W. A.; Hofman, A.; Brayne, C.; Breteler, M. M. B.; Clarke, M.; Copeland, J. R. M.; Dartigues, J. F.; Engedal, K.; Hagnell, O.; Heeren, T. J.; Jonker, C.; Lindesay, J.; Lobo, A.; Mann, A. H.; Molsa, P. K.; Morgan, K.; O'Connor, D. W.; da Silva Droux, A.; Sulkava, R.; Kay, D. W. K.; Amaducci, L. (1991) Frequency and distribution of Alzheimer's disease in Europe: A collaborative study of 1980–1990 prevalence rates. Annals of Neurology; 30: 381–390.

Roy, A. (1986) Depression, attempted suicide, and suicide in patients with chronic schizophrenia. Psychiatric Clinics of North America; 9: 193–206.

Rutter, M. (1989) Pathways from childhood to adult life. Journal of Child Psychology and Psychiatry; 30(1): 23–51.

Rutter, M.; Giller, H. (1983) Juvenile Delinquency: Trends and Perspectives. New York, NY: Penguin Books.

Rutter, M.; Tizard, J.; Whitmore, K. (1970) Education, Health and Behaviour. London, England: Longman.

Shaner, A.; Khalsa, M. E.; Roberts, L.; Wilkins, J.; Anglin, D.; Hsieh, S. C. (1993) Unrecognized cocaine use among schizophrenic patients. American Journal of Psychiatry; 150: 758–762.

Taylor, E. A.; Schachar, R.; Thorley, G.; Wieselberg, M. (1986) Conduct disorder and hyperactivity: I. Separation of hyperactivity and antisocial conduct in British child psychiatric patients. British Journal of Psychiatry; 149: 760–767.

Teri, L.; Wagner, A. (1992) Alzheimer's disease and depression. Journal of Consulting and Clinical Psychology; 60(3): 379–391.

Terry, R. D.; Masliah, E.; Salmon, D. P.; Butters, N.; DeTeresa, R.; Hill, R.; Hansen, L. A.; Katzman, R. (1991) Physical basis of cognitive alterations in Alzheimer's disease: Synapse loss is the major correlate of cognitive impairment. Annals of Neurology; 30: 572–580.

Velez, C. N.; Johnson, J.; Cohen, P. (1989) A longitudinal analysis of selected risk factors for childhood psychopathology. Journal of the American Academy of Child and Adolescent Psychiatry; 28(5): 861–864.

Vital Statistics of the United States. (1975) Suicide rates in the United States by age, sex, and color. Washington, DC: Mortality Statistics Branch.

Weiss, C.; Hechtman, L. (1986) Hyperactive Children Grown Up. New York, NY: The Guilford Press.

Weissman, M. M. (1988) Psychotherapy in the treatment of depression: New technologies and efficacy. In: W. H. Reid, Ed. Treatment of Psychiatric Disorders: Revised for the DSM-III-R. New York, NY: Brunner-Mazel; 1814–1823.

Weissman, M. M.; Bruce, M. L.; Lief, P. J.; Florio, L. P.; Holzer, C., III. (1991) Affective disorders. In: L. N. Robins and D. A. Regier, Eds. Psychiatric Disorders in America: The Epidemiological Catchment Area Study. New York, NY: The Free Press.

White, J. L.; Moffitt, T. E.; Earls, F.; Robins, L.; Silva, P. A. (1990) How early can we tell? Predictors of childhood conduct disorder and adolescent delinquency. Criminology; 24(4): 507–533.

Whitehouse, P. J.; Price, D. L.; Clark, A. W.; Coyle, J. T.; DeLong, M. R. (1981) Alzheimer disease: Evidence for selective loss of cholinergic neurons in the nucleus basalis. Annals of Neurology; 10: 122–126.

Whitehouse, P. J.; Price, D. L.; Struble, R. G.; Clark, A. W.; Coyle, J. T.; Delong, M. R. (1982) Alzheimer's disease and senile dementia: Loss of neurons in the basal forebrain. Science; 215: 1237–1239.

Winokur, G.; Tsuang, M. (1975) The Iowa 500: Suicide in mania, depression, and schizophrenia. American Journal of Psychiatry; 132: 650–651.

Wyatt, R. J. (1991) Neuroleptics and the natural course of schizophrenia. Schizophrenia Bulletin; 17: 325–351.

Zhang, M.; Katzman, R.; Kashani, J. H.; Salmon, D.; Jin, H.; Cai, G.; Wang, Z.; Qu, G.; Grant, I.; Yu, E.; Levy, P.; Klauber, M. R.; Liu, W. T. (1990) The prevalence of dementia and Alzheimer's disease in Shanghai, China: Impact of age, gender, and education. Annals of Neurology; 27: 428–437.

6

Risk and Protective Factors for the Onset of Mental Disorders

During the past 30 years a growing body of research has elucidated some of the risk factors that predispose children and
adults to mental disorder. Recent research has also helped to
change the concept of a risk factor from a fixed, specific circumstance or
life stress to a broader, more general phenomenon that may be modifiable, or malleable, and related to a developmental phase (Avison, 1992).
These findings have led to a shift in risk factor research in both emphasis
and complexity.

Risk factors are those characteristics, variables, or hazards that, if
present for a given individual, make it more likely that this individual,
rather than someone selected at random from the general population,
will develop a disorder (Werner and Smith, 1992; Garmezy, 1983). To
qualify as a risk factor, therefore, a variable must be associated with an
increased probability of disorder and must antedate the onset of
disorder. Variables that may be risk factors at one life stage may or may
not put an individual at risk at a later stage of development. Risk factors
can reside with the individual or within the family, community, or
institutions that surround the individual. They can be biological or
psychosocial in nature. Some risk factors play a causal role, although
this may not be known prior to an intervention study. Others merely
mark or identify the potential for a disorder rather than cause the
disorder, and for these, therefore, malleability is not an issue. For
example, unusual eye movement is often associated with and predates
schizophrenia. Its presence increases the likelihood that an individual
will develop schizophrenia, but any efforts to alter such eye movements

would be fruitless for preventing schizophrenia because it is not thought to have a causal role. The committee uses the term *marker* for both biological and psychosocial risk factors of this sort. Incorporated into this definition of risk factor is the concept of vulnerability, which is a predisposition to a specific disease process. Vulnerability traits are identifiable and measurable (and may sometimes be referred to as markers). They are not intrinsically the disease, but they may be necessary for a specific mental disorder to develop. Having vulnerability traits may increase an individual's risk for developing a disorder, but other risk factors also may be necessary for the illness to be expressed.

For years, mental health workers devoted their energies to the study of maladaptation and incompetence (Garmezy, 1983) as attempts were made to identify patterns of functioning in childhood that might portend the future development of mental disorders. Rutter (1985b) described this preoccupation as a "regrettable tendency to focus gloomily on the ills of mankind and all that can and does go wrong." But not everyone with risk factors goes on to develop a mental disorder, and the importance of protective factors is becoming more recognized. Recently, research has been directed toward understanding why some children appear to be resilient, and why they come to maturity relatively unscathed by the organic and psychosocial insults that prevent so many of their peers from achieving optimal intellectual, social, and emotional functioning (Werner and Smith, 1992). Werner and Smith (1992) defined resilience as "an unusual or marked capacity to recover from or successfully cope with significant stresses, of both internal and external origin." Theoretical explanations for the phenomenon of resilience (Rutter, 1985b; Garmezy, 1983) involve the interaction of risk factors, including individual vulnerability, and protective factors to explain why some are spared and others are not. Vulnerable individuals are considered to be those who, by virtue of genetic predisposition, chronic illness, hardship, deprivation, or abuse, are more susceptible to life stressors than others. Thus "they are at risk for failure to master, mature and adapt" (O'Grady and Metz, 1987). Rutter (1985b) defined protective factors as "those factors that modify, ameliorate or alter a person's response to some environmental hazard that predisposes to a maladaptive outcome." Protective factors seemingly function in a catalytic fashion. They do not necessarily foster normal development in the absence of risk factors, but they may make an appreciable difference on the influence exerted by risk factors. Protective factors also can reside with the individual or the family, community, or institutions and can be biological or psychosocial in nature.

Reviews of community surveys and longitudinal epidemiological studies have emphasized that each mental disorder is likely to have multiple risk factors (Hawkins, Catalano, and Miller, 1992; Werner and Smith, 1992; Offord, Boyle, and Racine, 1989; Rutter, 1989; Offord, Boyle, Szatmari, Rae Grant, Links, Cadman et al., 1987). Thus, in order to look for possible opportunities for intervention, it is necessary to identify as many risk and protective factors that impinge on individuals at different stages of development as possible. The process of critically examining risk factor research on mental disorders is part of the foundation for preventive interventions. Not all evidence from risk research is conclusive enough to warrant the design of a preventive intervention. Even where the evidence is strong, it is still worth seeking other potential markers and causal risk factors because targeting multiple risks may increase the success of a preventive intervention program.

This chapter examines the factors that current research indicates may potentially operate to predispose or protect against the occurrence of mental disorders. The examination proceeds first within a categorical framework organized around the five major mental disorders that are used as illustrations throughout this report—Alzheimer's disease, schizophrenia, alcohol abuse and dependence, depressive disorders, and conduct disorder. Because these are disorders in which the relative potential contribution of biological risk factors (including genetic vulnerability) and psychosocial risk factors (including individual, family, and community issues) varies greatly, as a group they provide an opportunity for a review of a wide range of diverse risk factors and the interplay among them. The discussion then moves away from a focus on specific disorders to a broad view of general risk and protective factors that are common to many disorders and dysfunctional states. The sequence of the disorders has been reversed in this chapter and emphasizes the range of risk factors along a continuum from heavily biological to heavily psychosocial.

ALZHEIMER'S DISEASE

Studies of epidemiology, biochemistry, pathology, and genetics have uncovered several biological risk factors related to Alzheimer's disease (AD), and there is limited evidence for the role of some psychosocial factors, particularly level of education. This section reviews knowledge about biological and psychosocial risk and protective factors for Alzheimer's disease and then discusses their implications for research and for prevention.

Biological Risk Factors

Genetic Vulnerability

Over the past decade, evidence that genetic factors play a major role in vulnerability to AD has accumulated. In a distinct minority of cases, AD begins early, in the fourth or fifth decade, rather than the more typical onset after age 70 or 75. This early onset, "presenile" form often clusters in families in a pattern consistent with inheritance of a single gene of major effect. (The pattern is most consistent with "autosomal dominant" inheritance, whereby 50 percent of the children of an affected parent are expected to inherit such a gene and develop the disease.) Breitner and colleagues have raised the question whether the absence of a familial pattern in the senile form of AD may be an artifact of "bias of ascertainment" (Breitner, Folstein, and Murphy, 1986a; Breitner, Murphy, and Folstein, 1986b). Because many first-degree relatives may have died of other causes before living through the period of risk, their loss leads to underestimates of the number who actually carry the gene. Using AD patients identified in nursing homes, Breitner and colleagues attempted to estimate the true prevalence among first-degree relatives (siblings and children) by taking a careful family history in a subpopulation marked by language disorders. If family history was ruled out only for cases in which both parents lived to at least age 85, they found that the risk for AD in first-degree relatives of AD patients approached 50 percent, consistent with autosomal dominant inheritance, even in cases of late onset (Breitner et al., 1986a; Breitner et al., 1986b). European case-control studies, however, showed that although family history was an important risk factor, it did not account for all cases (van Duijn, Clayton, Chandra, Fratiglioni, Graves, Heyman et al., 1991).

It is clear that there are several genetic forms of AD, but it is also clear that there are cases of "sporadic" AD that are not inherited. The relative prevalence of genetic and sporadic forms is subject to considerable debate among investigators. Investigators have turned to genetic studies, not only to identify the molecular events underlying AD, but also to ascertain the importance of environmental factors more precisely.

Twin Studies. Twin studies could theoretically be particularly useful in sorting among genetic and nongenetic contributions to the genesis of AD (Murphy and Breitner, 1992). One case report describes identical twins, only one of whom developed AD over a 20-year follow-up period (Renvoize, Mindham, Stewart, McDonald, and Wallace, 1986). This case of apparent twin discordance must be interpreted with some caution, however, as previous reports of discordance have proved to be premature. In one pair of identical twins initially reported as discordant, the second twin developed AD 13 to 15 years after her twin sister (Cook, Schneck, and Clark, 1981). AD in both twins could be a mere coincidence, or it could reflect factors that caused the age of onset to differ by more than a decade despite a genetic predisposition to AD. In surveys of twin studies, the age of onset may differ by as much as a decade between identical twins (Li, Silverman, and Mohs, 1991; Breitner, Murphy, Folstein, and Magruder-Habib, 1990; Nee, Eldridge, Sunderland, Thomas, Katz, Thompson et al., 1987). Because identical twins share their genes, if both do not develop AD, this is strong evidence of nongenetic factors.

At the very least, when the age of onset is different for a pair of identical twins, it indicates that environmental factors influence when symptoms begin, suggesting that prevention might work by delaying onset. In one twin study, for example, investigators found that symptoms of dementia began later among female than male twin pairs, an intriguing finding that merits further inquiry (Nee et al., 1987). The differing ages of onset between a pair of identical twins imply that even genetic factors underlying AD may be malleable to environmental interventions. Breitner notes that delaying onset of AD by only five years would reduce its clinical impact by half, because onset is typically delayed until late in life (Breitner, 1991). If the disease began five years later, many individuals would die before showing symptoms. Finding strategies to delay onset is thus a primary focus of epidemiological and other biomedical research.

Twin studies to date have been hampered by a bias, because the twins studied are likely to have volunteered. A more reliable population-based study that should not suffer from this flaw is under way, using a twin registry of U.S. veterans. This data set includes a heavy predominance of males, and clinical data are incomplete. This study cannot verify the preliminary finding that age of onset differs between the sexes, but its analysis should nonetheless illuminate the importance of many other nongenetic factors among identical and fraternal twins (Breitner, Welsh, Magruder-Habib, Churchill, Robinette, Folstein et al., 1990).

Studies of Down's Syndrome. Down's syndrome (DS), the most common genetically identified cause of mental retardation, has provided another line of evidence supporting genetic factors in the risk for AD (Coyle, Oster-Granite, and Gearhart, 1986). DS, or trisomy 21, results from having three copies, instead of the normal two, of all or part of chromosome 21, especially the distal end of its long arm. Thus DS does not result from "mutant genes" but rather from the altered gene expression from an abnormal gene copy number. Post mortem studies indicate that virtually all DS individuals develop the neuropathology of AD by the time they reach their fourth decade. The distribution and density of the pathological stigmata in DS brains are indistinguishable from AD. Furthermore, the DS brains with AD exhibit the same selective vulnerability of nerve cell populations. Nevertheless, some older DS individuals do not exhibit the cognitive deterioration expected on the basis of the microscopic findings in brain tissue, and thus do not fulfill the standard criteria for "dementia," which by definition entails cognitive decline.

Molecular Studies of Amyloid. Recent molecular biological studies have begun to shed light on the cellular processes leading to AD pathology by focusing upon amyloid (Mueller-Hill and Beyreuther, 1989). Amyloid in the senile plaque is an obvious target for analysis, because the density of senile plaques correlates both with cognitive impairment and with biochemical deficits in AD. Amyloid has been purified to homogeneity from the brains of individuals with AD or DS/AD, demonstrating that it is a peptide of approximately 42 amino acids. From the sequence of amino acids in amyloid, it is possible through molecular biological methods to clone the gene that contains the amyloid sequence. These studies demonstrate that amyloid is a breakdown by-product of a much larger protein (designated amyloid precursor protein, or APP) that is normally expressed on the surface of many cells in the body, but especially nerve cells in the brain's cerebral cortex. The gene encoding the APP protein is located on the long arm of chromosome 21 and can be processed inside cells into at least four proteins of varying length.

A critical question concerns the mechanisms that favor a breakdown pathway for APP that generates amyloid (Hardy and Higgins, 1992). In the case of DS, the three copies of the APP gene, due to its presence on chromosome 21, could result in a marked overexpression of APP in brain. As a consequence, amyloid might accumulate in the DS brain much more rapidly than normal. In AD, an aberrant enzyme that degrades or modifies APP and its metabolites could play a role. There are many possible explanations for how amyloid deposition relates to disease, and this will be a main target for AD research in coming years.

Preclinical studies suggest that aberrant addition of phosphate groups to the APP protein favors a metabolic route that generates amyloid instead of protein cleavage. One strategy for prevention focuses on delaying the degradation of APP. If amyloid accumulation is indeed a cause of cell death, then slowing its accumulation could delay this, and presumably also the onset of clinical dementia.

Genetic Mutations.   An obvious possible cause of abnormal disposition of APP is an alteration of the DNA constituting its gene—a mutation. Indeed, several families with autosomal dominant forms of presenile AD have been shown to have just such a mutation, localized to a specific position (codon 717) of the APP gene (Goate, Chartier-Harlin, Mullan, Brown, Crawford, Fidani et al., 1991). In other cases, a different mutation, at codon 670/671, has been found in the same gene, again associated with AD (Mullan, Crawford, Axelman, Houlden, Lilius, Winblad, and Lannfelt, 1992). Another mutation complex, affecting codons 713 and 715, was found in a 64-year-old woman with AD, but also in her 88-year-old mother and four siblings, all of whom were older than 62 and clinically unaffected (Carter, Desmarais, Bellis, Campion, Clerget-Darpoux, Brice et al., 1992). The significance of this double mutation is thus unclear, and it may represent a mere coincidence. Mutations in the APP account for only a very small percentage of early-onset familial AD cases, although they strongly suggest that the APP gene can be functionally related to AD in these few cases. This seems likely to prove but the first of many molecular aberrations that can lead to AD.

Genetic Heterogeneity.   There appear to be multiple genes that can cause AD in different families. The first report of linkage between AD and DNA markers appeared in 1987, implicating a region on chromosome 21, and was later confirmed by other groups (St. George-Hyslop, Haines, Farrer, Polinsky, Van Broeckhoven and Goate, 1990; St. George-Hyslop, Tanzi, Polinsky, Haines, Nee, Watkins et al., 1987). In addition to the very small fraction of familial cases associated with a mutation of the gene encoding the APP protein on chromosome 21 (Schellenberg, Anderson, O'dahl, Wisjman, Sadovnick, Ball et al., 1991), there is also evidence of a gene elsewhere on the same chromosome (Goate, Haynes, Owen, Farrall, James, Lai et al., 1989; St. George-Hyslop et al., 1987). Most of the evidence for another chromosome 21 gene, however, comes from a large Italian family that shows even stronger evidence of a gene on chromosome 14. A second chromosome 21 AD gene, in addition to the APP gene, is thus possible but by no means certain. A second gene on chromosome 21 may also modify the action of the APP gene or another gene, and hence show genetic linkage.

It was already clear in 1988 that the molecular defect among several different families with an inherited form of AD resided on sites other than chromosome 21 (Schellenberg, Bird, Wijsman, Moore, Boehnke, Bryant et al., 1988). Since that time, evidence has accumulated for another possible gene on chromosome 19 in a few families (Corder, Saunders, Strittmater, Schmechel, Gaskell, Small et al., 1993; Pericak-Vance, Bebout, Gaskell, Yamaoka, Hung, Alberts, and Walker, 1991), and a more common gene defect, perhaps accounting for most families with early onset, on chromosome 14 (Mullan, Houlden, Windelspecht, Fidani, Lombardi, Diaz et al., 1992; St. George-Hyslop, Haines, Rogaev, Mortilla, Vaula, Pericak-Vance et al., 1992; Van Broeckhoven, Backhovens, Cruts, DeWinter, Bruyland, Cras, and Martin, 1992). A few large families, called the Volga Germans for their common pattern of ethnic migration from Germany to Russia and thence to the United States early in this century, also have an inherited form of AD. In the Volga German families, the inheritance pattern is not consistent with any of the chromosomal locations associated with other families. This suggests one or more as yet undiscovered genes associated with AD or a mixture of genes on different chromosomes in the same family.

Continuing Investigation.   Viewed in aggregate, these studies indicate that AD is a common disorder with genetic heterogeneity, meaning that several genetic defects can cause a clinically and neuropathologically similar syndrome. AD can result from mutation in the APP gene, may possibly follow from overexpression of APP due to gene triplication (DS), and clearly can also be caused by mutations elsewhere in the human genome. AD may develop from one or more genes on chromosome 21 (the APP gene and perhaps one other), a gene on chromosome 14, perhaps another on chromosome 19, and one or more genes among the Volga German families. Because of the complexity of APP metabolism, there is reason to expect that mutations of genes encoding for enzymes that process amyloid protein could cause an accelerated rate of accumulation of amyloid, leading to AD. The clinical and pathological features of AD may also appear in response to entirely different biochemical defects not yet discovered. Those studying familial forms of AD hope to identify and isolate specific gene defects, which would lead to the protein those genes encode, and to possible clues about the causes of Alzheimer's disease.

The common conception that genetic disorders are resistant to intervention has proved untrue in many disorders. There are dietary treatments for phenylketonuria, and many genetic disorders require an environmental trigger. Twin studies, genetic linkage studies, and searches for specific genes not only provide logical paths for scientific investigation toward a causal explanation of AD, but also may provide clues for prevention, depending on what the genes do. Genetic studies to date have solidly established the role of genetic factors, but the implications for prevention are not yet clear.

History of Head Trauma

A history of head trauma has appeared as a risk factor for AD in several epidemiological studies (Henderson, Jorm, Korten, Creasey, McCusker, Broe et al., 1992; Mortimer, van Duijn, Chandra, Fratiglioni, Graves, Heyman et al., 1991; Graves, White, Koepsell, Reifler, van Belle, Larson, and Raskind, 1990; Amaducci, Fratiglioni, Rocca, Fieschi, Livrea, Pedone et al., 1986; French, Schuman, Mortimer, Hutton, Boatman, and Christians, 1985; Mortimer, French, Hutton, and Schuman, 1985; Heyman, Wilkinson, Stafford, Helms, Sigmon, and Weinberg, 1984). Recent studies show correlations with nonfamilial cases of AD, rather than familial cases (Henderson et al., 1992; Mortimer et al., 1991), suggesting it is an independent risk factor and may or may not contribute to dementia through an entirely different causal pathway from that of the genetic forms. These studies have rekindled interest in trauma as a cause of AD.

A clinical syndrome, *dementia pugilistica*, has long been described in the clinical literature (Mendez, 1993). Microscopic plaques and tangles are found at autopsy, but they are distributed more widely than in typical AD. Dementia pugilistica is most likely to occur among those who sustain repeated closed head injuries, especially boxers. Dementia typically begins several years after exposure to trauma. It is most common among those with a history of vascular disease, alcoholism, or low IQ (Mendez, 1993). Recent studies show a correlation between severe head injury and presence of plaques, which appear in one of three individuals subjected to repeated head trauma such as boxing (Clinton, Ambler, and Roberts, 1991; Roberts, Allsop, and Bruton, 1989).

Prevention of head trauma is itself a laudable goal. Head trauma can be reduced by use of seat belts and air bags in automobiles, wearing helmets while riding motorcycles or bicycles, and reducing exposure to events likely to result in trauma (e.g., boxing), and other measures. The immediate benefits include reduced risk of spinal cord injury and acute brain injury. Trauma, including head trauma, is a major cause of premature mortality, especially among young adults. Preventing AD several years hence may be but an additional, delayed, benefit from measures commendable in their own right. The association between repeated head trauma and dementia suggests that the sport of boxing carries a significant long-term risk.

Medical Risk Factors, Including Thyroid Disorders

Several other risk factors have been identified by one or more epidemiological studies. However, a recent study concluded that despite enormous efforts to gather clinical data on a large number of subjects, "we have been unable to identify any important candidate [medical] risk factors that may account for a substantial proportion of the cases of AD occurring in the community" (Kokmen, Beard, Chandra, Offord, Schoenberg, and Ballard, 1991). But there may be one exception. A recent review of several studies corroborated previous reports of an association with thyroid disorders (Breteler, van Duijn, Chandra, Fratiglioni, Graves, Heyman et al., 1991; Treves, 1991), although the effect was much smaller than that of family history or head trauma.

Maternal Age at Time of Birth

An even weaker association was found between AD and maternal age at time of birth, with AD prevalence increased among those born to either unusually young or unusually old mothers (Rocca, van Duijn, Chandra, Fratiglioni, Graves, Heyman et al., 1991). These preliminary results suggest future research directions.

Psychosocial Risk and Protective Factors

Educational Level

Several studies have shown a higher prevalence of dementia among those with less education, although findings are not entirely consistent from study to study. Projections of AD prevalence in the United States in 2050 yield estimates of 10.3 million cases of probable AD if the trend to increased education in the U.S. population is taken into account, but 15.4 million without this adjustment factor for education (Evans, Scherr, Cook, Albert, Funkenstein, Smith et al., 1990). Studies in Italy and China show more dementia among the less educated (Rocca, Bonaiuto, Lippi, Luciani, Turtu, Cavarzeran et al., 1990; Zhang, Katzman, Salmon, Jin, Cai, Wang et al., 1990; Amaducci et al., 1986), similar to previous North American and European studies. One recent community survey in Baltimore, Maryland, however, found the opposite effect, with higher AD prevalence among the more educated (Folstein, Bassett, Anthony,

Romanoski, and Nestadt, 1991). This effect was relatively weak and depended on a small number of cases in the higher-educated categories, and thus should be interpreted with some caution.

Katzman (1993) recently reviewed the literature on education and Alzheimer's disease, observing that several epidemiological criteria of causality have been met, but he still urges caution in interpreting results. He concluded that if education has the effect of increasing synaptic density in some brain regions, and if it is indeed loss of cells in these regions that predisposes to clinical dementia, then the epidemiological and biological data could be integrated into a plausible theory. The effect of education would not be to alter the underlying biological cause of cell loss, but rather to delay its clinically detectable effects, so that dementia does not ensue for an additional five or so years.

Smoking

Epidemiological case-control studies looking for associations between AD and smoking over the past decade have produced conflicting results. Graves and colleagues recently reported a meta-analysis of data from eight of these studies, which individually had reached different conclusions (Graves, van Duijn, Chandra, Fratiglioni, Heyman, Jorm et al., 1991). The reanalysis of pooled data disclosed a statistically significant inverse correlation between smoking and AD prevalence—that is, those who smoked more were less likely to have AD. The analysis included one study that had found a positive correlation (higher prevalence of AD among smokers), but the population in this study was unusual and even when cases from this study were included, the meta-analysis reached the same conclusion of an inverse correlation.

An association between reduced AD prevalence and smoking is an intriguing lead. It has some biological plausibility because nicotine, an active agent in tobacco products, binds to the acetylcholine receptors, whose loss is associated with AD. It is thus not unreasonable to postulate that smoking might delay onset of symptoms. Against this, however, the studies did not show a later onset in smoking than nonsmoking cases of AD, although one of the component studies from the Netherlands did find that when two or more family members developed AD, one of whom smoked and the others not, the onset was later for the smokers. This was based on a very small number of cases and is thus only a tantalizing but uncorroborated finding. The authors of the meta-analysis urge caution in interpreting the findings, as there are many possible confounding factors that could be controlled only by prospective longitudinal population-based studies, rather than case-control studies. Pursuing an AD-tobacco association is clearly a high priority in AD risk research.

Environmental Triggers

Alzheimer's disease exemplifies how basic biomedical research can address a complex disorder of unknown cause. For the most part, investigators have based molecular inquiry on clues derived from what is known about the pathology of AD, for example, the composition of plaques and tangles, or what is known about clinically similar disorders such as Parkinson's disease or Creutzfeldt-Jakob disease (CJD). CJD is a very rare dementia caused by an atypical transmissible agent (sometimes called a slow virus). Limited evidence suggests that some cases of AD may also be related to a transmissible agent (Manuelidis and Manuelidis, 1991). Following a different line of research, several reports of association with aluminum toxicity drew attention in the 1970s and 1980s, but a more recent study with a highly sensitive method suggests that findings in previous reports may have been laboratory artifacts (Landsberg, McDonald, and Watt, 1992). The high aluminum concentrations may have been due to the affinity of plaques and tangles for aluminum introduced during laboratory analysis, after the tissue was removed from the body, rather than the aluminum causing cell death.

If viruses or environmental toxins prove to be important in the causation of AD, then prevention measures would obviously follow. The evidence for these hypothetical environmental triggers, however, is not currently strong enough to warrant aggressive preventive measures.

Future Directions in Identification of Risk and Protective Factors

In a recent minireview, Drachman and Lippa (1991) listed 17 different causal hypotheses for AD, and each has been pursued by one or more research groups. Biomedical research on AD has flourished over the past decade. The federal research budget has risen from $3.9 million in 1976 (OTA, 1987) to an estimated $297 million in 1993 (DHHS, 1993). This profusion of funding has led to a dramatic rise in annual publications. A literature search for 1980 found 113 AD publications, whereas a similar search covering a 42-month period from 1989 to 1992, done as background for this report, found 4,189—almost 100 per month, and a more than tenfold increase in publication rate during the 1980s. Future research will entail a complex interplay among further biomedical research studies pursuing specific causal hypotheses, more refined epidemiological investigations to tease apart risk factors, and health services research aimed at improving services for those who develop AD.

Heterogeneity of cause is one highly plausible explanation for the inconsistency among epidemiological studies and the weak predictive power among those risk factors analyzed to date. Future studies may more successfully dissect out risk factors by segregating disease subtypes, perhaps through identifying genetic subgroups (those showing linkage to different chromosome regions, for example), or by separately analyzing cases arising from currently known risk factors such as head trauma or level of education.

Drugs to reverse the cognitive impairments of AD have been pursued vigorously for the past decade. One main line of attack has focused on drugs to sustain the action of the neurotransmitter acetylcholine. Farlow and colleagues recently conducted the largest clinical trial of the drug tacrine to date and reported that it measurably improved cognitive function in just over half the subjects, roughly equivalent to a six-month delay in the course of the disease (Farlow, Gracon, Hershey, Lewis, Sadowsky, and Dolan-Ureno, 1992). An editorial accompanying Farlow's publication suggested that the drug might prove clinically useful for a subset of patients who do not develop liver toxicity and are carefully monitored (Small, 1992). Drugs to address the loss of neuronal systems, using peptide transmitters, growth factors, and other possible approaches, remain of intense interest, but most are early in development and are being tested in exploratory clinical trials.

Hopes for prevention are pinned to understanding the biology of nerve cell death. Why do certain cells die? The discovery of hormones and growth factors that stimulate cell growth suggests that their absence may lead to cell death. Examples of genetically programmed cell death in nematode worms and other organisms also offer clues to possible reasons for the death of nerve cells. For the most part, these hypotheses have suggested lines for further research that may eventually suggest prevention strategies, but none is sufficiently advanced to merit even a prevention trial.

Advances in understanding how amyloid is deposited offer several strategies for intervening in the process (Katzman and Saitoh, 1991). Attention has turned recently to the development of drugs that could slow the formation of amyloid from APP or enhance the clearance of amyloid. Prophylactic administration of such drugs might be effective in slowing progression for patients in the early stages of AD or in preventing the onset of AD in individuals genetically at risk. Such pharmacological prevention is analogous to the use of cholesterol-lowering drugs in atherosclerosis, and the development of such drugs will be aided greatly by molecular biological studies to identify gene mutations that lead to AD vulnerability. Thus identification of these genes will permit gene-based diagnosis of AD vulnerability as well as lead to an understanding of the role of the mutant gene products in causing AD. Together, these current lines of investigation hold promise for the development of specific, pharmacological preventive interventions for those at genetic risk for AD.

Family Burden

The widely documented stress experienced by relatives caring for elderly, demented persons exacts a heavy toll. Several studies have sought to measure this impact on families, including the adverse effects on the caregiver's physical and mental health (George and Gwyther, 1986; Pratt, Schmall, and Wright, 1985). One of the determinants of distress in caregivers is depletion of their social support network, leaving them feeling abandoned, isolated, and without assistance and recognition. The Office of Technology Assessment noted a surprising lack of correlation between a patient's characteristics and behaviors and the caregiver's subjective experience of burden, although it is clear that coping skills and education can reduce that subjective experience (OTA, 1990). Caregivers differ markedly, as do the patients and the availability of support services. It is simplistic to assume that caregivers will respond consistently to any given intervention, but it is reasonable to assume that the availability of information and support services will reduce the stress and stress-related health effects among caregivers. Preventive intervention strategies for these high-risk family members—no matter what the nature of the prevailing mental disorder—therefore might include methods already in use, but inadequately evaluated, such as self-help support groups and psychoeducational programs (Falloon, Boyd, McGill, Razani, Moss, Gilderman, and Simpson, 1985; Bernheim, Lewine, and Beale, 1982; Vine, 1982). In addition to formal services, caregivers appear to benefit from group support, information, and the availability of someone they trust to answer questions when they need help (K. Maslow, personal communication, 1992; OTA, 1990). An improved care system may prevent the new incidence of stress-related disorders among caregivers. Better management of patients—particularly with regard to the troublesome behavioral symptoms of agitation, wandering, insomnia, and emotional outbursts—might also have positive effects for caregivers, although clinical literature to support this common-sense conclusion is surprisingly scant despite the intense assessment of family burden in recent years. This is a critical gap in research.

The study of care-related disability among caregivers continues to be an important area for research. The first wave of studies over the past decade has served mainly to describe differences among patients, caregivers, and the service system. This information is now laying the base for a second wave of more refined caregiver burden studies with more precise outcome measures, interventions, and service availability measures.

Findings and Leads

At this time, there is no research base sufficient to mount a preventive intervention campaign with potential AD victims. Research must continue to be focused on identification of risk factors, through research on genetics, continued basic research, and further epidemiological studies. It must also begin to identify the relative and attributable risks associated with each of these factors. The best hope for prevention in the near future lies in the research focused on delaying the onset of AD, either through education early in life or through the prophylactic use of drugs to improve cognitive function or to impede amyloid deposition in high-risk individuals. Although effective prevention often does not require a complete causal theory, it does require more robust risk and protective factor studies than exist for AD. The literature to date has netted three malleable factors—education, smoking, and head trauma— that are plausibly associated with AD. In all three cases, the reasons to change behavior are even stronger for other purposes than prevention of dementia. Reducing head trauma and promoting education are laudable social goals that may reduce future AD prevalence. Promoting smoking as a protective factor for AD is absurd given tobacco's serious health risks for cancer and heart disease. A more targeted prevention strategy depends either on discoveries that come from basic research or stronger epidemiological evidence of malleable risk factors than has been discovered to date. On the other hand, research trials on interventions to prevent stress-induced effects among caregivers of AD patients are warranted. Such studies will require rigorous methodology, including valid outcome measures.

SCHIZOPHRENIA

Schizophrenia is a heterogeneous disorder with different disease entities, subtypes, and pathological processes. Therefore the risk and protective factors associated with onset may be different for the various syndromes included within the disorder. Risk factors may bear different relationships to the three main domains of the psychopathology— psychosis as defined by hallucinations and delusions, dissociative thought processes, and primary negative symptoms such as emotional flatness. They may also have different patterns of heritability. On the other hand, they may be seriously confounded.

Biological Risk Factors

Genetic Vulnerability

Family Studies. The most prominent biological risk factor is heredity, although some legitimate controversy exists. Although there is wide-spread acceptance that genetic factors contribute to schizophrenia, two studies have questioned whether narrowly diagnosed schizophrenia is a familial disorder (Abrams and Taylor, 1983; Pope, Jones, Cohen, and Lipinski, 1982), claiming that earlier studies suffered from a lack of controls, bias in diagnoses, and inconsistent diagnostic criteria. In the 1980s, five careful studies reported a greater than fivefold increased risk in first-degree relatives (Kendler, Masterson, and Davis, 1985). Bolstered by more recent studies, this suggests genetic and/or shared environmental factors in families that increase the risk of schizophrenia (see Box 6.1). On the other hand, absence of a positive family history does not ensure freedom from risk. Positive family history shifts probabilities, but it is still not sufficiently clarifying except among identical twins, who actually share the same genetic material.

Twin Studies. An estimate of genetic influence can be established by using twin studies. The genetic contribution can be estimated by comparing concordance rates between monozygotic (identical) and dizygotic (fraternal) twin pairs. Kendler (1988) summarized 11 studies and derived a monozygotic mean concordance rate of 64 percent and a dizygotic mean concordance rate of 16 percent. This suggests a major role for genetic factors, although the estimate may seem high in light of the other, nontwin data. The fact that 36 percent of identical twins were discordant also clearly demonstrates the importance of nongenetic factors. Methodological issues include the assumption that monozygotic and dizygotic twins have an identical trait-relevant environment and the possibility of selection bias in the recruitment of monozygotic twins. Such criticisms are not supported by adoption studies. Twin studies have been updated (Gottesman, 1993), and there is now evidence that the risk to offspring of discordant monozygotic twins is remarkably similar. That is, the children of an unaffected identical twin have almost

BOX 6.1
Children of Parents with Schizophrenia:
Family History as a Risk Factor

The proportion of individuals with schizophrenia who marry is less than in the general population (25 to 47 percent for males and 39 to 82 percent for females), but the rate of reproduction among them has been increasing (from 58 percent of the general population rate in the 1930s to 70 percent in the 1960s), perhaps due to improvement in treatment (Erlenmeyer-Kimling et al., 1980) and to the remarkable diminution in the pattern of prolonged segregation by gender encountered during the era of long-term custodial care in public facilities.

The children of parents with schizophrenia are a high-risk group. First of all, they have an increased genetic vulnerability for schizophrenia. Second, their other parent is likely to have a mental disorder. The prevalence of assortative mating (i.e., the tendency of people to select as mates people with the same or similar characteristics) in schizophrenia has yet to be determined rigorously, but the best available data suggest it may be high. Rosenthal (1974) found that 58 percent of spouses of schizophrenic subjects themselves had a schizophrenic spectrum disorder. Fowler and Tsuang (1975), in a blind comparative study, found that 39 percent of spouses were psychiatrically disturbed, with alcoholism and personality disorders accounting for 70 percent of the problems. These additional disorders could have an additive effect on the genetic and/or psychosocial risk for the child. Third, capabilities of the schizophrenic parent to care adequately for the child may be adversely affected by the disorder, especially if the disorder is chronic and severe (Grunbaum and Gammeltoft, 1993).

Cohorts of children with at least one schizophrenic parent have been studied with a view toward understanding the premorbid state of this disorder and isolating factors that may either contribute to the onset of schizophrenia or serve as markers of children at high risk to express schizophrenia. Mednick and Silverton (1988) reviewed 22 studies in the literature and pointed out that the major logistical problem is the long time period between beginning to study the children and having them complete the risk period for developing the disorder.

Szatmari and Nagy (1990) reviewed the literature on children with schizophrenic parents and concluded that between 20 and 40 percent develop a mental disorder during their childhood, a rate that is very similar to that in children of parents with other mental disorders (Rutter and Quinton, 1984). Rarely, however, do these children develop childhood schizophrenia. Their adult outcome may be more influenced by genetic factors related to schizophrenia. Children who have two schizophrenic parents are at especially high risk (46 percent lifetime) for developing schizophrenia (Gottesman, 1991), but they are also at considerable risk for developing other mental disorders.

the same risk as the children of the affected twin. The risk in the offspring of schizophrenic identical twins is 16.8 percent; it is 17.4 percent in the unaffected twins' offspring (Gottesman and Bertelsen, 1989). This evidence that inheritance can "pass through" apparently asymptomatic, unaffected individuals suggests a strong genetic component but again clearly indicates that nongenetic factors are also involved.

Adoption Studies. Two strategies have been used to estimate genetic effects in adoptive families. One approach is to evaluate offspring of schizophrenic parents who have been adopted away from their biological parents into another environment and measure the rates at which such children develop schizophrenia. The second approach is to study the rearing, adoptive families of adopted children who have developed schizophrenia as adults. Heston (1966) studied adopted-away offspring of schizophrenic mothers and found a significant rate of schizophrenia in these children (10.4 percent prevalence, which became 16.6 when necessary age corrections were made), compared with children from unaffected mothers (no children with schizophrenia). A study by Rosenthal (1974) showed a similar result (13.9 percent from biologically affected families and 3.4 percent of controls), but the data did not achieve statistical significance. In a much larger Finnish study (Tienari, 1991a,b,c), 10.3 percent of schizophrenic women's children also became schizophrenic, even when raised by adoptive families, confirming Heston's results. Kety and co-workers, on the other hand, began their study with adoptees who grew up to be schizophrenic (Kety, Rosenthal, Wender, Schulsinger, and Jacobsen, 1978). The adoptees' adoptive and biological families were located and evaluated. Both schizophrenia and the schizophrenic spectrum disorders were significantly higher in the biological relatives than in the adoptive families. These results have been subject to extensive reanalysis, including careful diagnostic reevaluations (Kendler and Gruenberg, 1984). Taken as a body of work, these studies collectively indicate that the offspring of schizophrenic individuals have a greatly increased risk of developing schizophrenia and that schizophrenics do not transmit this vulnerability to their nonbiological families. This evidence points to a strong role for genetics as a risk factor. The genetic data also make clear that nongenetic factors, such as environmental influences and acquired brain damage, must have a role in accounting for the incidence of the disease (Gottesman and Bertelsen, 1989).

Linkage Studies. Linkage studies in schizophrenia using conventional markers and assuming a single major locus have been inconclusive.

With the development of polymorphic DNA markers, careful studies of specific candidate genes such as the D2 receptor (Moises, Gelerneter, Giuffra, Zarcone, Wetterberg, Civelli et al., 1991) and various regions of chromosomes 2, 5, 11, 12, and 22 have been examined. No reproducible linkage or association has been found (Waddington, Weller, Crow, and Hirsch, 1992). There are several possible reasons for the lack of progress in spite of the rapid increase in the power of molecular genetics. The limits of the mathematical models used to calculate the probability of linkage between a gene and the disorder mean that only one or two gene models are usually considered, and recent evidence suggests that this disorder is polygenic, involving several genes (Carter and Chung, 1980). If this is true, then linkage studies, at least of the type that have been undertaken so far, are of limited value. In addition, heterogeneity in the diagnosis of schizophrenia is probable, and this makes linkage studies considerably more difficult. The report of a linkage in Icelandic and British families by Sherrington and colleagues (Sherrington, Brynjolfsson, Petursson, Potter, Dudleston, Barraclough et al., 1988) had been thought to represent a case of heterogeneity because this linkage has not been reproduced in other studies (St. Clair, Blackwood, Muir, Bailie, Hubbard, Wright, and Evans, 1989; Kennedy, Giuffra, Moises, Cavalli-Sforza, Pakstis, Kidd et al., 1988; Detera-Wadleigh, Berrettini, Goldin, Boorman, Anderson, and Gershon, 1987). However, the Sherrington linkage has not held up with the addition of more informative markers.

Pregnancy and Birth Complications, Winter Births, and Viral Exposure

A recent study by Bracha and colleagues provides new evidence that second prenatal trimester insult may be associated with the expression of schizophrenia (Bracha, Torrey, Gottesman, Bigelow, and Cunniff, 1992). These researchers found that monozygotic twins discordant for schizophrenia had more differences in their fingerprints than normal twins. This finding suggests that disturbances occurred in the development of one of the fetuses that may be related to the fact that only one twin expressed his or her genetic predisposition toward schizophrenia.

In a variety of studies carried out with adult schizophrenics in the United States and Europe, an excess of obstetrical complications in the mothers of subjects who later became schizophrenic compared with control groups has been documented (McNeil, 1987). These complications appear to be related to infant anoxia during birth. Birth complications also appear to be associated with larger cerebral ventricles and may be negatively associated with a strong genetic history of schizophrenia in the family (Canon, Mednick, and Parnas, 1989). Thus individuals whose schizophrenia arises from brain trauma during birth may not have a genetic form of the illness. Such individuals are "phenocopies," because they have an illness that resembles one caused by genetic factors, but which arises from a nongenetic cause or in interaction with a subset of such factors. However, caution must be exercised in using birth complications as a risk factor to target in preventive interventions. A positive history for birth complications does not indicate whether an individual has suffered an insult to central nervous system development that is associated with the onset of schizophrenia, and a negative history for gestational and birth complications gives no assurance of this absence. It is also possible that genes associated with schizophrenia could cause gestational or birth complications. Finally, a recent, high-quality study by Done and colleagues had inconclusive results regarding birth trauma as a risk factor for the onset of schizophrenia (Done, Johnstone, Frith, Golding, Shepard, and Crow, 1991).

It has been suggested that there is an excess of winter births among schizophrenic patients (Dalen, 1988), but overall results of season-of-birth studies are highly inconsistent (Lewis, 1989). It has also been suggested that winter births of schizophrenics are related to maternal exposure to influenza. Barr, Mednick, and Munk-Jorgenson (1990) studied births in Finnish mothers exposed to the influenza epidemic in 1957 and found an increase in schizophrenic offspring among this cohort of births. However, population data from Scotland, England, and Wales failed to replicate this finding (O'Callaghan, Sham, Takei, Glover, and Murray, 1991; Kendell and Kemp, 1989). Furthermore, winter birth does not fit the viral hypothesis, which holds that maternal viral infection in the second trimester of pregnancy is related to higher rates of schizophrenia. If this were true, and if flu is more common in the winter months of January, February, and March, then children born in the spring should have higher rates of schizophrenia. To the degree that maternal or gestational viral infection might result in damage to the fetus's brain, these viruses could contribute to the development of schizophrenia, but there is no conclusive evidence for this, and at this time viral exposure cannot be considered a documented risk factor. Winter birth may be a risk factor, but season of birth does not provide evidence that any given individual will develop schizophrenia. Most winter-born schizophrenics presumably get schizophrenia for the same reason as nonwinter-born, and at this point it is impossible to determine which of the small minority have some other special risk associated with winter birth.

Biological Markers

The major biological markers under consideration to identify high-risk populations of children include (1) smooth pursuit eye tracking deficits (Holzman, Solomon, Levin, and Waternaux, 1984); (2) attentional deficits (Garmezy, 1978); (3) neurointegrative defects (Erlenmeyer-Kimling, Cornblatt, Freidman, Rutschmann, Simmons, and Devi, 1982); (4) electrodermal hyperresponsivity (Mednick and Schulsinger, 1968); and (5) increased cerebral ventricular size (DeLisi, Goldin, Hanovit, Maxwell, Kurtz, and Gershon, 1986). Like all risk factors, these markers do not necessarily mean that the disorder is or will be expressed. Although they may be apparent in high-risk children and some have been shown to be present in a high proportion of children who go on to develop schizophrenia (Erlenmeyer-Kimling, Rock, Squires-Wheeler, Roberts, and Yang, 1991; Erlenmeyer-Kimling et al., 1982), their presence does not necessarily predict the development of the disorder. Moreover, none of the markers have clearly established themselves as linked with a genetic vulnerability for schizophrenia, although a few remain viable candidates. (See the review by Hafner and Gattez, 1991.)

Smooth Pursuit Eye Tracking Deficits. One of the most investigated markers for schizophrenia is deviant smooth pursuit eye movements (Grove, Clementz, Iacono, and Katsanis, 1992; Clementz and Sweeney, 1990; Iacono, Bassett, and Jones, 1988; Holzman et al., 1984). When given the task of visually tracking a moving target, most individuals exhibit smooth, coordinated eye movements. Schizophrenics, however, show choppy disruptions in the tracking pattern. Although the nature of the link to schizophrenia is not clear, it has been a consistently replicated finding, and one that has attracted considerable attention. The marker is found in schizophrenics as well as their affected and unaffected family members (Iacono, 1985). This has led to speculation as to whether the marker reflects a genetic vulnerability to schizophrenia. The results, initially described by Holzman and colleagues (Holzman, 1983; Holzman, Proctor, and Hughes, 1973), have been widely replicated and suggest that between 50 and 85 percent of schizophrenic subjects, as well as 40 to 50 percent of their first-degree relatives, may have disrupted smooth pursuit movements, in contrast to a general population prevalence of 5 percent. Unfortunately, deficits in smooth pursuit eye tracking are induced by lithium administration (Levy, Dorus, Shaughnessy, Yasillo, Pandey, Janicak et al., 1985). Thus the weight of evidence suggests the marker is not specific for schizophrenia, but smooth pursuit eye tracking is clearly strongly associated with increased risk and may be a latent trait marker.

Attentional Deficits. Attentional deficits have also been suggested as possible markers with a linkage to schizophrenia. These deficits can also occur in other mental disorders, but the disturbance may be more pervasive in schizophrenics. In one study using a combined measure of attention and information processing, Cornblatt and Erlenmeyer-Kimling found that 27 percent of children of schizophrenics had impaired attention and information processing, compared with 11 percent of children from affectively ill parents (Erlenmeyer-Kimling and Cornblatt, 1992; Cornblatt and Erlenmeyer-Kimling, 1985). There are few data thus far on the specificity of the marker for subsequent development of schizophrenia.

Performance on a specific measure of focused and sustained attention, the continuous performance test (CPT), has received considerable attention as a possible marker for schizophrenia. Asarnow and colleagues showed that children of schizophrenic subjects performed significantly worse on this test than children of control subjects (Asarnow, Steffy, MacCrimmon, and Cleghorn, 1977). This finding has been replicated and extended to cohorts of schizophrenic patients. Nuechterlein and colleagues reviewed this work and suggested that because the abnormalities can be seen in actively psychotic patients, patients in relative remission, and children of schizophrenics, the CPT may represent a stable vulnerability marker (Nuechterlein, Dawson, Venture, Fogelson, Gitlin, and Mintz, 1990). Thus the CPT defect may reflect a trait marker with genetic potential, but a genetic analysis of this behavior has not been carried out.

Neurointegrative Defects. In infancy and early childhood, neurointegrative defects, including sensorimotor problems, visual motor defects, and soft neurological signs, may be a risk factor for the onset of schizophrenia (Marcus, Hans, Mirsky, and Aubrey, 1987; Mednick, Parnas, and Schulsinger, 1987; Erlenmeyer-Kimling et al., 1982; Marcus, Auerbach, Wilkinson, and Burack, 1981). In a review of nine prospective studies of infants at risk for schizophrenia, Fish and colleagues concluded that there is evidence that a schizophrenic genotype may be manifested in infants by a neurointegrative defect called pandysmaturation (Fish, Marcus, Hans, Auerbach, and Perdue, 1992). (Occurring during the first two years of life, pandysmaturation is the earliest manifestation of an enduring neurointegrative defect.) Again, there is little specificity in these clinical signs. For example, one small adult follow-up study of children with soft neurological signs found an excess of affective disorder, but not schizophrenia (Schaffer, Stokman, O'Connor, Shaffer, Barmack, Hess et al., 1986). Children with neurointegrative signs appear to be at higher risk for developing schizophrenia only if they have other risk factors for schizophrenia. Marcus and colleagues followed prospectively the offspring of schizophrenic parents and found that the group at highest risk had a schizophrenic parent, showed early neurointegrative deficits, and experienced troubled parenting (Marcus et al., 1987). Those children with schizophrenic parents and neurointegrative deficits who had positive parental experiences did not develop schizophrenia. This finding is of special importance to prevention research; it suggests placing greater attention on the parenting situation of high-risk children.

Electrodermal Hyperresponsivity. Electrodermal hyperresponsivity was proposed as a marker for schizophrenia in the Copenhagen high-risk project (Mednick et al., 1987) and was the variable used to choose a population of high-risk children for the Mauritius prevention project (Mednick, Venables, Schulsinger, Dalais, and Van Dusen, 1984). Electrodermal hyperresponsivity was first suggested by Mednick and Schulsinger (1968); subsequently, they suggested it was useful only for males. Subsequent studies suggested there is little evidence of a reproducible association between electrodermal hyperresponsivity and schizophrenia (Erlenmeyer-Kimling, Freidman, Cornblatt, and Jacobsen, 1985; Kugelmass, Marcus, and Schmueli, 1985).

Increased Cerebral Ventricular Size. Cerebral ventricular size has been shown to be enlarged in about 30 percent of schizophrenics. Evidence suggests that increased ventricular size is present early in the illness, and the enlargement is stable over time. The specificity of this variable is not clear, however. For example, patients with bipolar mood disorders also have increased ventricular size (Swayze, Andreasen, Alliger, Ehrhardt, and Yuh, 1990). Ventricular size, like many other attributes of bodily structures, is highly heritable. Twin studies have shown a slight increase in ventricular size for the schizophrenic monozygotic twin in twins selected to be discordant for schizophrenia (Revely, Revely, and Murray, 1984).

Psychosocial Risk Factors

Low Socioeconomic Status

Social status has been assessed in at least 25 epidemiological studies, most of which show heightened prevalence of risk for schizophrenia in the lower class (Eaton, 1974). This association could be the result of adversities and stresses connected to living in a lower social class, or it could result from downward mobility due to the disease's disability. There is evidence to support the idea that schizophrenia is linked to lower or lessened upward mobility (Turner and Wagenfield, 1967; Goldberg and Morrison, 1963). A study by Dohrenwend and co-workers supports a downward social drift hypothesis, which posits that schizophrenic individuals end up in lower social classes because of their disease-related impairments, rather than developing schizophrenia because of the stress of living in a low social class (Dohrenwend, Levav, Schrout, Schwartz, Naveh, Link et al., 1992). Thus poverty or low social class may be a consequence, rather than a cause, of this disease. There is, however, some highly speculative evidence that one consequence of extreme poverty— acute starvation during the first trimester of pregnancy—may play a role in the onset of schizophrenia, as demonstrated by Susser and Lin (1992) in a study of Dutch births following the famine of the winter of 1944–1945. However, serious but less severe starvation was not associated in one cohort, nor was starvation in the second and third trimester.

Disturbed Family Environment and Family Communicative Problems

An ongoing adoption study in Finland by Tienari (1992, 1991a,b), has given us the first evidence that family problems and communication disturbances within families may play a role in the onset of schizophrenia. This study demonstrates the overexpression of schizophrenia among a cohort of adoptees having biological mothers with the diagnosis of schizophrenia, confirming the role of genetic factors. The study also looks retrospectively at family environment and finds that 9 of the 13 adoptees (of a total of 138 adoptees with schizophrenic biological mothers) who expressed functional psychosis, which includes schizophreniform and delusional disorders, grew up in "severely disturbed" households. When the factors that can be reliably rated from contemporary discourse were examined, it was found that disrupted communication was the major risk factor predicting the onset of psychopathology. The authors have suggested that this supports a notion that genetic factors confer a vulnerability that requires an environmental trigger for the development of the disorder. Aside from a need for replication, the question of the role of a sick child in disrupting communication has not been fully addressed, and it appears that a higher proportion of families with children from schizophrenic mothers had "severe disturbances" than control families.

Serious Behavioral and Emotional Problems in Childhood

One precursor pattern in children who may develop schizophrenia is poor impulse control and aggression. These children have temper tantrums, are destructive, and receive frequent disciplinary action. This pattern is superimposed on the neurointegrative dysfunctions and attention deficits seen earlier in development. This pattern of behavior in children who would become schizophrenic was reported initially by Bender (1937) and has been confirmed by Emery, Weintraub, and Neale (1982) and Mednick and Schulsinger (1968).

Another precursor pattern is social withdrawal or awkwardness in interpersonal relations, diminished emotional expressiveness, and lack of feeling during childhood and adolescence. These problems define a population at high risk for the initial onset of schizophrenia during young adulthood (W. Carpenter, personal communication, 1993; Erlenmeyer-Kimling and Cornblatt, 1987; Garmezy, 1974; Mednick and Schulsinger, 1968).

Although there is some consistency in these two precursor behaviors exhibited by high-risk children who ultimately develop schizophrenia, there is little specificity. For example, the aggressive symptom pattern is also seen in a variety of other childhood disorders, such as attention deficit hyperactivity disorder, mood disorders, and conduct disorder. However, children who are aggressive *and* have a family history of schizophrenia have an increased likelihood of developing schizophrenia (Mednick and Silverton, 1988), so it may be the combination of risk factors that is most important.

Social Dysfunction

The contribution of social dysfunction, or social incompetence, as a risk factor in the onset of schizophrenia is not well understood. Whereas childhood behavior problems may be an expression of the disorder itself at an early developmental stage, social incompetence may relate to inherited genetic personality patterns, such as schizoid personality. In contrast, the role of social incompetence in the course and outcome of schizophrenia has been well established. For more than three decades, investigators have repeatedly replicated the strong predictive relationship of premorbid level of social incompetence or social maladjustment in areas such as occupation, education, peer friendships, and heterosexual intimacy to course and outcome (Strauss and Carpenter, 1974; Zigler and Phillips, 1961; Garmezy and Rodnick, 1959). The predictive correlations have been significant for a variety of measures of outcome, including symptomatic relapse, rehospitalization, and global ratings of improvement (Kokes, Strauss, and Klormann, 1977; Hersen and Bellack, 1976; Gittelman-Klein and Klein, 1969).

Substance Abuse

Because many substances, such as stimulants and PCP, can induce psychotic states that closely mimic schizophrenia, it has been postulated that recurrent drug abuse may lead to an increased risk of developing schizophrenia in vulnerable individuals. Bowers (1987) demonstrated that the increase in the proportion of schizophrenic patients admitted to Connecticut state hospitals paralleled an earlier increase in the level of drug abuse in Connecticut. To determine whether drug abuse could cause the expression of more schizophrenia, Bowers examined the family history of substance abusers with chronic psychosis. The greater the drug abuse, the less family history of schizophrenia was present (Bowers and Swigar, 1983), suggesting that high levels of drug abuse might lead to chronic illness without high levels of genetic vulnerability. In a study of first-episode schizophrenic patients, DeLisi et al. (1986) reported threefold higher levels of drug abuse in patients (35 percent) than in matched population controls (12 percent). Other researchers have also looked at the role of cannabis, hallucinogenics, and alcohol in the etiology of schizophrenia (Tien and Anthony, 1990; Andreasson, Allebeck, Engstrom, and Rydberg, 1987; Breakey, Goodell, Lorenz, and McHugh, 1974). This evidence suggests that schizophrenia-like illnesses may be precipitated by heavy drug abuse. It is possible that these individuals had precursor symptoms of schizophrenia and were self-medicating with these drugs, which then led to an exacerbation of the symptoms and acute onset of schizophrenia. The existence of uncontrolled variables, including type and duration of drug abuse, make this a hypothesis in need of rigorous testing.

Caregiver Burden

Schizophrenia in a family member can become a risk factor for stress-related disorders in other family members. Many factors affect caregiver burden, including financial difficulties, self-blame, degree of severity of the disease, social isolation, the caregiver's own health, the caregiver's coping skills, and the stigma attached to mental illness (Geiser, Hoche, and King, 1988; Fadden, Bebbington, and Kuipers, 1987).

The degree to which caregiver burden is linked with the development of stress-related problems such as depression, irregular sleeping and eating patterns, aggravated health problems, increased use of alcohol or tranquilizers, marital strain, and irritability is not well known. Several studies have found variability in caregivers' ability to cope (Oldridge and Hughes, 1992; Scottish Schizophrenia Research Group, 1985; Gibbons, Horn, Powell, and Gibbons, 1984). Oldridge and Hughes (1992) found that the levels of psychological distress of family members who care for a person with schizophrenia are about twice the level expected in the general population. Further risk studies are needed to determine which family members are most likely to experience these ill effects and what aspects of caregiver burden are the most frequent and the most malleable.

Findings and Leads

Although genetic vulnerability may predispose to schizophrenia, and may even be necessary in order for the disorder to appear, genetic factors by themselves cannot account for the illness. Many of the data are consistent with a developmental disorder that is set in place via genetic and biological factors early in life. This developmental pattern may be susceptible to psychosocial stress, which may trigger the symptomatic expression of the disorder or which may cross a threshold for disease expression.

For the last decade, research on the causes of schizophrenia has been focused on biological rather than psychosocial risk factors (Yank, Bentley and Hargrove, 1993; Gottesman, 1991). Results regarding the importance of most of these risk factors—both biological and psychosocial—remain equivocal. Only genetic factors have been demonstrated and quantified in repeated and varied experimental designs, but researchers are as yet unable to specify a mode of inheritance, a chromosomal localization of schizophrenia genes, or what function such genes might carry out. Hints with regard to factors that might affect onset, such as prenatal viral infection or food deprivation, are weak and nonspecific. The evidence for familial communicative disorders, neurointegrative defects in infancy, and prenatal developmental disturbance during the second trimester of gestation is preliminary and needs replication, as does the suggestion that substance abuse could play a role in the onset of schizophrenia. More work remains in identifying relative and attributable risk for all these factors.

Universal and selective interventions to prevent the onset of schizophrenia are not warranted at this time. Much more risk factor research is needed, and this must necessarily be limited to narrow populations based on positive ascertainment of risk factors. The best hope for identifying a group of individuals at high risk for the onset of schizophrenia is through the identification of a combination of risk factors whose relative and attributable risks are known.

To date, very few, if any, studies have attempted to examine carefully both environment and genetics. It is essential to know how genetic and environmental factors interact. This can best be done through interdisciplinary collaborative research. Some people in the field believe that such an understanding will be possible only when the genes associated with schizophrenia are characterized. On the other hand, it may be possible to identify genes of import only if there is a better understanding of the environment in which they function. Even if the gene or genes for subtypes of schizophrenia could be found, twin studies indicate that genetic vulnerability alone would not account for all the variance; there is a clear opening for other risk factors to operate.

The best hope now for prevention of schizophrenia lies with indicated preventive interventions targeted at individuals manifesting precursor signs and symptoms who have not yet met full criteria for diagnosis. The identification of individuals at this early stage, coupled with the introduction of pharmacological and psychosocial interventions, may prevent the development of the full-blown disorder.

The children of schizophrenic parents are at increased risk for emotional problems of many types, including schizophrenia, and preventive intervention research should continue to study this high-risk group. (Early efforts along these lines at the NIMH Prevention Research Branch have been discontinued.) The parents, spouses, and siblings of schizophrenic individuals can suffer an immense caregiver burden, both emotionally and financially, but as yet, little is known about specific risks within this family group or about the outcome of specific preventive interventions provided to them.

ALCOHOL ABUSE AND DEPENDENCE

Why some people continue to seek alcohol in the face of adverse consequences is not fully understood, and this puzzle marks an important area of study in alcohol research. The reinforcing properties of alcohol—those properties that produce euphoria—may explain, in part, why some people begin to drink. Drinking behavior cannot be explained solely by the direct pharmacological effects of alcohol, however. Genetic and psychological factors as well as the environment shape drinking behavior. Alcohol abuse and dependence arise through a complex interaction of biological risk factors, including genetic factors, and psychosocial risk factors, including personality features and contextual factors, involving the social environment in which an individual lives.

Biological Risk Factors

Genetic Vulnerability

Family Studies.   Family studies have clearly shown that alcohol dependence is familial. The evidence for genetic factors for alcohol abuse is less well substantiated (Schuckit, 1994, 1992). About 70 percent of alcoholics have a positive family history of alcoholism in first- or second-degree relatives (M. Schuckit, personal communication, 1993). Sons and daughters of alcoholics have a threefold to fourfold increased risk for developing this disorder (Schuckit, 1986; Cotton, 1979). This suggests that either the environment of an alcoholic family or the genetic contribution from parents influences the development of alcoholism. However, family studies by themselves cannot distinguish nature versus nurture influences on etiology.

Twin Studies.   The relative contribution of environment and genetics has been examined through twin studies as in the case of Alzheimer's disease and schizophrenia. If a trait has a high heritability, the concordance in monozygotic twins, who share 100 percent of their genes, will be greater than the concordance in dizygotic twins, who share only 50 percent. In general, this is what has been observed in the research (Hrubek and Omenn, 1981; Schuckit, 1981). A study with a small sample of psychiatric inpatients by Murray, Clifford, and Gurling (1983), however, showed no difference between monozygotic and dizygotic concordance using both male and female probands, so although the evidence from twin studies of the importance of genetic factors in the etiology of alcohol abuse and dependence is strong, it is not entirely conclusive.

Adoption Studies.   Adoption studies are another way to untangle the environmental and genetic contributions leading to the expression of a disease state. Adopted-away sons and daughters from alcoholic families who are raised by nonalcoholic adoptive parents have a significantly increased risk for alcohol abuse and dependence. This risk may be as high as three or fourfold (Goodwin, 1985; Bohman, Sigvardsson, and Cloninger, 1981; Cadoret, 1980; Cadoret and Gath, 1978; Goodwin, Schulsinger, Hermansen, Guze, and Winokur, 1973; Schuckit, Goodwin, and Winokur, 1972).

The data from Bohman, Sigvardsson, and Cloninger's (1981) large Swedish adoption study was used to hypothesize another step in the data analyses (Cloninger, Sigvardsson, Gilligan, von Knorring, Reich, and Bohman, 1989). They have postulated two forms of alcoholism with considerably different risk factors. The type I alcoholic begins drinking after age 25, infrequently demonstrates spontaneous alcohol-seeking behavior or serious legal problems due to drinking, shows psychological addiction and feels guilt over his or her alcohol use, and demonstrates a rather dependent, sentimental, and introverted personality. The type II alcoholic begins drinking well before age 25, is usually a male, demonstrates alcohol-seeking behavior, and has frequent legal problems due to drinking. These individuals do not show guilt or psychological dependence on alcohol. They demonstrate high novelty seeking and extroverted behavior. The type II alcoholic might have a higher genetic risk than the type I alcoholic.

Biological Markers

Finding potential markers for people susceptible to alcohol abuse and dependence has been the focus of a number of research studies. Biological markers may prove valuable in targeting high-risk populations for prevention trials.

Electrophysiological Markers. Event-related potentials, which are electrophysiological brain reactions to stimuli (Porjesz and Begleiter, 1983), have been studied in males with and without a family history of alcoholism. A low P_3 amplitude, a measure of one brain wave pattern, has been demonstrated in subjects with increased genetic risk (Begleiter and Porjesz, 1990). It occurs in at least one third of the sons of alcoholic fathers (Hill, Steinhauer, Park, and Zubin, 1990; Noble, 1990; O'Connor, Hesselbrock, Tasman, and DePalma, 1987; Begleiter, Porjesz, Bihari, and Kissin, 1984). Low P_3 amplitude has been replicated in other samples, even in alcoholics who are abstinent, suggesting its potential use as a trait marker.

Electroencephalograph synchrony, which appears to be under genetic control, has also been reported as a possible trait marker in women (Propping, 1980). This could prove to be the first marker that is specific for identifying women at risk.

Biochemical Markers. Studies of platelet enzymes have led to two potential markers of increased risk for alcohol abuse. First, stimulated adenylyl cyclase activity was found to be lower in a group of alcoholics than in nonalcoholics (Tabakoff, Hoffman, Lee, Saito, Willard, and De Leon-Jones, 1988). Second, monoamine oxidase (MAO) activity was found to be lower in alcoholics, and on further analysis the finding was shown to be specific to type II alcoholics (von Knorring, Bohman, von Knorring, and Oreland, 1985). This finding has been replicated in several laboratories (Pandey, Fawcett, Gibbons, Clark, and Davis, 1988; Tabakoff et al., 1988). MAO is an enzyme that is important in the metabolism of a variety of brain neurotransmitters that affect behavior, including dopamine, norepinephrine, epinephrine, and serotonin.

Decreased Sensitivity. Studies of individuals at high risk for alcohol abuse and dependence have also used challenge paradigms in which responses are measured to both placebos and ethanol. Results from some investigations (Moss, Yao, and Maddock, 1989; Lex, Lukas, Greenwald, and Mendelson, 1988; Savoie, Emory, and Moddy-Thomas, 1988; O'Malley and Maisto, 1985) suggest that in general these high-risk individuals may be less sensitive to the effects of alcohol than controls. They have less intense subjective feelings of intoxication following modest doses of alcohol (Schuckit, 1992). This is seen in such diverse measures as body sway, blood alcohol levels, and cortisol release following challenge. This again suggests that a genetic factor that decreases sensitivity to alcohol may play a role in the development of the illness. Schuckit (in press, 1994) has recently demonstrated that a low level of response to alcohol at age 20 was associated with a fourfold increased likelihood of future alcoholism in both sons of alcoholics and sons of controls.

Cognitive and Motor Functioning. There is some research that indicates that cognitive impairments are present in some children of alcoholic parents (Drejer, Theilgaard, Teasdale, Schulsinger, and Goodwin, 1985; Knop, Teasdale, and Schulsinger, 1985; Schaeffer, Parsons, and Yohman, 1984; Tarter, Hegedus, and Gaveler, 1984; Gabrielli and Mednick, 1983). The impairments are in lower verbal intelligence quotients, lower levels of reading comprehension, and problems with logic and abstract reasoning in achievement tests. These results have not been widely replicated. Some studies have found few differences on these measures when children of alcoholics are compared with controls (Drake and Valliant, 1988; Schuckit, Butters, Lyn, and Irwin, 1987), and the results that are found may pertain only to subgroups of children with multiple risk factors, such as those whose mothers had high-risk pregnancies and those with fetal alcohol effects.

Psychosocial Risk Factors

The majority of studies on psychosocial risk factors focus on adolescent onset. Many of the studies focus on the risk of initiating use, whereas the risk of escalating to abuse or heavy use has received less attention. Unfortunately, much of the work done in this area is cross-sectional, and so the results cannot distinguish factors associated with alcohol use from true risk factors that precede the onset of alcohol abuse or dependence. Because early and frequent use may lead to alcohol abuse, these factors are included in this review. Almost all of the studies on psychosocial risk factors fail to control for parental alcoholism or other mental disorder. Finally, many studies do not differentiate between alcohol use and other substance use.

Personality

There is little evidence that individuals at risk differ from controls on baseline measures of personality. The lack of evidence may at this time reflect methodological limitations in the studies that have been done or a true lack of association. However, there is one major exception to the lack of conclusiveness of personality measures—antisocial behavior. Antisocial behavior during childhood has been consistently related to alcohol problems in adulthood.

Difficulty in achievement-related activity among adolescents also has proved important, with studies documenting the following problems among those who later became alcoholic: poorer school performance, less productivity in high school, greater truancy, and greater incidence of dropping out (IOM, 1989). Aggressive behavior and the combination of aggressive behavior and shyness in the first grade have been found to predict heavy alcohol use at ages 16 and 17 (Kellam, Brown, and Fleming, 1982). Another study yielded similar results, indicating that males who were judged to be shy as children were least likely to become heavy alcohol users, but those who were rated as both shy and aggressive as children were most likely to develop drinking problems (McCord, 1988a,b). The relative risk of alcoholism has been found to be higher among males in their thirties who previously used alcohol with their peers when they were younger than 14 years of age (Hagnell, Isberg, Lanke, Rorsman, and Ohman, 1986). Males who later became alcoholic also had weaker interpersonal ties, ranging from being less considerate and less accepting of dependency to having a greater likelihood of leaving home early (IOM, 1989).

Cloninger (1987) has proposed an association between severe alcohol-related difficulties (in the type II alcoholism discussed earlier) and personality characteristics of high levels of novelty seeking and low levels of survival dependence and harm avoidance. These associations are all the more intriguing because the two disorders—alcohol abuse and dependence and antisocial personality disorder—probably have separate genetics.

Psychological factors such as low adaptability continue to influence alcohol use later in the life span. The probability of continued drinking and the eventual onset of alcohol abuse is higher if an individual is unable to develop alternative and more adaptive ways of coping with immediate situational demands, such as leaving home, changes in employment or marital status, retirement, or death of a spouse (IOM, 1989). In essence, the major determinants of problematic drinking may occur when the levels of external demand or strain are high and the individual is unable to cope with the stresses. The individual has high expectations that alcohol will produce the desired results, and he or she minimizes or denies the long-term negative consequences.

Contextual Factors

Factors external to the individual and arising in the broad social environment also affect the level of use and abuse of alcohol. The contextual factors that are strong predictors of use include community use patterns (Robins, 1984) and particularly peer group behavior (Barnes and Welte, 1986). Low socioeconomic status (Murray, Richards, Luepker, and Johnson, 1987) and neighborhood disorganization (Sampson, 1985) also contribute to increased risk for alcohol problems. Contextual factors also include the availability of alcohol, such as legality, enforcement, cost, and taxes (Hawkins, Catalano, and Miller, 1992). "Contrary to the prevalent view that prohibition failed, there is substantial evidence that it reduced alcohol consumption substantially" (Goldstein and Kalant, 1990, p. 1515). Beginning with Cook and Tauchen (1982), a series of studies have suggested that increasing taxes decreases consumption. Levy and Sheflin (1985) showed that a 1 percent tax increase decreased consumption by 0.5 percent. Of the contextual factors, laws controlling availability and taxes controlling price are the simplest to change.

Psychosocial Aspects of Parental Alcoholism

Parental alcoholism is associated with a constellation of other risk factors, and it is these factors plus the alcoholism itself that lead to poor outcomes in children—of which alcohol abuse is only one (see Box 6.2).

Protective Factors

Although much investigation has focused on identifying and assessing the magnitude of various risk factors involved in alcohol use, less is known about factors that may protect individuals from abusing alcohol.

BOX 6.2
Children of Parents with Alcohol Abuse and Dependence: Multiple Psychosocial Risk Factors for Their Development

Children growing up in families in which one or both parents are alcoholics face a wide range of problems (von Knorring, 1991). First of all, many attitudes, beliefs, and expectations concerning alcohol are formed early in life. Parental alcoholism adds pressures that may promote alcohol abuse. Children of alcoholics typically have early first-hand knowledge of alcohol; although many young children can identify various alcoholic beverages, researchers have found that there is a significant association between this ability and the level of drinking in the child's home. Some family dynamics reinforce the parent's abusive drinking, and children observe this and may internalize similar family norms. Studies have suggested that inadequate parenting—including lax supervision, an absence of parental demands, lack of parental interest or affection, and, most frequently, inadequate contact—is associated with increased risk of alcoholism (Zucker and Fitzgerald, 1991). It is not known whether this finding would hold if the study had controlled for other parental psychopathology, such as antisocial personality disorder, drug abuse, or depression.

Parental alcoholism also is associated with conflict and dysfunction in the family (Schulsinger, Knop, Goodwin, Teasdale, and Mikkelsen, 1986; Moos and Billings, 1982). Alcoholic families are less cohesive, less organized, less oriented toward intellectual or cultural pursuits, and more conflict-ridden (Clair and Genest, 1987). Children of alcoholics may have an increased risk of being neglected or abused (Zucker and Fitzgerald, 1991; Tarter et al., 1984; Lund and Landesman-Dwyer, 1979), but the evidence is not substantial. Children raised under such volatile circumstances may well be deficient in their socialization, and, also, a strong association between parental alcoholism and conduct disorder has been demonstrated (Steinhausen, Gobel, and Nestler, 1984).

Certain children in alcoholic families appear to be at particularly high risk. Children who have not experienced the cohesive impact of traditional family rituals during periods in which there is severe parental drinking are more likely to develop alcohol problems than are children from alcoholic families that have been able to maintain their rituals, such as those centering on dinner time, holidays, and vacations. In addition, boys with alcoholic fathers were more likely to become alcoholics themselves if the mother seemed to accept her husband's intoxicated behavior and to hold him in high esteem. These findings suggest that one developmental path to alcoholism may stem, in part, from family acceptance of an alcoholic parent's intoxicated behavior (IOM, 1989).

Positive Group Norms

Membership in structured, goal-directed peer groups that do not abuse alcohol may protect teenagers against adolescent substance abuse. The element that appears to be critical is a group norm that does not expect or approve of substance use (Hawkins, Catalano, and Miller, 1992).

Strong Attachments

Brook and colleagues identified two protective factors related to attachment that reduce risk for adolescent drug use (not alcohol use specifically) (Brook, Brook, Gordon, Whiteman, and Cohen, 1990). The first was a strong attachment, or bond, between parent and adolescent and the second was a strong attachment between adolescent and father, which potentiated the positive effects of other protective factors, such as positive maternal characteristics.

Genetic Factors Modifying Expression of the Disorder

There are four clearly delineated polymorphic genetic loci that appear to modify the expression of alcoholism. This is more detailed information on genetic factors than is available for any mental disorder other than Alzheimer's disease. These loci include three regions that are responsible for isozymes that catalyze the oxidation of acetaldehyde (the oxidation product of alcohol) and the region that encodes the dopamine D_2 receptor. The three loci encoding alcohol-metabolizing enzymes all can lead to an increase in the level of acetaldehyde following alcohol ingestion. Raised blood aldehyde levels are the basis of the flush reaction experienced by those carrying the appropriate genes. This reaction involves sweating, facial flushing, nausea, dizziness, and a feeling of faintness and is much more prevalent in Asian populations (Helzer, Canino, Yeh, Bland, Lee, Hwu, and Newman, 1990). Studies on Chinese, Japanese, and Korean populations show that these have between 30 and 50 percent expression of one of two inactive forms of aldehyde dehydrogenase, which leads to the flush reaction. In general, those affected with the flush reaction have much less tendency to abuse alcohol. This provides evidence that genetic factors can modify alcohol consumption and affect the expression of alcoholism. These factors can be modified by environmental factors, as shown by a study of men in Korea, where alcohol abuse is as high as in the West (Lee, Kwak, Yamamoto, Rhee, Kim, Han et al., 1990). Even here, those with aldehyde dehydrogenase deficiency tend to drink less than their non-affected counterparts; however, their level of abuse remains high due to cultural factors and peer pressure. This provides an interesting example of the power of environmental factors to overcome the inherent protection from alcoholism afforded by biological systems leading to acetaldehyde production.

In the case of the dopamine D_2 receptor, there is some limited evidence that the minor allele of the DRD2 gene on chromosome 11 is associated with alcoholism (Blum et al., 1990). Although this allele is not linked to the manifestation of alcoholism, it may be associated with the severity of the disease (Cloninger, 1991). Thus there may be genetic factors that can modify the expression of alcoholism even though they are not directly linked to the etiology of the disorder.

Findings and Leads

Alcohol abuse and dependence are genetically influenced disorders, and quantification of genetic risk has begun. Studies examining psychosocial risk factors for the onset of alcohol abuse and dependence have often failed to control for family history of alcoholism or other mental disorders, especially antisocial personality disorder and depression. As psychosocial risk factor research improves, more will become known about the relative and attributable risks associated with specific factors and with clusters of factors. It appears likely that it is the accumulation of both genetic and psychosocial risk factors that increases the risk for alcohol abuse and dependence. In particular, six risk factors are strongly associated with the onset of alcohol problems:

● Having a parent or other close biological relative with alcohol abuse or dependence. The mechanism may be genetic, psychosocial, or both.

● Having biological markers that are highly associated with later onset of alcohol dependence: (1) a low P_3 amplitude, which is a measure of a brain wave pattern (an electrophysiological marker); (2) a lower stimulated adenylyl cyclase activity or lower monoamine oxidase activity (a biochemical marker); and/or (3) a decreased sensitivity to the effects of alcohol.

● Demonstrating antisocial behaviors or a combination of aggressiveness and shyness during childhood.

● Having low adaptability and being unable to cope with immediate situational stresses, including adverse family conditions.

● Being exposed to community, neighborhood, or peer group norms that foster alcohol use and abuse.

● Having easy access to alcohol (resulting from low cost, low taxes, lenient laws, and/or minimal law enforcement).

Identification of high-risk populations should include these multiple risk factors whenever possible. Suitable preventive intervention trials could then be designed. For example, if individuals with biological markers could be identified before they use alcohol, they could be given information that might encourage them to abstain from alcohol. Also, without alcohol there would be, obviously, no alcohol abuse or dependence. Therefore control of availability has been and will continue to be a powerful prevention tool.

DEPRESSIVE DISORDERS

Major depression represents a profound biological dysregulation. Abnormalities in neurotransmitter function, the structure of sleep as measured by EEG studies, and regulation of neurohormonal response have been well documented. These can result in disturbances in eating, sleeping, energy, and attention, irritability, and distortions about the future, self-worth, and even about the value of life and living itself.

Major depression can result both from genetic influences and from severe and impairing traumatic life events. Animal models have elegantly demonstrated that a condition resembling severe depression that occurs in rats can result both from genetic influences and from environmental trauma and stress (Henn, Johnson, and Edwards, 1985). Thus, in the search for risk and protective factors, both classes of influence and their interactions are examined. Research has often focused solely on the broader category of mood disorders. In this review, evidence regarding mood disorders is used only when evidence on major depression is not available. When the older term "affective disorder" from DSM-III was used in the original research, that term is used here.

Biological Risk Factors

Genetic Vulnerability

In terms of genetic influences, an individual's risk for mood disorders becomes larger the larger the proportion of genes shared with a mood-disordered individual. Rates for mood disorders among monozygotic twins are about three times those for dizygotic twins. The rate of concordance for mood disorders for monozygotic twins is 0.50 for unipolar disorder (major depression) and 0.70 for bipolar disorder (Tsuang and Faraone, 1990). This emphasizes both the difference in heritability for unipolar and bipolar disorder and that environmental factors play a significant role. Studies of individuals with less severe forms of depression, that is, with symptoms that do not meet criteria for disorder, show considerably less heritability (Tsuang and Faraone, 1990).

Family Studies. Using family aggregation studies, estimates of lifetime morbidity risks in first-degree relatives of probands with major depression range from 0.18 to 0.30 for adults (Petersen, Compas, and Brooks-Gunn, 1992). Aggregated risk is generally higher in children than in adolescents and in adolescents than in adults. Rough estimates are about 0.50 for children and 0.35 for adolescents (Tsuang and Faraone, 1990). Thus the genetic loading for child and adolescent onset of major depression may be higher than that for adult onset. Current longitudinal studies suggest that early onset may be associated with more frequent episodes of major depression during childhood. Weissman and colleagues report that individuals with an onset of major depression prior to age 20 are more likely to have family members who are depressed than those whose first episode occurs after age 20 (Weissman, Gammon, John, Merikangas, Warner, Prusoff, and Sholomskas, 1987a). Although there is strong reason to support a genetic component to depression, the exact weight of genetic and psychosocial factors remains to be determined and the nature of the genetic transmission in depressive disorders remains to be elucidated. Segregation analyses have not been helpful in elucidating a mode of transmission in mood disorders.

Linkage Studies.   There is important work in progress regarding the forms of heritability of mood disorders. Most research has focused on bipolar disorder, but there has been some work regarding major depression. For example, Neiswanger and co-workers studied three extended families with unipolar affective illness and excluded linkage of this disorder to certain loci on chromosome 11 (Neiswanger, Slaugenhaupt, Hughes, Frank, Frankel, McCarty et al., 1990). A previous report of linkage to this region (Egeland, Gerhard, Pauls, Sussex, Kidd, Allen et al., 1987) also proved wrong when previously unaffected family members developed the illness (Pauls, Gerhard, Lacy, Hostetter, Allen, Bland et al., 1991).

Disease and Medication

Major depression frequently occurs in association with medical disorders and the use of certain medications. These depressions presumably occur because of disruption in neurotransmitter function that accompanies the underlying biological processes. Severe infections; tumors; endocrine conditions, including Cushing's disease, Addison's disease, hypothyroidism, hyperthyroidism, and diabetes mellitus; the use of medications such as reserpine and other antihypertensive agents, oral contraceptives, and various anticonvulsives; and the presence of anemia, electrolyte abnormality, and various metabolic disorders all are associated with the appearance of major depression.

Brain Injury

There is an association in children between brain injury and increased risk for mental disorders (Rutter, 1983). The mechanism involved in this association is poorly understood. However, it has long been observed that there is an association between various kinds of learning difficulties, in particular difficulties in learning to read, and subsequent problems with low self-esteem, which can predispose to depression.

Psychosocial Risk Factors

Severe and Traumatic Life Events

The presence of severe and traumatic events in an individual's life is associated with increased rates of major depression (Beardslee and Wheelock, in press; Coyne and Downey, 1991). Factors that have received the most attention include downward social mobility, loss of job, death of a spouse, child, or parent, divorce, and poverty. More recently, it has become clear that being the victim of child maltreatment carries with it a heavy risk for subsequent mental disorder including depression (Green, 1991). Although data are not definitive as yet, it is also likely that other severe traumas, such as being the victim of a violent crime or of a natural disaster, may predispose to depression (Coyne and Downey, 1991). In an examination of the connection between sexual assault and mental disorders in a community population, a strong association was found between history of assault and later onset of major depressive episodes (Burnam, Stein, Golding, Siegel, Sorenson, Forsythe, and Telles, 1988). There is an extensive literature to suggest that repeated negative experiences can lead to the development of a sense of helplessness, hopelessness, and low self-esteem, as well as to a sense of not being in control of one's surroundings. These overlapping conditions strongly predispose individuals to the development of depression (Petersen et al., 1992).

Whereas negative life circumstances, as described above, predispose to depression, the presence of close, intimate, supportive relationships appears to protect against it (Coyne and Downey, 1991). However, the nature of these relationships is complex. Perhaps the best model involves a major loss in childhood—the loss of a parent—and the development of subsequent depression. Brown and Harris (1989) have shown that adults who lost a parent in childhood and have become depressed not only have that risk factor, but also require a provoking agent in adulthood and the absence of good social support. In a series of studies of inner-city women in London who had lost a parent in child-hood, Brown and Harris (1989) demonstrated that those who did not have a close confiding relationship in adulthood and had unusually strong stressors developed depression. Those who had lost a parent in childhood but had good relationships and no such stressors did not develop depression. The authors also showed that the loss of care following the death of the parent was more important than the parental loss itself. Further studies established that lack of care in childhood following loss of a mother is associated with mood disturbance in adulthood. This influence is mediated by premarital pregnancy and marital dysfunction. Inadequate care increases the risk of early premarital pregnancy, which in turn increases the risk of marriage to an undependable partner. Marriage to such a partner, in addition to being low in intimacy, increases both the risk of serious life events like trouble with the law, threats of eviction, and poverty, and the risk of depression.

Accumulation of Stresses at a Time of Transition

Recent evidence in adolescent females indicates that the accumulation of stresses at a time of transition may place them at greater risk for developing depressive symptoms (Petersen et al., 1992). In trying to understand why the rates of disorder are so high in adolescent women, Petersen and colleagues have suggested that the combination of going through puberty and having a transition from one form of school to another (from primary to secondary school), along with a breakup of the family, form a constellation of risk factors that leads to increased rates of depression in this group. Clearly, the burdens of childrearing, when not adequately supported, predispose to depression (Weissman, Leif, and Bruce, 1987b). Downward social mobility and the lack of access to opportunities also can play a role in depression (Dohrenwend et al., 1992).

Sociodemographic Factors

Although in general, the foregoing risk factors are well established, detailed prospective studies of the influence of various risk factors over time and the mitigating effects of other variables, for the most part, have not been conducted in large samples. Two notable exceptions are the Epidemiologic Catchment Area (ECA) study (Anthony and Petronis, 1991) and the Alameda County study (Kaplan, Roberts, Camacho, and Coyne, 1987). Neither examined mood disorder in relatives, genetic influences, or the effect of severe trauma. They did, however, examine a variety of other influences. These studies excluded individuals who were depressed at the time of first assessment, so that these risk factors were for first onset of depression subsequent to first assessment. Using the ECA data base, the incidence of new cases of depression in a one-year period was assessed, and the factors from the first assessment that predicted the onset of new cases in that interval were examined. These factors dealt primarily with sociodemographic information. The major risk factors that predicted episodes of major depression were being female, being separated or divorced at initial assessment, and not having paid employment or a job with prestige. For less severe forms of depression, the effects of being separated or divorced and the diminished risk among working persons were also found.

In a follow-up study in the ECA catchment area, poverty was shown to have a profound impact on onset of new cases and thus to be a significant risk factor for depression (Bruce, Takeuchi, and Leaf, 1991). Using a general measure of mental disorder, 6 percent of all new cases of all types of mental disorder occurring in a six-month interval were the result of poverty. For depression specifically, 10 percent of new cases in that interval were attributed to poverty. By extrapolating from the sample at the New Haven site in the ECA study, Bruce and colleagues estimated that during the interval of the six-month interview period, 1,200 new episodes of major depression could be attributed to poverty (Bruce et al., 1991).

In a follow-up of approximately 7,000 Alameda County adults nine years after initial assessment, low education, presence of physical disability or other chronic medical conditions, poor perceived health, a strong sense of personal uncertainty, a move of residence, job loss, financial problems, and a sense of anomie and social isolation were all associated with increased risk for depressive symptoms at follow-up, while, interestingly, marital status was not (Kaplan et al., 1987).

Mental health services are underutilized by minority groups (Hough, Landsverk, Karno, Burnam, Timbers, Escobar, and Regier, 1987). This has implications for prevention. First, such groups may have a preference for preventive services that do not require that they identify themselves as psychiatric cases. Second, prevention programs should be organized so as not to make the mistake that treatment programs did, that is, to appear to be inaccessible or unacceptable to significant segments of the population, especially ethnic minorities.

Protective Factors

Across the life span, factors including good intelligence, easy temperament, and the presence of a supportive adult have all been shown to protect against the expression of psychopathology, including depression. In certain individuals whose parents suffer from depression, resiliency in late adolescence is associated with good interpersonal relationships, a strong sense of self, and a clear understanding of self and of the parent's illness (Beardslee and Podorefsky, 1988). In fact, most studies show that during adolescence the majority of children of parents with mood disorder are functioning reasonably well. At any one point in time, complex interaction between risk and protective factors operates in children of depressed parents, and an understanding of these factors across the developmental course highlights opportunities for prevention (see Box 6.3).

Findings and Leads

Depression is a common disorder that is seriously impairing and has multiple etiologies. It is associated with a series of other disorders and conditions that predispose to poor outcome. In particular, five risk factors are likely to be associated with the onset of depression:

- Having a parent or other close biological relative with a mood disorder. The mechanism may be genetic, psychosocial, or both.
- Having a severe stressor such as a loss, divorce, marital separation, unemployment, job dissatisfaction, a physical disorder such as a chronic medical condition, a traumatic experience, or, in children, a learning disorder.
- Having low self-esteem, a sense of low self-efficacy, and a sense of helplessness and hopelessness.
- Being female.
- Living in poverty.

It is appropriate to consider the possibility of programs to prevent the emergence of depression because of the substantial knowledge base about depression, the frequency of the disorder, and the costs associated with it.

Approaches that have targeted the prevention of clinical depression in high-risk adults or the prevention of depressive symptoms for those at high risk because of a major loss have all shown some promise (see Chapter 7 for illustrations of numerous preventive intervention research programs on depression). Definitive evidence of the prevention of the initial episode of major depressive disorder is not available at this time. Problems have included lack of large enough sample sizes, lack of adequate follow-up, and lack of valid measurement of symptoms and disorders. The most successful efforts to date have been able to show reductions in depressive symptomatology in high-risk groups rather

BOX 6.3
Children of Parents with Mood Disorders:
Opportunities for Prevention

Having a parent with a serious mood disorder is the single largest risk factor for initial onset of depression in childhood and adolescence and, because it involves both genetic and psychosocial risk factors, is among the largest risk factors for depression across the life span. A brief review of the literature on children of parents with depression is in order both to look at how this risk factor operates and to illuminate opportunities for prevention.

Documentation of the Risk Factor

For decades, it has been well established that severe mental disorder in parents is associated with increased rates of mental disorder in offspring. Recently, a series of rigorous empirical studies have been conducted using standard diagnostic instruments with the children of parents with serious mood disorders (Beardslee and Wheelock, in press; Downey and Coyne, 1990). The majority of these studies focused on parental major depression, but some focused on bipolar disorder, and therefore the more inclusive term mood disorder is used here. These studies are the result both of the recognition of childhood depression as a discrete entity and of the awareness that such children are themselves at heightened risk, particularly for depression. There is a clear consensus in the empirical research literature that children of parents with mood disorders fare much more poorly than subjects in comparison samples. A series of studies conducted by different investigators in different sites, but with similar designs, have conclusively established that the rates of adolescent depression in offspring of parents with mood disorders are at least several times higher than in children of parents with no disorder. These rates often reach 30 percent by the end of adolescence (Downey and Coyne, 1990). Children in these families also manifest impairments in adaptive and social functioning, as well as school and medical problems. Moreover, youngsters who experience depression or other serious psychopathology are largely unrecognized and untreated (Keller, Lavori, Beardslee, Wunder, and Ryan, 1991). These findings parallel findings of underrecognition and undertreatment of childhood disorders in epidemiological studies and studies of pediatric practice (Beardslee, Salt, Porterfield, Rothberg, van DeVelde, Swatling et al., 1993b). They also parallel the corresponding finding in adults that depression is underrecognized and undertreated. There is also substantial literature to indicate that children of parents with severe mood disorder are at considerable risk for a variety of poor developmental outcomes from birth to age five (Beardslee and Wheelock, in press; Downey and Coyne, 1990).

Most of the studies of the impact of parental mood disorder on children have been conducted using clinically referred parents. Extension of studies to nonreferred samples has demonstrated the same powerful effect of parental mood disorder on child outcome (Beardslee, Keller, Lavori, Staley, and Sacks, 1993a).

(continued)

Parental Mood Disorders: A Constellation of Risk Factors

The strong association between parental mood disorder and poor child outcomes is not a simple relationship. Parental mood disorder is associated with a number of other risk factors, and it is this entire constellation, including parental mood disorder, that leads to poor outcomes in children. This has important implications both for understanding etiology and for fashioning preventive intervention approaches.

In children with a depressed parent, the risk of developing depressive symptoms or disorders is greatly heightened by the presence of other associated mental disorders in the parent, depressive disorder in both parents, greater chronicity and severity of the parental disorder, the presence of divorce, and disturbances in parenting (Beardslee and Wheelock, in press; Downey and Coyne, 1990). These factors suggest particular groups for targeting. Adults with mood disorder have high co-morbidity with other disorders, in particular anxiety disorders and substance abuse. Given the phenomenon of assortative mating (i.e., the tendency of people to select as mates people with the same or similar characteristics), there is a much higher than chance rate of depression in the spouse of an individual identified with mood disorder. Hence youngsters are likely to be exposed both psychosocially and genetically to depressive disorder in both parents. Moreover, there is a higher rate of divorce and marital dysfunction in individuals with mood disorder, and these are risk factors for psychopathology in children independent of depression. Finally, there is overwhelming evidence that severe depression, regardless of its cause, profoundly impairs interpersonal relationships and imposes a heavy interpersonal burden on the family.

There are numerous interactional studies examining the patterns of relationship between depressed mothers and their young children that demonstrate profound disturbances in parenting (Beardslee and Wheelock, in press). The two psychosocial factors that have received the most attention across a wide range of studies of children of parents with mood disorders are (1) interferences with the ability to parent and (2) the presence of severe marital discord and divorce (Rutter, 1990).

Need to Study Multiple Outcomes

It is important to frame outcomes for children in developmentally appropriate terms. Outcomes reflecting depression in children from birth to age five are not diagnosable depressive disorders but impairments in cognitive functioning, psychosocial development, and attention. Depressive symptoms exhibited by school-age children are more variable but often involve interpersonal relationships, some depressive symptomatology, and some mental disorders. From early adolescence on, impairments can be classed in terms of the major diagnostic categories in DSM-III-R. For depression in one parent, the outcomes are quite variable. Some children develop anxiety disorders, some have school problems, and some develop depressive symptoms or disorders. Thus, at least for children and adolescents, preventive interventions targeting a single risk factor need to consider not a single diagnosis but a range of outcomes and a range of diagnoses.

(continued)

Preventive Intervention Research

Children of parents with mood disorders present a particular opportunity for prevention because the risk to them is well documented. Interventions must be informed by a knowledge of the specific developmental level of the child and also must involve parents and other caretakers. Interventions that enhance parenting skills, apply cognitive behavioral techniques used with adults (Muñoz, 1987), or promote understanding in adolescence are encouraging. Another approach helps parents focus on the future of the children, helps the children better understand the illness experience of the parent, and enhances resiliency in the children. Initial results of this approach to strengthening families in adversity have proved promising (Beardslee et al., 1993b).

than documenting prevention of onset of major depression. This area is one of the most promising for continued preventive intervention research.

CONDUCT DISORDER

Conduct disorder has the earliest average age of onset of the five illustrative disorders in this report. It is an important disorder on several accounts. It is the disorder most frequently referred to child psychiatric clinics. It is hard to treat. It has a significant level of persistence into adult life and is a precursor to many other dysfunctions that give rise to impairment in adult life, including alcoholism and schizophrenia (Robins, 1966). There are at least two subtypes of conduct disorder—early onset and adolescent onset.

Biological Risk Factors

Genetic Vulnerability

The role of genetic influences in the development of conduct disorder has been difficult to sort out. The families in which conduct problems arise often are disorganized and have a parent who exhibits either antisocial behavior or substance abuse. Thus the problem clearly runs in families, but the families also create environments that may result in conduct problems. There have not been twin and adoption studies of conduct disorder as there have been for the other illustrative disorders. In part, this is because conduct disorder is a relatively new diagnosis, appearing in the DSM for the first time in 1968. However, estimates of heritability can be obtained from adults with antisocial disorder. It is a safe assumption that the adults with these problems did exhibit conduct disorder in childhood, but they are not representative of the entire group of individuals who have conduct disorder, many of whom will not go on to show full-scale antisocial behavior or criminality. Adult twin studies have demonstrated higher concordance for monozygotic over dizygotic twins in criminal behavior (Christiansen, 1977a,b). The use of adopted-away samples is an even better way to approach the question, but these studies are limited. Cadoret, Cain, and Crowe (1983) studied several adopted samples and concluded that both genetic and environmental forces play a role in the expression of antisocial behavior. In a large-scale Danish study of criminality, Mednick, Gabrielli, and Hutchings (1984) came to a similar conclusion that a genetic predisposition played a role in the development of criminal behavior. In 1986, Mednick and co-workers reported that biological fathers and male adoptees have much higher rates of criminality than adoptive fathers (Mednick, Moffitt, Gabrielli, and Hutchings, 1986). More recently, DiLalla and Gottesman (1989) reported that a heritable contribution to adult criminality appears more clearly established than to conduct disorder and delinquency.

Some studies thus support a role for genetic factors, but the data are inconsistent, inconclusive, and suffer from instability of diagnosis and other methodological flaws.

Physiological Abnormalities

It has been proposed that physiological abnormalities underlie the symptoms of impulsivity and the failure to inhibit aggressive behaviors. Earls (in press) has reviewed the potential physiological processes in conduct disorder that might be under a degree of genetic control, and thus in part might explain the heritability of antisocial behavior, assuming that such heritability proves accurate upon future investigations. The most well-replicated physiological influence is disturbance of the autonomic nervous system, demonstrated by low heart rate, decreased amplitude and slow recovery of skin conductance, and slow EEG wave activity. Other possible, but not well-studied, influences include central neurotransmitter systems, dietary or metabolic influences, the effects of gonadal hormones, abnormal levels of platelet monoamine oxidase, and low levels of plasma dopamine B hydroxylase. Rutter and Giller (1983) have suggested that the autonomic features support a biological basis for the reported reduced anxiety and impaired passive avoidance following punishment in antisocial individuals.

Gender

Conduct disorder has been repeatedly shown to be more common in boys than in girls. In the Isle of Wight studies (Rutter, Tizard, and Whitmore, 1970), the rate of conduct disorder, using a much broader definition than that in DSM-III-R, in 10- and 11-year-olds showed a boy:girl ratio of 3.8:1. Similarly, in the Ontario Child Health Study (Offord et al., 1987), the rates for boys and girls 6 to 11 years were 6.5 and 1.8 percent, respectively. In early adolescence the rate in boys (9.1 percent) was found to be almost four times the rate in girls (Offord and Boyle, 1988). However, in the same study it was found that the ratio of conduct disorder in 15- and 16-year-olds approached 1 because of the later onset of conduct disorder in girls (Offord and Waters, 1983). It is still not clear whether the different ratios at the earlier ages are due to constitutional differences reflected in behavioral differences (Earls, 1987) or to differences in socialization, resulting in different learning experiences and expectations for boys than girls. What is clear is that the difference in ratios between boys and girls occurs early. In studies of young children, the precursors of conduct disorder—early behavioral problems, including oppositional behavior—are also more likely to occur in boys than girls (Earls and Jung, 1987; Richman, Stevenson, and Graham, 1982).

Early Temperamental Difficulties

Temperament refers to those aspects of personality that show some consistency across time (Kazdin, 1992). Differences in temperament are based on individual characteristics such as activity level, responsiveness, consistency of mood, and social adaptability (Chess and Thomas, 1977). "Easy to manage" children are characterized by a happy disposition, adaptability to change, and a willingness to approach new stimuli. Children who are temperamentally difficult and have mentally ill parents are more than twice as likely as children with easy temperaments and mentally ill parents to be the target of parental anger and criticism (Rutter and Quinton, 1984). Children who are difficult are more likely to show later behavioral problems than children who are less difficult (Reitsma-Street, Offord, and Finch, 1985; Earls, 1981). Greenberg, Speltz, and DeKlyen (1993) point out that data from the Bloomington Longitudinal Study (Bates, Bayles, Bennet, Ridge, and Brown, 1991) show that mothers' reports of infant difficultness at six months and infant resistance to control at one year significantly predicted maternal reporting of externalizing behavior problems at ages 3, 6, and

8 years. The intermediate variable was coercive mother-child interaction during the preschool years. It is the combination of infant difficulty with family stress or dysfunction that has been found to contribute to later behavior problems (Maziade, Coté, Bernier, Boutin, and Thivierge, 1989). Conversely, easy temperament appears to act as a protective factor in these circumstances. Although these results are encouraging, the evidence for temperament as a risk or protective factor for conduct disorder is still incomplete.

Hyperactivity

There is considerable co-morbidity between attention deficit hyperactivity disorder (ADHD) and conduct disorder. In the Ontario Child Health Study, 40 percent of ADHD children in 1983 also showed symptoms of conduct disorder four years later (Offord, Boyle, Racine, Fleming, Cadman, Blum et al., 1992). The difference between those with both disorders and those who remained attention deficit disordered but did not develop co-morbid conduct disorder was the level of family functioning (Offord et al., 1992). Families who are able to provide a supportive, consistent environment with expectable limits presumably allow these children to develop enough prosocial skills that they can function reasonably well in school and with their peers.

Cognitive and Neuropsychological Deficits

There has been considerable debate as to whether conduct disorder precedes or follows from low intelligence, language dysfunction, or neuropsychological deficits. There is some evidence that cognitive and linguistic problems precede the behavior problems (White, Moffitt, and Silva, 1989; Beitchman, Nair, Clegg, Patel, Ferguson, Pressman, and Smith, 1986). It has been suggested that cognitive deficits, poor language comprehension, and impulsivity in aggressive children and adolescents may be related to dysfunctions in the left frontal lobe of the brain (Gorenstein, Mammato, and Sandy, 1989). The specific deficits that are seen include inability to plan, concentrate, rechannel potentially harmful behaviors, and learn from the negative consequences of behavior (Moffitt, 1993; Moffitt and Henry, 1991).

Cognitive deficits understandably lead to school underachievement, which has been consistently associated with conduct disorder. In the Isle of Wight study (Rutter et al., 1970), one third of the 10- and 11-year-olds who were severely delayed in reading showed evidence of conduct disorder, and, conversely, one third of the conduct disordered children were at least two years delayed in their reading after allowing for IQ differences. These associations held even after controlling for family size and social class. There are four major hypotheses concerning the overlap between underachievement and conduct disorder: (1) underachievement leads to externalizing behavior, (2) externalizing behavior leads to underachievement, (3) hypotheses 1 and 2 occur simultaneously, and (4) underlying variables are the actual cause in both problems. All four hypotheses need further exploration to derive explanatory models with sufficient rigor, complexity, and validity to handle the diversity of causal factors (Hinshaw, 1992).

Chronic Ill Health

Children with chronic ill health, if they also have a functional physical limitation (any sensory, physical disorder, or disability that interferes with functioning), have been found to have three times the incidence of conduct disorder as healthy peers (Cadman, Boyle, Offord, Szatmari, Rae Grant, Crawford, and Byles, 1986). Children with chronic ill health without disability have been found to have twice the incidence of conduct disorder (Cadman et al., 1986). Chronic conditions affecting the central nervous system place the child at even higher rates of risk; children with central nervous system damage have five times the incidence of conduct disorder, according to studies by Rutter (1977) and Brown and colleagues (Brown, Chadwick, Shaffer, Rutter, and Traub, 1981). It is not known whether brain damage exerts its effect primarily through the presence of cognitive disability per se or through the resulting difficult temperament on the part of the infant.

Psychosocial Risk Factors

Precursor Symptoms in the Child

Identification of patterns of early precursor symptoms may lead to identification of children and adolescents who are at especially high risk for developing conduct disorder. Beginning at ages four to six, aggression predicts later delinquency (Loeber and Dishion, 1983). When aggression is combined with other behavioral characteristics, however, the predictive power increases. A combination of aggressiveness and shyness appears to be predictive of conduct disorder as well as drug abuse (Farrington and West, 1990; Moskowitz and Schwartzman, 1989; McCord, 1988a,b; Kellam, Brown, Rubin, and Einsminger, 1983). Farrington and colleagues from the Cambridge Study in Delinquent Development found that there was a tendency for shyness to act as a protective factor against delinquency and crime for nonaggressive boys but as an aggravating factor for aggressive boys (Farrington, 1989, 1987; Farrington, Gallagher, Morley, St. Ledger, and West, 1985). Another pattern that may predict conduct disorder is the combination of aggressiveness with peer rejection (Andersson, Bergman, and Magnusson, 1989). Finally, early substance abuse correlates with adolescent onset of conduct disorder (Robins, 1980).

The number of symptoms appears to be a better indication of the potential for serious disorder than the pattern at any one point in time (Robins and Ratcliff, 1980; Robins and Wish, 1977). Likewise, the earlier the first symptoms appear, the higher the risk may be for subsequent conduct disorder, and early onset of the disorder has been consistently linked to poorer outcomes, including serious and chronic antisocial behavior (Farrington, Loeber, Elliott, Hawkins, Kandel, Klein et al., 1990; Loeber, Brinhaupt, and Green, 1990; Tolan, 1987; Loeber and Dishion, 1983; Robins, 1966).

Family Adversity

The importance of parental psychopathology as a cause of conduct disorder has been addressed in numerous studies, but as mentioned earlier, the influences of nature versus nurture have not been sorted out. A review of studies conducted from 1975 to 1985 found that criminal and alcoholic parents have a greatly increased risk of having children with conduct disorder (West and Prinz, 1987). In a large longitudinal case comparison study of 518 single-parent and 502 two-parent families, Avison (1992) found that children with externalizing problems directed toward others had mothers who were likely to score more than twice as high on measures of psychological distress and were twice as likely to have experienced problems with alcohol or to have had a major depressive episode. The same study identified that maternal alcohol problems have the greatest effect on the behaviors of younger boys.

Other studies have found that maternal antisocial personality has a profound negative effect on a child (Frick, Lahey, Hartdagen, and Hynd, 1989; Lahey, Russo, Walker, and Piacentini, 1989). Alcoholism and antisocial personality disorder in the father, combined with low socioeconomic status, are highly correlated with conduct disorder in the child (Earls, Reich, Jung, and Cloninger, 1988). The mechanism may be primarily through the poor parenting environment provided or through a genetic component. Children of alcoholics appear to have an elevated rate of truancy, more contacts with the police, and more substance abuse and are more likely to drop out of school (West and Prinz, 1987). In addition to the influence of parental behaviors and psychopathology, it has been found that there can be a potentiation of antisocial behavior among brothers (Jones, Offord, and Abrams, 1980). However, the presence of sisters in a family tends to suppress antisocial behavior (Reitsma-Street et al., 1985).

Weiss and Hechtman (1986) studied 75 young adults and 45 normal controls matched initially on age, gender, IQ, and socioeconomic status. At 10- and 15-year follow-up into adulthood, the 25 percent of hyper-active adolescents who demonstrated significant antisocial behavior had higher initial ratings of aggressive behavior and family psychopathology.

Marital discord in families has been persistently found to predict disruptive behavior problems in boys, especially in combination with maternal depression (Rutter and Giller, 1983). It is the extent of discord and overt conflict, regardless of whether parents are separated, that is associated with the risk for antisocial behavior (Hetherington, Cox, and Cox, 1982). Grych and Fincham (1991) recently reviewed studies of marital conflict and children's adjustment, concluding that 15 of 19 relevant studies support the association between parental discord and children's psychopathology. Some studies have documented this link more specifically for conduct disorder (Jouriles, Murphy, and O'Leary, 1989). Furthermore, the effects of witnessing marital violence have recently been shown to predispose boys to use violence as a means of conflict resolution (Jaffe, Hurley, and Wolfe, 1990).

Other dysfunctional parenting practices, especially harsh, erratic, and abusive forms of discipline, also predispose to the development of conduct disorder. Patterson, Reid, and their colleagues have carefully documented how aversive behavior on the part of both child and parent, combined with parental inconsistency, create negative reinforcement patterns in which child aggression and coercion (increasingly demanding interaction) are reinforced (Patterson, DeBarysh, and Ramsey, 1989; Patterson, Chamberlain, and Reid, 1982). The combination of inadequate supervision, parental criticism, harsh and inconsistent discipline, and rejecting attitudes toward the child have been described by Patterson, Reid and their colleagues to have a specific, independent association with antisocial behavior in children.

On the basis of studies by several investigators (Widom, 1989a,b; Carmen, Rieker, and Mills, 1987; Lane and Davis, 1987), Earls (in press) has concluded that there is a strong association between child maltreatment and delinquency and adult crime in later years. Dodge and colleagues found that children who had been physically abused in infancy had clinically significant symptoms by the age of six but that not all of the children had aggressive symptoms (Dodge, Bates, and Pettit, 1990). Some symptoms, especially those of girls, were of an internalizing nature, directed inwards. Approximately 25 percent of the abused or neglected children became delinquent, a rate double that in nonabused controls. The antisocial behavior apparently begins very early. Children who have been physically abused tend to behave in more aggressive ways than children who have not (Cicchetti and Carlson, 1989; Widom, 1989a,b). Lewis (1992) described a lack of empathy in abused toddlers, which she suggested reflects their conditioned ability to insulate themselves from any stimuli that might evoke their own painful experiences. The long-term effects of physical abuse and neglect seem to be greatest among those who have aggressive parents and became aggressive themselves (McCord, 1983).

Community Risk Factors

Indicators of socioeconomic disadvantage, such as poverty, overcrowding, and poor housing, have been shown to be associated with an increased risk of childhood conduct problems (Hawkins, Catalano, and Miller, 1992). Socioeconomic disadvantage appears to have its effect due to the aggregation of risk factors, that is, the number of life stresses and daily hassles that inevitably have an impact on family interactions and relationships in a way that changes what Rutter has termed the "under the roof culture" of the family (including family cohesiveness, parental responsiveness, and limit setting) (Rutter, 1985a). This effect occurs predominantly in urban settings. Offord and colleagues found that low income was one of the most significant risk factors for the onset of conduct disorder, but it had its effect on children aged 4 to 11, not on adolescents (Offord, Alder, and Boyle, 1986). In an exceptionally lengthy risk study—a 30-year follow-up to measures taken in the first five years of life—Kolvin and co-workers demonstrated that low socioeconomic status of a child's family at age 5 is a powerful risk factor (Kolvin, Miller, Fleeting, and Kolvin, 1988). Of the 31 percent of males who committed either a juvenile or an adult offense, only 5 percent came from the higher socioeconomic groups, I and II, whereas 26 percent came from group III and 42 percent from groups IV and V.

Sociological studies have shown that urban areas typically have higher rates of delinquency. In Rutter's classic studies comparing children living in the Isle of Wight with those in inner London, it was found that the rates of conduct disorder were twice as high in London. Within cities with high crime rates, there is marked variation by neighborhood (Sampson, 1985), with rates varying by a factor as large as five (Rutter and Giller, 1983). High-delinquency neighborhoods are those areas in which there is social disintegration with a high rate of social problems, including high rates of adult crime, substance abuse, infant mortality, low birthweight, and child maltreatment.

In socially disorganized communities a significant decline in the proportion of older, long-time male residents leads to an increase in youths becoming members of delinquent gangs. Having an antisocial peer group plays a part in the acquisition and maintenance of aggressive behavior. Some reports support the idea that if antisocial youth leave an antisocial peer group and join a more prosocial group their level of antisocial behavior may diminish (Osborn and West, 1980; Knight and West, 1975). Despite the risk effects that tend to congregate in large urban areas, certain high schools, which emphasize academic achievement and personal responsibility and reward prosocial behavior, have been found to reduce the risk of antisocial behavior in their students (Rutter, Maughan, Mortimore, Ouston, and Smith, 1979). On the other hand, evidence suggests that being apprehended by the police escalates antisocial behavior in youth with conduct disorder, possibly because contact with law enforcement may lead to increased antiauthoritarian attitudes (Offord, 1989).

Accumulation of Risk Factors

Studies have consistently confirmed that as the number of adverse conditions accumulates, the risk of conduct disorder increases proportionately (Blantz, Schmidt, and Esser, 1991; Rutter, 1978). Moffitt (1990) reported that the presence of family adversity—including low education, psychiatric illness, substance abuse, and criminality in the parent; marital distress and family violence; and poverty and overcrowding—at age 5 was a significant predictor of teenage delinquency in children who showed hyperactivity and disruptive behavior problems in early childhood. The correlates of conduct disorder reported in the Ontario Child Health Study (Offord et al., 1992) indicate that the three most significant risk factors exerting independent effects on conduct disorder were family dysfunction (relative odds = 3.1), parental mental disorder (relative odds = 2.2), and low income. Low income had its effect on children aged 4 to 11 years (relative odds = 3.7) but not on adolescents. Farrington (1991) found that inadequate parental discipline and school failure, combined with economic disadvantage and family criminality, predicted juvenile convictions.

Greenberg, Speltz, and DeKlyen (1993) have suggested that there are four domains of risk that are necessarily interrelated to produce early-onset conduct disorder. These are (1) contributions from the child's organic, biological difficulties (such as difficult temperament and abnormal psychophysiology); (2) factors in the family ecology and family adversity, disruption, and stress; (3) ineffective parental management and socialization; and (4) problems in early parent-child relations (such as insecure attachment in infancy and the preschool years).

It appears that it is the transactional interaction between factors in the child (such as genetic and temperamental factors) and factors in the family environment (any factor that produces a lack of responsivity in the primary caretaker) that produces aggressiveness in early childhood. Aggressive children are apt to be rejected by parents, peers, and teachers. This sets up further negative interaction cycles.

Just as the accumulation of risk factors influences outcomes in childhood, it also influences outcomes further on in the life cycle. A 25-year follow-up study of children with attention deficit hyperactivity disorder by Hechtman has suggested that a combination of measures influence outcome in adulthood (Hechtman, 1991; Weiss and Hechtman, 1986). These include (1) individual personal characteristics (such as IQ, health, and temperament); (2) family parameters (such as socioeconomic status, family composition, mental health of family members, emotional climate of the home, and childrearing practices); and (3) the larger social and physical environment.

Protective Factors

The protective factors that reduce the chance that a child at risk will develop conduct disorder include good intelligence; easy disposition; an ability to get along well with parents, siblings, teachers, and peers; an ability to do well in school; having friends; being competent in non-school skill areas (Rae Grant, Thomas, Offord, and Boyle, 1989); and having a good relationship with at least one parent and with other important adults (Werner and Smith, 1992).

The presence of a positive warm bond between parent and child in early childhood can lead to greater compliance and reciprocity. This good relationship allows the child to empathize with another person's affective state, and, according to Minde (1992), is an essential prerequisite for prosocial behavior. In contrast, aggressive children tend to misperceive frustration in others as hostility directed toward them, and then respond aggressively (Dodge, 1980). Involvement in extracurricular activities for which recognition is received (Rae Grant et al., 1989), the support of other significant adults in the community (Werner and

Smith, 1992), prosocial peer groups, and good schools that foster academic success, responsibility, and self-discipline (Rutter et al., 1979) all are associated with a diminished risk of conduct disorder and more favorable outcomes, even for adolescents living in high-risk situations. Hawkins and colleagues have emphasized the role of social bonding, which refers to attachment, commitment, and adherence to the values of others (Hawkins and Lam, 1987; Hawkins and Weis, 1985). This occurs in the contexts of family, school, and peer relationships.

Good schools have been found to have a profound protective effect on students at the secondary level. Rutter et al. (1979) has described these as emphasizing academic work, reinforcing good work and behavior, providing good working conditions for students, having consistent teacher expectancies, making teachers available to deal with problems, and according responsibility to students.

Findings and Leads

Much still remains unknown about conduct disorder, including its subtypes, the risk factors involved in its onset, and the protective factors in the child, family, and community that lead to more favorable outcomes. Both prospective, longitudinal studies that begin early in life and well-designed efforts at prevention are needed for progress to occur (Tonry, Ohlin, and Farrington, 1990).

It is the accumulation of risk factors and the interaction among them rather than any specific risk factor that is important in the onset of conduct disorder. The transactional interaction between the individual child and his or her environment over time is the ecological crucible in which the pathways to the development of a range of positive or negative childhood and adult outcomes are forged. During the early years of development, the family environment is of greater importance. As children develop and move outside the family, influences from peers, the school, and the community assume increasing importance and should be targeted for intervention studies. Preventive intervention programs must address these multifactorial risks across social settings. Knowledge will grow from research on the relative and attributable risks associated with single risk factors as well as clusters of risk factors.

The lack of twin and adoption studies in conduct disorder is a major research gap. Such data could contribute toward understanding the roles of genetic as well as environmental influences.

Because early onset has been consistently linked with poorer outcomes, preventive interventions should increasingly focus on the youngest age groups possible, especially preschoolers.

The transition from antisocial behaviors in adolescence to similar behaviors in adulthood especially warrants careful longitudinal study. The range of outcomes should include both psychiatric and nonpsychiatric adult dysfunctions in order to elucidate the various pathways during this transitional period (Earls, in press). Studies of those individuals who do not carry over their antisocial behaviors into adulthood are warranted, for they could lead to clues about protective factors and possibly preventive interventions.

RISK AND PROTECTIVE FACTORS COMMON TO MANY DISORDERS

It has become evident that even though some risk factors may be specific to a particular disorder, other risk factors are common to many disorders. A continuing emphasis solely on the identification of risk factors unique to *specific* mental disorders is not likely to be productive. The low incidence of some mental disorders, such as schizophrenia, makes predictions based on the occurrence of presumed risk factors especially difficult. Instead, there may be greater value in clarifying the role of those risk factors that appear to be common to many mental disorders, especially in view of the frequent co-morbidity of these disorders.

Individual risk factors during childhood can lead to a state of vulnerability in which other risk factors may have more effect. For example, a prematurely born, low-birthweight baby may be more vulnerable than a full-term, healthy sibling in a suboptimal family environment (see Box 6.4 for a description of low birthweight as a general risk factor). Similarly, a child may be vulnerable to parent-child interaction difficulties by reason of a difficult temperament, a chronic physical illness, neurophysiological deficits, or below-average intelligence. Low IQ is associated with several mental disorders. Research also has shown links between early language disabilities and the later development of severe behavior disorders (Dattilo and Camarata, 1991; Camarata, Hughes, and Ruhl, 1988; Carr and Durand, 1985; Donnellan, Anderson, and Mesaros, 1984). Gender is another important genetic factor (Rutter, 1979). In the prenatal period and first 10 years of life, boys are more likely than girls to be vulnerable to both physical and psychosocial stressors. In the second decade, girls appear to be more vulnerable to psychosocial stressors, and in early adulthood men once again appear to be more vulnerable (Werner and Smith, 1992).

Factors in the family that constitute significant risk factors for increased childhood psychopathology include severe marital discord, social disadvantage, overcrowding or large family size, paternal crimi-

---

BOX 6.4
Low Birthweight as a General Risk Factor

The vulnerability of low-birthweight children to a range of poor health outcomes including suboptimal intelligence has long been identified and has been recently reexamined in a large-scale study that included 676 low-birthweight children (under 2,500 grams) (McGauhey, Starfield, Alexander, and Ensminger, 1991). Twenty-five percent of the normal-birthweight children versus 36 percent of the low-birthweight children lived in a high-risk social environment, defined as stressful life events and a cumulative social environment risk index of ongoing stressful life conditions. Low-birthweight children were consistently more likely to have worse outcomes when exposed to a high-risk social environment than similar normal-birthweight children. However, low-birthweight children were not more likely than normal-birthweight children to have poor health outcomes in either a low- or moderate-risk social environment. Low-birthweight children were found to be consistently more likely to have poor outcomes in the presence of a high-risk social environment; thus a high-risk social environment doubled the risk of school failure and behavior problems for normal-birthweight children but quadrupled these risks for low-birthweight children (McGauhey et al., 1991).

Outcomes for very low birthweight infants (under 1,500 grams) are even more problematic. These infants are at risk not only because of their prematurity but also because of the complications of this state and the potential attachment problems associated with a long stay in an intensive neonatal care unit. Transactional interaction with family factors in this group remains an important topic for research.

---

nality, maternal mental disorder, and admission into the care of the local authorities, that is, child welfare services (Rutter, 1979). Community factors that impinge on children include social disadvantage, particularly the experience of being part of a welfare family. This is not simply due to income levels; with income controlled, rates of impairment have been found to be significantly higher for children from low-income welfare families than for children from low-income nonwelfare families (Offord et al., 1987). Living in subsidized housing (Rutter, 1981) and living in an area that has a high rate of community disorganization have also been found to increase the risk for mental disorders in childhood. Community institutions such as schools can either enhance or detract from intellectual and social growth and development and thus can function as a community risk or protective environment for children and adolescents (Rutter et al., 1979).

Although protective factor research has made major advances, it is less well developed than risk factor research, and several conceptual and methodological issues remain inadequately resolved (Luthar, 1993).

There is evidence, however, that a core set of individual characteristics and sources of support can buffer the effects of both biological and psychosocial risk factors during childhood.

Positive temperament, above-average intelligence, and social competence can contribute to individual resilience (Rutter, 1985b; Rutter et al., 1970). Children who are easygoing and responsive call forth the best from their parents and from peers, teachers, and other adults. Above-average intelligence may allow a child not only to do well in school but also to develop problem-solving skills and a sense of perspective and psychological differentiation from the family or community, fostering the growth of the autonomy and independence necessary for optimal adult functioning. Social competence includes the ability to get along with others. In adolescence, having a sense of coherence and an internal locus of control orientation (that is, a personal sense of being able to take charge of one's life) has been cited as a protective factor (O'Grady and Metz, 1987).

Smaller family structure, that is, not more than four children in the family and spacing of more than two years between siblings, has been found to be protective (Werner and Smith, 1992). In early childhood, having a close relationship with a parent who is responsive and accepting is very important (see Box 6.5 for a description of the quality of interaction with parents as a general protective factor). For older children, supportive parents, good sibling relationships, and adequate rule setting by parents have been found to be protective (Werner and Smith, 1982). A supportive relationship with one parent was found to provide a substantial protective effect for children living in severely discordant, unhappy homes (Rutter, 1985b).

Protective community factors include the relationships that children develop outside the family, with peers, significant other adults, and any available external support system such as church, youth groups, school, and recreational activities, all of which build competence and provide children with success (Jones and Offord, 1989; Werner, 1989; Werner and Smith, 1982). Good secondary schools positively affect academic achievement and, subsequently, vocational outcome. They also reduce the rates of truancy, school dropout, and juvenile court appearances for children in disadvantaged areas (Rutter, 1979).

In the Kauai Longitudinal Study, three clusters of protective factors differentiated the resilient group from other high-risk youth who developed serious and persistent problems in childhood and adolescence (Werner and Smith, 1992). These were (1) at least average intelligence and temperamental attributes that elicit positive responses from family members and strangers; (2) good relationships with parents or parent

---

BOX 6.5
Quality of Interaction with Parents as a General Protective Factor

There is consistent evidence that the nature and quality of children's interaction with their parents affect their school performance, social competence, and interpersonal behaviors (Amato, 1989; Dornbusch, 1989). Behavior problems in the preschool years appear to vary with the extent to which parents are emotionally available to respond to their children's needs (Gotlib and Avison, 1993; Lee and Gotlib, 1991). Adequate parents are generally sensitive to their children's cues in relation to their developmental needs (Rutter, 1989). Emde (1989) has suggested that this sensitivity includes both physiological and psychological regulation of the infant's needs. Empathic responsiveness facilitates the sharing of feelings and expressions of positive social behaviors (Easterbrooke and Emde, 1988). Minde (1991) emphasized that a further parental activity related to sensitive responsiveness is the function of discipline. Normal parents encourage self-control in a child by regulating the expression of feelings. Bowlby and others have convincingly shown that the quality of the tie or attachment between parent and infant plays an important part in the overall social and emotional functioning of a child (Bowlby, 1988).

The quality of the early mother-child relationship may be affected by a number of variables, including the mother's own experience in childhood (Main and Hesse, 1990) and the presence of mental disorders (especially depression). Psychiatrically disturbed parents are generally more preoccupied with themselves and thus are less responsive to their children (Minde, 1991).

A close relationship between the child and parents during the first five years of life is especially important because primary attachment relationships are developed during this period. Children who experience multiple changes in parental figures are therefore at risk for psychosocial problems.

---

substitutes, which encourage trust, autonomy, and initiative; and (3) an external support system that rewards competence and provides a sense of coherence. Resilient children were reported to grow into competent, confident, and caring adults.

In general, protective factors in adulthood fall into two broad groupings—(1) those that arise from the buffering effects of social support available to the individual and (2) personality factors or personal characteristics that affect the individual's ability to cope with stress (O'Grady and Metz, 1987).

MODELS FOR UNDERSTANDING RISK AND PROTECTIVE FACTOR INTERACTION

Understanding that risk and protective factors are common to many disorders is only a first step. It is also essential to understand that these factors do not function in isolation; instead, there exists a dynamic interaction among them that undergoes modification and change throughout an individual's life span.

Three possible models for the ways in which risk and protective factors interact to produce competence in children are the compensatory model, the challenge model, and the protective model—all adapted from Garmezy, Masten, and Tellegen (1984).

In the compensatory model, risk factors, including genetic vulnerability and stresses, combine additively and can potentiate each other. Usually, it is the aggregation of risk factors rather than presence of any single risk factor that impairs development. This is not to say that all risk factors have equal weight; they probably do not. For example, genetic vulnerability may account for more of the attributable risk for schizophrenia than any other risk factor. However, generally, multiple risks potentiate each other. Sameroff (1987) found that children reared in families with seven or more risk factors scored 30 IQ points below children from families with no risk factors. Infancy risk factors appear to be magnified synergistically when family environments in childhood are negative or when a child is subjected to stressful life events (O'Grady and Metz, 1987).

It is evident that adverse conditions in a child's environment do not necessarily produce adverse outcomes. However, it is becoming increasingly clear that a combination of risk factors in the child and risk factors in the family environment, particularly if these are multiple, predispose the individual to negative outcomes. Rutter and Quinton (1977) suggested that a fourfold increase in the amount of stress in childhood produced a 24-fold increase in the incidence of later mental disorder. Studies have consistently demonstrated a relationship between the number and severity of life events and behavior problems. Findings for adults are similar, but research findings are less plentiful (O'Grady, 1983).

The challenge model describes a curvilinear relationship in which stress as a risk factor enhances competence as long as it is not excessive. This phenomenon has been described as one of "steeling" or "inoculation" (Werner and Smith, 1982; Anthony, 1974). Murphy and Moriarty (1976) have suggested that successive, moderately challenging experiences strengthen coping capacities. The protective model suggests that protective factors modulate or buffer the impact of risk factors by, for instance, improving coping, adaptation, and competence building.

The concept of causal or etiological chains is helpful in understanding risk and protective factor interaction. Robins (1970) first described this concept as a process in which one event calls forth another in a chain that leads to an outcome. For example, consider a causal chain involving a mother and her infant:

Depressed mother ⟶ unresponsive parenting by the mother ⟶ lack of language stimulation by the mother during the child's early years ⟶ language delay in the child ⟶ learning difficulties in the child ⟶ cognitive disorder in the child.

Robins suggested that one could intervene at any point along the causal chain. Intervening at the weakest link, however, might be the most productive strategy. For example, an intervention could be aimed at improving parental responsiveness by treating the mother's depression or by providing another responsive adult in the environment to interact with the infant. In some ways, this chain is too simplistic; for example, it could continue snowballing for many years, and it does not take into account that several chains can be operating simultaneously.

Sameroff (1987) modified Robins's concept of unidirectional causal chains to include a temporal framework that is bidirectional, emphasizing reciprocal interactions between the child and the environment. In other words, how things turn out is a complex result of the interaction between the child and the family environment early in life and the child and the peer, school, and community environment in later childhood. The patterns of interaction between the child's personal attributes and risk and protective factors in the family, school, and community environments are not linear, but are interwoven—like the threads in a Jacquard tapestry—in patterns of increasing complexity. Initially, parents develop a pattern of interaction with their infants that is dependent on many factors, including their own childhood experiences, marital relationships, and the quality of their social support systems. Factors related to the child may include gender, health status, physical maturity, and temperament. Infants change the nature of their parents' responses to them, and thus the interactions change. Parents in turn have an impact on their children. Research on child maltreatment has provided illustrations of this more complex conceptualization of causal chains (see Box 6.6).

As they grow older, children carry the patterns of interaction and expectation learned in the family environment into their relationships with other adults and peers. These interactions will mold further relationship experiences and be molded by them, changing the developmental trajectory in positive or negative directions.

Things go wrong when the family environment is not able to meet the needs of the child, either because the child is too impaired or temperamentally difficult or because the parents lack responsiveness owing to their own lack of nurturing, mental disorder, or overwhelming environmental distress. Sameroff and Chandler (1975) have described this as the "continuum of the caretaking casualty"; at one end of this continuum is

BOX 6.6
Child Maltreatment

Research on child maltreatment was stimulated in the early 1960s by reports of the "battered child" syndrome in the medical literature (Kempe, Silverman, Steele, Droegemueller, and Silver, 1962). Since that time, research studies in this field have generally focused on four types of child maltreatment: physical abuse, sexual abuse, emotional maltreatment, and child neglect.

Child maltreatment serves as a useful illustration of the complexities associated with identifying and addressing risk and protective factors in an etiological chain encompassing both social problems and mental disorders. It is both a social problem, with its own set of risk and protective factors, and a risk factor in itself for several mental disorders.

Etiology

Although several key variables or risk factors have been associated with child maltreatment, such as poverty, a parental history of abusive experiences, and parental psychopathology, research on the causes of child abuse and neglect suggests that no single variable can adequately explain the origins of child maltreatment. The results of etiological studies are often conflicting, and the predictive power of single or combined variables, such as the individual characteristics of the parent, child, or environment alone, is limited. For example, although a strong association has been shown between poverty and child abuse, the relationship is complex—most poor parents clearly are not abusive, and poverty alone is not a sufficient or even a necessary antecedent for child maltreatment.

Models of child maltreatment have evolved from isolated cause-and-effect models to approaches that consider multiple pathways and interactive effects among factors that contribute to child maltreatment. Recognizing the importance of situational factors has led to the development of contemporary multicausal interactive models that emphasize the sociocultural context of child maltreatment. Child maltreatment is now described less as an individual disorder or psychological disturbance, and more as a symptom of an extreme disturbance of childrearing, often within a context of other serious family problems, such as alcoholism or antisocial behavior (Wolfe, 1991; Burgess, 1979; Starr, 1979). Although studies of abusive and nonabusive parents have not detected significant personality differences, research on the interactions of abusive and nonabusive family processes has yielded important distinctions. Abusive parents have unrealistic expectations of their children, tend to view their own children's behavior as extremely stressful, and view themselves as inadequate or incompetent parents (Wolfe, 1991).

The information in this box is based in part on *Understanding Child Abuse and Neglect* (CBASSE, 1993).

(continued)

Child Maltreatment as a Risk Factor for Mental Disorders

Although research has suggested a relationship between child abuse and neglect and a variety of psychosocial and mental disorders, considerable uncertainty and debate remain about the effects of child victimization on children, adolescents, and adults. For example, the majority of children who are abused do not show signs of extreme disturbance. The consequences of abuse or neglect may not become apparent until the child becomes an adolescent or an adult, and thus the connections between the experience of abuse and the short- or long-term consequences may be diffuse and uncertain.

In addition, it is often difficult to separate the experience of child victimization from other traumatic experiences that may affect the life of a child. Child maltreatment often occurs within a family context or social environment characterized by multiple problems, including poverty, violence, substance abuse, and unemployment, and the process of distinguishing the consequences of behaviors that are associated directly with the experience of child maltreatment from those that result from other social disorders and family dysfunctions is a challenging task. For example, several studies suggest that the child's experience of witnessing violence toward siblings or parents may be as harmful as the experience of victimization itself (Faller, 1988; Rosenberg, 1987; Rosenbaum and O'Leary, 1981).

Studies of physical child abuse and child neglect consistently highlight physical aggression and antisocial behavior among the outcomes associated with these forms of child maltreatment (Kaufman and Cicchetti, 1989; Walker, Downey, and Bergman, 1989; Rohrbeck and Twentyman, 1986; Hoffman-Plotkin and Twentyman, 1984; Salzinger, Kaplan, Pelcovitz, Samit, and Kreiger, 1984; Perry, Doran, and Wells, 1983). Evidence from longitudinal studies indicates continued problems of aggression and anger (Egeland and Stroufe, 1981b) and the development of conduct disorder (Rogeness, Amrung, Macedo, Harris, and Fisher, 1986). Maltreated children also appear to be less competent that their peers in social interactions (Strauss and Gelles, 1990; Howes and Espinosa, 1985). In physically abused children, lack of social competence may be manifest in withdrawal or avoidance (Kaufman and Cicchetti, 1989), whereas in other children, it appears as fear, anger, or aggression (Main and George, 1985).

The consequences of neglect can be especially severe and powerful in the early stages of child development. Drotar (1992) notes that maternal detachment and lack of availability may harm the development of bonding and attachment between child and parent, affecting the neglected child's emotional state, expectations of adult availability, problem solving, social relationships, and ability to cope with new or stressful situations (Aber and Allen, 1987; Main and George, 1985).

A prospective study of mothers who were psychologically unavailable to their infants compared their children to physically abused, neglected, verbally rejected, and control group children from the same high-risk sample (Egeland and Stroufe, 1981a). The results indicated that children in all maltreatment groups functioned poorly and their functioning deteriorated over time (Erickson, Egeland, and Pianta, 1989). Nearly all the children in this study whose mothers were psychologically unavailable were anxiously attached at 18

(continued)

months of age, and these children demonstrated a nearly 40-point decline in performance on the Bayley Scales of Infant Development between 9 and 24 months.

Clinical samples of maltreated children have reported a high incidence of suicide attempts and self-mutilation (Green, 1978). Comparison studies of physically abused and nonphysically abused children have indicated heightened levels of depression, hopelessness, and lower self-esteem (Allen and Tarnowski, 1989; Kazdin, Moser, Colbus, and Bell, 1985) and greater emotional difficulties in older children (Kinard, 1982, 1980). Kaufman (1991) found that a disproportionate number of maltreated children met diagnostic criteria for one of the major mood disorders.

Inappropriate sexual behavior, such as frequent and overt self-stimulation, inappropriate sexual overtures toward other children and adults, and play and fantasy with sexual content, are the most commonly studied symptoms in studies that compare sexually abused children to children in control groups (Kendall-Tackett, Williams, and Finkelhor, 1993). Although sexually inappropriate behavior would seem relatively specific to sexual abuse, Deblinger and colleagues compared reports of inappropriate sexual behaviors across groups of children who experienced different forms of maltreatment and found approximately the same percentage of sexually inappropriate behavior in physically abused (17 percent) as in sexually abused children (18 percent) (Deblinger, McLeer, Atkins, Ralphe, and Foa, 1989). Kendall-Tackett et al. (1993) have found that sexually abused children were more symptomatic than their nonabused counterparts in terms of fear, nightmares, post-traumatic stress disorder (PTSD), withdrawn behavior, neurotic mental illness, cruelty, delinquency, sexually inappropriate behavior, regressive behavior, and other general problem behaviors. Estimates of sexually abused children diagnosed as meeting the DSM-III-R criteria for PTSD range from 21 percent (Deblinger et al., 1989) to 48 percent (McLeer, Deblinger, Atkins, Foa, and Ralphe, 1988).

The majority of abused children do not become delinquent, and the majority of delinquents were not abused as children. Prospective studies estimate the incidence of delinquency in adolescents who have been abused or neglected to be about 20 to 30 percent (Widom, 1989a). There have been numerous retrospective studies linking childhood maltreatment, especially sexual abuse, to specific forms of adult psychopathology, including mood disturbance, post-traumatic stress, self-injurious behavior, substance abuse, somatization, eating disorders, multiple personality disorder, and interpersonal violence. As with all retrospective studies, the validity of recall information is of questionable value.

Prevention of Child Maltreatment

Most programs to prevent child maltreatment have lacked methodological rigor, and their findings are equivocal. However, two research programs—the Prenatal/Early Infancy Project in Elmira, New York (see Chapters 7 and 11) and the Children and Youth Program (Hardy and Streett, 1989) have met with significant success and have demonstrated a reduction in child maltreatment.

an adaptive family environment that can meet the needs of the organically damaged or temperamentally difficult infant, and at the other end is the disordered family environment that cannot meet the needs of the least distressed, most healthy, normal, temperamentally easy newborn. In between are the majority of average environments that provide "good enough" parenting.

In discussing the ways in which early events might be linked to later outcomes, Rutter (1989) emphasized that not only continuities but also discontinuities are found between events in childhood and subsequent adult outcomes. Some risk pathways turn into more adaptive routes because of adventitious happenings. For example, a child from a dysfunctional family who is physically abused and then placed in a foster home has started on a life course of negative events. However, a continuous negative cycle is not predetermined; the course could be altered by an especially good relationship with the foster parents. This relationship could produce a discontinuity in the life course that had been expected prior to placement. Rutter (1989) has demonstrated that children at risk early in life who subsequently had good school experiences were three times more likely to show planning in their choice of life career or marital partner than those who had poor school experiences. Similarly, for women earlier at risk because of institutional experiences, the presence of marital support was found to lead to good social functioning and good parenting, in contrast with those who did not receive good marital support (Quinton and Rutter, 1988).

Werner and Smith (1982) have suggested that the interaction of risk and protective factors is a balance between the power of the person and the power of the social and physical environment. A balance is necessary throughout life, although different factors vary in importance at different developmental stages. These authors suggested that constitutional factors are more important during infancy and childhood and interpersonal factors are more important during adolescence. However, certain genetic vulnerabilities may not be potentiated until later in the life span. For example, schizophrenia usually appears in later adolescence, and Alzheimer's disease appears late in life. Adaptation at all ages appears in large part to be a function of the individual's ability to elicit predominately positive responses from others in his or her environment.

MAJOR FINDINGS AND PROMISING LEADS

Mental health outcomes depend on the interactions of risk and protective factors in the child, the family, and the wider environment. The nature, timing, severity, and length of particular risk factors and the gender, age, and cultural identity of the individual are all key variables in determining mental health outcomes.

It appears that most risk and protective factors, other than genetic factors, are not specific to a single disorder. Much remains to be learned about both risk and protective factors and their interaction. Therefore, at this time the most fruitful approach for preventive interventions may be to use a risk reduction model that includes the enhancement of protective factors and to aim at clusters or constellations of risk and protective factors. Markers can be used to identify high-risk populations, but the interventions will be aimed at those causal and malleable risk factors that appear to have a role in the expression of several mental disorders. Identification of relative and attributable risks associated with various clusters of risk factors could greatly facilitate preventive intervention research.

Risk factors, including markers, should always be reviewed in relation to their rate of occurrence in the normal population. A given risk factor may not be unique to those individuals who will eventually develop a mental disorder. It may be quite prevalent in normal populations and thus will not—by itself—be especially useful in identifying individuals at risk. For example, increased cerebral ventricular size occurs in many individuals with schizophrenia, but it also occurs in about 4 percent of persons without the disorder. Screening a general population for ventricular size would identify more nonschizophrenics than preschizophrenics. A similar lack of specificity would probably result from screening for many, if not most, other risk factors—such as aggressiveness, poverty, and life stress—in general populations. Thus these factors are best used in combinations. It is the accumulation of risk factors, with appropriate weighting of the relative importance of each factor, that will yield the targets with the most potential for prevention of later onset of mental disorder(s).

The task in preventive interventions is to decrease risk and/or increase protection in the individual, the family environment, and the wider environment with which the individual comes into contact. But not all risk factors need to be reduced. Even reducing some in a multirisk situation is likely to result in more advantageous outcomes. Because of developmental changes, the timing of the reduction of risk may be even more critical than the number of risk factors addressed. Conversely, if the number of protective factors can be increased in the individual, family, and community, then resilience is likely to be increased and the disorder may be avoided.

General risk factors may lend themselves to universal preventive interventions consonant with broad community mental health efforts that focus on public education and social welfare. Risk factors specific to a particular group of people can be addressed in selective preventive interventions. Individuals with early behavioral symptoms or markers are potential recipients of indicated preventive interventions. Risk reduction would seem to be a promising approach for prevention. The question that remains is whether it is being widely and successfully used. This issue is addressed in Chapter 7, which reviews illustrative preventive intervention research programs.

REFERENCES

Aber, J. L.; Allen, J. P. (1987) The effects of maltreatment on young children's socioemotional development: An attachment theory perspective. Developmental Psychology; 23: 406–414.

Abrams, R.; Taylor, M. A. (1983) The genetics of schizophrenia: A reassessment using modern criteria. American Journal of Psychiatry; 140: 171.

Allen, D.; Tarnowski, K. (1989) Depressive characteristics of physically abused children. Journal of Abnormal Child Psychology; 17: 1–11.

Amaducci, L. A.; Fratiglioni, L.; Rocca, W. A.; Fieschi, C.; Livrea, P.; Pedone, D.; Bracco, L.; Lippi, A.; Gandolfo, C.; Bino, G. (1986) Risk factors for clinically diagnosed Alzheimer's disease. Neurology; 36: 922–931.

Amato, P. R. (1989) Family processes and the competence of adolescents and primary school children. Journal of Youth and Adolescence; 18: 39–53.

Andersson, T.; Bergman, L. R.; Magnusson, D. (1989) Patterns of adjustment, problems, and alcohol abuse in early adulthood: A prospective longitudinal study. Development and Psychopathology; 1: 119–131.

Andreasson, S.; Allebeck, P.; Engstrom, A.; Rydberg, U. (1987) Cannabis and schizophrenia: A longitudinal study of Swedish conscripts. Lancet; 2(8574): 1483–1486.

Anthony, E. J. (1974) The syndrome of the psychologically invulnerable child. In: E. J. Anthony and C. Koupernik, Eds. The Child and His Family: Children at Psychiatric Risk. Vol. 3. New York, NY: John Wiley and Sons; 99–121.

Anthony, J. C.; Petronis, K. R. (1991) Suspected risk factors for depression among adults 18–44 years old. Epidemiology; 2: 123–132.

Asarnow, R. F.; Steffy, R. A.; MacCrimmon, D. J.; Cleghorn, J. M. (1977) An attentional assessment of foster children at risk for schizophrenia. Journal of Abnormal Psychology; 86: 267.

Avison, W. R. (1992) Risk factors for children's conduct problems and delinquency: The significance of family milieu. Paper presented at the American Society of Criminology Annual Meeting, New Orleans, LA.

Barnes, G. M.; Welte, J. W. (1986) Patterns and predictors of alcohol use among 7–12th grade students in New York State. Journal of Studies on Alcohol; 47(1): 53–62.

Barr, C. E.; Mednick, S. A.; Munk-Jorgenson, P. (1990) Exposure to influenza epidemics during gestation and adult schizophrenia. Archives of General Psychiatry; 47: 869–874.

Bates, J. E.; Bayles, K.; Bennet, D. S.; Ridge, B.; Brown, M. M. (1991) Origins of externalizing behavior problems at eight years of age. In: D. J. Pepler and K. H. Rubin, Eds. The Development and Treatment of Childhood Aggression. Hillsdale, NJ: Lawrence Erlbaum Associates; 93–120.

Beardslee, W. R.; Keller, M. B.; Lavori, P. W.; Staley, J.; Sacks, N. (1993a) The impact of parental affective disorder on depression in offspring: A longitudinal follow-up in a non-referred sample. Journal of the American Academy of Child and Adolescent Psychiatry; 32(4): 723–730.

Beardslee, W. R.; Podorefsky, D. (1988) Resilient adolescents whose parents have serious affective and other psychiatric disorders: Importance of self-understanding and relationships. American Journal of Psychiatry; 145(1): 63–69.

Beardslee, W. R.; Salt, P.; Porterfield, K.; Rothberg, P. C.; Van de Velde, P.; Swatling, S.; Hoke, L.; Moilanen, D. L.; Wheelock, I. (1993b) Comparison of preventive interventions for families with parental affective disorder. Journal of the American Academy of Child and Adolescent Psychiatry; 32(2): 254–263.

Beardslee, W. R.; Wheelock, I. (in press) Children of parents with affective disorders: Empirical findings and clinical implications. In: W. R. Reynolds and H. F. Johnston, Eds. Handbook of Depression in Children and Adolescents. New York, NY: Plenum Publishers.

Begleiter, H.; Porjesz, B. (1990) Neuroelectric processes in individuals at risk for alcoholism. Alcohol and Alcoholism; 25(2–3): 251–256.

Begleiter, H.; Porjesz, B.; Bihari, B.; Kissin, B. (1984) Event-related brain potentials in boys at risk for alcoholism. Science; 227: 1493–1496.

Beitchman, J. H.; Nair, R.; Clegg, M.; Patel, P. G.; Ferguson, B.; Pressman, E.; Smith, A. (1986) Prevalence of speech and language disorders in 5-year-old kindergarten children in the Ottawa-Carleton region. Journal of Speech and Hearing Disorders; 51(2): 98–110.

Bender, L. (1937) Behavior Problems in the Children of Psychotic and Criminal Parents. General Psychology Monograph. 19; 229.

Bernheim, K.; Lewine, R.; Beale, C. (1982) The Caring Family: Living with Chronic Mental Illness. New York, NY: Random House.

Blantz, B.; Schmidt, M. H.; Esser, G. (1991) Familial adversities and child psychiatric disorders. Journal of Child Psychology and Psychiatric Disorders; 32(6): 939–950.

Blum, K.; Noble, E. P.; Sherida, P. J.; Montgomery, A.; Ritchie, T.; Jagadeeswaran, P.; Nogami, H.; Briggs, A. H.; Cohn, J. B. (1990) Allelic association of human dopamine D2 receptor gene in alcoholism. Journal of the American Medical Association; 263: 2055–2060.

Bohman, M.; Sigvardsson, S.; Cloninger, R. (1981) Maternal inheritance of alcohol abuse: Cross-fostering analysis of adopted women. Archives of General Psychiatry; 38: 965–969.

Bowers, M. B., Jr. (1987) The role of drugs in the production of schizophreniform psychosis and related disorders. In: H. Y. Meltzer, Ed. Psychopharmacology: The Third Generation of Progress. New York, NY: Raven Press; 819–823.

Bowers, M. B., Jr.; Swigar, M. E. (1983) Vulnerability to psychosis associated with hallucinogen use. Psychiatry Research; 9(2): 91–97.

Bowlby, J. (1988) A Secure Base: Clinical Application of Attachment Theory. London, England: Routledge.

Bracha, H. S.; Torrey, E. F.; Gottesman, I. I.; Bigelow, L. B.; Cunniff, C. (1992) Second-trimester markers of fetal size in schizophrenia: A study of monozygotic twins. American Journal of Psychiatry; 149(10): 1355–1361.

Breakey, W. R.; Goodell, H.; Lorenz, P. C.; McHugh, P. R. (1974) Hallucinogenic drugs as precipitants of schizophrenia. Acta Psychiatrica Scandinavica; 69: 162–174.

Breitner, J. C. S. (1991) Clinical genetics and genetic counseling in Alzheimer disease. American College of Physicians; 115(8): 601–606.

Breitner, J. C. S.; Folstein, M. F.; Murphy, E. A. (1986a) Familial aggregation in Alzheimer dementia—I. A model for the age-dependent expression of an autosomal dominant gene. Journal of Psychiatric Research; 20: 31–43.

Breitner, J. C. S.; Murphy, E. A.; Folstein, M. F. (1986b) Familial aggregation in Alzheimer dementia—II. Clinical genetic implications of age-dependent onset. Journal of Psychiatric Research; 20: 45–55.

Breitner, J. C. S.; Murphy, E. A.; Folstein, M. F.; Magruder-Habib, K. M. (1990) Twin studies of Alzheimer's disease: An approach to etiology and prevention. Neurobiological Aging; 11: 641–648.

Breitner, J. C. S.; Welsh, K. A.; Magruder-Habib, K. M.; Churchill, C. M.; Robinette, C. D.; Folstein, M. F.; Murphy, E. A.; Priolo, C. C.; Brandt, J. (1990) Alzheimer's disease in the National Academy of Sciences registry of aging twin veterans. Dementia; 1: 297–303.

Breteler, M. M. B.; van Duijn, C. M.; Chandra, V.; Fratiglioni, L.; Graves, A. B.; Heyman, A.; Jorm, A. F.; Kokmen, E.; Kondo, K.; Mortimer, J. A.; Rocca, W. A.; Shalat, S. L.; Soininen, H.; Hofman, A. (1991) Medical history and the risk of Alzheimer's disease: A collaborative re-analysis of case-control studies. International Journal of Epidemiology; 20: S36–S42.

Brook, J. S.; Brook, D. W.; Gordon, A. S.; Whiteman, M.; Cohen, P. (1990) The psychosocial etiology of adolescent drug use: A family interactional approach. Genetic, Social, and General Psychology Monographs. Washington, DC: Heldref Publications; 116(No. 2).

Brown, G.; Chadwick, O.; Shaffer, D.; Rutter, M.; Traub, M. (1981) A prospective study of children with head injuries: III. Psychiatric sequelae. Psychological Medicine; 11: 63–78.

Brown, G. W.; Harris, T. O. (1989) Depression. In: G. W. Brown and T. O. Harris, Eds. Life Events and Illness. New York, NY: Guilford Press; 49–94.

Bruce, M. L.; Takeuchi, D. T.; Leaf, P. J. (1991) Poverty and psychiatric status: Longitudinal evidence from the New Haven Epidemiologic Catchment Area Study. Archives of General Psychiatry; 48: 470–474.

Burgess, R. L. (1979) Child abuse: A social interactional analysis. In: B. B. Lahey and A. Kazdin, Eds. Advances in Clinical Child Psychology. New York, NY: Plenum Press; 142–172.

Burnam, M. A.; Stein, J. A.; Golding, J. M.; Siegel, J. M.; Sorenson, S. B.; Forsythe, A. B.; Telles, C. A. (1988) Sexual assault and mental disorders in a community population. Journal of Consulting and Clinical Psychology; 56(6): 843–850.

CBASSE (Commission on Behavioral and Social Sciences and Education). (1993) Understanding Child Abuse and Neglect. Panel on Research on Child Abuse and Neglect, National Research Council. Washington, DC: National Academy Press.

Cadman, D.; Boyle, M. H.; Offord, D. R.; Szatmari, P.; Rae Grant, N.; Crawford, J. W.; Byles, J. A. (1986) Chronic illness and functional limitation in Ontario children: Findings of the Ontario Child Health Study. Canadian Medical Association Journal; 135: 761–767.

Cadoret, R. J. (1980) Development of alcoholism in adoptees raised apart from alcoholic biologic relatives. Archives of General Psychiatry; 37: 561–563.

Cadoret, R. J.; Cain, C. A.; Crowe, R. R. (1983) Evidence for gene-environment interaction in the development of adolescent antisocial behavior. Behavior Genetics; 13(3): 301–310.

Cadoret, R. J.; Gath, A. (1978) Inheritance of alcoholism in adoptees. British Journal of Psychiatry; 132: 252–258.

Camarata, S. M.; Hughes, C.; Ruhl, K. (1988) Children with mild to moderate behavior disorders: A population at risk for language impairment. Language, Speech, and Hearing in Schools; 19: 191–200.

Canon, T. D.; Mednick, S. A.; Parnas, J. (1989) Genetic and perinatal determinants of structural brain deficits in schizophrenia. Archives of General Psychiatry; 46: 883–889.

Carmen, E.; Rieker, P. P.; Mills, T. (1987) Victims of violence and psychiatric illness. American Journal of Psychiatry; 141: 378–383.

Carr, E. G.; Durand, V. M. (1985) Reducing behavior problems through functional communication training. Journal of Applied Behavior Analysis; 18: 111–126.

Carter, C. L.; Chung, C. S. (1980) Segregation analysis of schizophrenia under a mixed genetic model. Human Heredity; 30(6): 350–356.

Carter, D. A.; Desmarais, E.; Bellis, M.; Campion, D.; Clerget-Darpoux, F.; Brice, A.; Agid, Y.; Jailliard-Serradt, A.; Mallet, J. (1992) More missense in amyloid gene. Nature Genetics; 2: 255–256.

Chess, S.; Thomas, A. (1977) Temperament and the parent-child interaction. Pediatrics Annals; 6(9): 574–582.

Christiansen, K. O. (1977a) A review of studies of criminality among twins. In: S. A. Mednick and K. O. Christiansen, Eds. Biosocial Bases of Criminal Behavior. New York, NY: Gardner Press.

Christiansen, K. O. (1977b) A preliminary study of criminality among twins. In: S. A. Mednick and K. O. Christiansen, Eds. Biosocial Bases of Criminal Behavior. New York, NY: Gardner Press.

Cicchetti, D.; Carlson, V. (1989) Child Maltreatment: Theory and Research on the Causes and Consequences of Child Abuse and Neglect. Cambridge, England: Cambridge University Press.

Clair, D.; Genest, M. (1987) Variables associated with the adjustment of offspring of alcoholic families. Journal of Studies on Alcohol; 48: 345–355.

Clementz, B. A.; Sweeney, J. A. (1990) Is eye movement dysfunction a biological marker for schizophrenia? A methodological review. Psychological Bulletin; 108(1): 77–92.

Clinton, J.; Ambler, M. W.; Roberts, G. W. (1991) Post-traumatic Alzheimer's disease: Preponderance of a single plaque type. Neuropathology and Applied Neurobiology; 17: 69–74.

Cloninger, C. R. (1991) D2 dopamine receptor gene is associated but not linked with alcoholism. Journal of the American Medical Association; 266: 1823–1834.

Cloninger, C. R. (1987) A systematic method for clinical description and classification of personality variants. A proposal. Archives of General Psychiatry; 44(6): 573–588.

Cloninger, C. R.; Sigvardsson, S.; Gilligan, S. B.; von Knorring, A. F.; Reich, T.; Bohman, M. (1989) Genetic heterogeneity and the classifications of alcoholism. In: E. Gordis, B. Tabakoff, and M. Linnoila, Eds. Alcohol Research from Bench to Bedside. New York, NY: Haworth Press; 3–16.

Cook, P. J.; Tauchen, G. (1982) The effect of liquor taxes on heavy drinking. Bell Journal of Economics; 13: 379–390.

Cook, R. H.; Schneck, S. A.; Clark, D. B. (1981) Twins with Alzheimer's disease. Archives of Neurology; 38: 300–301.

Corder, E. H.; Saunders, A. M.; Strittmater, W. J.; Schmechel, D. E.; Gaskell, P. C.; Small, G. W.; Roses, A. D.; Haines, J. L.; Pericak-Vance, M. A. (1993) Gene dose of Apolipoprotein E Type 4 allelle and the risk of Alzheimer's disease in late onset families. Science; 261: 921–923.

Cornblatt, B.; Erlenmeyer-Kimling, L. (1985) Global attentional deviance as a marker of risk for schizophrenia: specificity and predictive validity. Journal of Abnormal Psychology; 94: 470.

Cotton, N. S. (1979) The familial incidence of alcoholism. Journal of Studies on Alcohol; 40: 89–116.

Coyle, J. T.; Oster-Granite, M. L.; Gearhart, J. D. (1986) The neurobiologic consequences of Down Syndrome. Brain Research Bulletin; 16: 773–787.

Coyne, J. C.; Downey, G. (1991) Social factors and psychopathology: Stress, social support, and coping processes. Annual Review of Psychology; 42: 401–425.

Dalen, P. (1988) Schizophrenia, season of birth, and maternal age. British Journal of Psychiatry; 153: 727–733.

Dattilo, J.; Camarata, S. M. (1991) Facilitating conversation through self-initiated augmentative communication treatment. Journal of Applied Behavior Analysis; 24: 369–378.

Deblinger, E.; McLeer, S. V.; Atkins, M. S.; Ralphe, D. L.; Foa, E. (1989) Post-traumatic stress in sexually abused, physically abused, and nonabused children. Child Abuse and Neglect; 13: 313–408.

DeLisi, L. E.; Goldin, L. R.; Hanovit, J. R.; Maxwell, M. E.; Kurtz, D.; Gershon, E. S. (1986) A family study of the association of increased ventricular size with schizophrenia. Archives of General Psychiatry; 43(2): 148–153.

Detera-Wadleigh, S. D.; Berrettini, W. H.; Goldin, L. R.; Boorman, D.; Anderson, S.; Gershon, E. S. (1987) Close linkage of c-Harvey-ras-1 and the insulin gene to affective disorder is ruled out in three North American pedigrees. Nature; 325: 806–808.

DHHS (Department of Health and Human Services). (1993) Public Health Service. Department of Health and Human Services: Fiscal Year 1994 Supplemental Budget Data (Moyer Material). Washington, DC: DHHS; Vol. XI.

DiLalla, L. J.; Gottesman, I. I. (1989) Heterogeneity of causes for delinquency and criminality: Lifespan perspectives. Development and Psychopathology; 1: 339–349.

Dodge, K. A. (1980) Social cognition and children's aggressive behavior. Child Development; 51(1): 162–170.

Dodge, K. A.; Bates, J. E.; Pettit, G. (1990) Mechanisms in the cycle of violence. Science; 250: 1678–1683.

Dohrenwend, B. P.; Levav, I.; Schrout, P. E.; Schwartz, S.; Naveh, G.; Link, B. G.; Skodol, A. E.; Stueve, A. (1992) Socioeconomic status and psychiatric disorders: The causation-selection issue. Science; 255: 946–951.

Done, D. J.; Johnstone, E. C.; Frith, C. D.; Golding, J.; Shepard, P. M.; Crow, T. J. (1991) Complications of pregnancy and delivery in relation to psychosis in adult life: Data from the British Perinatal Mortality Survey Sample. British Medical Journal; 302: 1576–1580.

Donnellan, A. M.; Anderson, J. L.; Mesaros, R. A. (1984) An observational study of stereotypic behavior and proximity related to the occurrence of autistic child-family member interactions. Journal of Autism and Developmental Disorder; 14(2): 205–210.

Dornbusch, S. M. (1989) The sociology of adolescence. In: W. R. Scott and J. Blake, Eds. Annual Review of Sociology. Vol. 15. Palo Alto, CA: Annual Reviews Inc.; 233–259.

Downey, G.; Coyne, J. C. (1990) Children of depressed parents: An integrative review. Psychological Bulletin; 108: 50–76.

Drachman, D. A.; Lippa, C. F. (1991) The etiology of Alzheimer's disease: The pathogenesis of dementia. The role of neurotoxins. Annals of the New York Academy of Sciences; 648: 176–186.

Drake, R. E.; Valliant, G. E. (1988) Predicting alcoholism and personality disorder in a 33-year longitudinal study of children of alcoholics. British Journal of Addiction; 83: 799–807.

Drejer, K.; Theilgaard, A.; Teasdale, T. W.; Schulsinger, F.; Goodwin, D. W. (1985) A prospective study of young men at high risk for alcoholism: Neuropsychological assessment. Alcoholism; 9: 498–502.

Drotar, D. (1992) Prevention of neglect and nonorganic failure to thrive. In: D. J. Willis, E. W. Holden, and M. Rosenberg, Eds. Prevention of Child Maltreatment: Developmental and Ecological Perspectives. New York, NY: John Wiley and Sons; 115–149.

Earls, F. (in press) Oppositional-defiant and conduct disorders. In: M. Rutter, E. Taylor, and L. Hersov, Eds. Child and Adolescent Psychiatry. 3rd ed. Oxford, England: Blackwell Scientific Publishers.

Earls, F. (1987) Annotation on the familial transmission of child psychiatric disorder. Journal of Child Psychology and Psychiatry; 28(6): 791–802.

Earls, F. (1981) Temperament characteristics and behavior problems in three-year-old children. Journal of Nervous and Mental Disease; 169: 367–373.

Earls, F.; Jung, K. (1987) Temperament and home environment characteristics as causal factors in the early development of childhood psychopathology. Journal of the American Academy of Child and Adolescent Psychiatry; 26(4): 491–498.

Earls, F.; Reich, W.; Jung, K.; Cloninger, C. R. (1988) Psychopathology in children of alcoholic and antisocial parents. Alcoholism: Clinical and Experimental Research; 12: 481–487.

Easterbrooke, A.; Emde, R. N. (1988) Marital and parent-child relationships: The role of affect in the family system. In: R. Hinde and J. Stevenson-Hinde, Eds. Relationships Within Families: Mutual Influences. Oxford, England: Oxford University Press.

Eaton, W. W. (1974) Residence, social class, and schizophrenia. Journal of Health and Social Behavior; 15(4): 289–299.

Egeland, B.; Stroufe, L. A. (1981a) Attachment and early maltreatment. Child Development; 52: 44–52.

Egeland, B.; Stroufe, L. A. (1981b) Developmental sequelae of maltreatment in infancy. In: New Directions for Child Development, 11. Developmental Perspectives on Child Maltreatment. San Francisco, CA: Jossey-Bass Publishers; 77–92.

Egeland, J. A.; Gerhard, D. S.; Pauls, D. L.; Sussex, J. N.; Kidd, K. K.; Allen, C. R.; Hostetter, A. M.; Housman, D. E. (1987) Bipolar affective disorders linked to DNA markers on chromosome 11. Nature; 325(6107): 783–787.

Emde, R. N. (1989) The infant's relationship experience: Developmental and affective aspects. In: A. Sameroff and R. N. Emde, Eds. Relationship Disturbances in Early Childhood: A Developmental Approach. New York, NY: Basic Books.

Emery, R. E.; Weintraub, S.; Neale, J. M. (1982) Effects of marital discord on the school behavior of children of schizophrenic, affectively disordered and normal parents. Journal of Abnormal Child Psychology; 10: 215.

Erickson, M. F.; Egeland, B.; Pianta, R. (1989) The effects of maltreatment on the development of young children. In: D. Cicchetti and V. Carlson, Eds. Child Maltreatment: Theory and Research on the Causes and Consequences of Child Abuse and Neglect. Cambridge, England: Cambridge University Press; 647–684.

Erlenmeyer-Kimling, L.; Cornblatt, B. (1992) A summary of attentional findings in the New York High-Risk Project. Journal of Psychiatric Research; 26(4): 405–426.

Erlenmeyer-Kimling, L.; Cornblatt, B. (1987) High risk research in schizophrenia: A summary of what has been learned. Journal of Psychiatric Research; 21: 401–411.

Erlenmeyer-Kimling, L.; Cornblatt, B.; Freidman, D.; Marcuse, Y.; Rainer, J. D.; Rutschmann, J. (1980) A prospective study of children of schizophrenic parents. International Journal of Rehabilitation Research; 3(1): 90–91.

Erlenmeyer-Kimling, L.; Cornblatt, B.; Freidman, D.; Rutschmann, J.; Simmons, S.; Devi,

S. (1982) Neurological, electrophysiological and attentional deviations in children at risk for schizophrenia. In: H. A. Nasrallah and F. Henn, Eds. Schizophrenia as a Brain Disease. New York, NY: Oxford University Press; 61.

Erlenmeyer-Kimling, L.; Freidman, D.; Cornblatt, B.; Jacobsen, R. (1985) Electrodermal recovery data on children of schizophrenic parents. Psychiatric Research; 14(149).

Erlenmeyer-Kimling, L.; Rock, D.; Squires-Wheeler, E.; Roberts, S.; Yang, J. (1991) Early life precursors of psychiatric outcomes in adulthood in subjects at risk for schizophrenia or affective diorders. Psychiatry Research; 39(3): 239–256.

Evans, D. A.; Scherr, P. A.; Cook, N. R.; Albert, M. S.; Funkenstein, H. H.; Smith, L. A.; Hebert, L. E.; Wetle, T. T.; Branch, L. G.; Chown, M.; Hennekens, C. H.; Taylor, J. O. (1990) Estimated prevalence of Alzheimer's disease in the United States. Milbank Quarterly; 68: 267–289.

Fadden, G.; Bebbington, P.; Kuipers, L. (1987) The burden of care: The impact of functional psychiatric illness on the patient's family. British Journal of Psychiatry; 150: 285–292.

Faller, K. C. (1988) Child Sexual Abuse. New York, NY: Columbia University Press.

Falloon, I. R. H.; Boyd, J. L.; McGill, C. W.; Razani, J.; Moss, H. B.; Gilderman, A. M.; Simpson, G. M. (1985) Family management in the prevention of morbidity of schizophrenia. Archives of General Psychiatry; 42: 887–896.

Farlow, M.; Gracon, S. I.; Hershey, L. A.; Lewis, K. W.; Sadowsky, C. H.; Dolan-Ureno, J. (1992) A controlled trial of Tacrine in Alzheimer's disease. Journal of the American Medical Association; 268(18): 2523–2529.

Farrington, D. P. (1991) Antisocial personality from childhood to adulthood. The Psychologist: Bulletin of the British Psychological Society; 4: 389–394.

Farrington, D. P. (1989) Early predictors of adolescent aggression and adult violence. Violence Victim; 4(2): 79–100.

Farrington, D. P. (1987) Epidemiology. In: H. C. Quay, Ed. Handbook of Juvenile Delinquency. New York, NY: John Wiley and Sons; 33–61.

Farrington, D. P.; Gallagher, B.; Morley, L.; St. Ledger, R. J.; West, D. J. (1985) Cambridge study in delinquent development: Long-term follow-up (First annual report to the Home Office, August 31, 1985). Cambridge, England: Cambridge University Press.

Farrington, D. P.; Loeber, R.; Elliott, D. S.; Hawkins, J. D.; Kandel, D. B.; Klein, M. W.; McCord, J.; Rowe, D. C.; Tremblay, R. E. (1990) Advancing knowledge about the onset of delinquency and crime. In: B. B. Lahey and A. E. Kazdin, Eds. Advances in Clinical Child Psychology. Vol. 13. New York, NY: Plenum Press; 283–342.

Farrington, D. P.; West, D. J. (1990) The Cambridge study in delinquency development: A long-term follow-up of 411 London males. In: H. J. Kerner and G. Kaiser, Eds. Criminality, Personality, Behavior, and Life History. Berlin, Germany: Springer-Verlag.

Fish, B.; Marcus, J.; Hans, S. L.; Auerbach, J. G.; Perdue, S. (1992) Infants at risk for schizophrenia: Sequellae of a genetic neurointegrative defect. A review and replication analysis of pandysmaturation in the Jerusalem Infant Development Study. Archives of General Psychiatry; 49: 221–235.

Folstein, M. F.; Bassett, S. S.; Anthony, J. C.; Romanoski, A. J.; Nestadt, G. R. (1991) Dementia: Case ascertainment in a community survey. Journal of Gerontology; 46: M132-M138.

Fowler, R. C.; Tsuang, M. (1975) Spouses of schizophrenics: A blind comparative study. Comprehensive Psychiatry; 16: 339–342.

French, L. R.; Schuman, L. M.; Mortimer, J. A.; Hutton, J. T.; Boatman, R. A.; Christians,

B. (1985) A case-control study of dementia of the Alzheimer type. American Journal of Epidemiology; 121: 414–421.

Frick, P. J.; Lahey, B. B.; Hartdagen, S.; Hynd, G. W. (1989) Conduct problems in boys: Relations to maternal personality, marital satisfaction, and socioeconomic status. Journal of Clinical Child Psychology; 18(2): 114–120.

Gabrielli, W. F., Jr.; Mednick, S. A. (1983) Intellectual performance in children of alcoholics. Journal of Nervous and Mental Disorders; 171(1): 444–447.

Garmezy, N. (1983) Stressors of childhood. In: N. Garmezy and M. Rutter, Eds. Stress, Coping and Development in Children. New York, NY: McGraw-Hill; 43–84.

Garmezy, N. (1978) Attentional processes in adult schizophrenia and children at risk. Journal of Psychiatric Research; 14(3): 3–34.

Garmezy, N. (1974) Children at risk: The search for antecedents of schizophrenia. Schizophrenia Bulletin; 55–125.

Garmezy, N.; Masten, A.; Tellegen, A. (1984) The study of stress and competence in children. Child Development; 55: 97–111.

Garmezy, N.; Rodnick, E. (1959) Premorbid adjustment and performance in schizophrenia: Implications for interpreting heterogeneity in schizophrenia. Journal of Nervous and Mental Disease; 129: 450–466.

Geiser, R.; Hoche, L.; King, J. (1988) Respite care for the mentally ill patients and their families. Hospital and Community Psychiatry; 39(3): 291–295.

George, L. K.; Gwyther, L. P. (1986) Caregiver well-being: A multidimensional examination of family caregivers of demented adults. The Gerontologist; 26: 253–259.

Gibbons, J. S.; Horn, S. H.; Powell, J. M.; Gibbons, J. L. (1984) Schizophrenic patients and their families. British Journal of Psychiatry; 144: 70–77.

Gittelman-Klein, R.; Klein, D. F. (1969) Premorbid social adjustment and prognosis in schizophrenia. Journal of Psychiatric Research; 7: 35–53.

Goate, A. M.; Chartier-Harlin, M.; Mullan, M.; Brown, J.; Crawford, F.; Fidani, L.; Giuffra, L.; Haynes, A.; Irving, N.; James, L.; Mant, R.; Newton, P.; Rooke, K.; Roques, P.; Talbot, C.; Pericak-Vance, M.; Roses, A.; Williamson, R.; Rossor, M.; Owen, M.; Hardy, J. (1991) Segregation of a missense mutation in the amyloid precursor protein gene with familial Alzheimer's disease. Nature; 349: 704–706.

Goate, A. M.; Haynes, A. R.; Owen, M. J.; Farrall, M.; James, L. A.; Lai, L. Y. C.; Mullan, M. J.; Roques, P.; Rossor, M. N.; Williamson, R.; Hardy, J. A. (1989) Predisposing locus for Alzheimer's disease on chromosome 21. Lancet; I(8634): 352–355.

Goldberg, E. M.; Morrison, S. L. (1963) Schizophrenia and social class. British Journal of Psychiatry; 109: 785–802.

Goldstein, A.; Kalant, H. (1990) Drug policy: Striking the right balance. Science; 249: 1513–1521.

Goodwin, D. W. (1985) Alcoholism and genetics. Archives of General Psychiatry; 42: 171–174.

Goodwin, D. W.; Schulsinger, F.; Hermansen, L.; Guze, S. B.; Winokur, G. (1973) Alcohol problems in adoptees raised apart from alcoholic biological parents. Archives of General Psychiatry; 28: 238–243.

Gorenstein, E. E.; Mammato, C. A.; Sandy, J. M. (1989) Performance on inattentive-overactive children on selected measures of prefontal-type function. Journal of Clinical Psychology; 45(4): 619–632.

Gotlib, I. H.; Avison, W. R. (1993) Children at risk for psychopathology. In: C. G. Costello, Ed. Basic Issues in Psychopathology. New York, NY: Guilford Press; 271–319.

Gottesman, I. I. (1993) The origins of schizophrenia: Past as prologue. In: R. Plomin and

G. E. McClearn, Eds. Nature, Nurture, and Psychology. Washington, DC: American Psychological Association Books.

Gottesman, I. I. (1991) Schizophrenia Genesis: The Origins of Madness. New York, NY: W. H. Freeman and Company.

Gottesman, I. I.; Bertelsen, A. (1989) Confirming unexpressed genotypes for schizophrenia: Risks in the offspring of Fischer's Danish identical and fraternal discordant twins. Archives of General Psychiatry; 46: 867–872.

Graves, A. B.; van Duijn, C. M.; Chandra, V.; Fratiglioni, L.; Heyman, A.; Jorm, A. F.; Kokmen, E.; Kondo, K.; Mortimer, J. A.; Rocca, W. A.; Shalat, S. L.; Soininen, H.; Hofman, A. (1991) (for the EURODEM Risk Factors Research Group). Alcohol and tobacco consumption as risk factors for Alzheimer's disease: A collaborative reanalysis of case-control studies. International Journal of Epidemiology; 20(Suppl. 2): S48-S57.

Graves, A. B.; White, E.; Koepsell, T. D.; Reifler, B. V.; van Belle, G.; Larson, E. B.; Raskind, M. (1990) The association between head trauma and Alzheimer's disease. American Journal of Epidemiology; 131: 491–501.

Green, A. H. (1991) Child sexual abuse and incest. In: M. Lewis, Ed. Child and Adolescent Psychiatry: A Comprehensive Textbook. Baltimore, MD: Williams & Wilkins; 1019–1030.

Green, A. H. (1978) Psychopathology of abused children. Journal of the American Academy of Child Psychiatry; 17: 92–103.

Greenberg, M. T.; Speltz, M. L.; DeKlyen, M. (1993) The role of attachment in the early development of disruptive behavior problems. Development and Psychopathology; 5: 191–214.

Grove, W. M.; Clementz, B. A.; Iacono, W. G.; Katsanis, J. (1992) Smooth pursuit ocular motor dysfunction in schizophrenia: Evidence for a major gene. American Journal of Psychiatry; 149(10): 1362–1368.

Grunbaum, L.; Gammeltoft, M. (1993) Young children of schizophrenic mothers. American Journal of Orthopsychiatry; 63(1): 16–27.

Grych, J. H.; Fincham, F. D. (1991) Marital conflict and children's adjustment: A cognitive contextual framework. Psychological Bulletin; 108: 267–290.

Hafner, H.; Gattez, W. F. (1990) Search for the Causes of Schizophrenia, Vol. 2. New York, NY: Springer-Verlag.

Hagnell, O.; Isberg, P.; Lanke, J.; Rorsman, B.; Ohman, R. (1986) Predictors of alcoholism in the Lundby Study. III. Social risk factors for alcoholism. European Archives of Psychiatry and Neurological Science. 235(4): 197–199.

Hardy, J. A.; Higgins, G. A. (1992) Alzheimer's disease: The amyloid cascade hypothesis. Science; 256: 184–185.

Hardy, J. B.; Streett, R. (1989) Family support and parenting education in the home: An effective extension of clinic-based preventive health care services for poor children. The Journal of Pediatrics; 115(6): 927–931.

Hawkins, J. D.; Catalano, R. F.; Miller, J. Y. (1992) Risk and protective factors for alcohol and other drug problems in adolescence and early adulthood: Implications for substance abuse prevention. Psychological Bulletin; 112(1): 64–105.

Hawkins, J. D.; Lam, T. (1987) Teacher practices, social development, and delinquency. In: J. D. Burchard and S. N. Burchard, Eds. Prevention of Delinquent Behavior. Newbury Park, CA: Sage Publications; 241–274.

Hawkins, J. D.; Weis, J. G. (1985) The social development model: An integrated approach to delinquency prevention. Journal of Primary Prevention; 6(2): 73–97.

Hechtman, L. (1991) Resilience and vulnerability in long term outcome of attention deficit disorder. Canadian Journal of Psychiatry; 36: 415–421.

Helzer, J.; Canino, G.; Yeh, E. K.; Bland, R. C.; Lee, C. K.; Hwu, H. G.; Newman, S. (1990) Alcoholism—North America and Asia. Archives of General Psychiatry; 47(4): 313–319.

Henderson, A. S.; Jorm, A. F.; Korten, A. E.; Creasey, H.; McCusker, E.; Broe, G. A.; Longley, W.; Anthony, J. C. (1992) Environmental risk factors for Alzheimer's disease: Their relationship to age of onset and to familial or sporadic types. Psychological Medicine; 22: 429–436.

Henn, F. A.; Johnson, A.; Edwards, E. (1985) Melancolia in rodents: Neurobiology and pharmacology. Psychopharmacology Bulletin; 21: 443–446.

Hersen, M.; Bellack, A. S. (1976) Social skills training for chronic patients: Rationale, research findings and future directions. Comprehensive Psychiatry; 17: 559–580.

Heston, L. L. (1966) Psychiatric disorders in foster home reared children of schizophrenia mothers. British Journal of Psychiatry; 112(819).

Hetherington, E. M.; Cox, M.; Cox, R. (1982) Effects of divorce on parents and children. In: M. Lamb, Ed. Non-traditional families. Hillsdale, NJ: Lawrence Erlbaum Associates; 223–285.

Heyman, A.; Wilkinson, W. E.; Stafford, J. A.; Helms, M. J.; Sigmon, A. H.; Weinberg, T. (1984) Alzheimer's disease: A study of epidemiological aspects. Annals of Neurology; 15: 335–341.

Hill, S.; Steinhauer, S.; Park, J.; Zubin, J. (1990) Event-related potential characteristics in children of alcoholics from high density families. Alcohol Clinical and Experimental Research; 14: 6–16.

Hinshaw, S. P. (1992) Externalizing behavior problems: Academic causal relationships and underlying mechanisms. Psychological Bulletin; Vol. III(I): 127–155.

Hoffman-Plotkin, D.; Twentyman, C. (1984) A multimodal assessment of behavioral and cognitive deficits in abused and neglected preschoolers. Child Development; 55: 794–802.

Holzman, P. S. (1983) Smooth pursuit eye movements in psychopathology. Schizophrenia Bulletin; 9(1): 33–36.

Holzman, P. S.; Proctor, L. R.; Hughes, D. W. (1973) Eye-tracking patterns in schizophrenia. Science; 181(95): 179–181.

Holzman, P. S.; Solomon, C. M.; Levin, S.; Waternaux, C. S. (1984) Pursuit eye movement dysfunctions in schizophrenia, family evidence for specificity. Archives of General Psychiatry; 41(136).

Hough, R. L.; Landsverk, J. A.; Karno, M.; Burnam, M. A.; Timbers, D. M.; Escobar, J. I.; Regier, D. A. (1987) Utilization of health and mental health services by Los Angeles Mexican Americans and non-Hispanic whites. Archives of General Psychiatry; 44: 702–709.

Howes, C.; Espinosa, M. P. (1985) The consequences of child abuse for the formation of relationships with peers. Child Abuse and Neglect; 9: 397–404.

Hrubec, Z.; Omenn, G. S. (1981) Evidence of genetic predisposition to alcohol cirrhosis and psychosis: Twin concordances for alcoholism and its biological end points by zygosity among male veterans. Alcohol Clinical and Experimental Research; 5: 207–212.

Iacano, W. G. (1985) Psychophysiological markers of psychopathology: A review. Canadian Journal of Psychiatry; 46: 883–889.

Iacano, W. G.; Bassett, A. S.; Jones, B. D. (1988) Eye tracking dysfunction associated with partial trisomy of chromosome 5 and schizophrenia. Archives of General Psychiatry; 45: 1140–1141.

IOM (Institute of Medicine). (1989) Community approaches and perspectives from other health fields. In: Prevention and Treatment of Alcohol Problems: Research Opportunities. Washington, DC: National Academy Press; 109–127.

Jaffe, P. G.; Hurley, D. J.; Wolfe, D. (1990) Children's observations of violence: I. Critical issues in child development and intervention planning. Canadian Journal of Psychiatry; 35(6): 466–470.

Jones, M. B.; Offord, D. R. (1989) Reduction of antisocial behavior in poor children by nonschool skill-development. Journal of Child Psychology and Psychiatry; 30(5): 737–750.

Jones, M. B.; Offord, D. R.; Abrams, N. (1980) Brothers, sisters and antisocial behavior. British Journal of Psychiatry; 136: 139–145.

Jouriles, E. N.; Murphy, C. M.; O'Leary, K. D. (1989) Effects of maternal mood on mother-son interaction patterns. Journal of Abnormal Child Psychology; 17(5): 513–525.

Kaplan, G. A.; Roberts, R. E.; Camacho, T. C.; Coyne, J. C. (1987) Psychosocial predictors of depression: Prospective evidence from the Human Population Laboratory Studies. American Journal of Epidemiology; 125: 206–220.

Katzman, R. (1993) Views and reviews: Education and the prevalence of dementia and Alzheimer's disease. Neurology; 43: 13–20.

Katzman R.; Saitoh, T. (1991) Advances in Alzheimer's disease. FASEB; 5: 278–286.

Kaufman, J. (1991) Depressive disorders in maltreated children. Journal of the American Academy of Child and Adolescent Psychiatry; 30: 257–265.

Kaufman, J.; Cicchetti, D. (1989) The effects of maltreatment on school-age children's socioemotional development: Assessments in a day camp setting. Developmental Psychology; 15: 516–524.

Kazdin, A. E. (1992) Overt and covert antisocial behavior: Child and family characteristics among psychiatric inpatient children. Journal of Child and Family Studies; 1: 3–20.

Kazdin, A.; Moser, J.; Colbus, D.; Bell, R. (1985) Depressive symptoms among physically abused and psychiatrically disturbed children. Journal of Abnormal Psychology; 94: 298–307.

Kellam, S. G.; Brown, C. H.; Fleming, J. P. (1982) Social adaptation to first grade and teenage drug, alcohol and cigarette use. Journal of School Health; 52(5): 301–306.

Kellam, S. G.; Brown, C. H.; Rubin, B. R.; Einsminger, M. E. (1983) Paths leading to teenage psychiatric symptoms and substance use: Developmental epidemiologic studies in Woodlawn. In: S. B. Guze, F. J. Earls, and J. E. Barratt, Eds. Childhood Psychopathology and Development. New York, NY: Raven Press; 17–51.

Keller, M. B.; Lavori, P. W.; Beardslee, W. R.; Wunder, J.; Ryan, N. (1991) Depression in children and adolescents: New data on "undertreatment" and a literature review on the efficacy of available treatments. Journal of Affective Diorders; 21(3): 163–171.

Kempe, C. H.; Silverman, B.; Steele, B.; Droegemueller, W.; Silver, H. K. (1962) The battered child syndrome. Journal of the American Medical Association; 181: 105–112.

Kendell, R. E.; Kemp, I. W. (1989) Maternal influenza in the etiology of schizophrenia. Archives of General Psychiatry; 46(10): 878–882.

Kendall-Tackett, K. A.; Williams, L.; Finkelhor, D. (1993) The impact of sexual abuse on children: A review and synthesis of recent empirical studies. Psychological Bulletin; 113: 164–180.

Kendler, K. S. (1988) The genetics of schizophrenia: An overview. In: M. T. Tsuang and J. C. Simpson, Eds. Handbook of Schizophrenia, Vol. 3. New York, NY: Elsevier Science; 437.

Kendler, K. S.; Gruenberg, A. M. (1984) An independent analysis of the Copenhagen sample of the Danish adoption study of schizophrenia: VI. The pattern of psychiatric illness, as defined by DSM-III in adoptees and relatives. Archives of General Psychiatry; 41: 555–564.

Kendler, K. S.; Masterson, C. C.; Davis, K. L. (1985) Psychiatric illness in first-degree relatives of patients with paranoid psychosis, schizophrenia, and medical illness. British Journal of Psychiatry; 147: 524–531.

Kennedy, J. L.; Giuffra, L. A.; Moises, H. W.; Cavalli-Sforza, L. L.; Pakstis, A. J.; Kidd, J. R.; Castiglione, C. M.; Sjorgen, B.; Wetterberg, L.; Kidd, K. K. (1988) Evidence against linkage of schizophrenia to markers on chromosome 5 in a northern Swedish pedigree. Nature; 336: 167–170.

Kety, S. S. (1983) Observations on genetic and environmental influences in the etiology of mental disorders from studies on adoptees and their relatives. In: S. S. Kety, L. P. Rowland, R. L. Sedman, and S. W. Matthysse, Eds. Genetics of Neurological and Psychiatric Disorders. New York, NY: Raven Press.

Kety, S. S. (1988) Schizophrenic illness in the families of schizophrenic adoptees: Findings from the Danish national sample. Schizophrenia Bulletin; 14: 217–222.

Kety, S. S.; Rosenthal, D.; Wender, P. H.; Schulsinger, F.; Jacobsen, B. (1978) The biological and adoptive families of adopted individuals who become schizophrenic. In: L. C. Wynne, R. L. Cromwell, and S. Matthysse, Eds. The Nature of Schizophrenia. New York, NY: John Wiley and Sons; 25–37.

Kinard, E. M. (1982) Experiencing child abuse: Effects on emotional adjustment. American Journal of Orthopsychiatry; 52: 82–91.

Kinard, E. M. (1980) Emotional development in physically abused children. American Journal of Orthopsychiatry; 50: 686–696.

Knight, B. J.; West, D. J. (1975) Temporary and continuing delinquency. British Journal of Criminology; 15: 43–50.

Knop, J.; Teasdale, T. W.; Schulsinger, F. (1985) A prospective study of young men at high risk for alcoholism: School behavior and achievement. Journal of Studies on Alcohol; 46: 273–278.

Kokes, R. F.; Strauss, J. S.; Klormann, R. (1977) Premorbid adjustment in schizophrenia. Schizophrenia Bulletin; 3: 186–213.

Kokmen, E.; Beard, C. M.; Chandra, V.; Offord, K. P.; Schoenberg, B. S.; Ballard, D. J. (1991) Clinical risk factors for Alzheimer's disease: A population-based case-control study. Neurology; 41(9): 1393–1397.

Kolvin, F. J.; Miller, J. W.; Fleeting, M.; Kolvin, P. A. (1988) Social and parenting factors affecting criminal-offence rates: Findings from the Newcastle thousand family study (1947–1980). British Journal of Psychiatry; 152: 80–90.

Kugelmass, S.; Marcus, J.; Schmueli, J. (1985) Psychophysiological reactivity in high risk children. Schizophrenia Bulletin; 11(1): 66–73.

Lahey, B. B.; Russo, M. F.; Walker, J. L.; Piacentini, J. C. (1989) Personality characteristics of the mothers of children with disruptive behavior disorders. Journal of Consulting and Clinical Psychology; 57(4): 512–515.

Landsberg, J. P.; McDonald, B.; Watt, F. (1992) Absence of aluminum in neuritic plaque cores in Alzheimer's disease. Nature; 360: 65–68.

Lane, T. W.; Davis, G. E. (1987) Child maltreatment and juvenile delinquency: Does a relationship exist? In: J. D. Burchard and S. N. Burchard, Eds. Prevention of Delinquent Behavior: Primary Prevention of Psychopathology. Newbury Park, CA: Sage Publications; 122–138.

Lee, C. K.; Kwak, Y. S.; Yamamoto, J.; Rhee, H.; Kim, Y. S.; Han, J. H.; Choi, J. O.; Lee, Y. H. (1990) Psychiatric epidemiology in Korea: Part II. Urban and rural differences. Journal of Nervous and Mental Disease; 178(4): 247–252.

Lee, C. M.; Gotlib, I. H. (1991) Family disruption, parental availability and child adjustment: An integrative review. In: R. J. Prinz, Ed. Advances in the Behavioral Assessment of Children and Families. Vol. 5. London, England: Kingsley Publishers.

Levy, D. L.; Dorus, E.; Shaughnessy, R.; Yasillo, N. J.; Pandey, G. N.; Janicak, P. G.; Gibbons, R. D.; Gaviria, M.; Davis, J. M. (1985) Pharmacologic evidence for specificity of pursuit dysfunction to schizophrenia. Lithium carbonate associated with abnormal pursuit. Archives of General Psychiatry; 42(4): 335–341.

Levy, D.; Sheflin, N. (1985) The demand for alcoholic beverages: An aggregate time-series analysis. Journal of Public Policy and Marketing; 4: 47–54.

Lewis, D. O. (1992) From abuse to violence: Psychological consequences of maltreatment. Journal of the American Academy of Child and Adolescent Psychiatry; 31(3): 383–391.

Lewis, M. S. (1989) Age incidence and schizophrenia: Part I. The season of birth controversy. Schizophrenia Bulletin; 15: 59–73.

Lex, B. W.; Lukas, S. E.; Greenwald, N. E.; Mendelson, J. H. (1988) Alcohol-induced changes in body sway in women at risk for alcoholism: A pilot study. Journal of Studies on Alcohol; 49: 346–356.

Li, G.; Silverman, J. M.; Mohs, R. C. (1991) Clinical genetic studies of Alzheimer's disease. The Psychiatric Clinics of North America; 14(2): 267–286.

Loeber, R.; Brinhaupt, V. P.; Green, S. M. (1990) Attention deficits, impulsivity, and hyperactivity with or without conduct problems: Relationships to delinquency and unique contextual factors. In: R. J. McMahon and R. Peters, Eds. Behavior Disorders of Adolescence: Research, Intervention and Policy in Clinical and School Settings. New York, NY: Plenum Press.

Loeber, R. T.; Dishion, T. (1983) Early predictors of male delinquency: A review. Psychological Bulletin; 93: 68–99.

Lund, C. A.; Landesman-Dwyer, S. (1979) Pre-delinquent and disturbed adolescents: The role of parental alcoholism. Currents in Alcoholism; 5: 339–348.

Luthar, S. S. (1993) Annotation: Methodological and conceptual issues in research on childhood resilience. Journal of Child Psychology and Psychiatry; 34(4): 441–453.

McCord, J. (1988a) Alcoholism: Toward understanding genetic and social factors. Psychiatry; 51(2): 131–141.

McCord, J. (1988b) Identifying developmental paradigms leading to alcoholism. Journal of Studies on Alcohol; 49(4): 357–362.

McCord, J. (1983) A forty year perspective on effects of child abuse and neglect. Child Abuse and Neglect; 7: 265–270.

McGauhey, P. J.; Starfield, B.; Alexander, C.; Ensminger, M. E. (1991) Social environment and vulnerability of low birth weight children: A social-epidemiological perspective. Pediatrics; 88(5): 943–953.

McLeer, S. V.; Deblinger, E.; Atkins, M. S.; Foa, E. B.; Ralphe, D. L. (1988) Post-traumatic stress disorder in sexually abused children: A prospective study. Journal of the American Academy of Child and Adolescent Psychiatry; 27(5): 650–654.

McNeil, T. F. (1987) Perinatal influences in the development of schizophrenia. In: H. Helmenche and F. A. Henn, Eds. Biological Perspectives of Schizophrenia. Chichester, NY: John Wiley and Sons.

Main, M.; George, C. (1985) Response of abused and disadvantaged toddlers to distress in agemates: A study in the daycare setting. Developmental Psychology; 21: 407–412.

Main, M.; Hesse, E. (1990) Adult lack of resolution of attachment-related trauma related to infant disorganized/disoriented behavior in the Ainsworth strange situation: Linking parental states of mind to infant behavior in a stressful situation. In: M. T. Greenberg,

206 / Reducing Risks for Mental Disorders

D. Cicchetti, and M. Cummings, Eds. Attachment in the Preschool Years: Theory, Research and Intervention. Chicago, IL: University of Chicago Press; 339–426.
Manuelidis, E. E.; Manuelidis, L. (1991) Search for a transmissible agent in Alzheimer's disease: Studies of human buffy coat. Current Topics in Microbiology and Immunology; 172: 275–280.
Marcus, J.; Auerbach, J.; Wilkinson, L.; Burack, C. M. (1981) Infants at risk for schizophrenia. The Jerusalem Infant Development Study. Archives of General Psychiatry; 38(6): 703–713.
Marcus, J.; Hans, S. L.; Mirsky, A. F.; Aubrey, A. (1987) A review of NIMH-Israeli kibbutz study and the Jerusalem Infant Development Study. Schizophrenia Bulletin; 13(425): 425–438.
Maziade, M.; Coté, R.; Bernier, H.; Boutin, P.; Thivierge, J. (1989) Significance of extreme temperament in infancy for clinical status in pre-school years: I. British Journal of Psychiatry; 14: 535–543.
Mednick, S. A.; Gabrielli, W. F., Jr.; Hutchings, B. (1984) Genetic influences in criminal convictions: Evidence from an adoption cohort. Science; 224(4651): 891–894.
Mednick, S. A.; Moffitt, T.; Gabrielli, W.; Hutchings, G. (1986) Genetic factors in criminal behavior: A review. In: D. Olweus, J. Block, and M. Radke-Yarrow, Eds. Development of Antisocial and Prosocial Behavior: Research Theories and Issues. New York, NY: Academic Press.
Mednick, S. A.; Parnas, J.; Schulsinger, F. (1987) The Copenhagen High-Risk Project, 1962–86. Schizophrenia Bulletin; 13(3): 485–495.
Mednick, S.; Schulsinger, F. (1968) Some premorbid characteristics related to breakdown in children with schizophrenic mothers. In: D. Rosenthal and S. Kety, Eds. Transmission of Schizophrenia. New York, NY: Pergamon Press.
Mednick, S. A.; Silverton, L. (1988) High risk studies of the etiology of schizophrenia. In: M. T. Tsuang and J. C. Simpson, Eds. Handbook of Schizophrenia, Vol. 3. New York, NY: Elsevier Science; 543.
Mednick, S. A.; Venables, P. H.; Schulsinger, F.; Dalais, C.; Van Dusen, K. (1984) A controlled study of primary prevention: The Mauritius Project. In: N. F. Watt, E. J. Anthony, L. C. Wynne, and J. E. Rolf, Eds. Children at Risk for Schizophrenia: A Longitudinal Perspective. Cambridge, England: Cambridge University Press.
Mendez, M. F. (1993) Miscellaneous causes of dementia. In: P. J. Whitehouse, Ed. Dementia. Philadelphia, PA: F. A. Davis; 343–346.
Minde, K. (1992) Aggression in preschoolers: Its relation for socialization. Journal of the American Academy of Child and Adolescent Psychiatry; 31: 5.
Minde, K. (1991) The effect of disordered parenting on the development of children. In: M. Lewis, ed. Child and Adolescent Psychiatry. A Comprehensive Textbook. Baltimore, MD: Williams & Wilkins; 394–407.
Moffitt, T. E. (1993) The neuropsychology of conduct disorder. Development and Psychopathology; 5: 135–151.
Moffitt, T. E. (1990) Juvenile delinquency and attention deficit disorder: Boys' developmental trajectories from age 3 to age 15. Child Development; 61: 893–910.
Moffitt, T. E.; Henry, B. (1991) Neuropsychological studies of juvenile delinquency and juvenile violence. In: J. S. Milner, Ed. Neuropsychology of Aggression. Boston, MA: Kluwer Academic Publishers; 67–91.
Moises, H. W.; Gelernter, J.; Giuffra, L. A.; Zarcone, V.; Wetterberg, L.; Civelli, O.; Kidd, K. K.; Cavalli-Sforza, L. L.; Grandy, D. K.; Kennedy, J. L. (1991) No linkage between D2 dopamine receptor gene region and schizophrenia. Archives of General Psychiatry; 48(7): 643–647.

Moos, R. H.; Billings, A. G. (1982) Children of alcoholics during the recovery process: Alcoholic and matched control families. Addictive Behavior; 7: 155–163.

Mortimer, J. A.; French, L. R.; Hutton, J. T.; Schuman, L. M. (1985) Head injury as a risk factor for Alzheimer's disease. Neurology; 35: 264–267.

Mortimer, J. A.; van Duijn, C. M.; Chandra, V.; Fratiglioni, L.; Graves, A. B.; Heyman, A.; Jorm, A. F.; Kokmen, E.; Kondo, K.; Rocca, W. A.; Shalat, S. L.; Soininen, H.; Hofman, A. (1991) Head trauma as a risk factor for Alzheimer's disease: A collaborative re-analysis of case-control studies. International Journal of Epidemiology; 20: S28–S35.

Moskowitz, D. S.; Schwartzman, A. E. (1989) Painting group portraits: Studying life outcomes for aggressive and withdrawn children. Journal of Personality; 57(4): 723–746.

Moss, H. B.; Yao, J. K.; Maddock, J. M. (1989) Responses by sons of alcoholic fathers to alcoholic and placebo drinks: Perceived mood intoxication and plasma prolactin. Alcohol Clinical and Experimental Research; 13: 252–257.

Mueller-Hill, B.; Beyreuther, K. (1989) Molecular biology of Alzheimer's disease. Annual Review of Biochemistry; 58: 287–307.

Mullan, M.; Crawford, F.; Axelman, K.; Houlden, H.; Lilius, L.; Winblad, B.; Lannfelt, A. (1992) A pathogenic mutation for probable Alzheimer's disease in the APP gene at the N-terminus of b-amyloid. Nature Genetics; 1: 345–347.

Mullan, M.; Houlden, H.; Windelspecht, M.; Fidani, L.; Lombardi, C.; Diaz, P.; Rossor, M.; Crook, R.; Hardy, J.; Duff, K.; Crawford, F. (1992) A locus for familial early-onset Alzheimer's disease on the long arm of chromosome 14, proximal to the (ALT 224) 1-antichymotrypsin gene. Nature Genetics; 2: 340–342.

Muñoz, R. F. (1987) Depression Prevention: Research Directions. Washington, DC: Hemisphere Publishing.

Murphy, E. A.; Breitner, J. C. S. (1992) Threshold model in the genetics of age-dependent disease in twins: I. General principles as applied to Alzheimer disease. American Journal of Medical Genetics; 42: 842–850.

Murphy, L. B.; Moriarity, A. E. (1976) Vulnerability, coping and growth: From infancy to adolescence. New Haven, CT: Yale University Press.

Murray, D. M.; Richards, P. S.; Luepker, R. V.; Johnson, C. A. (1987) The prevention of cigarette smoking in children: Two and three-year follow-up comparisons of four prevention strategies. Journal of Behavioral Medicine; 10(6): 595–611.

Murray, R. M.; Clifford, C. A.; Gurling, H. M. (1983) Twin and adoption studies. How good is the evidence for a genetic role? Recent Developments in Alcohol; 1: 25–48.

Nee, L. E.; Eldridge, R.; Sunderland, T.; Thomas, C. B.; Katz, D.; Thompson, K. E.; Weingartner, H.; Weiss, H.; Julian, C.; Cohen, R. (1987) Dementia of the Alzheimer type: Clinical and family study of 22 twin pairs. Neurology; 37: 359–363.

Neiswanger, K.; Slaugenhaupt, S. A.; Hughes, H. B.; Frank, E.; Frankel, D. R.; McCarty, M. J.; Chakravarti, A.; Zubenko, G. S.; Kupfer, D. J.; Kaplan, B. B. (1990) Evidence against close linkage of unipolar affective illness to human chromosome 11p markers HRAS1 and INS and chromosome Xq marker DXS52. Biological Psychiatry; 28: 63–72.

Noble, E. P. (1990) Alcoholic fathers and their sons: Neurophysiological, electrophysiological, personality and family correlates. In: H. Begleiter and R. Cloninger, Eds. Banberry Report 33: Genetics and the Biology of Alcoholism. New York, NY: Cold Springs Harbor Laboratory.

Nuechterlein, K. H.; Dawson, M. E.; Venture, J.; Fogelson, D.; Gitlin, M.; Mintz, J. (1990) Testing vulnerability models: Stability of potential vulnerability indicators across clinical state. In: H. Hafner and W. F. Gottaz, Ed. Search for the Causes of Schizophrenia, Vol. II. New York, NY: Springer-Verlag: 177.

O'Callaghan, E.; Sham, P.; Takei, N.; Glover, G.; Murray, R. M. (1991) Schizophrenia after prenatal exposure to 1957 A2 influenza epidemic. Lancet; 337(8752): 1248–1250.

O'Connor, S.; Hesselbrock, V.; Tasman, A.; DePalma, N. (1987) P3 amplitudes in two distinct tasks are decreased in young men with a history of paternal alcoholism. Alcohol; 4: 169–173.

Offord, D. R. (1989) Conduct disorder: Risk factors and prevention. In: Prevention of Mental Disorders, Alcohol and Other Drug Use in Children and Adolescents. OSAP Prevention Monograph—2: DHHS Pub. No. (ADM) 89–1646: 273–307.

Offord, D. R.; Alder, R. J.; Boyle, M. H. (1986) Prevalence and sociodemographic correlates of conduct disorder. American Journal of Social Psychiatry; 6: 272–278.

Offord, D. R.; Boyle, M. H. (1988) The epidemiology of antisocial behavior in early adolescents, aged 12 to 14. In: M. D. Levine and E. R. McAnarney, Eds. Early Adolescent Transitions. Lexington, MA: D. C. Heath and Co.; 245–259.

Offord, D. R.; Boyle, M. H.; Racine, Y. (1989) Ontario Child and Health Study: Correlates of Disorder. Journal of the American Academy of Child and Adolescent Psychiatry; 28: 856–860.

Offord, D. R.; Boyle, M. H.; Racine, Y. A.; Fleming, J. E.; Cadman, D. T.; Blum, H. M.; Byrne, C.; Links, P. S.; Lipman, E. L.; Macmillan, H. L. (1992) Outcome, prognosis and risk in a longitudinal follow-up study. Journal of the American Academy of Child and Adolescent Psychiatry; 31(5): 916–923.

Offord, D. R.; Boyle, M. H.; Szatmari, P.; Rae Grant, N. I.; Links, P. S.; Cadman, D. T.; Byles, J. A.; Crawford, J. W.; Blum, H. M.; Byrne, C.; Thomas, H.; Woodward, C. A. (1987) Ontario Child Health Study: Six month prevalence of disorder and rates of service utilization. Archives of General Psychiatry; 44: 832–836.

Offord, D. R.; Waters, B. G. (1983) Socialization and its failure. In: M. D. Levine, W. B. Carey, A. C. Crocker, and R. T. Gross, Eds. Developmental-Behavioral Pediatrics. Philadelphia, PA: W. B. Saunders; 650–682.

O'Grady, D. D. (1983) Protective factors contributing to resilience in children at high risk for psychological disorder. Ann Arbor, MI: University Microfilms International.

O'Grady, D.; Metz, J. R. (1987) Resilience in children at high risk for psychological disorder. Journal of Pediatric Psychology; 12: 3–23.

Oldridge, M. L.; Hughes, I. C. T. (1992) Psychological well-being in families with a member suffering from schizophrenia: An investigation into long-standing problems. British Journal of Psychiatry; 161: 249–251.

O'Malley, S. S.; Maisto, S. A. (1985) Effects of family drinking history and expectancies on response to alcohol in men. Journal of Studies on Alcohol; 46: 289–297.

Osborn, S. G.; West, D. J. (1980) Do delinquents really reform? Journal of Adolescence; 3: 99–114.

OTA (Office of Technology Assessment). (1990) Confused Minds, Burdened Families: Finding Help for People With Alzheimer's and Other Dementias. U.S. Congress; Washington, DC: Government Printing Office; OTA-BA-403.

OTA (Office of Technology Assessment). (1987) Losing a Million Minds: Confronting the Tragedy of Alzheimer's Disease and Other Dementias. U.S. Congress; Washington, DC: Government Printing Office; OTA-BA-323.

Pandey, G. N.; Fawcett, J.; Gibbons, R.; Clark, D. C.; Davis, J. M. (1988) Platelet monoamine oxidase activity. Psychiatry Research; 7(325): 15–24.

Patterson, G. R.; Chamberlain, P.; Reid, J.B. (1982) A comparative evaluation of a parent training program. Behavior Therapy; 13: 638–650.

Patterson, G. R.; DeBarysh, B. D.; Ramsey, E. (1989) A developmental perspective on antisocial behavior. American Psychologist; 44: 329–335.

Pauls, D. L.; Gerhard, D. S.; Lacy, L. G.; Hostetter, A. M.; Allen, C. R.; Bland, S. D.; LaBuda, M. C.; Egeland, J. A. (1991) Linkage of bipolar affective disorders to markers on chromosome 11p is excluded in a second lateral extension of Amish pedigree 110. Genomics; 11(3): 730–736.

Pericak-Vance, M. A.; Bebout, J. L.; Gaskell, P. C., Jr.; Yamaoka, L. H.; Hung, W. Y.; Alberts, M. J.; Walker, A. P. (1991) Linkage studies in familial Alzheimer disease: Evidence for chromosome 19 linkage. American Journal of Human Genetics; 48: 1034–1050.

Perry, M. A.; Doran, L. D.; Wells, E. A. (1983) Developmental and behavioral characteristics of the physically abused child. Journal of Clinical Child Psychology; 12: 320–324.

Petersen, A. C.; Compas, B. E.; Brooks-Gunn, J. (1992) Depression in Adolescence: Current Knowledge, Research Directions, and Implications for Programs and Policy. New York, NY: Carnegie.

Pope, H. G.; Jones, J. M.; Cohen, B. M.; Lipinski, J. F. (1982) Failure to find evidence of schizophrenia in first degree relatives of schizophrenia probands. American Journal of Psychiatry; 138: 826.

Porjesz, B.; Begleiter, H. (1983) Brain dysfunction and alcohol. In: B. Kissin and H. Begleiter, Eds. The Pathogenesis of Alcoholism. New York, NY: Plenum Press; 415.

Pratt, C. C.; Schmall, V. L.; Wright, S. (1985) Burden and coping strategies of caregivers to Alzheimer's disease patients. Family Relations; 34: 27–33.

Propping, P. (1980) Genetic aspects of alcohol action on the electroencephalogram (EEG). Advances in Experimental Medical Biology; 126: 589–602.

Quinton, D.; Rutter, M. (1988) Parental Breakdown: The Making and Breaking of Intergenerational Links. Aldershot, England: Gower Publishing.

Quinton, D.; Rutter, M. (1985) Family pathology and child psychiatric disorder: A four year prospective study. In: A. R. Nicol, Ed. Longitudinal Studies in Child Psychology and Psychiatry. Chichester, England: John Wiley and Sons; 91–134.

Rae Grant, N.; Thomas, B. H.; Offord, D. R.; Boyle, M. H. (1989) Risk, protective factors, and the prevalence of behavioral and emotional disorders in children and adolescents. Journal of the American Academy of Child and Adolescent Psychiatry; 28(2): 262–268.

Reitsma-Street, M.; Offord, D. R.; Finch, T. (1985) Pairs of same-sexed siblings discordant for antisocial behaviour. British Journal of Psychiatry; 146: 415–423.

Renvoize, E. B.; Mindham, R. H. S.; Stewart, M.; McDonald, R.; Wallace, D. R. D. (1986) Identical twins discordant for presenile dementia of the Alzheimer type. British Journal of Psychiatry; 149: 509–512.

Revely, A. M.; Revely, M. A.; Murray, R. M. (1984) Cerebral ventricular enlargement in non-genetic schizophrenia: A controlled twin study. British Journal of Psychiatry; 144(89): 89–93.

Richman, N.; Stevenson, J.; Graham, P. J. (1982) Pre-school to School: A Behavioural Study. London, England: Academic Press.

Roberts, G. W.; Allsop, D.; Bruton, C. (1989) The occult aftermath of boxing. Neuropathology and Applied Neurobiology; 15: 273–274.

Robins, L. N. (1984) The natural history of adolescent drug use. American Journal of Public Health; 74: 656–657.

Robins, L. N. (1980) The natural history of drug abuse. Acta Psychiatrica Scandinavica; 62(Suppl. 284): 7–20.

Robins, L. N. (1970) Follow-up studies investigating childhood disorders. In: E. H. Hare and J. K. Wing, Eds. Psychiatric Epidemiology. London, England: Oxford University Press.

Robins, L. N. (1966) Deviant Children Grown Up: A Sociological and Psychiatric Study of Sociopathic Personality. Baltimore, MD: Williams & Wilkins.

Robins, L. N.; Ratcliff, K. S. (1980) Childhood conduct disorders and later arrest. In: L. N. Robins, P. J. Clayton, and J. K. Wing, Eds. The Social Consequences of Psychiatric Illness. New York, NY: Brunner/Mazel; 248–263.

Robins, L. N.; Wish, E. (1977) Childhood deviance as a developmental process: A study of 223 urban men from birth to 18. Social Forces; 56: 448–473.

Rocca, W. A.; Bonaiuto, S.; Lippi, A.; Luciani, P.; Turtu, F.; Cavarzeran, F.; Amaducci, L. (1990) Prevalence of clinically diagnosed Alzheimer's disease and other dementing disorders: A door-to-door survey in Appignano, Marcerata Province, Italy. Neurology; 40: 626–631.

Rocca, W. A.; van Duijn, C. M.; Chandra, V.; Fratiglioni, L.; Graves, A. B.; Heyman, A.; Jorm, A. F.; Kokmen, E.; Kondo, K.; Mortimer, J. A.; Shalat, S.; Soininen, H.; Hofman, A. (1991) Maternal age and Alzheimer's disease: A collaborative re-analysis of case-control studies. International Journal of Epidemiology; 20: S21–S27.

Rogeness, G.; Amrung, S.; Macedo, C.; Harris, W.; Fisher, C. (1986) Psychopathology in abused and neglected children. Journal of the American Academy of Child Psychiatry; 25: 659–665.

Rohrbeck, C.; Twentyman, C. (1986) Multimodal assessment of impulsiveness in abusing, neglecting, and nonmaltreating mothers and their preschool children. Journal of Consulting and Clinical Psychology; 54: 231–236.

Rosenbaum, A.; O'Leary, K. D. (1981) Children: The unintended victims of marital violence. American Journal of Orthopsychiatry; 51: 692–699.

Rosenberg, M. S. (1987) New directions for research on the psychological maltreatment of children. American Psychologist; 42: 166–171.

Rosenthal, D. (1974) The concept of subschizophrenic disorders. In: S. A. Mednick, F. Schulsinger, J. Higgins, and B. Bell, Eds. Genetics, Environment and Psychopathy. Amsterdam, The Netherlands: North-Holland Publishing Company.

Rutter, M. (1990) Commentary: Some focus and process considerations regarding effects of parental depression on children. Developmental Psychology; 26(1): 60–67.

Rutter, M. (1989) Pathways from childhood to adult life. Journal of Child Psychology and Psychiatry; 30(1): 23–51.

Rutter, M. (1985a) Family and school influences on behavioural development. Journal of Child Psychology and Psychiatry; 26: 349–368.

Rutter, M. (1985b) Resilience in the face of adversity: Protective factors and resistance to psychiatric disorder. British Journal of Psychiatry; 147: 598–611.

Rutter, M. (1983) Introduction: Concepts of brain dysfunction syndromes. In: M. Rutter, Ed. Developmental Neuropsychiatry. New York, NY: Guilford Press; 1–14.

Rutter, M. (1981) Stress, coping and development: Some issues and some questions. Journal of Child Psychology and Psychiatry; 22(4): 323–356.

Rutter, M. (1979) Protective factors in children's responses to stress and disadvantage. In: M. W. Kent and J. E. Rolf, Eds. Primary Prevention of Psychopathology, Vol. 3: Social Competence in Children. Hanover, NH: University Press of New England.

Rutter, M. (1978) Family, area, and school influences in the genesis of conduct disorders. In: L. A. Hersov and M. Berger, Eds. Aggression and Anti-social Behaviour in Childhood and Adolescence. London, England: Pergamon Press; 95–114.

Rutter, M. (1977) Brain damage syndromes in childhood: Concepts and findings. Journal of Child Psychology and Psychiatry; 18: 1–21.

Rutter, M.; Giller, H. (1983) Juvenile Delinquency: Trends and Perspectives. New York, NY: Penguin Books.

Rutter, M.; Maughan, B.; Mortimore, P.; Ouston, J.; Smith, A. (1979) 15000 Hours: Secondary Schools and Their Effects on Children. Cambridge, MA: Harvard University Press.

Rutter, M.; Quinton, D. (1984) Parental psychiatric disorders: Effects on children. Psychological Medicine; 14: 853–880.

Rutter, M.; Quinton, D. (1977) Psychiatric disorder: Ecological factors and concepts of causation. In: H. McGurk, Ed. Ecological Factors in Human Development. Amsterdam, The Netherlands: North-Holland Publishing Co.

Rutter, M.; Tizard, J.; Whitmore, K. (1970) Education, Health and Behaviour. London, England: Longman Publishing Group.

St. Clair, D.; Blackwood, D.; Muir, W.; Bailie, D.; Hubbard, A.; Wright, A.; Evans, H. J. (1989) No linkage of chromosome 5q11-q13 markers to schizophrenia in Scottish families. Nature; 339: 305–309.

St. George-Hyslop, P. H.; Haines, J. L.; Farrer, L. A.; Polinsky, R.; Van Broeckhoven, C.; Goate, A. (1990) Genetic linkage studies suggest that Alzheimer's disease is not a single homogeneous disorder. Nature; 347: 194–197.

St. George-Hyslop, P.; Haines, J.; Rogaev, E.; Mortilla, M.; Vaula, G.; Pericak-Vance, M.; Foncin, J.-F.; Montesi, M.; Bruni, A.; Sorbi, S.; Rainero, I.; Pinessi, L.; Pollen, D.; Polinsky, R.; Nee, L.; Kennedy, J.; Macciardi, F.; Rogaeva, E.; Liang, Y.; Alexandrova, N.; Lukiw, W.; Schlumpf, K.; Tanzi, T.; Tsuda, T.; Farrer, L.; Cantu, J. M.; Duara, R.; Amaducci, L.; Bergamini, L.; Gusella, J.; Roses, A.; Crapper McLachlan, D. (1992) Genetic evidence for a novel familial Alzheimer's disease locus on chromosome 14. Nature Genetics; 2: 330–334.

St. George-Hyslop, P. H.; Tanzi, R. E.; Polinsky, R. J.; Haines, J. L.; Nee, L.; Watkins, P. C.; Myers, R. H.; Feldman, R. G.; Pollen, D.; Drachman, D.; Growdon, J.; Bruni, A.; Foncin, J. F.; Salmon, D.; Frommelt, P.; Amaducci, L.; Sorbi, S.; Piacentini, S.; Stewart, G. D.; Hobbs, W. J.; Conneally, P. M.; Gusella, J. F. (1987) The genetic defect causing familial Alzheimer's disease maps on chromosome 21. Science; 235: 885–890.

Salzinger, S; Kaplan, S.; Pelcovitz, D.; Samit, C.; Kreiger, R. (1984) Parent and teacher assessment of children's behavior in child maltreating families. Journal of the American Academy of Child Psychiatry; 23: 458–464.

Sameroff, A. J. (1987) Transactional risk factors and prevention. In: J. A. Steinberg and M. M. Silverman, Eds. Preventing Mental Disorders: A Research Perspective. Rockville, MD: Department of Health and Human Services; 76.

Sameroff, A. J.; Chandler, M. J. (1975) Reproductive risk and the continuum of caretaking casualty. In: F. D. Horowitz, M. Hetherington, and S. Scarr-Salopatek, Eds. Review of Child Development Research. Vol. 4. Chicago, IL: University of Chicago Press; 187–244.

Sampson, R. J. (1985) Neighborhood and crime: The structural determinants of personal victimization. Journal of Research on Crime and Delinquency; 22: 7–40.

Savoie, T. M.; Emory, E. K.; Moddy-Thomas, S. (1988) Acute alcohol intoxication in socially drinking female and male offspring of alcoholic fathers. Journal of Studies on Alcohol; 49: 430–435.

Schaeffer, K. W.; Parsons, O. A.; Yohman, J. R. (1984) Neuropsychological differences between male familial and nonfamilial alcoholics and nonalcoholics. Alcohol Clinical Experimental Research; 8(4): 347–351.

Schaffer, D.; Stokman, C. S.; O'Connor, P. A.; Shaffer, S.; Barmack, J. E.; Hess, S.; Spalten, D.; Schonfeld, I. S. (1986) Early soft neurological signs and later psychopathology. In: L. Erlenmeyer-Kimling and N. E. Miller, Eds. Life Span Research on the Prediction of Psychopathology. Hillsdale, NJ: Lawrence Erlbaum; 31.

Schellenberg, G. D.; Anderson, L.; O'dahl, S.; Wisjman, E. M.; Sadovnick, A. D.; Ball, M. J.; Larson, E. B.; Kukull, W. A.; Martin, G. M.; Roses, A. D.; Bird, T. D. (1991) APP717, APP693, and PRIP gene mutations are rare in Alzheimer disease. American Journal of Human Genetics; 49: 511–517.

Schellenberg, G. D.; Bird, T. D.; Wijsman, E. M.; Moore, D. K.; Boehnke, M.; Bryant, E. M.; Lampe, T. H.; Nochlin, D.; Sumi, S. M.; Deeb, S. S.; Beyreuther, K.; Martin, G. M. (1988) Absence of linkage of chromosome 21q21 markers to familial Alzheimer's disease. Science; 241: 668–671.

Schuckit, M. A. (in press) Low level of response to alcohol as a predictor of future alcoholism. American Journal of Psychiatry.

Schuckit, M. A. (1994) A clinical model of genetic influences in alcohol dependence. Journal of Studies on Alcohol; 55(1): 5–17.

Schuckit, M. A. (1992) Advances in understanding the vulnerability to alcoholism. In: C. P. O'Brien and J. H. Jaffe, Eds. Advances in Understanding the Vulnerability to Alcoholism. New York, NY: Raven Press; 93–108.

Schuckit, M. A. (1986) Alcoholism and affective disorders: Genetic and clinical implications. American Journal of Psychiatry; 143: 140–147.

Schuckit, M. A. (1981) Twin studies on substance abuse: An overview. In: L. Gedda, P. Parisi, and W. Nance, Eds. Twin Research 3: Epidemiological and Clinical Studies. New York, NY: Alan R. Liss; 61–70.

Schuckit, M. A.; Butters, N.; Lyn, L.; Irwin, M. (1987) Neuropsychological deficits and the risk for alcoholism. Neuropsychopharmacology; 1: 45–53.

Schuckit, M. A.; Goodwin, D. A.; Winokur, G. A. (1972) A study of alcoholism in half-siblings. American Journal of Psychiatry; 128: 1132–1136.

Schulsinger, F.; Knop, J.; Goodwin, D. W.; Teasdale, T. W.; Mikkelsen, U. (1986) A prospective study of young men at high risk for alcoholism. Archives of General Psychiatry; 43(8): 755–760.

Scottish Schizophrenia Research Group. (1985) First episode schizophrenia (IV): Psychiatric and social impact on the family. British Journal of Psychiatry; 150: 340–344.

Sherrington, R.; Brynjolfsson, J.; Petursson, H.; Potter, M.; Dudleston, K.; Barraclough, B.; Wasmuth, J.; Dobbs, M.; Gurling, H. (1988) Localization of a susceptibility locus for schizophrenia on chromosome 5. Nature; 336: 164–167.

Small, G. (1992) Tacrine for treating Alzheimer's disease. Journal of the American Medical Association; 268(18): 2564–2565.

Starr, R. H. (1979) Child abuse. American Psychologist; 34(10): 872–878.

Steinhausen, H. C.; Gobel, D.; Nestler, V. (1984) Psychopathology in the offspring of alcoholic parents. Journal of the American Academy of Child and Adolescent Psychiatry; 23(4): 465–471.

Strauss, J. S.; Carpenter, W. T. (1974) The prediction of outcome in schizophrenia. Archives of General Psychiatry; 31: 37–42.

Strauss, M. A.; Gelles, R. J. (1990) Physical Violence in American Families: Risk Factors and Adaptations to Violence in 8145 Families. New Brunswick, NJ: Transaction Publishers.

Susser, E. S.; Lin, S. P. (1992) Schizophrenia after prenatal exposure to the Dutch Hunger Winter of 1944–1945. Archives of General Psychiatry; 49(12): 983–988.

Swayze, V. W., II; Andreasen, N. C.; Alliger, R. J.; Ehrhardt, J. C.; Yuh, W. T. (1990) Structural brain abnormalities in bipolar affective disorder: Ventricular enlargement and focal signal hyperintensities. Archives of General Psychiatry; 47(11): 1054–1059.

Szatmari, P.; Nagy, J. (1990) Children of schizophrenic parents: A critical review of issues in prevention. Journal of Preventive Psychiatry and Allied Disciplines; 4(4): 311–327.

Tabakoff, B.; Hoffman, P.; Lee, J.; Saito, T.; Willard, B.; De Leon-Jones, F. (1988) Differences in platelet enzyme activity between alcoholics and nonalcoholics. New England Journal of Medicine; 318: 134–139.

Tarter, R. E.; Hegedus, A. M.; Gaveler, J. S. (1984) Hyperactivity in sons of alcoholics. Journal of Studies on Alcohol; 46: 259–261.

Tien, A. Y.; Anthony, J. C. (1990) Epidemiological analysis of alcohol and drug use as risk factors for psychotic experiences. Journal of Nervous and Mental Disease; 178: 473–480.

Tienari, P. (1992) Biological and psychosocial factors: Interaction between genetic vulnerability and rearing environment. In: A. Werbert and J. Cullberg, Eds. Psychotherapy of Schizophrenia: Facilitating and Obstructive Factors. Oslo, Norway: Scandinavian Press.

Tienari, P. (1991a) Cross-fostering. A research strategy for clarifying the role of genetic and experiental factors in the etiology of schizophrenia. In: S. Torgersen, P. Abrahamsen, and T. Sorenson, Eds. Psychiatry at the Crossroads Between Social Science and Biology. Oslo, Norway: Norwegian University Press; 122–133.

Tienari, P. (1991b) Genes, family environment or interaction. Findings from an adoption study. In: E. Kringlen, N. J. Lavik, and S. Torgensen, Eds. Etiology of Mental Disorders. Oslo, Norway: Department of Psychiatry, Vindern, University of Oslo; 33–48.

Tienari, P. (1991c) Interaction between genetic vulnerability and family environment: The Finnish adoptive family study of schizophrenia. Acta Psychiatrica Scandinavica; 84(5): 460–465.

Tolan, P. H. (1987) Implications of age of onset for delinquency risk. Journal of Abnormal Child Psychology; 15(1): 47–65.

Tonry, M.; Ohlin, L.; Farrington, D. (1990) Human Development and Criminal Behavior: New Ways of Advancing Knowledge. New York, NY: Springer-Verlag.

Treves, T. A. (1991) Epidemiology of Alzheimer's disease. Psychiatric Clinics of North America; 14: 251–265.

Tsuang, M. T.; Faraone, S. V. (1990) Summary and conclusions. In: M. T. Tsuang and S. V. Faraone, Eds. The Genetics of Mood Disorders. Baltimore, MD: The Johns Hopkins University Press; 166–176.

Turner, R. J.; Wagenfield, M. O. (1967) Occupational mobility and schizophrenia. American Sociological Review; 32: 104–113.

Van Broeckhoven, C.; Backhovens, H.; Cruts, M.; De Winter, G.; Bruyland, M.; Cras, P.; Martin, J-J. (1992) Mapping of a gene predisposing to early-onset Alzheimer's disease to chromosome 14q24.3. Nature Genetics; 2: 335–339.

van Duijn, C. M.; Clayton, D.; Chandra, V.; Fratiglioni, L.; Graves, A. B.; Heyman, A.; Jorm, A. F.; Kokmen, E.; Kondo, K.; Mortimer, J. A.; Rocca, W. A.; Shalat, S. L.; Soininen, H.; Hofman, A. (1991) Familial aggregation of Alzheimer's disease and related disorders: A collaborative re-analysis of case-control studies. International Journal of Epidemiology; 20: S13–S20.

Vine, P. (1982) Families in Pain. New York, NY: Pantheon Books.

von Knorring, A.-L. (1991) Annotation: Children of alcoholics. Journal of Child Psychology and Psychiatry; 32(3): 411–421.

von Knorring, A.-L.; Bohman, M.; von Knorring, L.; Oreland, L. (1985) Platelet MAO activity as a biological marker in subgroups of alcoholism. Acta Psychiatrica Scandinavica; 72(52): 51–58.

Waddington, J. L.; Weller, M. P.; Crow, T. J.; Hirsch, S. R. (1992) Schizophrenia, genetic retrenchment, and epidemiologic renaissance. The Sixth Biennial Winter Workshop on Schizophrenia, Badgastein, Austria, January 26-February 1, 1992. Archives of General Psychiatry; 49(12): 990–994.

Walker, E.; Downey, G.; Bergman, A. (1989) The effects of parental psychopathology and maltreatment on child behavior: A test of the diathesis-stress model. Child Development; 60: 15–24.

Weiss, C.; Hechtman, L. (1986) Hyperactive Children Grown Up. New York, NY: Guilford Press.

Weissman, M. M.; Gammon, G. D.; John, K.; Merikangas, K. R.; Warner, V.; Prusoff, B. A.; Sholomskas, D. (1987a) Children of depressed parents: Increased psychopathology and early onset of major depression. Archives of General Psychiatry; 44: 847–853.

Weissman, M. M.; Leif, P.; Bruce, M. L. (1987b) Single parent women. Social Psychiatry; 22: 29–36.

Werner, E. E. (1989) High risk children in young adulthood: A longitudinal study from birth to 32 years. American Journal of Orthopsychiatry; 59: 72–81.

Werner, E. E.; Smith, R. S. (1992) Overcoming the Odds: High Risk Children from Birth to Adulthood. New York, NY: Cornell University Press.

Werner, E. E.; Smith, R. S. (1982) Vulnerable but Invincible: A Longitudinal Study of Resilient Children and Youth. New York, NY: McGraw-Hill.

West, M. O.; Prinz, R. J. (1987) Parental alcoholism and childhood psychopathology. Psychological Bulletin; 102(2): 204–218.

White, J. L.; Moffitt, T. E.; Silva, P. A. (1989) A prospective replication of the protective effects of IQ in subjects at high risk for juvenile delinquency. Journal of Clinical and Consulting Psychology; 57: 719–724.

Widom, C. S. (1989a) The cycle of violence. Science; 244: 160–166.

Widom, C. S. (1989b) Does violence beget violence? A critical examination of the literature. Psychological Bulletin; 106(1): 3–28.

Wolfe, D. A. (1991) Preventing Physical and Emotional Abuse of Children. New York, NY: Guilford Press.

Yank, G. R.; Bentley, K. J.; Hargrove, D. S. (1993) The vulnerability-stress model of schizophrenia: Advances in psychosocial treatment. American Journal of Orthopsychiatry; 63(1): 55–69.

Zhang, M.; Katzman, R.; Salmon, D.; Jin, H.; Cai, G.; Wang, Z.; Qu, G.; Grant, I.; Yu, E.; Levy, P.; Klauber, M. R.; Liu, W. T. (1990) The prevalence of dementia and Alzheimer's disease in Shanghai, China: Impact of age, gender, and education. Annals of Neurology; 27: 428–437.

Zigler, E.; Phillips, L. (1961) Social competence and outcome in psychiatric disorders. Journal of Abnormal and Social Psychology; 63: 264–271.

Zucker, R. A.; Fitzgerald, H. E. (1991) Early developmental factors and risk for alcohol problems. Alcohol, Health and Research World; 15(1): 5–10.

7

Illustrative Preventive Intervention Research Programs

Although preventive intervention research is still a relatively young field and formidable tasks lie ahead, the past decade has brought encouraging progress. At present, there are many intervention programs that rest on sound conceptual and empirical foundations, and a substantial number are rigorously designed and evaluated. From a mental health perspective, these interventions are consistent with—even though they do not prove—the hypothesis that serious psychological problems can be avoided by preventive action before the onset of a diagnosable disorder.

In this chapter the committee selects a limited number of these interventions to illustrate a range of promising program approaches to achieving diverse prevention goals. This review of preventive interventions is based on three principles presented in earlier chapters in this report: (1) Prevention of the initial onset of mental disorders can be accomplished through intervention programs aimed at risk reduction, which can include both reduction of causal risk factors and enhancement of protective factors. The goal is to address malleable, or modifiable, risk and protective factors related to the onset of disorders, including precursor symptoms, to reduce the incidence of mental disorders or at least to delay their onset. However, even if the interventions fail to prevent a disorder, they may have some effect on reducing the severity or duration of the disorder. (2) Preventive intervention programs can be successfully implemented at all three levels—universal, selective, and indicated—described in Chapter 2. (3) Preventive intervention programs can be initiated throughout the life span.

The committee reviewed numerous prevention programs that were supported by federal agencies and private foundations. A wide net was cast in soliciting nominations, but the search could not be exhaustive. A majority of the prevention programs that currently exist are service programs and demonstrations that have not incorporated rigorous research methodologies. Even those that have an evaluation component usually have not used rigorous standards for assessment of effectiveness. Thus the nation is spending billions of dollars on programs whose effectiveness is not known. Most of the prevention programs discussed in this chapter meet the criteria listed below, including the use of a randomized controlled trial design. Such a high standard lends credence to the results of these studies. These program illustrations demonstrate that rigorous protocols can be applied to complex interventions, yielding tangible outcomes.

Many of the prevention programs that were reviewed used quasi-experimental designs. Where their findings provide some confirmatory evidence for a study with a randomized controlled trial design, or where their findings provide new leads in areas where there have been no randomized controlled studies, the information is briefly discussed in the chapter. Also, three well-known service projects that have not been rigorously evaluated are presented to highlight the potential for applying experimental designs to preventive interventions created by practitioners. All prevention program titles are in italics. Titles of programs that met the criteria for use as full illustrations are preceded by an asterisk. These illustrative programs are also listed in Table 7.1 and are abstracted in more detail in the background materials (program abstracts are available as indicated in Appendix D).

The programs target different age groups and are arranged here in developmental sequence from gestation through old age. As individuals move from one stage to the next, the developmental tasks facing them change, as does the nature of the risk and protective factors. This life course presentation serves to emphasize the importance of continuity and integration of interventions across the entire life span. Prevention programs that lasted for several years and bridged successive developmental phases or had effects on more than one generation are presented in this chapter at the earliest developmental phase. At the end of each section, several findings and leads that emerged from the review of programs addressing that age group are listed. The order of the points does not imply priority, and the list is not meant to be comprehensive but rather to illustrate the sorts of patterns, problems, and directions for future work that can be learned from such a perspective.

CRITERIA FOR EXAMINING PREVENTIVE INTERVENTION PROGRAMS DESCRIBED IN THE LITERATURE

As a basis for selecting the illustrative preventive intervention research programs, the committee formulated six criteria. The criteria pertain to (1) the risk and protective factors addressed, (2) the targeted population group, (3) the intervention itself, (4) the research design, (5) evidence concerning the implementation, and (6) evidence concerning the outcomes. Each of these criteria is described in detail below. In addition, Figure 7.1 displays these criteria in a format that may be useful to the reader in future examinations of published prevention programs.

Description of the Risk and Protective Factors Addressed

A well-documented description of the risk and protective factors addressed in the preventive intervention and how they relate to developmental tasks of the targeted group is a critical scientific first step. Without such specification, the rationale for identifying any group for intervention will be difficult to provide. Furthermore, the accumulation of data about well-documented risk and protective factors is essential to the design of preventive interventions, and the identification of malleable, or modifiable, risk factors is crucial to the success of prevention efforts built on the risk reduction model.

In identifying risk and protective factors, the causal status of the risk or protective factor is crucial. Some risk factors may not be causal but are nevertheless useful for identifying and targeting high-risk populations. The risk factors used to target the population may not always be the risk factors that one is attempting to modify through an intervention.

Although definitive scientific evidence of the causal role that a risk or protective factor plays in the development of mental disorder is seldom available until an intervention is tried, certain critical pieces of evidence should be in place. For example, there should be epidemiological evidence to suggest that the risk or protective factor is statistically correlated with the incidence or prevalence of the disorder itself. Furthermore, evidence that the risk or protective factor precedes the disorder is an important indication that the factor has at least a potential role in causation. Also, there may be a dosage effect, that is, the stronger the risk factor, the more disorder. In addition, the mechanism or process through which the risk or protective factor potentially operates should be specified. For example, a protective factor may affect risk either directly by operating on the antecedent risk factor itself or indirectly by affecting the strength of the relationship between the risk factor and

Program Name

Reference(s):

Investigator(s):

1. Description of the Risk and Protective Factors Addressed	2. Description of the Targeted Population Group	3. Description of the Intervention Program	4. Description of the Research Methodologies	5. Description of the Evidence Concerning Implementation	6. Description of the Evidence Concerning Outcomes
Documentation	Universal, selective, or indicated	Goals and Content	Methods of recruitment	Exposure of target group to intervention	Changes in status of risk and/or protective factors
Relationship to developmental task	Evidence that group is at risk for disorder or problem	Protocols	Sample size	Fidelity of delivery in accordance with design	Evidence of reduction of new cases
Causal status	Sociodemographic variables	Personnel delivering the intervention	Randomization		Evidence of delay of onset
Status in malleability		Site	Baseline measures		Side effects
Correlation with incidence and prevalence		Institutional or cultural content	Statistical analysis		Benefit-cost and cost-effectiveness analyses
		Ethical considerations	Attrition of subjects		
		Equipment or instrumentation			
		Method of delivery and techniques			
		Duration and extent			
		Multiple components			

FIGURE 7.1 A framework for examining preventive interventions. This format might be used as a worksheet in determining the methodological rigor of a specific program.

some mental health outcome. A protective factor may also operate by affecting some mediating mechanism that stands causally between the risk factor and the development of mental disorder.

Ultimately, it is important that the risk and protective factors addressed in the prevention program be explicitly identified and established as risk and protective factors in rigorous scientific studies. As scientific evidence converges on particular sets of risk and protective factors, interventions addressing them become more plausible and more likely to succeed.

Description of the Targeted Population Group

A description of the characteristics of the targeted group is another critical ingredient. As described in Chapter 2, universal preventive interventions are provided to entire populations; selective preventive interventions are targeted toward groups or individuals with high lifetime or high imminent risk; and indicated preventive interventions are targeted toward high-risk individuals on the basis of the individual's minimal, but detectable, behavioral symptoms that could later develop into a full-blown mental disorder, or the individual's biological markers that identify him or her as being at especially high risk.

Because our knowledge of precursor signs and symptoms of mental disorders is only preliminary (for example, no standardized lists of these exist), it is often difficult in practice to distinguish between selective and indicated interventions. We are just beginning to understand which risk factors contribute in a general way to multiple disorders and which are actually precursor symptoms for a single disorder. For example, in the causal chain leading to conduct disorder, aggressive behaviors at ages 4 to 6 are stable predictors of later problems and could be used to trigger an indicated intervention. Farther along the chain, at ages 9 to 11, academic difficulties also begin to stabilize as predictors of later conduct disorder and substance abuse. At this point the academic problems are not just a general risk factor for multiple disorders; they are also a precursor symptom for conduct disorder and can also be used to target an indicated population. The committee believes that the exercise in distinguishing between selective and indicated targeted populations is a useful one—and has attempted to do it for the illustrations given here—for it allows us to see more clearly where past efforts have been directed and how successful they have been. In addition, the distinction provides clues as to what degree of specification of targeted group tends to produce the best outcomes.

Specifying the targeted group is important for evaluating the degree to which the group actually displays the purported risk factors, for evaluating the actual and potential impact of the intervention, and for replicating the intervention. For example, scientific evidence should be provided to indicate that the group targeted actually is a group at risk for a particular disorder, cluster of disorders, or problem, and, if known, the degree to which the group is at risk should also be provided.

The targeted group should be described not only in terms of its risk and protective factors but also in terms of a combination of sociodemographic variables, including such characteristics as gender, age, race, socioeconomic status, living conditions, exposure to major life transitions, and family configuration. The number of participants and the distribution of sociodemographic characteristics in various experimental and control conditions should also be specified. Finally, because of potential effects on outcomes, there should be a description of the recruitment process and the consent process.

Description of the Intervention Program

All too often, treatment interventions as well as preventive interventions lack adequate description. This lack of specification is sometimes due to restrictions imposed by journal publication formats. In other cases, adequate descriptions of intervention protocols, including documents such as intervention manuals and training programs for delivery of the intervention, are simply missing. This is a danger signal, impeding evaluation.

Adequate descriptions of the goals and content of the intervention, and of the personnel delivering the intervention, including their professional qualifications and/or training for the delivery of the intervention, are needed. Detailed descriptions of the intervention site, including information on physical surroundings; the institutional and cultural context; special ethical considerations; and special physical aspects of the environment, including equipment or instrumentation, are other elements.

The actual methods of delivery must also be described, including the use of any special techniques, such as media devices and learning exercises. In addition, there must be a clear indication of the duration and extent of the intervention, including the prescribed length of exposure to the intervention by individuals or groups, whether booster sessions after the main intervention are required, and if so, at what intervals.

Finally, many preventive interventions have multiple components that are designed to work in an additive, sequential, or interactive fashion. Each of the components, modules, or stages ought to be described in enough detail that replication is possible.

Description of the Research Methodologies

The choice of research methodologies is a major issue in examining preventive interventions and the research trials designed to determine their outcomes. It heavily determines whether evidence is compelling that a preventive intervention could have produced its intended effect.

The ideal research design in a preventive trial is a randomized controlled trial of adequate size embedded in a longitudinal study. However, a variety of other designs, including group comparisons such as pretest-posttest, and quasi-experimental designs such as interrupted time series and regression discontinuity, are often employed. Such designs may be particularly necessary for large-scale community interventions. Although such designs have the potential for yielding useful data, they are less desirable than true randomized experimental designs. Such designs also require detailed descriptions of comparison groups, including methods of recruitment and any other information that might allow evaluation of comparison groups.

The research design should include appropriate use of statistical methods and account for attrition of participants through appropriate use of weighting procedures, statistical modeling of attrition effects, or the conservative use of full randomized designs even where attrition has taken place (Kraemer, 1992; Cohen, 1988; see also commissioned paper by Kraemer and Kraemer in the background materials, available as indicated in Appendix D).

Even when randomized assignment is possible, attrition is still a threat. It is frequently still necessary to confirm that randomized assignment has had its intended effects by comparing experimental and control groups on sociodemographic characteristics and other characteristics in addition to the outcomes. Furthermore, designs that employ appropriate and sufficient baseline measures, such as data on intelligence, personality, and physical health, are highly desirable because variables that appear extraneous are potentially significant. Inclusion of such measures has become standard practice for the evaluation of most randomized trials.

Description of the Evidence Concerning the Implementation

How well the intended objectives and processes of the intervention were actually implemented needs to be examined even when an adequate, detailed description of the intervention program is available. The critical issue is whether the intervention was delivered in accordance with its design. It is important to assess the degree to which targeted participants actually were exposed to the intervention and, wherever possible, the degree to which there were variations in exposure or dosage. The degree to which the intervention was delivered with fidelity can be determined if evidence is provided through various program data collected by external observers, through detailed program archives documenting contacts with participants, or through knowledge obtained from participants who were targets of the intervention.

Description of the Evidence Concerning the Outcomes

The final element to be examined is the outcomes. Most fundamentally, evidence should be provided that risk or protective factors have been changed. Without at least preliminary evidence that the intervention was successful in reducing risk factors or increasing protective factors, or in showing that protective factors reduced the strength of the relationship between risk factors and outcomes or affected some hypothesized mediating process, the claim that the intervention had an effect on some aspect of the causal chain leading to disorder becomes less convincing.

Other obvious sources of evidence of preventive effects would be an actual reduction in the observed rate of new cases of disorder or a delayed onset of disorder in the experimental group. It is entirely possible for a trial to provide evidence that the incidence of a particular disorder was reduced or the onset was delayed without clearly showing the mechanism of action by which the effect occurred. Accordingly, trials should, if possible, identify evidence not only on rates and age of onset of disorder but also on effects on risk or protective factors.

Still other outcomes are important to assess. These include the identification of unanticipated side effects, data regarding the costs and benefits of the intervention, and any benefit-cost or cost-effectiveness analyses conducted as part of the intervention evaluation. However, information on side effects and benefits and costs rarely has been included in published reports. Increasingly, it should become a standard part of the evidence on outcomes.

A DEVELOPMENTAL PERSPECTIVE

With these criteria in mind, the committee reviewed the preventive intervention research using, as an organizing conceptual framework, an understanding of human development throughout the life span. As mentioned above, each developmental phase brings new tasks to be accomplished; each is accompanied by potential biopsychosocial risk factors as well as opportunities for growth. Just as each individual is continually changing and evolving, risk and protective factors emerge and disappear over time or, if present for a long time, may express themselves differently. Likewise, outcome variables may need to vary through developmental stages. Figure 7.2 illustrates the conceptual framework of the life course of human development, with developmental tasks and corresponding social relationships and settings, such as family of orientation and peer group, which are the appropriate targets and contexts for preventive interventions. (See Table 7.1 for a summary of research programs corresponding to this life course framework.)

INTERVENTIONS FOR INFANTS

In infancy, the biopsychosocial risk factors that can hinder development include, but are not limited to, preventable infections, disease, or injuries that can cause brain damage, neurodevelopmental disorders, or behavioral disorders; problems of parent-infant attachment or parenting; deprivation of cognitive and language stimulation; economic deprivation; and child maltreatment. The corresponding protective factors of robust health and "good-enough" parenting—coupled with adequate nutrition and shelter—encourage the physical, intellectual, and emotional growth of the child.

In recent years, there have been notable increases in infants and children at risk for developmental impairments, and in infants and children already showing such problems (Rickel and Allen, 1987). Unemployment, deteriorating neighborhoods, increased violence, and lack of access to medical care have all contributed to this problem (see Chapter 6 on risk and protective factors). The Center for the Study of Social Policy (1992) concluded that our nation has failed to keep pace with the needs of its youngest citizens: over the 1980s child poverty expanded, births to unmarried teens climbed, more children were living in families with only one parent, and more babies were being born at risk because they were underweight.

Although the larger societal and structural issues will require societal and macroeconomic solutions, a number of creative and comprehensive programs have shown that it is possible to address the adverse effects on mothers and children of the heightened risks caused by these social changes. Preventive intervention strategies that have been used during infancy to target babies and their parents include high-quality prenatal

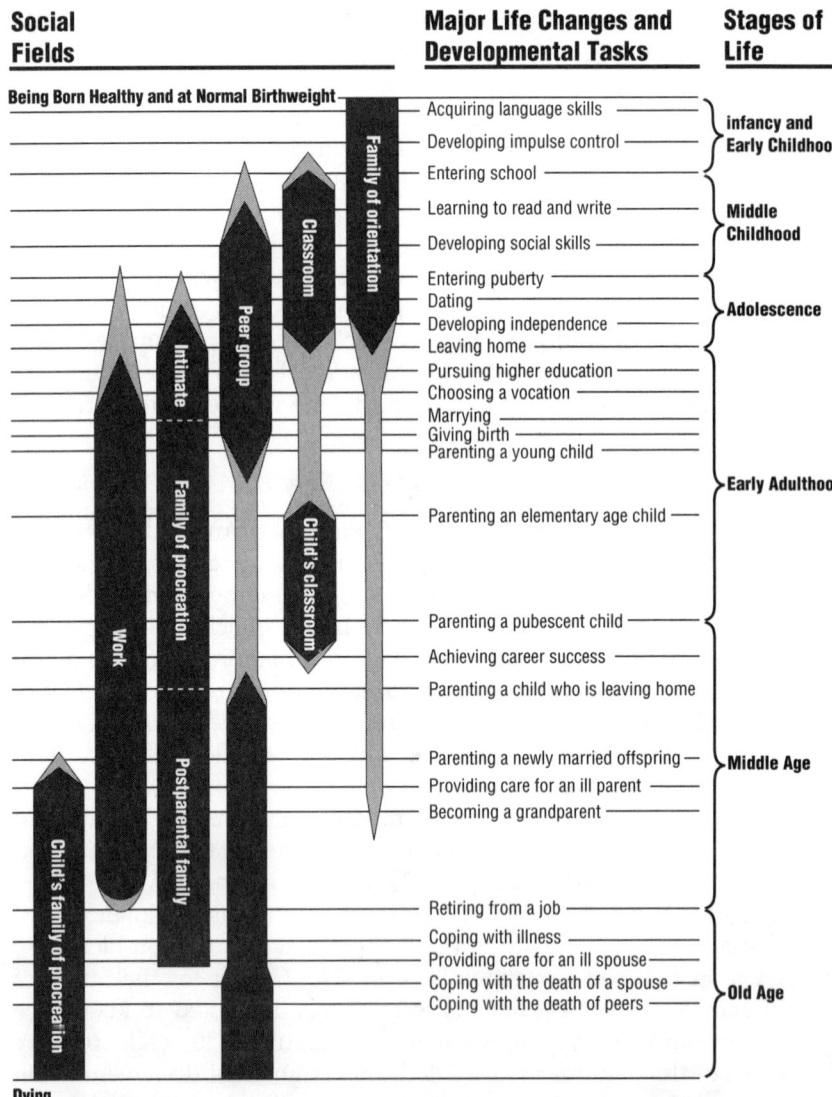

FIGURE 7.2   Developmental tasks and social fields for preventive interventions over the life course. Source: Adapted from Kellam, S. G.; Branch, J. D.; Agrawal, K. C.; Ensminger, M. E. (1975) Mental Health and Going to School. Chicago, IL: University of Chicago Press.

and perinatal care, childhood immunization, regular home visitation, parenting education, promotion of healthy parent-infant interaction, appropriate cognitive and language stimulation, well-baby health care, family support, and center-based infant day care.

Physical Health Interventions with Applications to Mental Health

High-Quality Prenatal and Perinatal Care

Prenatal and perinatal care provide examples of universal preventive interventions directed at the entire population of pregnant women for the protection of the developing fetus and the newborn baby. There is a strong general health promotion and wellness aspect to prenatal care, but such care is also known to prevent prematurity and low birthweight, as well as specific disabilities and disorders in newborns.

There is general agreement that all pregnant women should receive early, regular, and comprehensive prenatal care. In *Healthy People 2000: National Health Promotion and Disease Prevention Objectives* (DHHS, 1991), the U.S. Public Health Service affirmed that ensuring all infants a healthy start in life and enhancing the health of their mothers must be a top priority in the 1990s if we are to ensure the future health of the nation. Despite this consensus, however, there continue to be large numbers of women in the United States who do not receive prenatal care. Teenage mothers, mothers who are members of disadvantaged minorities, and unmarried mothers all tend to receive prenatal care that is late or inadequate, or they receive no prenatal care at all (IOM, 1985). Well-established medical guidelines define the timing and protocol for appropriate prenatal care, but frequently these are not followed for these high-risk groups (IOM, 1985).

Lack of prenatal care has important implications for mental disorders. Inadequate or absent prenatal care is the main cause of a mixed group of preventable disorders that appear in low-birthweight babies. In the United States, there are disproportionately high rates of low-birthweight babies in some racial and ethnic groups, particularly among African-Americans (Center for the Study of Social Policy, 1992). Low-birthweight babies constitute about 60 percent of all infant deaths. Those babies that survive often do so with major lifelong disorders, such as mental retardation and cerebral palsy, as well as behavioral, emotional, and learning problems (IOM, 1985). There is also some preliminary limited evidence that pregnancy and birth complications may play a role in later development of schizophrenia (see Chapter 6). Improving prenatal and perinatal care and delivering this care to all pregnant

TABLE 7.1 Illustrative Preventive Intervention Programs Using Randomized Controlled Trial Design

	Targeted Population Group/Sample Size When Project Began	Risk Factors Addressed	Outcomes (for total intervention group or subgroups)	Principal Investigator(s) and Year(s)
Infants				
Prenatal/Early Infancy Project	Selective/ N=394	Economic deprivation, maternal prenatal health and damaging behaviors, poor family management practices	Improved maternal diet and reduced smoking during pregnancy, fewer preterm deliveries, higher-birthweight babies, less child abuse	Olds, 1988, 1986
Tactile/Kinesthetic Stimulation	Selective/ N=40	Preterm delivery, low birthweight	Better physical and mental development of infants	Field, 1986
Early Intervention for Preterm Infants	Selective/ N=60	Teenage parenthood, low socioeconomic status, preterm delivery	Better parenting behaviors and attitudes of mothers, better cognitive competence, better physical development, better temperament of infants	Field, 1980
Infant Health and Development Program	Selective/ N=985	Low birthweight, poor family management practices, academic failure, early behavior problems	Better cognitive competence, fewer behavior problems	Ramey, 1990
Carolina Abecedarian Project	Selective/ N=107	Academic failure, lack of readiness for school, economic deprivation, low commitment to school	Better cognitive competence, lower rates of retention in grade in school	Horacek and Ramey, 1987

Young Children

Program	Type/N	Risk factors	Outcomes	Citation
Houston Parent-Child Development Center	Selective/N=~700	Economic deprivation, academic failure, early behavior problems, poor family management practices	Better family management practices, fewer behavior problems	Johnson, 1991, 1990
Mother-Child Home Program of Verbal Interaction Project	Selective/N=156	Academic failure, economic deprivation, poor family management practices, early behavior problems	Better family management practices, better cognitive competence	Levenstein, 1992, 1984
Parent-Child Interaction Training	Indicated/N=105	Economic deprivation, early behavior problems, poor family management practices, maternal depressive symptoms	Lower rates of attention deficits and conduct problems	Strayhorn, 1991
High/Scope Preschool Curriculum Comparison Study (including Distar)	Selective/N=68	Academic failure, early behavior problems, economic deprivation	Better cognitive competence	Weikart and Schweinhart, 1992, 1986
Perry Preschool Program (using High/Scope curriculum)	Selective/N=123	Academic failure, economic deprivation, early behavior problems, low commitment to school	Better cognitive competence, greater achievement and school completion, better vocational outcomes, fewer conduct problems and arrests	Weikart and Schweinhart, 1987, 1984
I Can Problem Solve: Interpersonal Cognitive Problem-Solving Program	Selective/N=219 (N=60 in pilot study)	Economic deprivation, poor impulse control, early behavior problems	Better cognitive problem-solving skills, fewer behavior problems	Shure and Spivack, 1982, 1979

Elementary-Age Children

Program	Type/N	Risk factors	Outcomes	Citation
Assertiveness Training Program (program 1)	Universal/N=343	Early behavior problems, academic failure	Improved social assertiveness, improved academic performance	Rotheram, 1982

(continued)

TABLE 7.1 (Continued)

	Targeted Population Group/Sample Size When Project Began	Risk Factors Addressed	Outcomes (for total intervention group or subgroups)	Principal Investigator(s) and Year(s)
Assertiveness Training Program (program 2)	Indicated/ N=101	Early behavior problems, academic failure	More assertive behavior, better school achievement, fewer behavior problems	Rotheram, 1982
Children of Divorce Intervention Program	Selective/ N=75	Marital conflict and separation, early conduct problems	Lower anxiety, fewer learning problems, better adjustment	Pedro-Carroll and Cowen, 1989, 1986, 1985
Family Bereavement Program	Selective/ N=72	Child bereavement, poor family management practices, early behavior problems	Lower levels of symptoms of depression and conduct disorder	Sandler, 1992
Social Skills Training	Selective/ N=28	Peer rejection, early conduct problems	Less peer rejection, better interpersonal skills	Bierman, 1986
Social Relations Intervention Program	Indicated/ N=86	Early behavior problems (aggression), peer rejection, impulsivity	Less aggression, less peer rejection, more prosocial behavior	Lochman, in press
Montreal Longitudinal-Experimental Study	Indicated/ N=172	Poor family management practices, peer rejection, academic failure, early behavior problems, violence on television	Less aggressive behavior, less delinquent behavior, better school achievement	Tremblay, 1992, 1991
Community Epidemiological Preventive Intervention: Mastery Learning and Good Behavior Game	Universal/ N=2314	Academic failure, aggressive and antisocial behavior, concentration problems, depressive symptoms, shy behavior	Less aggressive and shy behavior, better cognitive competence—especially among those with early depressive symptoms	Kellam and Rebock, 1992

Program	Type/N	Risk factors	Outcomes	Citation
Academic Tutoring and Social Skills Training	Selective/N=40	Academic failure, peer rejection, early behavior problems, early depressive symptoms	Better cognitive competence, less peer rejection	Coie and Krehbiel, 1984
Seattle Social Development Project	Universal/N=908	Poor family management practices, early behavior problems, low commitment to school, academic failure	Better family management practices and family bonding, greater attachment to school, lower rates of delinquency and drug use initiation	Hawkins and Catalano, 1988
Adolescents				
Changing Teaching Practices	Selective/N=1166	Low commitment to education, academic failure, behavior problems	Greater attachment and commitment to school, lower rates of school suspension for misbehavior	Hawkins, 1988
Positive Youth Development Program	Universal/N=282	Early drug use onset, favorable attitudes toward drugs, social influences to use	Better coping skills, better stress management strategies, better conflict resolution and impulse control, less excessive alcohol use	Caplan and Weissberg, 1992
Adolescent Alcohol Prevention Trial	Universal/N=3011	Attitudes favorable to the use of drugs, social influences to use, early onset of drug use	Lower rates of tobacco, alcohol, and marijuana use, lower prevalence of problem alcohol use and drunkenness	Hansen and Graham, 1991
ALERT Drug Prevention	Universal/N=6527	Social influences to use, early onset of drug use, attitudes favorable to the use of drugs	Lower rates of tobacco, alcohol, and marijuana use	Ellickson and Bell, 1990
Alcohol Education Project	Universal/N=2536	Favorable attitudes toward alcohol consumption, early onset of alcohol use, association with alcohol-consuming friends, community norms favorable toward alcohol use	Less initiation of alcohol use, increased knowledge about alcohol, decreased use among those drinking prior to study	Perry et al., 1989

(continued)

TABLE 7.1 (Continued)

	Targeted Population Group/Sample Size When Project Began	Risk Factors Addressed	Outcomes (for total intervention group or subgroups)	Principal Investigator(s) and Year(s)
Midwestern Prevention Project	Universal/ N=5065	Social influences to use, early onset of drug use, attitudes favorable to the use of drugs	Lower rates of tobacco, alcohol, and marijuana use	Pentz, 1989
Behaviorally Based Preventive Intervention	Indicated/ N=80	Academic failure, early behavior problems, alienation from family, low commitment to school	Less conduct problems and delinquency	Bry, 1992
Intervention Campaign Against Bully-Victim Problems	Universal/ N=2400	Aggressive behavior, poor family management practices, favorable attitudes toward bullying/aggression	Less bullying, less delinquent behavior, more attachment to school	Olweus, 1991
Adults				
Prevention and Relationship Enhancement Program (PREP):An Empirically Based Preventive Intervention Program for Couples	Universal/ N=135	Couple relationship problems	Better marital adjustment, less divorce, less physical violence	Markman, 1992
University of Colorado Separation and Divorce Program	Selective/ N=153	Marital separation/divorce, anxiety, depression, childrearing problems, economic problems	Fewer symptoms of anxiety and depression, better vocational outcomes	Bloom and Hodges, 1985, 1982

Program	Type/N	Risk Factors	Outcomes	Citation
Perceived Personal Control Preventive Intervention for a Caesarean Birth Population	Selective/ N=70	Caesarean delivery, depressive symptoms	Lower levels of postpartum depression, more rapid physical and psychological recovery	Tadmor and Brandes, 1988, 1984
Prenatal/Early Infancy Project	Selective/ N=394	Single parent status, school dropout, economic hardships, joblessness, subsequent pregnancy	Better vocational adjustment, fewer second pregnancies, better educational achievement	Olds, 1988
Caregiver Support Program for Coping with Occupational Stress	Selective/ N=247	Occupational stress, distress, anxiety, depression	Lower psychological distress, better job satisfaction	Heaney, 1992
JOBS Project for the Unemployed: Michigan Prevention Research Center	Selective/ N=928	Involuntary job loss, anxiety, depression, alcohol abuse, marital stress	Fewer depressive symptoms, higher pay, cost-effective outcomes	Vinokur, Price, Caplan, and van Ryn, 1992, 1991
San Francisco Depression Prevention Research Project: A Randomized Trial with Medical Outpatients	Selective/ N=150	Depressive symptoms, medical problems, low income, minority status in public primary care setting	Lower levels of depressive symptoms	Muñoz, 1993, 1990, 1987
Projecto Bienestar: An Intervention for Preventing Depression in Hispanic Immigrant Women in the Community	Selective/ N=399	Low income, immigrant minority status, distress, depressive symptoms	Fewer depressive symptoms	Vega, 1990, 1987
Peer- and Professionally-Led Groups to Support Family Caregivers	Selective/ N=56	Caregiver burden, anxiety, depression	Lower levels of psychiatric symptoms, including anxiety and depression, better coping skills	Toseland, 1990, 1989

Elderly

Program	Type/N	Risk Factors	Outcomes	Citation
Widow-to-Widow: A Mutual Help Program for the Widowed	Selective/ N=162	Widowhood, bereavement, depression, anxiety, social isolation	Fewer depressive symptoms, less social withdrawal	Vachon, 1982, 1980, 1979

women may decrease developmental risks associated with the later onset of many mental disorders.

Interventions with high-risk groups should use the broad definition of prenatal care recommended by the U.S. Public Health Service Expert Panel on the Content of Prenatal Care (USPHS, 1989). Going beyond the traditional guidelines for prenatal care, the panel argued that all pregnant women, as a minimum, should receive general information about the physiological and emotional changes of pregnancy as well as fetal growth and development. In addition, they should receive education regarding positive maternal health behaviors and habits, psychosocial preparation for childbirth, and education and support for effective parenting and family behaviors (USPHS, 1989). There was specific emphasis on the identification of and intervention for behavior disorders likely to produce child maltreatment and/or family violence.

In 1988 the Institute of Medicine assessed the barriers to adequate prenatal care and reviewed 31 intervention programs nationwide, all of which were selective programs directed at high-risk groups (IOM, 1988). Programs studied were categorized according to one of five areas of major emphasis: (1) reducing financial obstacles, (2) increasing the basic capacity of the prenatal care system, (3) improving institutional practices to make services more accessible and acceptable, (4) casefinding, and (5) providing social support. Few of these programs used randomization techniques or other strong research designs to assess program effects. Selection bias, in particular, flawed most evaluations. Moreover, because many of the programs were complex, it was difficult to distinguish the specific impact of individual elements. The IOM committee concluded that although several types of programs can succeed in bringing women into prenatal care and maintaining their participation, the success of many programs has been modest, often because they have become embedded in a complicated, fragmented network of maternity services characterized by pervasive financial and institutional obstacles to care (IOM, 1988). Access barriers were identified in all five categories. A significant finding was that casefinding and social support are the most effective means of increasing early and continuing use of prenatal care and compliance with health recommendations among mothers most at risk of absent or inadequate prenatal care (IOM, 1988).

Immunization

Childhood immunization, like prenatal care, is an example of a universal preventive intervention directed at the entire population even though it is given to individuals. Immunization is an example of the traditional public health model—in which each vaccine can confer long-lasting, often lifetime, protection against a specific physical disease. Currently, infants and children can and should be immunized against poliomyelitis, diphtheria, pertussis, tetanus, measles, mumps, rubella, *Haemophilus influenzae* type b (Hib) to protect children from meningitis, and hepatitis B. For example, when children are not immunized for Hib and meningitis occurs, there is the possibility of long-term negative effects on the brain, resulting in neurodevelopmental problems, mental retardation, learning disability, and psychological and behavioral disorders (Plotkin and Mortimer, 1988).

In the United States, widespread vaccination on appropriate schedules has produced a dramatic drop in the number of cases of the previously common childhood diseases, and their associated high mortality, morbidity, and sequelae. These declines are reported at 97 percent or more since the year the maximum number of cases for each disease was reported (Peter, 1992).

The cost-effectiveness of vaccination is well documented (Hinman, 1988). In 1983 the measles-mumps-rubella vaccine program had a cost-benefit ratio of 14:1, leading to a total saving of $1.4 billion (White, Koplan, and Orenstein, 1985). A study of pertussis vaccine showed that $2.10 is saved for each $1.00 spent on pertussis vaccination (Hinman and Koplan, 1985).

Currently, there is an immunization crisis in the United States, signaled by recurrent measles epidemics. Because measles is the most contagious of the vaccine-preventable diseases, its resurgence acts as a sentinel that warns of a breakdown in the overall immunization rates for other diseases. Epidemiological studies find that the source of the problem lies in the failure to achieve adequate immunization rates among children in the first two years of life. Rates are well below the 1990 national objective of 90 percent of children with completed immunizations by the second birthday (Cutts, Zell, Mason, Bernier, Dini, and Orestein, 1992; CDC, 1991). The failures of preschool immunization are most notable in inner-city and minority populations. In the inner-city areas, typically, fewer than 50 percent of the two-year-olds have been appropriately vaccinated, and African-American and Hispanic children are at highest risk (CDC, 1992, 1991, 1990).

In 1991 the National Vaccine Advisory Committee identified four major reasons for the low immunization rates among preschool children: (1) missed opportunities for vaccination, (2) deficiencies in the public health care delivery system, (3) lack of access to care, and (4) inadequate public awareness of the importance of immunizations. To ensure that immunizations reach all high-risk groups, specially designed selective interventions may be needed. These interventions should take the above problems of access into account.

Programs Aimed at Improving Parenting and Reducing Risks for Infants

In addition to the universal, widely implemented programs just discussed, there are some specific, experimentally designed preventive interventions targeted at infants and their families. The *Prenatal/Early Infancy Project* is an example of a comprehensive program intended to prevent a wide range of maternal and child problems often associated with poverty (Olds, Henderson, Tatelbaum, and Chamberlin, 1988, 1986). It is a selective program targeted to a high-risk geographical area, with high rates of poverty and child maltreatment, in the semirural Appalachian region of New York. The sample consisted of 394 women, most of whom were white, who entered the program at no later than 25 weeks of pregnancy. At registration, 47 percent were 19 years old or younger, 62 percent were unmarried, and 61 percent were from the lowest socioeconomic group. Violence, drug abuse, and alcoholism were common. Many women reported having been abused as children.

The specific goals were to reduce the mothers' prenatal health-damaging behaviors, enhance parenting skills, give social support to mothers, encourage the use of existing community resources, help the mothers achieve desired educational and occupational goals, and reduce unwanted or inappropriate additional pregnancies. Olds expected that these objectives for the mothers could be attained through a home nurse visitation program. He also expected highly desirable outcomes for the children, including reduction in prematurity and low birthweight, decreases in accidents and infectious diseases, improvement in cognition and language development, decreases in psychological and behavioral problems, reduction in child abuse and neglect, and facilitation of healthy growth and nutrition.

The intercorrelated nature of the biological and psychosocial factors were also recognized. As previously stated, unwed and teenage mothers are at greater risk of having low-birthweight and premature babies. There is increasing understanding that the established higher likelihood of adverse developmental, learning, and behavioral outcomes for low-birthweight and premature babies is largely mediated by adverse childrearing factors, such as poorly educated parents, poverty, isolation of the family, and a stressful environment (Rose, Feldman, Rose, Wallace, and McCarton, 1992; Sameroff and Chandler, 1975).

The intervention was a randomized clinical trial. Women were randomly assigned to one of four groups: (1) developmental screening of the children at one and two years of age and referral for services, (2) developmental screening and transportation to well-child care clinics, (3) home nurse visitation during pregnancy, and (4) home nurse visitation during pregnancy and until children were two years old.

The program design was conceptually based on the "ecological" model (Bronfenbrenner, 1979), which posits interdependence among social systems that operate simultaneously at the level of the marital and parent-child dyads, the family as a whole, and the larger socioeconomic influences of the community. The intervention strategy relied on home nurse visitation during critical phases of the life cycle of a family— pregnancy and the first two years of the infant's life. The home visits, which the mother's primary support person was encouraged to attend, were biweekly at first and tapered off to every six weeks by two years of age.

The design of the program permitted evaluation of the relative effects of specific elements of intervention for both the whole sample and those subsets defined as being at risk. For the evaluation of the postnatal outcomes, groups 1 and 2 were combined into one control group for purposes of analysis and compared with group 4 as the experimental condition, referred to here as "nurse-visited." It was found that during pregnancy, nurse-visited mothers made better use of medical and other formal services than the control group. The nurse-visited mothers experienced greater social support, improved their diets more, and reduced their cigarette smoking. The greatest impact on infant's birthweight and mother's length of pregnancy was for nurse-visited young teenagers. They had a 75 percent reduction in preterm delivery. For the women who were at highest risk (poor, unmarried, and teenage), there was a reduction in the incidence of verified cases of child abuse, a drop from 19 to 4 percent among those who were nurse-visited (Olds and Kitzman, 1990). (For outcomes with the mothers, see the discussion in the section below on interventions for adults.)

Unfortunately, community-level implementation of the Prenatal/Early Infancy Project by one public health department was unsuccessful (see Box 11.1 in Chapter 11). The program is now, however, being replicated by Olds in an urban area in another part of the country with a different high-risk group, minority mothers, to test the generalizability of the intervention.

In an intense 10-day selective preventive intervention program, the *Tactile/Kinesthetic Stimulation* study, Field and colleagues demonstrated positive outcomes for preterm, low-birthweight babies (Field, Schanberg, Scafidi, Bauer, Vega-Lahr, Garcia et al., 1986). In a randomized controlled trial, the infants who received tactile, kinesthetic stimulation gained significantly more weight—47 percent more per day—than infants in the control group. The infants in the intervention group also were alert and awake more during the awake/sleep behavioral observation, scored significantly higher on the Brazelton subscales of mature habituation, orientation, motor, and range of scale behavior, and were hospitalized significantly fewer days after the onset of the intervention period. This last outcome has positive implications for benefit-cost analyses.

In the *Early Intervention for Preterm Infants* study, Field and colleagues had targeted preterm neonates whose mothers were African-American, unmarried, less than 19 years of age, and of low socioeconomic status based on education and occupation (Field, Widmayer, Stringer, and Ingatoff, 1980). The selective preventive intervention, which consisted of home visits by a two-person team—a trained interventionist and a teenage African-American work study student—aimed to prevent developmental delays in the infants by teaching mothers about caretaking practices and enhancing parent-infant interactions. At four months, the infants who had been randomly assigned to the intervention group had significantly better weight and length and higher scores on the Denver Developmental Screening test. At eight months the results still held, with the intervention infants exhibiting significantly higher mental scores on the Bayley Scales of Infant Development. Additionally, these infants had significantly lower blood pressures.

The *Infant Health and Development Program* is a selective preventive intervention focused on preventing or reducing the health problems, developmental disabilities, and learning and behavioral problems associated with low birthweight (Infant Health and Development Program, 1990; Kraemer and Fendt, 1990). This eight-site randomized clinical trial was designed to evaluate the efficacy of a multicomponent program consisting of pediatric care, child development activities, and family support services. It is a good example of the use of a multicenter clinical trial design applied to research in human development. It is also a well-designed prospective study that illustrates the feasibility of applying a standard comprehensive intervention in diverse community sites.

This kind of ambitious multisite design was desirable and ready to be tested because a number of previous small studies had demonstrated the efficacy of early intervention for improving the developmental, cognitive, and behavioral outcomes for low-birthweight babies. These previous studies, however, were limited by small numbers of subjects at single sites and lack of long-term follow-up. There was, nevertheless, sufficient relevant experience with home visitation programs for parent education and with high-quality center-based infant day care to adopt those materials as curricula for the multisite program. Thus, building on the previous studies, the multisite intervention was designed as the first intervention for low-birthweight babies to include both home visitation and center-based components.

A total of 985 infants, each with a birthweight of 5½ pounds (2,500 grams) or less and a gestational age of 37 weeks or less, participated in the study. Two birthweight groups of the 985 infants were defined to assess possible differential responses: heavier babies (weighing 2,001 to 2,500 grams) and lighter babies (weighing less than 2,000 grams). Within each weight group, one third of the subjects were randomly assigned to an experimental group, and two thirds to a control group. The experimental and control groups both received the same high-quality pediatric surveillance, which included periodic medical, developmental, and social (family) assessments, with referrals for services as needed. The experimental group received two additional components: (1) Home visits by educators to teach parents about the specialized, curriculum-based child development activities they were to administer, and also to supervise curriculum-based problem solving by the parents for self-identified problems. The home visits were weekly during the baby's first year and biweekly until 36 months. (2) Participation by the children in a center-based child development program from the ages of 12 to 36 months for teacher-administered, curriculum-based developmental activities five days per week. Transportation to and from the center was provided. In addition, parenting groups met bimonthly for education and support.

The major finding was that the experimental group achieved significantly higher cognitive scores than the control group at 36 months of age (correcting for prematurity). There was also a marked difference in the response of the heavier and the lighter babies to the intervention. For the heavier babies, the IQ scores in the experimental group were, on average, 13.2 points higher than in the control group. For the lighter babies, results were also positive and significant, but not as great. The IQ scores were 6.6 points higher in the lighter-weight experimental group than for their control counterparts.

For the total control group, both heavier and lighter babies, over 18 percent had IQ scores below 70 (the mental retardation range), and almost 50 percent were below 85. The intervention was not effective for any of the study infants with birthweights of 1,500 grams or less. In this lowest-weight group (used only for analysis purposes), there was virtually no difference between the experimental and the control groups in the proportion who tested at IQ of 70 or below.

There were small but significant intervention effects at age 36 months in behavioral competence. The intervention had a positive effect, especially with infants of mothers with low education levels. Mothers in the intervention group reported that there were fewer serious behavior problems but more minor problems.

Longer-term follow-ups have been planned, and results pertaining to academic achievement and behavioral problems in school will be available soon as a measure of the durability of the effects of this infancy and early childhood intervention. This carefully designed program will soon be scaled up into larger field trials by the Centers for Disease Control and Prevention, with support from The Robert Wood Johnson Foundation. The issue of program effectiveness will be a high priority.

Horacek and co-workers demonstrated the utility of early and continued intervention to prevent developmental delays and promote academic success among children at risk by virtue of economic and social deprivation (Horacek, Ramey, Campbell, Hoffman, and Fletcher, 1987). In the *Carolina Abecedarian Project*, they randomly assigned socially and economically deprived children at infancy to experimental or control groups. A composite of risk indicators, including low level of family education, low family income, low parental and sibling IQ, and evidence of family psychopathology or social maladaptation, was used to identify children at risk for school failure. The intervention included (1) year-round, center-based full-day care for children beginning at 8 to 12 weeks of age and continuing until kindergarten entry, (2) a toy-lending library to permit continuity of learning from center to home, (3) a home visitation program, and (4) parent group meetings. At kindergarten entry, 96 of the original 111 subjects were randomly assigned again to school-age experimental and control conditions, which continued for three years. This design allowed comparison of the effects of early versus late versus combined intervention on children's cognitive and social development. Some children received both the preschool and the school-age intervention, some received only the preschool or the school-age intervention, and some received no intervention.

The intervention significantly reduced the number of children repeating a grade in school, and it improved the children's test scores in reading and math. Effects were greatest for children who received both the early and the school-age intervention phases. In spite of the fact that the children came from environments predictive of academic failure, they achieved a rate of advancement to the next grade nearly equal to that of an average-risk comparison group constituted for the study. For children who received only one intervention phase, those who received the preschool intervention performed better than those who received the school-age intervention.

Evidence from a Quasi-Experimental Study

The *Family Development Research Program* served a poor, predominantly African-American sample of 108 families with incomes of less than $5,000 in which mothers had less than a high school education and a history of semiskilled or unpaid work (Lally, Mangione, and Honig, 1988). Over 85 percent of the participating families were single-parent, female-headed households. This selective study retained a large proportion of families; thus differential attrition was not a major threat to its conclusions.

The multicomponent intervention was provided from the last trimester of the mother's pregnancy through age five for the child. The intervention included a weekly home visit by a "child development trainer" who sought to serve as a friend and advisor on important family issues. The home visitor sought to foster a positive, supportive mother-child relationship, encouraged the family to take an active role in the child's development, and helped the family make contacts with local service agencies. In addition, child care and early educational enrichment were provided in a community center for children from six months to five years of age.

A 10-year follow-up study revealed that children who participated in the intervention had less involvement with the juvenile justice system than did the comparison group (6 percent versus 22 percent), and when they were involved with juvenile justice, their delinquent behavior was less serious. In addition, there were positive effects on school achievement, but these were for girls only (Lally, Mangione, Honig, and Wittner, 1988).

Unfortunately, the study used a quasi-experimental design. The matched comparison group was constituted when subjects were three years old, so obviously there was no random assignment to groups. Such a design prevents the elimination of many alternative hypotheses regarding sources of observed group differences.

An Example from Prevention Services

Healthy Start in Hawaii, a selective intervention program for families at risk of child abuse, is similar in concept and content to the Prenatal/Early Infancy Project described above. Healthy Start, however, was initiated by the Maternal and Child Health Branch of the Hawaii Health Department in 1985 not as a research project but as a statewide service project. In 1990 the U.S. Advisory Board on Child Abuse described the program as "clearly the star" of U.S. home visitation programs (U.S. Advisory Board on Child Abuse and Neglect, 1990).

Healthy Start registers pregnant women and mothers with babies up to three months old and serves them until the child is five years old. It uses 15 selection factors to screen for at-risk status. In 1992, Healthy Start was screening 55 percent of the population, and by 1995 it expects to screen 90 percent. About 20 percent of those screened are found to be at risk.

Program elements include early identification of at-risk families, community-based home visiting by laypersons (not nurses as in the Prenatal/Early Infancy Project), linkage to primary health care services and a "medical home," and linkage and coordination with community services. The goals of the program are to provide (1) adequate prenatal and primary well-child health care; (2) quality child care in infancy and early childhood; (3) parental competence and promotion of child development through parent education, infant stimulation, home visitors, and social support; (4) links to medical and community services and (5) continuity of funding so that clients and providers both experience reliability of service provision.

Since the inception of the program, the rates of child abuse and neglect in Hawaii have been slowly decreasing, but it is impossible to determine how much of this is due to the program. A rigorous evaluation is needed. Such an evaluation should provide a detailed analysis of the screening factors that best detect high risk, the implementation, cost-effectiveness, and the child outcomes, including developmental progress, language proficiency, school readiness, and an array of behavioral outcomes, as well as data on rates of child abuse and neglect. However, the ideal way of determining program effectiveness would be a randomized controlled trial with multiple outcome measures.

Findings and Leads

On the basis of the review of interventions for infants, the following points emerge:

- Infants born to high-risk mothers and children at high risk of not being immunized could benefit from preventive interventions that reduce financial, institutional, and other access barriers.
- Home nurse visitation can be an effective means of influencing

maternal and child outcomes. In some programs, it may be most effective with the at-risk mothers who are the hardest to reach and most distrustful and may have relatively little effect on mothers who are not at risk.

• Provision of intensive and prolonged center-based early childhood education, combined with home visitation to families, can prevent cognitive developmental delays and academic failure in children at risk.

• It is possible to adhere to a rigorous protocol for a complex, comprehensive human development study across several sites that show great diversity in their characteristics. Even with rigorous protocols, appropriate care in implementation can lead to low attrition rates and positive responses from the participants.

• Highly regarded service programs, such as Healthy Start in Hawaii, can be mined for useful leads on which to base more rigorously designed research studies. Such studies could provide more powerful evidence regarding the outcomes of the programs and could improve the effectiveness of these preventive services.

INTERVENTIONS FOR YOUNG CHILDREN

During early childhood, two examples of important developmental tasks that must be achieved to lower risk for adverse mental health outcomes are (1) the acquisition of language skills to prepare the child to read and write and (2) the development of impulse control (Hawkins and Catalano, 1992). Achieving these tasks has a significant benefit for the ongoing social and cognitive development of the child. Failure at these tasks has been associated with later behavioral and school maladjustment, as well as with the development of mental health problems (Hawkins and Catalano, 1992).

Recent preschool preventive interventions have addressed several risk factors that are related to these developmental tasks, as well as to the development of mental and behavior problems. Risk factors and precursor symptoms that have been addressed in promising interventions during childhood include economic deprivation, poor family management practices, cognitive or developmental delays, school failure, and early behavior problems.

Prevention efforts that address these risk factors during early childhood have adopted a number of approaches, including (1) center-based early childhood education, in which preschool programs are designed to enhance social competence and cognitive development; (2) home visitation to provide a variety of support and educational services; (3) parenting training and education to teach skills in caregiving and effective behavior management; (4) family support services, which provide survival-focused support; and (5) policy initiatives that address issues of child safety, health, and education. Most programs have combined two or more of these approaches in multicomponent interventions.

Dramatic increases in the proportion of children living in poverty have stimulated research on the developmental outcomes associated with growing up in poverty. As mentioned above, children from poor families are at heightened risk for mental health problems, as well as other problem behaviors (Farrington, Loeber, Elliott, Hawkins, Kandel, Klein et al., 1990). The risk poor children face has been addressed in two ways. First, poverty has been used as a selection criterion in choosing target populations for early childhood intervention. Second, some programs have directly addressed the financial, housing, and other economic needs of poor families in addition to addressing the child's risk for later problems (e.g., Infant Health and Development Program, 1990; Lally, Mangione, and Honig, 1988; Lally, Mangione, Honig, and Wittner, 1988; Andrews, Blumenthal, Johnson, Kahn, Ferguson, Lasater et al., 1982). Virtually all the programs reviewed in this section have focused on reducing risk for children raised in poverty.

Programs Aimed at Improving Parenting and Enhancing Child Development

Multicomponent programs that add center-based child care and early education to their parenting components can be introduced at this phase of development as well as during infancy. The *Houston Parent-Child Development Center* program provides another example of the effectiveness of these augmented approaches (Johnson, 1991, 1990; Johnson and Walker, 1987). The Houston Parent-Child Development Center recruited Mexican-American families in poverty who had one-year-old children with no neurological impairments or chronic illnesses. Because mothers were required to participate extensively, the project did not include families whose mother's employment might interfere with their participation. Eligible volunteers recruited from door-to-door surveys were randomly assigned to experimental or control conditions.

The two-year selective preventive intervention included 20 to 30 home visits of 1½ hours duration during the first year, which focused on mother-child interaction, recognized the child's developmental status, and used the home as an environment for learning. In addition, four weekend workshops were offered on special topics to ensure participation of fathers, 90 percent of whom were present in participating families.

During the second year, children attended nursery school four mornings per week, and mothers attended three-hour classes at the center four mornings per week for eight months. Class topics included home management (including health and budgeting) and child development and management issues. Monthly evening sessions for mothers and fathers were offered on special topics, including sex education, family planning, and driver education. The center explicitly sought to serve as a support system for participating mothers and families. Cultural relevance and bilingual format were included in the program design.

At 36 months, mothers showed significantly positive effects of the program. They used more praise and less criticism, and there was more positive mother-child interaction. Few differences were observed in children's behavior during the preschool period, but at follow-up, when children were aged 8 to 11 (in grades 2 to 5), intervention children were rated by teachers as more prosocial and engaging in less acting out and problem behavior, including less impulsive and disruptive behavior and less fighting. The program did not affect measured intelligence.

Overall, this intervention made extensive time demands on mothers. Approximately 550 hours of family participation was expected. Unfortunately, about half of the intervention participants had left by the end of the program, in part because of the high mobility of the Mexican-American families in the sample and also perhaps because full participation consumed so many hours that it almost completely prevented the mother from having a job. This high attrition rate presents a major difficulty in evaluating program effectiveness, which perhaps could have been avoided had these cultural and logistic issues been considered.

The *Mother-Child Home Program of Verbal Interaction Project* targeted economically disadvantaged, single mothers of low educational attainment who had two-year-old children (Levenstein, 1992; Madden, O'Hara, and Levenstein, 1984). The selective preventive intervention design involved trained home visitors (either paid paraprofessionals or unpaid volunteers), who visited mothers and their children twice per week for 30 minutes when the child was aged two to four. Home visitors followed cognitive curricula that employed books and toys. They played with the child and mother together, modeling the verbal curriculum and helping the mother to improve her skills to enhance the child's development. Visitors were trained to involve the mother and to pull gradually away from the interaction, allowing the mother and child to play together. On average, more than 35 visits were made each year to intervention families.

Compared with evaluation-only and control groups, the experimental group of children improved significantly in IQ at two-year follow-up and scored significantly better on achievement and IQ tests in grades 5 and 8. The investigators found evidence of improvement in maternal childrearing behavior, including verbal interaction, following the intervention. Improvements in the mother's childrearing behavior by the time the child reached age four were linked to the child's later positive classroom attitudes and behavior as rated by first-grade teachers. Moreover, younger siblings of intervention children entering the program in later years had significantly higher IQ scores (by eight points), suggesting the possibility that what the mother learned about parenting enhanced the cognitive development of her younger children also.

As in many field studies, influences other than the intervention affected the outcomes. For example, 94 percent of the parents in the experimental group and 75 percent of the parents in the control group reported that their children attended preschool programs after the intervention. These programs may have affected performance in grades 5 and 8. A low rate of acceptance (52 percent) by those who were offered an opportunity to be in the study may have introduced self-selection. In addition, the subject randomization process used in later years of the study also may have introduced self-selection of more highly educated and intelligent mothers into the study sample. Nonetheless, this multi-year intervention study indicates the promise of a home-delivered curriculum focused on improving maternal skills to facilitate the cognitive development of the child.

Parent-child interaction has also been targeted during early childhood through indicated preventive interventions. Strayhorn and Weidman (1991) reported the results of a study, *Parent-Child Interaction Training*, in which low-income parents who identified one or more behavioral problems in their children were recruited from Head Start and other sources. They were randomly assigned to the experimental or the control group. Participants were 64 percent African-American, and a majority were single female heads of household. Over 41 percent of the mothers evidenced mild or greater depression on the Beck Depression Inventory. Parents in the experimental group were offered four to five two-hour group sessions with instruction and role playing on parenting skills, including behavioral management. They were also trained in play and conducted individual play sessions with their children, attending sessions until they reached "criterion."

Although parental participation in the intervention varied, group comparisons at one-year follow-up revealed significant improvements in experimental subjects when compared with controls on teacher-rated attention deficit/hyperactivity and on behavior as rated by teachers on the Behar behavior questionnaire. Again, analyses suggested that improved parenting practices following intervention predicted better child outcomes one year later. Conclusions are limited by attrition, the absence of baseline data for the experimental and control children, and some changes in patterns of significant findings from posttest to one-year follow-up. Nevertheless, these results suggest the promise of interventions aimed at enhancing parents' skills in behavioral management and in verbal interaction with their children during prosocial play when such interventions are offered to economically deprived parents of children evidencing early behavior problems in the home.

Other programs have aimed at helping children develop the skills to meet the demands of schooling. Many of these center-based programs have also included parent-focused components such as home visitation. In the *High/Scope Preschool Curriculum Comparison Program* (Weikart, Schweinhart, and Larner, 1986), the highly structured Distar model (a programmed learning approach wherein the teacher initiates activities and the children respond (Carnine, Carnine, Karp, and Weissberg, 1988)), the child-directed experiential approach of the High/Scope Cognitive Curriculum (Hohmann, Banet, and Weikart, 1979), and the nursery school program based on psychoanalytic theory produced similar improvement in cognitive performance through age 10 when combined with educational home visits by teachers. Differences in long-term effects on behavior were found as a function of the curriculum approach that was adopted (Schweinhart and Weikart, 1992). Subjects exposed to the Distar teacher-led, programmed-learning approach were twice as likely as subjects in other early childhood education groups ($p < .05$) to report involvement in delinquent acts (e.g., violence, drug abuse, and status offenses) at 10-year follow-up (when they were age 15). The effect size for the overall delinquency score ranged from 0.48 to 0.60. This difference was attributed by the investigators to the fact that the Distar program, which was primarily academic, gave little attention to the social behavior of the children, whereas the two other curriculum approaches did.

The *Perry Preschool Program* used the High/Scope curriculum and focused on enhancing the intellectual and social development of three- and four-year-old African-American children from backgrounds of extreme poverty. The selective preventive intervention, begun in 1962, consisted of daily participation in preschool over a one- to two-year period and weekly home visits by trained teachers. The experimental intervention was associated with positive effects on academic performance and social adjustment when randomly assigned experimental and control subjects were followed up and compared at age 19 (Berrueta-Clement, Schweinhart, Barnett, Epstein, and Weikart, 1984). Attendance in the Perry Preschool Program was associated with a lower rate of deviant behavior and greater social competence in adolescence and early adulthood (Schweinhart, 1987). In primary school the Perry Preschool children demonstrated lower rates of aggression, disobedience, disruptive behavior, lying, stealing, and profanity (an average of 2.3 offenses per person, compared with 3.2 for the no-preschool group). At age 15 the Perry Preschool group reported fewer acts of misconduct, and at age 19 they reported fewer violent acts and less police contact (an average of 1.2 arrests per person, compared with 2.3 for the no-preschool group). Only 31 percent of the preschool group had been arrested at least once by age 19, compared with 51 percent of the no-preschool group. By age 19, experimental preschool participants had lower arrest rates and fewer lifetime arrests, as well as lower rates of self-reported fighting, than control subjects. They also had higher rates of secondary school completion, lower rates of placement in special education classes, and higher grade point averages than their control counterparts (Berrueta-Clement et al., 1984).

Programs Aimed at Enhancing Social Competence

The evidence linking aggression and other behavior problems in childhood with increased risk of later mental disorders has led to the development of educational strategies designed to enhance the social competence of youngsters. These interventions are based, in part, on the hypothesis that aggressive and disruptive children are deficient in basic, teachable, interpersonal skills (Spivack and Shure, 1974) and that acquiring these skills can reduce the risk of childhood psychopathology and later mental disorders.

Social competence interventions seek to enhance children's capacities to coordinate cognition, affect, and behavior so that they can respond adaptively to social tasks and challenges (Weissberg, Caplan, and Sivo, 1989). These interventions have focused on four skill areas: (1) self-management or self-control, (2) communication, (3) decision making and problem solving, and (4) resisting negative and limiting social influences.

One of the original programs to enhance social competence, Shure and Spivack's *I Can Problem Solve: An Interpersonal Cognitive Problem-Solving (ICPS) Program,* was targeted to economically disadvantaged four- and five-year-old African-American children from federally funded Head Start day care centers and kindergarten classrooms in inner-city Philadelphia. The curriculum includes a manual of scripted lessons of games and interpersonal dialogues provided daily for 20 minutes over a three- to four-month period. It also includes 10 to 12 lessons that introduce the language and basic concepts for thinking about alternative solutions to problems and about the consequences of actions, approximately 20 lessons that teach children to recognize and be sensitive to the feelings of others, and approximately 15 lessons teaching problem-solving processes for generating several possible solutions in a social situation and thinking about the likely consequences of each solution. Each lesson is delivered to small groups of nursery school or kindergarten children by a classroom teacher trained in the curriculum. Teachers are taught an important informal communication method called "problem solving dialoguing" to provide children with opportunities to use their new skills in social situations arising in the classroom or on the playground.

In testing the curriculum, Shure and Spivack chose not to restrict the intervention to children who were already showing skills deficits, but rather to provide it to all urban children from families in poverty attending intervention day care centers and intervention kindergartens, thus making it a selective preventive intervention.

A complicated design, small numbers, and substantial attrition (39 percent lost in year two) hampered the study. Nevertheless, the results provided empirical support for the efficacy of enhancement of social competence through training in interpersonal problem-solving skills at ages four and five in urban day care and school settings. Shure and Spivack (1988, 1982, 1980) reported that social competence training produced durable effects on social behavior. Children trained in nursery school were rated as significantly better than untrained controls on measures of adjustment at the end of the intervention and again one year later when rated by kindergarten teachers. These effects were observed in those at highest risk. For children trained in kindergarten, 70 percent of those previously rated as impulsive were rated as adjusted, compared with 6 percent of the impulsive controls. The investigators showed that acquisition of skills to generate alternative solutions and consequential thinking skills predicted behavioral adjustment at post-test.

The results suggest that providing a social competence curriculum to inner-city disadvantaged children before first grade can help to reduce aggressive and socially inappropriate behaviors predictive of later mental health problems. By the spring of kindergarten, only 30 percent of children in control classrooms were rated by their teachers as normally adjusted, compared with 77 to 85 percent of the children in the three experimental groups exposed to different lengths and combinations of intervention at ages four and five.

The investigators had first conducted a pilot test of the use of the ICPS curriculum by inner-city African-American mothers in poverty (Shure and Spivack, 1982). Twenty mothers of four-year-old children who showed observable behavioral difficulties in nursery school and 20 matched controls were studied in an indicated preventive intervention. The findings demonstrated that mothers could be trained to teach their children ICPS lessons at home. Children in the experimental group improved significantly more than controls on measures of interpersonal skills and behavioral adjustment. Moreover, the improvement in behavior generalized to the classroom, as reflected in teacher ratings of behavioral adjustment.

Findings and Leads

• Multicomponent interventions that address multiple risk factors have proved effective in improving the family management practices of low-income parents and in facilitating the cognitive and social development of children of low-income, low-birthweight, and low-education backgrounds, preparing them for successful entry into the primary grades. There is also some evidence that multicomponent early childhood interventions have shown effects in promoting prosocial behavior and preventing behavior problems.

• Preventive interventions designed to enhance social competence through teaching interpersonal problem-solving skills at ages four and five in urban day care and school settings and through parents training their children in these skills at home have produced durable effects on conduct problems in children.

• Early childhood interventions can have positive long-term effects on academic performance and social adjustment. Achieving enduring effects through adolescence, a period of great risk for onset of mental disorders, by intervening in early childhood is a noteworthy possibility.

• All of these early childhood interventions are characterized by intensity. In most of the programs, services were provided daily over periods of several years, often involving frequent visits to families' homes. All of the effective early childhood programs reviewed here recognize the role of parents in the continuing development of children, and all involve parents on some level, whether through home visitation or center-based programs. All of the programs worked to involve parents in supporting the cognitive and behavioral development of their children. Some provided parents with supports for handling financial, housing, and other material problems as well. These successful interventions typically involved multiple intervention components focused on multiple risk factors for later disorders.

● Early childhood interventions, delivered with fidelity and quality, clearly can reduce risks for later disorders in children from at-risk families. Data are not yet available regarding the effects of these early childhood interventions on the incidence of a wide range of diagnosable disorders, including, but not limited to, substance abuse disorders, conduct disorder, depressive disorders, and schizophrenia.

INTERVENTIONS FOR ELEMENTARY-AGE CHILDREN

Middle to late childhood (ages 5 to 12) is a period of rapid cognitive and social development. Most children learn to read and to interact in ways that gain social approval from peers during this period. Children who cannot perform academic tasks at grade level by grade 4 and/or who develop social incompetence, impulsivity, and aggressive behavior during this period are at high risk for developing mental disorders, especially substance abuse, conduct disorder, and depressive disorders.

In addition, the family environment may contribute to risk during this period. Poor parenting practices, high levels of conflict in the family, and a low degree of bonding between children and parents appear to increase the risk for mental disorders.

Preventive interventions at this period have focused on the children, with less attention to parents. The children, now developmentally more advanced, are capable of engaging in more verbal interventions. High-risk factors for children, including early behavior problems, have been addressed through enhancement of social competence and academic achievement. Intensive family preservation services have provided crisis intervention for families where children are at risk for out-of-home placement.

Programs Aimed at Enhancing Parenting Skills and Family Functioning

Universal interventions seeking to enhance parenting skills, such as courses on parenting complete with books and video tapes, have been popularized over the past two decades. Unfortunately, virtually no controlled studies have examined the effects of these relatively widely disseminated programs, either in terms of risk reduction or in terms of the prevention of mental disorders or related health and behavior problems. A number of experimental treatment studies, however, have demonstrated the effectiveness of parenting skills training during early and middle childhood to reduce antisocial behaviors in children meeting diagnostic criteria for disorder. (See Chapter 8; also see Dumas, 1989;

McMahon and Wells, 1989; Fraser, Hawkins, and Howard, 1988; Kazdin, 1987; for reviews.)

An Example from Prevention Services:
Family Preservation Services

In a related but separate area, public and private providers of children's services have initiated intensive family preservation services for families whose children are at risk for out-of-home placement. These short-term crisis interventions are delivered to families in their homes toward the goal of stabilizing the family—by improving family functioning and linking the family to sustaining sources of support—to the point that out-of-home placement of the child is not necessary. These programs are both a response to evidence that out-of-home placement is predictive of more negative social, health, and mental health outcomes and therefore is a risk factor for mental disorders and a response to the rising costs of foster care, congregate care, and institutional care for children removed from their families. Reducing the risk of out-of-home placement might reduce the subsequent onset of mental disorders.

The *Homebuilders Program* in Tacoma, Washington, pioneered the development of intensive family preservation services. In programs based on the Homebuilders model, workers deliver a variety of clinical and material services in the home setting. The services are of short duration (90 days or less) and intensive (a minimum of 8 to 10 hours of face-to-face client contact per week). The mental health status of the parents and children is not assessed.

Early uncontrolled evaluations of intensive family preservation services reported significant cost savings resulting from avoidance of out-of-home placements (Kinney, Madsen, Fleming, and Haapala, 1977), stimulating legislative and administrative interest in the intervention. Currently, intensive family preservation services are being implemented in child welfare, juvenile justice, and mental health systems.

The most rigorous evaluation of intensive family preservation services was a New Jersey study in which 214 eligible families were randomly assigned to family preservation services using the Homebuilders model or to a control group that received existing community services (Feldman, 1991a,b). In spite of an attempted random assignment, there was a significantly higher percentage of whites in the family preservation group (51.3 percent) than in the control group (33 percent). Excellent implementation data indicate that the intervention was conducted in accordance with the Homebuilders model. Both experimental and control groups were at risk for out-of-home placement; just under 20 percent had experienced a prior out-of-home placement. Over 86 percent were from poverty. Most were referred as a result of the child's out-of-control behavior; one quarter were referred because of abuse, neglect, or risk thereof.

At the termination of this intervention, children had entered placement in only 6 percent of experimental families, compared with 16.5 percent of control families. A series of comparisons suggest that families receiving preservation services functioned better than control families when the intervention ended, an indication that the services had improved social support systems for families, reduced family conflict, and strengthened family bonding. The difference in the percentages of children entering placement from experimental and control families persisted over time through multiple follow-ups to 12 months after termination, at which time placement rates were 42.7 percent for the experimental group and 56.7 percent for the control group. These results suggest that even though intensive family preservation services are effective in avoiding some out-of-home placements in the short-term, their long-term results are less impressive.

Programs Aimed at Enhancing Social Competence

In the *Assertiveness Training Program,* a universal preventive intervention, Rotheram, Armstrong, and Booraem (1982) trained college students to lead assertiveness training sessions with a sample of 60 percent white, 35 percent Chicano, and 5 percent African-American fourth-, fifth-, and sixth-grade students from predominantly working-class homes in California. An experimental study comparing assertiveness training against a placebo control intervention demonstrated effects at one-year follow-up on both social competence and academic achievement. In addition to this universal program, an indicated preventive intervention study was done with 101 children targeting four groups: underachievers, disruptive students with conduct problems, children with multiple problems related to achievement and conduct, and exceptional children without major problems. In this study, effects appeared to be least strong among children evidencing multiple problems at baseline (Rotheram, 1982).

Social competence components also have been included in interventions designed for populations selected for intervention because of exposure to specific risk factors or stressors during childhood, including parental divorce, parental substance abuse, and parental depression.

Children from homes broken by marital discord are at risk for conduct disorder and substance abuse disorders (Baumrind, 1983; Penning and

Barnes, 1982; Robins, 1980). Pedro-Carroll and Cowen (1985), in their *Children of Divorce Intervention Program (CODIP)*, sought to reduce risk and enhance adaptation among children of divorce. They developed a curriculum of 10 one-hour weekly sessions for children in grades 4 through 6 whose parents had divorced. The curriculum included a component focused on understanding feelings about divorce and divorce-related anxieties, a cognitive skills-building component for resolving interpersonal conflicts, and a component dealing with skills for controlling anger. A team of two trained facilitators led the school-based intervention.

This selective preventive intervention was first tested with children from white middle-class families in four suburban schools. Participants were recruited through letters and phone calls to parents. Parental consent was necessary for participation. Parents of participants had been separated for an average of 23.6 months. Participants were matched by gender, grade, length of time since parental separation, and other preadjustment measures before being randomly assigned to the experimental group or control group that received a delayed intervention.

At posttest, two weeks following program completion, teachers rated experimental participants as being significantly better adjusted than control subjects on two measures of the Classroom Adjustment Rating Scale (CARS)—shy-anxious behaviors and learning problems. Teachers also rated participants as significantly more socially competent at posttest than controls on the Health Resources Inventory (HRI), which includes indicators of adaptive assertiveness, peer sociability, and frustration tolerance. Similarly, experimental children rated themselves as significantly less anxious than controls at posttest. Further, at posttest, parents of intervention children rated them as significantly less maladjusted than did parents of controls on a scale including items on peer relationships, school performance, and feelings about divorce. These findings were replicated in a less rigorously designed study by Pedro-Carroll and colleagues (Pedro-Carroll, Cowen, Hightower, and Guare, 1986).

Alpert-Gillis, Pedro-Carroll, and Cowen (1989) subsequently extended the program to 16 45-minute sessions and tested it with second- and third-grade children in an urban setting. About 31 percent of participating children were nonwhite. The curriculum was revised to reflect the sociocultural population of urban children targeted. Unfortunately, they used a quasi-experimental design; that is, the experimental group was recruited by a different procedure than the comparison group, and there was no random assignment to the two groups. Greater emphasis was placed on teaching children ways to cope with the problem of infrequent contact with noncustodial parents and to seek support from extended family members and other caring adults. In addition, curriculum materials were selected to portray families of diverse ethnic backgrounds. The definition of divorce was also expanded to include the termination of a common-law relationship or a long-standing live-in partnership if the mother reported a separation. Participants' parents had separated an average of 3.75 years before the intervention.

Pretest comparisons with a group of children from intact families showed both the experimental and the comparison groups of children of divorce were significantly less well adjusted. At posttest, one to four weeks following the intervention, experimental children evidenced significant improvements when compared with comparison groups on (1) self-ratings on the Children's Divorce Adjustment Scale, which assesses coping skills and attitudes toward family, parents, and self; (2) parent ratings of children's feelings, behaviors, and problem-solving skills; and (3) teacher ratings of children's competence, including assertiveness, frustration tolerance, and peer social skills.

The findings from the original study, receiving some support from the second study, suggest that a relatively brief social competence intervention can produce immediate reductions in anxiety, adjustment problems, and behavior problems among both middle-class white children and poor and working-class, urban, multiethnic children who have experienced parental divorce or separation. Longer-term effects of the intervention have not been investigated. The results to date suggest the promise of selective preventive interventions focusing on the enhancement of social competence during the elementary grades for children who have recently experienced parental separation.

Other investigators are also seeking to reduce risk and enhance adaptation of children of divorce (see Grych and Fincham, 1992, for a review; Gwynn and Brantley, 1987; Stolberg and Garrison, 1985; Kalter, Pickar, and Lesowitz, 1984). In addition, Sandler and colleagues, in the *Family Bereavement Program, sought to improve the mental health of children who had experienced the death of a parent within the past two years (Sandler, West, Baca, Pillow, Gersten, Rogosch et al., 1992). They did this by attempting to enhance the family environment. The intervention group received a three-session family grief workshop and 13 highly structured sessions from a family advisor who had personally experienced a bereavement similar to the deaths experienced by the families. Parent reports indicated that the intervention group improved on symptoms related to depression and conduct disorder, especially for the older children. This finding suggests the need to target programs to children's different developmental needs.

More targeted social competence interventions have been designed for populations of children with risk factors for later disorders, such as peer rejection or early aggressive behavior. Bierman's (1986) program, *Social Skills Training*, examined the impact of a social skills training program that involved role playing naturalistic interactions between a target child and peer partners. This selective intervention was targeted at 11-year-olds who had low peer acceptance and were deficient in conversation skills. Children were randomly paired with two same-gender peers and assigned to one of two experimental conditions: social skills training or peer experience. On short-term follow-up, the social skills training showed an overall positive effect on conversational skill acquisition and peer response.

Lochman and co-workers tested an expanded social competence curriculum, the *Social Relations Intervention Program*, with a sample of 86 African-American fourth-grade children identified through sociometric ratings as the most socially rejected and physically aggressive in their classrooms and then randomly assigned to intervention and control groups (Lochman, Coie, Underwood, and Terry, in press). The indicated intervention, based on earlier quasi-experimental work (Lochman and Curry, 1986), consisted of positive social skills training to promote prosocial behaviors and cognitive-behavioral training to decrease anti-social reflexive responses and foster adaptive social problem solving. The curriculum included 26 30-minute individual sessions and 8 small-group sessions. It had four components: social problem-solving training, positive play training, group entry skills training, and training on coping with anger (including how to identify and reduce impulsive behavior and how to use self-talk to regulate behavior). Sessions were held twice weekly at school from early October to late April, for a total of 12 to 18 sessions, by a team of psychology graduate students and a university psychologist.

Small samples, nonequivalent comparison groups, and substantial attrition posed threats to this study, but teacher-rated aggression and rejection were significantly lower among a subgroup of rejected-aggressive children who had received the intervention than among rejected-aggressive children in schools not offered the intervention. One year later, for those remaining in the study, significantly lower teacher ratings of aggression and higher teacher ratings of prosocial behavior were observed in the aggressive-rejected subsample. The intervention appeared to have little effect on the behaviors or ratings of rejected children not also identified as aggressive.

Lochman (1992) followed up several of these aggressive boys in a quasi-experimental study of the longer-term effects of the anger-coping curriculum. Thirty-one boys rated by their teachers as aggressive and disruptive in grades 4, 5, and 6 were compared with 52 boys in other schools rated by either teachers or peers as aggressive. The intervention was followed by significant short-term improvements in rates of substance use, general behavioral deviance, and classroom behavior as measured by observational data and self-reports from the two groups. Three years following the intervention, boys exposed to the school-based intervention had lower rates of drug and alcohol involvement and higher levels of social problem-solving skills, although not lower rates of delinquency or classroom behavior problems. However, a subset of 12 who received booster sessions in the year following the original intervention, combined with five parent training workshops, also showed enduring effects on passive off-task classroom behavior three years after the intervention.

Building explicitly on the treatment interventions developed by Patterson and colleagues (Patterson, Reid, Jones, and Conger, 1975), Tremblay and colleagues at the University of Montreal designed a two-year indicated intervention program for disruptive seven-year-old boys, the *Montreal Longitudinal-Experimental Study* (Tremblay, McCord, Boileau, Charlebois, Gagnon, LeBlanc, and Lariveet, 1991). It combined home-based training for parents in family management skills, offered once every two weeks for a two-year period, with social skills training delivered in schools to disruptive boys within small groups of prosocial male peers. Parents received an average of 17 parenting sessions over the two-year period, and 19 training sessions were provided to the children over the same time. Sessions for the children focused on initiating social interaction, improving interpersonal skills, making verbal requests, following rules, handling anger, and mastering "look and listen" techniques for regaining self-control.

A field experiment tested the intervention with a sample of 172 boys from low-socioeconomic areas of Montreal who were assessed by their teachers at the end of kindergarten as highly disruptive. Boys were randomly assigned to one of three groups: experimental (received intervention); observational (received attention but no intervention); and control. Teacher ratings indicated that boys in the experimental group became significantly less aggressive than boys who did not receive the intervention. This difference lasted through the most recently reported follow-up at age 12, three years following intervention. Further, significantly more control boys were retained in a lower school grade or placed in special classes, schools, or institutions. Twice as many control boys (44 percent) as boys in the experimental group (22 percent) were rated as having serious adjustment problems at age 12. Moreover, significantly more control boys had initiated minor delinquency by age 12 (Tremblay, Vitaro, Bertrand, LeBlanc, Beauchesne, Boileau, and David, 1992; Tremblay et al., 1991).

Programs Aimed at Enhancing Academic Achievement

Apparently reciprocal relationships between achievement and early depression have led some researchers to explore interventions focused on the promotion of academic achievement as a preventive intervention (Kellam and Rebok, 1992). Similarly, the evidence that poor academic achievement predicts both later drug abuse and delinquency (Hawkins, Catalano, and Miller, 1992) has led to the investigation of enhancement of academic competence as a component of preventive interventions.

Several intervention studies have focused on the enhancement of academic competence during the elementary grades. The use of certain methods of instruction in classrooms has been shown in experimental studies to improve achievement. Several studies have linked achievement gains to the amount of active instruction and direct supervision of learning provided by teachers (Brophy and Good, 1986). Some intervention trials have trained teachers in the use of effective instructional methods, including the use of interactive and "mastery" teaching methods, in which teachers frequently monitor students' performance. Teachers are trained to use the results of these frequent assessments to adjust instruction or provide more intensive support, such as tutoring or cooperative learning groups, to increase the academic and cognitive development of all students, including those at risk of poor achievement.

An experimental community-based study, *Community Epidemiological Preventive Intervention: Mastery Learning and Good Behavior Game,* of mastery learning methods in first grade in 19 ethnically and sociodemographically mixed public schools in Baltimore, Maryland, found positive effects on reading achievement (Kellam and Rebok, 1992). Moreover, virtually all of the reading gains occurred among students initially showing depressive symptoms and among those with initially low reading scores, suggesting that this universal intervention may have greater benefits for those at risk for depressive disorders. In addition, the Good Behavior Game program had positive effects on aggressive and shy behavior, with the largest effects found for the most aggressive children.

Learning and achievement problems have also been addressed in tandem with peer rejection through selective interventions targeted at children with both risk factors. Individual tutoring has been shown to produce significant improvements in reading and math achievement among low-achieving, socially rejected fourth graders in *Academic Tutoring and Social Skills Training,* and effects on reading scores remained at one-year follow-up (Coie and Krehbiel, 1984).

Hawkins, Catalano, and their colleagues implemented the *Seattle Social Development Project* with first graders in eight Seattle, Washington, public schools (Hawkins, Catalano, Morrison, O'Donnell, Abbott, and Day, 1992). The initial universal preventive intervention program lasted four years, from the first through the fourth grade. It was a multicomponent intervention and sought to reduce risks in family, school, and peer environments. Although participating schools were chosen on the basis of high crime in their catchment areas (and therefore the intervention might be designated as selective), the program focused on all children rather than on identified at-risk children. One school implemented the program with all students, and one school served as a full control school. The students in the remaining six schools were randomly assigned to experimental and control classrooms. The intervention included teacher training and supervision to modify classroom instruction and classroom management practices in grades 1 through 4, training and supervision of first-grade teachers in the use of Shure and Spivack's (1988) Interpersonal Cognitive Problem Solving Curriculum (see the section above on early childhood), and parent training in grades 1, 2, and 3. Teachers were trained in proactive classroom management, effective instructional methods, and cooperative learning (Hawkins, Doueck, and Lishner, 1988; Hawkins and Lam, 1987). Parents were offered two programs. The first, offered when children were in first grade, was a skills-training program focused on management of children's behavior (Hawkins, Catalano, Jones, and Fine, 1987). The second, "How to Help Your Child Succeed in School," offered when children were in second and third grades, focused on providing parental support for academic development (Hawkins et al., 1987).

Results of assessments were reported shortly after the children entered fifth grade (Hawkins et al., 1992). Fewer children in the experimental group than in the control group reported having initiated delinquent behavior and alcohol use. Children from the experimental group also reported more positive results than control group children for parent management, family communication, family involvement, attachment to family, school rewards, school attachment, school commitment, and achievement tests.

An Example from Prevention Services: School Reorganization

Academic achievement can also be enhanced through a preventive intervention aimed at altering the organization of a school. The *School*

Development Program was created by Comer and colleagues at the Yale Child Study Center as a demonstration of a prevention service that was evaluated initially by quasi-experimental methods and only later by a randomized controlled trial (Comer, 1985). The organizational development model that was used focuses on broadening the involvement of those who have a stake in the school. It creates a school management team, a mental health team, and a program to encourage and support parent involvement. Parents, teachers, and administrators play active and meaningful roles in all these groups, and the result is an enhanced sense of "ownership" of the school's programs.

The School Development Program was first applied in two inner-city elementary schools serving predominantly low-income African-Americans in New Haven, Connecticut, beginning in 1968. Comer (1988) reported positive gains in student academic achievement and in standardized reading and math tests compared with national norms over a 12-year period after implementation of the program. A follow-up study of children from intervention schools and a matched comparison group found higher reading and math scores, school grades, and social competence scores among the children in the intervention schools (Cauce, Comer, and Schwartz, 1987). After further testing with increasingly more rigorous design, the School Development Program is now being used in more than 100 schools throughout the country, and The Rockefeller Foundation has awarded funding for national dissemination of the intervention. A randomized controlled study of the intervention, supported by the MacArthur Foundation, is currently under way in Prince Georges County, Maryland (Jessor, 1993). Such a rigorous design is especially difficult in community intervention of this scale, but the study may yield valuable information regarding the efficacy of the intervention.

Evidence from Quasi-Experimental Studies

Elias and colleagues extended and elaborated on Shure and Spivack's (1988) Interpersonal Cognitive Problem Solving Curriculum for use with children in grades 4 and 5 to prepare them to handle the transition to middle school more effectively (Elias, Gara, Ubrlaca, Rothbaum, Clabby, and Schuyler, 1986). Quasi-experimental analyses with a sample of white children from predominantly working-class homes suggested some small but lasting effects on indicators of psychopathology six years later (Elias, Gara, Schuyler, Brandon-Muller, and Sayette, 1991).

Interventions to enhance social competence have been included in programs offered in settings beyond the school, including after-school programs for latchkey children (Ross, Saavedra, Shur, Winters, and

Felner, 1992), after-school programs for children in public housing (Jones and Offord, 1989), and programs offered through Boys and Girls Clubs in public housing (Schinke, Orlandi, and Cole, 1992). Nonexperimental results suggest that providing well-designed opportunities for active learning and practice of cognitive, interpersonal, and problem-solving skills to children from economically deprived backgrounds during late childhood and early adolescence in after-school programs might contribute to the development of social competence and reduce behavior problems.

Alterations in teaching methods have been combined with other intervention elements to increase achievement among students at risk by virtue of extreme economic deprivation. In a predominantly African-American school in which 76 percent of the children were eligible for federally funded free lunch, Slavin and colleagues in the *Success for All* program, which had a quasi-experimental design, sought to bring all students up to grade level in reading by the end of third grade (Slavin, Madden, Karweit, Livermon, and Dolan, 1990). The project provided half-day preschool and full-day kindergarten focused on language development, academic readiness, and improved self-concept. In grades 1 through 3, pull-out programs and special education programs were replaced with an intensive interactive reading program supplemented by reading tutoring for students needing extra assistance. In addition, a team of two social workers provided family support, and a parent liaison worker provided parent education and encouraged parents to become involved in the child's education. Two inner-city schools serving predominantly African-American and low-income children were matched. Matched pairs of students from each school at grade levels K through 3 were compared. At the end of one year of intervention, children in the intervention school had higher scores on reading tests, with greatest effects found for students with the lowest 15 percent at baseline. The results were hampered by lack of clarification about how schools were assigned to the experimental and control groups.

Findings and Leads

● Intensive family preservation services appear to be an effective short-term mechanism for reducing risk of out-of-home placement, stabilizing families in crisis, and developing family competences and supports. However, long-term results are less impressive, and outcome data related to mental health for children and their parents are not available. More rigorous research designs of service programs such as this one could yield valuable information.

- Preventive interventions to enhance social competence for children of elementary age can be effective in reducing early behavior problems predictive of risk for several mental disorders. Whether delivered to whole classrooms of high-risk children or targeted to individual children referred for early behavior problems, social competence curricula have produced significant reductions in early risk factors associated with later onset of conduct disorder, depressive disorders, and substance abuse disorders. Although the evidence is not conclusive, these interventions appear to produce larger and more consistent effects on behavior when begun in the early elementary grades, when followed by booster sessions or offered continuously for more than a year, and when combined with parent training interventions that enlist adult caretakers in more effectively managing child behavior.

- The use of specific instructional methods in classrooms and individual tutoring interventions for low achievers holds promise for reducing academic failure among those at risk for mental disorders. Some selective interventions focused on enhancing academic achievement appear to have the greatest effects with those at greatest risk when subgroups have been analyzed separately (Kellam and Rebok, 1992; Slavin et al., 1990). It is plausible that ensuring the academic success of all children through the use of effective instructional methods in the classroom will reduce academic failure as a risk factor for depressive disorders, conduct disorder, and substance abuse. Unfortunately, few studies have moved beyond short-term follow-ups of effects on risk factors for these disorders.

- Because multiple risk factors have been implicated in the etiology of most, if not all individual disorders, including conduct disorder, substance abuse disorders, and mood disorders, investigators have designed multicomponent interventions focused on reducing risks in several domains (including family, school, and peer environments) by using efficacious risk reduction components. Program results suggest that such designs are highly promising. For example, when guided by a common theory that specifies common aims and principles for a preventive intervention in different domains, teacher and parent training programs offered together can strengthen prosocial involvements and reduce early-appearing health and behavior problems.

- Current preventive intervention research designs, such as those for children of divorce, could be applied to other groups of high-risk children. For example, work has begun in designing and fielding interventions for children of alcoholics (e.g., Springer, Phillips, Phillips, Cannady, and Derst-Harris, 1992; Emshoff, 1990), but these have not yet been well evaluated. Work has also begun with children whose parents are depressed. Parental depression itself is among the strongest predictors of depression in offspring (Petersen, Compas, Brooks-Gunn, Stemmler, Ey, and Grant, 1993; see Box 6.3 in Chapter 6). Clinical and education interventions for multiple family members based on etiological studies of resilient adolescents exposed to parental depression have been developed (Beardslee, Salt, Porterfield, Rothberg, van de Velde, Swatling et al., 1993; Beardslee, Hoke, Wheelock, Rothberg, van de Velde, and Swatling, 1992; Beardslee, 1990), and rigorous testing of the effects of these interventions on children's behaviors and psychopathology is currently under way.

INTERVENTIONS FOR ADOLESCENTS

Biological events associated with puberty have come to symbolize the transition from childhood to adolescence. This period between childhood and adulthood has become more prolonged as the age of puberty has decreased in industrialized nations (now beginning for girls on average at age 12½ years) and the entry into full-time productive adult roles has been delayed by educational decisions. Hamburg (1992) has described the developmental risk factors that are associated with adolescence, including the exploratory behavior that is central to early adolescence. For example, children today appear to be at greatest risk for the initiation of substance use and delinquent behaviors indicative of conduct disorder from ages 12 to 15.

The early initiation of delinquent behaviors or substance use has been shown to be strongly predictive of antisocial personality or substance abuse disorders. Thus efforts to prevent conduct disorder and substance abuse disorders during adolescence have focused largely on reducing the incidence of disorders by preventing early onset. Even though the co-morbidity of numerous disorders, including substance abuse, conduct, and mood disorders, has been well established (Elliott, Huizinga, and Menard, 1989; Jessor and Jessor, 1977), the preponderance of research on preventive interventions for adolescents has been disorder-specific, focusing for the most part on the prevention of substance abuse, or to a lesser extent, on the prevention of conduct disorder. Virtually no prevention programs during adolescence have focused on the prevention of depressive disorders or depressive symptoms (Muñoz, 1993a) or schizophrenia, in spite of the fact that the incidence of depressive disorders increases during this period (Petersen et al., 1993) and the initial onset of schizophrenia often occurs in late adolescence. Few prevention studies targeting adolescents have measured the effects of intervention on the incidence of multiple disorders.

Prevention efforts during adolescence have received less attention than have efforts to treat individuals who already have these disorders. Given the disorder-specific nature of much prevention research during this period, it is useful to review interventions that have focused specifically on the prevention of substance abuse or conduct disorder. First, however, a program is presented that focused on academic performance and behaviors more generally.

Program Aimed at Enhancing Academic Achievement and School Behavior

There is some evidence from the Seattle Social Development Project (discussed in the section on the elementary period above) that, when implemented in middle-school classrooms in grade 7, the selective interventions of teacher and parent training are particularly effective in changing the school behavior of adolescents who are at elevated risk by virtue of low achievement. Hawkins, Doueck, and Lishner (1988), in their study *Changing Teaching Practices*, conducted a selective preventive intervention research program in which seventh-grade students in three schools were randomly assigned to one of 15 experimental or 18 control classrooms. Teachers were also randomly assigned to experimental or control classrooms. One additional school was assigned to be a full control school, and another to be a full experimental school. The intervention included teacher training in proactive classroom management, effective instructional methods, and cooperative learning methods. After one year, the full experimental and control groups were compared (Hawkins and Lam, 1987). A separate investigation focused on intervention effects on low achievers, defined as those students who received a math achievement score in the lower three stanines (bottom 23 percent) on the California Achievement Test in the spring of sixth grade. Although the students from the experimental group did not report different rates of delinquency or drug use, low achievers in experimental classrooms were significantly more attached and committed to school and significantly less likely to have been suspended from school than their control counterparts. This effect was significant only among low achievers, and not in the general population.

Programs Aimed at Preventing Substance Abuse

The evidence that early first use of substances is predictive of later substance abuse disorder (Kandel, Yamaguchi, and Chen, 1992; Robins and Przybeck, 1985) suggests the goal of preventing, or at least delaying, initiation in hopes of preventing later abuse. Substance abuse prevention research has focused largely on preventing the initiation of substance use or reducing use among those who have initiated use early. To accomplish this goal, prevention researchers have tested school curricula focusing on enhancing social competence, providing social influence resistance training, and promoting norms against drug use. The risk factors addressed by these programs include the early age of onset, social influences to use drugs, including drug-using peers, and norms and attitudes favorable to alcohol or other drug use. In addition, interventions to change laws and norms regulating alcohol and other drug behaviors have also been assessed for effects on adolescents.

Enhancing Social Competence

Social competence curricula have been developed that include specific content on prevention of substance use. The *Positive Youth Development Program* combined training in general social competence with information on substance abuse and on how to apply the skills to situations involving alcohol and drug use (Caplan, Weissberg, Grober, Sivo, Grady, and Jacoby, 1992). Participants were students in an urban middle school (90 percent African-American, 8 percent Hispanic, 2 percent mixed race) and in a suburban middle school (99 percent white, 1 percent Hispanic). The 20-session curriculum was provided in two 50-minute sessions per week by university-based health educators who worked with teachers in classrooms randomly assigned to the intervention training.

Regardless of setting, exposure to the curriculum was associated with better impulse control and conflict resolution skills, as rated by teachers, and with lower scores on a self-reported measure of intent to use alcohol. It was also associated with lower rates of self-reported heavy alcohol use among intervention students than among control students, although no significant differences between groups were found in the incidence (rates of initiation) of alcohol, marijuana, or tobacco use.

Providing Social Influence Resistance Training and Promoting Norms Against Drug Use

Many approaches to drug abuse prevention in the schools have been tried. To date, consistently effective interventions have included at least two components: (1) classroom-based training in skills to identify and resist influences to use drugs and (2) encouragement to adopt norms against drug use during adolescence. Social influence resistance training (Ellickson and Bell, 1990; Hansen, Johnson, Flay, Graham, and Sobel,

1988) provides instruction, modeling, and role play for students to learn to identify and resist influences to use drugs. Curricula promoting norms against drug use (Hansen and Graham, 1991; Ellickson and Bell, 1990; Perry, 1986) have included portrayals of drug use as socially unacceptable, identification of short-term negative consequences of drug use, provision of evidence that drug use is less prevalent among peers than children may think, encouragement for children to make public commitments to remain drug free, and in some cases the use of peer leaders to teach the curriculum.

Nearly all curricula include information on the prevalence and effects of alcohol and other drug use. However, this component alone does not appear sufficient to change the drug and alcohol behavior of youth (Hansen, 1992; Schinke, Botvin, and Orlandi, 1991; Stuart, 1974; Weaver and Tennant, 1973).

The combination of social influence resistance and normative change content in school curricula has produced modest significant reductions during early adolescence in the onset and prevalence of cigarette smoking, alcohol, and marijuana use across a number of experimental studies conducted by a variety of investigators (Ellickson and Bell, 1990; Hansen et al., 1988; McAlister, Perry, Killen, Slinkard, and Maccoby, 1980; see Hansen, 1992, for a recent review.)

Hansen and Graham (1991) have examined the relative contribution of the two components in a universal four-condition experimental study, the *Adolescent Alcohol Prevention Trial*, of 3,011 seventh-grade students at 12 junior high schools. The study population was 44 percent white and 54 percent minority (e.g., African-American, Hispanic, and Asian-Americans). Schools were stratified by size, test scores, and ethnic composition, and randomized to the following conditions: (1) an information program about the social and health consequences of alcohol and drug use; (2) a resistance training program on how to identify and resist peer and advertising pressure to use alcohol and drugs; (3) a normative education program geared toward remedying students' false perceptions about the prevalence and acceptability of alcohol and drug use among their same-age peers (methods used included discussing topics in class, completing and reviewing interviews with nondrinkers, developing positive friendships, establishing nondrinking as a positive quality, and writing and videotaping antialcohol rap songs); and (4) a shortened combination of information, resistance training, and normative education.

Results, which were analyzed at the classroom level on data collected in the year following intervention, suggested that normative change was the active ingredient in the curricula. Overall, those classrooms that received the normative education program had significantly reduced rates of alcohol consumption ($p < .001$), marijuana use ($p < .001$), and cigarette smoking ($p < .05$), compared with classrooms that did not (groups 1 and 2). Analyses were conducted of program effects on prevalence and incidence using dichotomous measures of alcohol, cigarette, and marijuana use. For alcohol use, the greatest effect was on the delay in the age of onset of ever being drunk; the incidence of drunkenness in classrooms not exposed to the normative change component increased 11 percent, compared with an increase of 4 percent for those exposed to that component. There was also a greater increase in prevalence of problem alcohol use in the groups not exposed to the component (an increase of 2.4 percent) than in the normative education groups (which increased 0.3 percent).

Exposure to the normative change component had a similar effect on the use of marijuana. Classrooms that did not receive that component demonstrated an increased prevalence of marijuana use, compared with the normative education classrooms (an increase of 6.2 versus 2.2 percent). Hansen and Graham (1991) have suggested that previously reported positive effects of peer resistance skills-training programs may have been due to the normative education components included in these programs. It appears that the enhancement of social norms against tobacco, alcohol, and marijuana use in adolescence is an essential component of school curricula seeking to prevent the early onset of alcohol and other drug use as a strategy for preventing substance abuse disorders.

Ellickson and Bell (1990) reached a similar conclusion in another universal program, when, at one-year follow-up, the initial effects on alcohol use from their social influence resistance training, *ALERT Drug Prevention,* had disappeared. They speculated that social influence training is less effective in preventing alcohol use than tobacco and marijuana use because a normative consensus has not been established around the use of alcohol.

There is some evidence that the use of peer leaders from the student population to share in the teaching of the substance abuse prevention curriculum is more effective than teacher-led conditions (Botvin, Baker, Filazzola, and Botvin, 1990a; Klepp, Halper, and Perry, 1986; Murray, Johnson, Luepker, and Mittelmark, 1984; McAlister, 1983). Peer leaders may be effective in stimulating classroom norms antithetical to drug use.

Perry and colleagues, in a four-country pilot study conducted under the auspices of the World Health Organization, attempted to delay the onset of alcohol use in eighth and ninth graders and to reduce the use of alcohol by those already involved with it (Perry, Grant, Ernberg,

Florenzano, Langdon, Myeni et al., 1989). Twenty-five schools were randomly assigned to one of three conditions: peer-led education, teacher-led education, or control. The teacher-led and peer-led curricula (five sessions) were identical in content, except for the fact that the peer-led program took place in small groups, whereas the teacher-led program was conducted with the classroom as a whole. Self-report data at one-month follow-up showed that peer-led programs for teenage drinkers and nondrinkers were significantly more effective in preventing or reducing alcohol use than programs taught by teachers.

Although attention to the establishment of a clear consensus regarding norms is apparently an important component of substance abuse prevention programs, this strategy has some limitations and risks. For example, Ellickson and Bell (1990) found that although their curriculum was effective in preventing tobacco use among those who were not tobacco users in grade 7, the program had counterproductive effects on those already smoking. Smokers at baseline who were exposed to the curriculum actually smoked more at posttest than their control counterparts. It is plausible that explicit campaigns to show drug use as nonnormative behavior isolate or alienate those who already engage in that behavior. Ellickson and Bell found that these individuals were already at risk for mental health problems by virtue of high levels of family conflict, problems in parent-child communication, early delinquency, low achievement, and low commitment to school (truancy).

Multicomponent Interventions

The establishment through public policy of clear normative standards regarding alcohol and other drugs appears important in preventing or at least delaying the onset of drug use. Peers, family members, the community, and the media all influence the development of an adolescent's norms and attitudes regarding behavior. Some drug abuse prevention programs have combined school-based curriculum interventions with interventions focused on parents, community leaders, and the media to promote greater normative clarity and consistency in the adolescent's social environment.

Pentz and colleagues tested a multicomponent communitywide program, The *Midwestern Prevention Project*, involving a curriculum of social influence resistance skills training and normative change content for students in grades 6 and 7 (Pentz, Dwyer, MacKinnon, Flay, Hansen, Wang, and Johnson, 1989). A 10-session school-based universal intervention provided information on the health consequences and prevalence of substance use and taught assertiveness and social resistance skills. This was combined with homework assignments to be conducted with parents; booster sessions in the year after the initial intervention; organizational and training opportunities for parents in positive parent-child communication and in reviewing school policies; training of community leaders to organize drug abuse prevention task forces; and news coverage via newspaper articles, short television clips, and a press conference. The multicomponent program produced lower rates of weekly cigarette smoking (down 8 percent), alcohol use (down 4 percent), and marijuana use (down 3 percent) after the second year of intervention, and significantly lower prevalence of monthly cigarette (down 6 percent) and marijuana (down 3 percent) use three years after the initial school intervention, although the prevalence of alcohol use was not significantly reduced at this measurement point (Johnson, Pentz, Weber, Dwyer, Baer, MacKinnon, Hansen, and Flay, 1989). The comprehensive intervention appears to have been effective in lowering tobacco and marijuana use prevalence among those at risk because of exposure to parental drug use, drug-using peers, and early initiation of use.

This study's conclusions are tempered by methodological consider-ations. Only 8 of the 42 participating schools were randomly assigned to experimental and control conditions. In the other 34 schools, the assignment was based on the flexibility of the principal and his or her willingness to reschedule classes to accommodate the intervention. Additionally, students in different grades were compared in the quasi-experimental nonequivalent comparison group design. The results of a more controlled trial of the multicomponent intervention conducted by Pentz and her colleagues in Indiana have not been reported in full. Nevertheless, the results reported to date indicate multiple drug use behaviors were reduced by the combination of curriculum and mobili-zation of parents, community members, and the media to promote norms consistent with those provided in the curriculum.

Policy Initiatives

Substance abuse disorders depend on the availability of substances and on the prevalence of substance use in the population. Current policy-focused prevention strategies seek to limit the availability of drugs through prohibition of drugs such as marijuana and cocaine, taxation on alcohol at purchase (Levy and Sheflin, 1985), raising the minimum drinking age (Joksch, 1988; Saffer and Grossman, 1987; Cook and Tauchen, 1984; Kreig, 1982), and restrictions on how alcohol is sold (Holder and Blose, 1987). The legal status of a substance is associated with the prevalence of its use in the population. Alcohol, an intoxicant legal for adults to purchase and use, is the substance most widely used by both adults and adolescents. Alcohol abuse and alcoholism are, in turn, the most prevalent substance abuse disorders.

With respect to alcohol, increases in taxes on alcohol at purchase have been shown to produce immediate and sharp decreases in liquor consumption rates and cirrhosis mortality (Cook and Tauchen, 1982). Similarly, increased alcohol availability resulting from the privatization of wine sales has been shown to result in at least short-term increases in alcohol consumption (Wagenaar and Holder, 1991). However, longer time series analyses conducted by Mulford, Ledolter, and Fitzgerald (1992) have suggested that the increased consumption following privatization of sales is only temporary. Long-term sales trends in one state tracked for 10 years were unaffected by the change in distribution system approximately midway through the period.

Increasing the legal age for drinking alcohol to 21 years has been shown to be associated with lower levels of alcohol use among high school seniors and recent high school graduates, and with lowered involvement in alcohol-related fatal crashes among drivers under 21 (O'Malley and Wagenaar, 1991). Lower levels of alcohol use persisted into the early twenties, beyond the legal drinking age.

Investigation of another policy measure to limit alcohol availability, restricting how alcohol is sold, has shown that allowing patrons to purchase distilled spirits by the drink increased the consumption of distilled spirits and the frequency of alcohol-related car accidents (Holder and Blose, 1987).

Evidence from a Quasi-Experimental Study

As noted above, components on alcohol and other drugs have been included in some social competence curricula (Caplan et al., 1992). Conversely, the work of Botvin and colleagues in substance abuse prevention has combined (1) training in skills to resist social influences to use drugs with (2) a focus on the development of general social competences, including verbal and nonverbal communication skills, skills for social interaction with same- and opposite-sex peers, assertiveness skills, and skills for coping with anxiety (Botvin et al., 1990a; Botvin, Baker, Tortu, and Botvin, 1990b). A recent evaluation suggested the promise of this approach when led by peers, but the evaluation highlighted the importance of the fidelity or integrity of implementation of curricula-based interventions (Botvin et al., 1990a). Only about 62 percent of the trained experimental teachers in their study implemented

60 percent or more of the curriculum content. This finding has clear implications for the dissemination of preventive interventions.

Programs Aimed at Preventing Conduct Disorder

Conduct disorder involves frequent, persistent, and patterned antisocial behaviors, including delinquent behaviors, whether against property (e.g., burglary, fire-starting) or persons (e.g., fighting, violent behavior, rape), as well as other problem behaviors (e.g., lying, running away). (For more detailed descriptions of conduct disorder, see Chapters 5 and 6.) During adolescence, conduct disorder increases in prevalence and affects current functioning. Conduct-disordered behaviors that become integrated into the behavior patterns of the individual during adolescence predict antisocial personality in adulthood, indicate risk for other disorders (including mood disorders and schizophrenia), and affect adult functioning and opportunities.

Risk factors associated with the development and diagnosis of conduct disorder include early aggressive behavior, school failure, criminal and alcoholic behavior of parents, poor family management practices (e.g., inconsistent discipline, poor monitoring), and family conflict (Kazdin, 1990). These factors are often well established before the onset of adolescence. During early adolescence, as with substance use, peer influences and norms conducive to antisocial behaviors increasingly and strongly predict involvement in delinquent and other problem behaviors (Elliott et al., 1989).

In contrast to substance abuse prevention, the preponderance of the evaluated efforts to prevent conduct disorder have focused on individuals at risk rather than on community or school populations. For example, preventive interventions effective in preventing conduct disorder during adolescence have focused on 12- to 15-year-olds at risk by virtue of academic or behavioral problems and by virtue of an older sibling's involvement in status offenses.

A family-focused treatment intervention in an experimental study demonstrated positive effects in preventing delinquent behaviors in siblings of 13- to 16-year-olds who had committed minor delinquent offenses or had been declared ungovernable by the juvenile court (Alexander and Parsons, 1980, 1973). The intervention combined behavior management skills training techniques for parents with communications skills training. The brief family systems intervention significantly altered patterns of communication within experimental families and resulted in statistically significant preventive effects on younger siblings. A 2½- to 3½-year follow-up of the juvenile court records of the younger siblings of the originally targeted participants found that 20 percent of the younger siblings in families that received the short-term family systems intervention were referred to court, compared with 43 to 63 percent of the younger siblings in families that received other experimental or control conditions (Klein, Alexander, and Parsons, 1977).

Some indicated preventive interventions that have shown positive effects in preventing delinquency have involved both family and school intervention. Bry's (1982) three-year indicated preventive intervention, *Behaviorally Based Preventive Intervention*, targeted adolescents with academic and behavior problems at school. Samples of seventh-grade students with low academic motivation, alienation from family, and several school discipline referrals were identified in a low-income urban school and a middle-income suburban school. Within schools, participants were placed in matched pairs on the basis of sixth-grade academic records and randomly assigned to receive the intervention or serve as controls. The intervention consisted of the use of positive reinforcements for desirable school behavior. Weekly report cards were used to monitor student behavior in the classroom as reported by teachers. Program staff met weekly with intervention students to discuss report cards. Positive reports elicited praise and approval from staff, and negative reports elicited discussions of how to win more approval from teachers. Parents were routinely informed of students' progress through phone calls, letters, and home visits. Booster sessions were also provided every two weeks over a period of two years following the initial intervention, although attendance at booster sessions was low. Nevertheless, the intervention appeared to prevent later delinquency as measured both by self-reports of criminal behavior at one-year follow-up and by court records at five-year follow-up. Ten percent from the intervention group, compared with 30 percent from the control group, had accumulated a court file.

Evidence from Quasi-Experimental Studies: Altering School Organization and Social Environments

School transitions represent a time of risk for increased symptoms of psychological problems. Both substance use and antisocial behaviors increase in prevalence following transitions from elementary to middle or junior high school and from middle school to high school. There is evidence that the structure of schooling itself may affect these changes in behavior following school transitions (Hamburg, 1992). Comprehensive recommendations for changing the structure of education, especially in middle schools, have been made (Carnegie Council on Adolescent Development, 1989).

Gottfredson and Gottfredson (1992) also have focused on changes in school organization and management in testing interventions to prevent delinquency and substance abuse in secondary schools. (See similar work by Comer in the section on interventions in the elementary period.) An important ingredient in the Gottfredsons' work is a focus on providing a method for school stake-holders to reorganize the school to make it more effective in the social and cognitive development of all students. The method involves a systematic assessment of school problems carried out by a school improvement team of teachers, parents, school administrators, community agencies, students, and district-level staff. The team reviews school policy, climate, instruction, and organization and plans and implements changes. The intervention is called the *Program Development Evaluation* method (Gottfredson, 1984).

Gottfredson (1986) evaluated an intervention that included the establishment of an organizational structure to facilitate shared decision making and management in schools, the use of curriculum and specialists trained to respond to student concerns, academic innovations including cooperative learning, reading and test taking programs, and career exploration. In addition, direct services were provided to a randomly assigned subsample of high-risk students in participating schools. After three years, students in experimental schools reported lower rates of drug use, delinquent behavior, and alienation, and higher rates of attachment to school, higher educational expectations, and a greater belief in school rules than students in comparison schools. However, although the direct services for selected high-risk students improved their school achievement (promotion and graduation rates), these services did not produce significant effects on the delinquent behaviors of the high-risk students over and above the effects of the organizational intervention in the school (Gottfredson and Gottfredson, 1992; Gottfredson, 1986).

Gottfredson has evaluated the method in inner-city Baltimore, Maryland, and in Charleston, South Carolina. The Baltimore study showed significant decreases in rebellious behavior and negative student attitudes toward school following use of the method (Gottfredson, 1988). An evaluation of the method in six Charleston schools found that, in comparison with control schools, those using the method improved significantly in classroom order, classroom organization, and clarity of rules (Gottfredson, Karweit, and Gottfredson, 1989).

Another broad intervention targeted the school environment at a particular developmental phase. Felner and colleagues focused on the restructuring of schools through the *School Transitional Environmental Project (STEP)* designed to address the risks associated with the transition from middle school to high school, including academic failure and low commitment to school (Felner, Ginter, and Primavera, 1982; Felner and Adan, 1988). The intervention had two components: (1) reorganizing the school environment to alleviate stressors associated with the transition and (2) redefining the role of homeroom teachers to give them more central roles as counselors and mediators between students and the school administration. The goal of STEP was to enhance adjustment through a school restructuring program that assigned project students to one of four experimental homerooms. The homeroom teachers were given more responsibility to meet the administrative, counseling, and guidance needs of their students. The students in the experimental groups were assigned to take their core academic courses (math, English, social studies, and science) together, and all the experimental classrooms were in close proximity to enhance feelings of belonging and social support among a more stable cohort of peers. The underlying hypothesis was that by changing the role of school personnel and the overall social ecology of the high school environment to increase levels of social support available to students and reduce the confusion and complexity of the new school environment, both academic and personal adjustment would be enhanced.

The effectiveness of STEP, a selective preventive intervention, was examined with a sample of 185 ninth graders (65 in the experimental group and 120 in the control group) from a primarily minority, lower-income high school. The experimental sample was selected randomly from the entering ninth-grade population who had met all requirements for the eighth grade and who had not been identified as needing special mental health services. The control group was matched on age, gender, and race with the experimental group, but there was no random assignment to the groups. Three-year follow-up data collected at the end of high school revealed lower school dropout rates for the students in the experimental group (21 versus 43 percent of controls) (Felner and Adan, 1988). Positive effects on two indexes of school adjustment, namely, grade point average ($p < .05$) and absenteeism ($p < .05$), were observed following the intervention and were maintained through grade 10. In addition, project students rated the school environment as demonstrating greater order, rule clarity, teacher control, and innovation ($p < .01$), suggesting that reported changes in behavior and academic performance reflected changes in the school environment associated with the intervention. These results show the promise of interventions aimed at the risk factors associated with school transitions. They also suggest that throughout primary and secondary school, having a close relationship with a supportive teacher may be a significant protective factor against academic and mental health problems. Felner has now combined the school restructuring components of STEP with curriculum changes suggested by the Carnegie Council and applied the program in 50 schools with 22,000 children (R. Felner, personal communication, 1993).

Others have taken a more comprehensive approach by targeting the broader social environments of the school, family, and community, seeking to spread the prevention message throughout the social environments affecting the adolescent. Olweus's *Intervention Campaign Against Bully-Victim Problems* was designed to prevent bullying among children and adolescents in Norway (Olweus, 1991). The primary emphasis of the multicomponent prevention program was to educate the community, families, and school personnel on the scope of the bully-victim problem, and potential solutions. The intervention program was implemented as a nationwide campaign. The components of the program included (1) an educational booklet on the bullying problem distributed to all schools, (2) parent education (in the form of a booklet) on the bullying problem and possible solutions, (3) a 25-minute video with stories about the lives of "bullied children," which was available for rent or sale, and (4) a self-report questionnaire to be completed by the children in the program.

The universal preventive intervention was evaluated by using a quasi-experimental cohort sequential design, and time-lagged comparisons were made between age-equivalent groups. The sample consisted of 2,400 students in grades 4 through 7 from 42 primary and secondary schools. Using self-reports of "being bullied" and "bullying others," the findings indicated a 50 percent reduction in the levels of bully-victim problems at both the 8-month and the 20-month follow-up assessments. Youths also reported a reduction in reports of antisocial behavior (e.g., vandalism, theft, truancy) and an increased satisfaction with school life. Although the design does not rule out potential sources of influence, the fact that children reported a reduction in bullying, victimization, and other antisocial behavior following the intervention suggests the potential benefit of interventions seeking to reduce violence by establishing commonly shared concerns regarding antisocial behavior and discouraging such behavior in the media, schools, and homes.

Evidence from a Quasi-Experimental Study: Programs Aimed at Violence Prevention

The emergence of concern with violence as a major public health problem (Rosenberg and Mercy, 1991; Sullivan, 1991; see also Chapter 3) has led to the development of interventions focused on preventing violent behaviors included in the diagnostic criteria for conduct disorder. In this area the emerging prevention strategies bear some resemblance to prevention programs targeting substance abuse. That is, the preventive interventions focus on changing norms regarding violent behavior and providing skills to solve problems without violence. Social competence promotion in problem solving and developmentally appropriate social interaction have been included in school-based curricula seeking to prevent violence. However, the committee is aware of no published controlled studies of classroom-based prevention curricula focused explicitly on preventing violence, although some studies are under way.

To date, methodological problems, including quasi-experimental designs, have thwarted a clear assessment of the effectiveness of community-based intervention programs to prevent violence in the United States. For example, the *Violence Prevention Project (VPP)*, a comprehensive prevention program using a community-based model for the prevention of youth violence, recently reported data from an evaluation study of the intervention (Hausman, Spivak, Prothrow-Stith, and Roeber, 1992). The curriculum included a 10-session community-based "Violence Prevention Curriculum for Adolescents" and a mass media normative change campaign involving television, posters, T-shirts, and brochures. The results indicated little difference in exposure to the intervention between youths in control neighborhoods and youths in experimental neighborhoods. About 55 percent of both experimental and control youths self-reported exposure to the intervention. The results underscore the importance of monitoring implementation and program exposure in evaluating preventive interventions. They also leave open the question of whether combined interventions focused on establishing norms opposed to violence are effective in actually preventing it.

Findings and Leads

• Prevention of early substance use has been shown to be a logical and effective strategy for the prevention of substance abuse disorders. There is evidence that the incidence of substance use can be reduced by school curricula that promote norms antithetical to substance use and teach skills to resist social influences to use drugs. The promotion of clear norms against use appears to be a key component of these interventions. There is also evidence that promoting explicit norms against use in family, school, and community settings through multi-component communitywide interventions holds promise for preventing early substance use. However, normative change strategies may be counterproductive with some of those at highest risk by virtue of their exposure to multiple biopsychosocial risk factors. For example, adolescents who have been exposed to parental alcoholism and violence and who have already initiated use of alcohol themselves may react to normative change campaigns by increasing their substance use. This possibility suggests that combining risk reduction interventions introduced earlier in development with norm-focused interventions during adolescence might be a useful approach.

• There is also evidence that preventive interventions that seek to restrict the availability of alcohol and other substances through higher taxation, raising the legal age of drinking, or limiting how liquor is distributed may reduce both the rates of alcohol consumption and the adverse consequences associated with alcohol use, including alcohol-related accidents.

• During adolescence, initiatives focused on the nature and structure of schooling and school experiences themselves may have mental health promotion or disorder prevention potential. Few of these interventions have been evaluated for effects on conduct or other mental disorders, but a number have shown effects in reducing risk factors. Examples include efforts to promote broader academic success during adolescence.

• The concept of school reorganization and the leads from Comer's and the Gottfredsons' studies suggest the promise of efforts to empower school communities at both the elementary and the secondary levels to regain control of the cognitive and social development agenda of their schools. Intervention trials that focus on identifying how the school and its community can be more effective in reducing risks for and enhancing protective processes against the development of psychopathology may be particularly useful.

• There is some evidence from Norway that preventive interventions can change community norms regarding aggression. The extent to which such a normative consensus can be created regarding the prevention of violence in this country, given the diversity of race, culture, and class, remains to be demonstrated.

• Attention to fidelity and integrity of implementation is critical to the success of a prevention program.

INTERVENTIONS FOR ADULTS

Movement from adolescence to adulthood changes the developmental tasks facing the individual as well as the nature of the risk and protective factors. As various life domains in adulthood, such as family and work life, begin to exert their separate influences, developmental tasks become more differentiated (see Figure 7.2). These tasks include establishing and maintaining committed relationships as well as successful childbearing and effective parenting. Assuming and maintaining occupational roles are also crucial, not only because work can provide a sense of mastery and satisfaction, but also because paid employment provides material support for the developing adult and his or her family. For some adults—particularly poor, single parents—coping with chronic stressors such as financial hardship and lack of emotional support for their parental role also complicates their efforts to perform these tasks successfully and places them at increased risk.

In adulthood, psychosocial risk factors that increase the likelihood of mental health problems correspond closely to these developmental tasks. Marital conflict and divorce, unsupported childbirth and childrearing, stressful work roles and occupations, involuntary job loss, chronic poverty, and discrimination all constitute critical risk factors in adulthood, particularly among those with psychosocial or biological vulnerabilities.

However, there are corresponding protective factors that, when incorporated into systematic preventive intervention efforts, can help to reduce the likelihood of mental disorder. These include problem-solving skills, the availability of responsive social and medical services, and social, material, and emotional support from friends, family, and others. Work supervisors, health personnel, teachers, spouses, and others can be potent sources of either support or stress or both. In addition, a variety of social skills, including the ability to cope with one's emotions, to control the demands of work and mobilize supportive co-workers, to use job seeking skills, and to nurture spouse and family support, all are protective factors that can help safeguard mental health.

The following review of a number of prevention programs focuses on five major areas of adult life where preventive trials have reduced risk factors and enhanced protective factors in the course of adult development. These include programs aimed at (1) the development and maintenance of marital relationships, as well as programs for coping with marital separation; (2) the special stresses of childbearing and childrearing; (3) occupational stress and job loss; (4) preventing depressive disorders among adults at risk because of poverty and minority status; and (5) supporting adult children who provide care for ill parents.

Programs Aimed at the Marital Relationship

The marital relationship can be a major protective factor or stressor, especially for vulnerable individuals. Two preventive programs are described below. One is aimed at enhancing marital relationships, and the other is intended to cope with the risks associated with separation and divorce.

Enhancing Marital Relationships

Destructive marital conflict and marital distress are major risk factors for many forms of interpersonal and psychological dysfunction and psychopathology (Coie, Hawkins, Ramsey, and Watt, 1991). Specifically, marital distress has been associated with higher rates of depression in adults and also related to the development of conduct disorder in children (see Chapter 6). Markman (1984) has argued that destructive conflict among spouses, marital distress, and the effects of divorce constitute a major social problem that costs billions of dollars per year.

Markman and colleagues have developed the *Prevention and Relationship Enhancement Program (PREP)*, designed to prevent distress and divorce in couples who are already married or planning marriage (Renick, Blumberg, and Markman, 1992). PREP, a universal preventive intervention, is based on the identification of and intervention with variables that are most predictive of later distress and relationship satisfaction. Couples who are not currently experiencing relationship difficulties are taught skills identified by research as predicting satisfying and healthy relationships. They are also taught how to thwart those behaviors that predict later marital distress. The central principle underlying the program is that the constructive handling of disagreements can prevent later distress. Furthermore, PREP assumes that opportunities in a relationship should be created to control conflicts and handle problems before they get too large.

Earlier research on which PREP is based (Markman, 1984, 1981, 1979; Gottman, Markman, and Notarius, 1977) suggested that distressed and nondistressed couples communicate differently. Distressed couples were found to engage in negative escalation during discussions, whereas nondistressed couples exited at the beginning stages of negative interaction cycles (Gottman et al., 1977). Furthermore, longitudinal studies (Markman, 1984, 1981, 1979) indicate that the quality of communication before marriage and before the development of distress in the relationship is one of the best predictors of future marital distress.

The PREP intervention takes one of two formats. In the extended version, couples attend six 2- to 2½-hour weekly sessions in groups of four to eight couples. They hear lectures on communication skills and then privately practice their new communication skills to discuss issues in their relationship. The communications consultant acts as a coach to help the couple master these new skills. In the second format, groups of 20 to 40 couples hear the same lectures at a weekend retreat and then use their private rooms to practice their skills on their own.

At the 1½-year follow-up, PREP couples report greater relationship satisfaction and fewer relationship problems. At three years, they report fewer sexual difficulties and less problem intensity. At four years, PREP husbands report better relationship satisfaction than controls and show less dominance, conflict, and overall negative communication. At five years, husbands report greater relationship satisfaction, show less denial and negative escalation, and use more problem-solving behaviors. In addition, at five years, 19 percent of control couples had divorced, whereas only 8 percent of PREP couples had done so. Furthermore, PREP couples reported fewer instances of physical violence with their spouse than did control couples across the three-, four-, and five-year follow-ups (Markman, Renick, Floyd, Stanley, and Clements, 1993).

Most of the evaluation findings for the PREP program have focused on reduction of risk factors rather than specific mental health outcomes, and an improved version of this study would also assess mental health outcomes. This program has been disseminated both in Europe and in the United States and has been adopted for use by clergy, who often provide premarital counseling.

Coping with Separation and Divorce

The epidemiology of divorce as well as stressful life events theory (Bloom, 1985) suggests that marital separation and divorce constitute major stressful life events with major impacts on health and mental health. Epidemiological research conducted in Pueblo, Colorado, as well as a review of the research literature (Bloom, Asher, and White, 1978), indicates that marital separation is associated with higher levels of distress, anxiety, and depression and higher rates of admission to psychiatric inpatient facilities.

Five specific categories of risk can be identified in the literature associated with marital separation and divorce. They include (1) weakened support systems, (2) problems with childrearing and single parenting, (3) legal and financial issues, (4) housing and homemaking problems, and (5) education and occupational problems, particularly for the female spouse in joining or rejoining the labor force.

Bloom and Hodges developed the *University of Colorado Separation and Divorce Program* specifically to address these risk factors and to enhance protective factors (Bloom, Hodges, Kern, and McFaddin, 1985; Bloom,

Hodges, and Caldwell, 1982). This intervention is aimed at newly separated persons who are engaged in the task of negotiating the transition to single life with new occupational and childrearing responsibilities. It is not aimed at improving preexisting marital relationships. Participants had separated because of marital discord and had been separated no longer than 6 months. Bloom and Hodges (1988) followed a number of guidelines in designing the selective program. Principles included the use of a clear program rationale, focus on newly separated persons, specified duration and eligibility requirements, use of a university site so as to avoid defining marital separation as an illness, economical program delivery, a goal of education and competence enhancement, and attempts to be comprehensive in the range of services.

The Separation and Divorce Program was coordinated by a number of program representatives, each of whom worked with 15 newly separated persons. Information in coping with a wide variety of life domains was provided by subject matter specialists, who provided two-hour workshops with groups of participants. Program areas included socialization, childrearing and single parenting, housing and homemaking, employment and education, and legal and financial issues, all designed to enhance coping skills and mobilization of support.

After four years of follow-up in a well-designed and well-executed randomized trial, a number of positive impacts on mental health could be observed. Experimental group members were significantly higher in adjustment, had fewer separation-related problems, and reported significantly greater separation-related benefits than controls. Positive program effects, including lower levels of psychiatric symptoms, were still evident after four years. Preventive effects included reductions in maritally related sources of distress as well as in symptoms of anxiety and depression (Bloom et al., 1985).

The Separation and Divorce Program has been documented with a series of research papers and also a clear and well-documented program manual, which includes details of rationale, design, data collection, and examples from the point of view of participants and staff members.

Programs Aimed at the Challenges of Childbearing and Childrearing

Childbearing and childrearing present major challenges that can affect the well-being of women and their children. Below are two prevention programs that promise to reduce risks associated with insufficiently supported childbearing and childrearing.

Coping with the Stresses of Caesarean Childbirth

Women who deliver children by caesarean section are more likely than control populations to develop postnatal depressive symptoms (Kendell, Rennie, Clark, and Dean, 1981). In addition, the emotional difficulties encountered by women delivering by caesarean birth (CB) are accentuated by hospital practices and attitudes of the hospital staff (Cohen, 1977; Donovan, 1977). Tadmor (1988) reported that CB mothers were not usually well prepared for the event and were cast into the role of surgical patient rather than mother. They were also often separated for longer periods from their children and their new babies, and they may not have received adequate support from their spouse.

The specific psychological and developmental tasks confronted by the CB mother include acquiring a realistic appraisal of the reasons for the caesarean birth and a share in the decision-making process. In addition, she faces the task of dealing with the loss of the natural childbirth process and with the negative feelings associated with caesarean birth. Other psychological tasks include establishing an attachment to the baby and dealing with the physiological limitations imposed by the caesarean birth.

Tadmor and Brandes developed the *Perceived Personal Control (PPC) Preventive Intervention for a Caesarean Birth Population*, a selective prevention program, to enable the CB mother to accomplish the specific psychological tasks associated with caesarean births and to enhance her coping skills so that she can ensure a positive outcome and deal successfully with any future caesarean births (Tadmor, Brandes, and Hofman, 1988; Tadmor and Brandes, 1984). The underlying theoretical framework of the intervention is the perceived personal control crisis model developed most specifically by Caplan (1977) and Caplan and Killilean (1976). The premise of this model was that the availability of a coping response that mediates between the individual's appraisal of some event and his or her responses to it is a critical protective factor that will produce a generalized measure of resistance to stressors.

The intervention begins with an anticipatory guidance session, which helps to familiarize the CB couple with the medical environment and the sequence of steps through which they will pass. They receive detailed information with respect to the course, safety, and duration of the caesarean birth, anesthesia, and the physiological and emotional reactions they can anticipate. During the birth itself, the father actively provides emotional support to the mother. A variety of efforts to enhance the possibility of immediate bonding between infant and parents are engaged. After delivery, the mother and father are given full care of the baby under supervision.

The program was evaluated in a randomized controlled trial. Mothers completed questionnaires on the fourth or fifth postpartum day, and there were follow-ups at 6 and 12 months after the caesarean birth to assess physiological and psychological recovery and to document the implementation of the intervention model, beneficial effects of the model, duration of full breast-feeding, and response to crises.

Results indicated that the program had a number of impacts. Experimental mothers were released from the hospital sooner than controls, initiated independent care of the baby sooner, and continued nursing longer. After day one, experimental mothers requested less medication than controls, and experimental fathers showed closer attachment to the babies than control fathers. Experimental mothers also had a more rapid psychological recovery from the caesarean birth, and distress was reduced.

The PPC intervention is designed to be implemented only in a community institution such as a general hospital. Resistance in the hospital by medical and nursing staff is a major potential limitation. Implementation requires dealing with a complex network of interlocking events and may impose additional burdens on the staff as well as on the mental health worker who implements the program. Furthermore, continuous training has to be provided for new physicians and nurses who join the department.

Enhancing Personal Development of New Mothers

The *Prenatal/Early Infancy Project* is a comprehensive selective preventive intervention designed to prevent a wide range of maternal and child problems often associated with poverty (Olds et al., 1988; Olds et al., 1986). It is a unique program in that it targeted both children and mothers and measured outcomes for both generations. The design of the study and the outcomes related to improved parenting and reducing risks for the children were presented in the section "Interventions for Infants" earlier in this chapter. Discussion here is limited to intervention strategies and outcomes related to the mothers' personal development.

The Prenatal/Early Infancy Project was based on the assumption that nurse home visitors are in an ideal position to identify and change factors in the family environment that interfere with maternal health habits and personal accomplishments in the area of work, education, and family planning. Beginning during pregnancy, nurses attempted to form effective and supportive relationships with the women by emphasizing the women's personal strengths. Nurses encouraged the women to clarify plans for completing education, returning to work, and bearing additional children. Nurses stressed that the decision to return to school and seek employment after delivery should be made after full consideration of the women's own best interests as well as the babies'. Nurses helped interested women find appropriate jobs or job placement services and plan for child care. They also advised them about job interviews and showed them and their partners birth control devices, discussing the advantages of different methods of family planning.

Results of a randomized controlled trial evaluating the effect of the nurse visiting program on outcomes for the mothers showed reduction in a number of risk factors. Among women who had not graduated from high school when registered for the study, 59 percent of the nurse-visited and 27 percent of the comparison group had either graduated or enrolled in an educational program by six months postpartum.

Between birth and the 22-month follow-up, the nurse-visited, poor, unmarried older women had worked 2½ times longer than their counterparts in the control group, who were not nurse-visited. Qualitative analysis of the employment data indicated that by the 46-month interview, most of the women who worked held unskilled labor and service positions; some held semiskilled jobs; and a few were in clerical or sales positions. Nurse-visited, poor, unmarried older women reported that they received more help from other families with child care and were on public assistance 157 fewer days than the poor, unmarried older women in the control group, a 40 percent reduction. This effect, however, did not extend into the two-year period following the end of the intervention at 24 months postpartum. Subsequent pregnancies were reduced in the nurse-visited, poor, unmarried group, with the women having one third fewer subsequent pregnancies than the poor, unmarried women in the control group.

Programs Aimed at Occupational Stress and Job Loss

Work and unemployment represent areas of risk for adults. Occupational stress on the one hand and job loss on the other represent critical points for preventive intervention. Two preventive programs are described below, one aimed at a stressful work role, the other at vulnerable persons who have recently experienced job loss.

Occupational Stress and Coping

In work life and more generally, the beneficial and protective factors of social support on health are well documented (Israel and Rounds,

1987; Cohen and Wills, 1985; Berkman, 1984; House, 1981). Social support has been associated with longer life (Berkman, 1984), compliance with health regimens, higher levels of psychological well-being, decreased morbidity (Cohen and Wills, 1985; House, 1981), and more rapid recovery from serious physical illness and injury. In addition, a variety of studies have shown that social support can buffer the adverse consequences of stress. Although the mechanisms are not yet entirely understood, low levels of social support have been firmly established as a risk factor for poor mental and physical health (Berkman, 1984).

House (1981) and Thoits (1986) have suggested that social support can protect employees from the deleterious effects of exposure to unmodifiable or unavoidable work place stressors. Mechanisms through which social support may provide its positive effects include helping employees to modify stressful situations, develop new appraisals of stressful situations, and decrease the emotional upset associated with problematic situations.

The *Caregiver Support Program* (Heaney, 1992) is a selective prevention program designed to help one particular occupational group, house managers and direct caregivers of the mentally ill and developmentally disabled in group homes. Caregivers work long hours on multiple and rotating shifts, with mental patients who are sometimes assaultive. Their job responsibilities include helping clients with activities for daily living, carrying out behavioral programming, accompanying clients on community outings, and coping with a variety of unscheduled demands and tasks, sometimes in relative social isolation. The low levels of social support, high levels of burden and work demands, and inadequate material and informational resources for coping with the task of caregiving all constitute risk factors for psychological distress (Heaney, 1992).

The Caregiver Support Program was designed to train house managers and caregivers to cope more effectively in their stressful work environment. Six weekly or biweekly training sessions, involving analysis and strengthening of social networks, developing effective staff training skills, and work group problem solving, as well as maintaining new skills and occupational self-esteem, were delivered to house managers and at least one other member of each group home support team. Training sessions were facilitated by a pair of trainers, and training protocols were highly specified and delivered with high reliability.

A randomized controlled trial evaluating the Caregiver Support Program showed changes in risk factors, with the strongest effects occurring as improvements in supervisor support, reductions in supervisor undermining, and higher levels of contact with and positive feedback from supervisors in the experimental group. In addition, the program reduced depressive symptoms and somatization among employees most at risk for leaving their jobs.

As with many work place interventions where participation is voluntary, there is likely to be substantial variation in exposure to the actual intervention, even in a randomized experiment. Statistical models can estimate the interaction between characteristics associated with participation and actual exposure to the intervention to estimate experimental effects, but differential selection into or out of exposure to the intervention remains an issue. The effects of the intervention were probably reduced by the incomplete implementation associated with the "train-the-trainer" approach, in which only house managers and one direct care staff person per home were primarily exposed to the training intervention. Thus the effects of exposure to the Caregiver Support Program represent a lower-bound estimate of the program's impact.

Coping with Job Loss and Reemployment

There is substantial epidemiological evidence that unemployment is associated with higher levels of mental health problems, particularly symptoms of depressive and anxiety disorders (Kessler, Turner, and House, 1988). Furthermore, involuntary job loss is a stressful life event that produces a range of subsequent crises, including financial hardship and family conflict. Some epidemiological evidence suggests that in addition to higher levels of anxiety and depressive disorders, unemployment rates are associated with higher levels of alcohol abuse, child abuse, marital conflict, and a variety of other related mental health problems (Gordus, 1984). These data are of mixed quality, but more recent, community-based epidemiological studies by Kessler and colleagues indicate a higher relative risk of high levels of symptoms of depressive disorders and anxiety disorder in unemployed groups than in steadily employed groups (Kessler et al., 1988; Kessler, House, and Turner, 1987).

The process of job seeking itself is stressful, but the process can be enhanced by protective factors that reduce the likelihood of lowered motivation, discouragement, and prolonged unemployment. Such protective factors include the acquisition of effective job-seeking skills and strong social support during the job-seeking process.

The *JOBS Project for the Unemployed* was a selective preventive intervention designed to help job losers cope with the stresses of job loss and setbacks in the job search process, as well as seek social support and develop and use job-searching skills leading to more rapid reemployment in high-quality jobs (Price, van Ryn, and Vinokur, 1992; Vinokur,

Schul, and Price, 1992; Caplan, Vinokur, Price, and van Ryn, 1989; Vinokur, van Ryn, Gramlich, and Price, 1991).

The intervention was based on the theory of self-efficacy; that is, the knowledge that one can succeed is a motivational force for attempting difficult behaviors. The target group for the JOBS intervention was recent job losers who had applied for unemployment insurance from the various offices of the Michigan Employment Security Commission. It was delivered to groups of 18 to 20 persons in the form of a training program with eight three-hour sessions over two weeks. Trainers were trained intensively before program delivery, and the intervention was monitored closely by observers during delivery. Pairs of trainers delivered a standard curriculum to job losers, including components on (1) skills training and support for dealing with obstacles to reemployment, (2) identifying sources of job leads, (3) finding job leads and social networks, (4) conducting an information interview, (5) handling emotions related to unemployment, (6) practicing and rehearsing interviews, (7) thinking like an employer, and (8) evaluating a job offer.

The impact of the JOBS project was evaluated in a randomized controlled trial. Two and one-half years after the completion of the randomized trial, people in the experimental group showed significant reductions in depressive symptoms (Price et al., 1992). Furthermore, participants obtained higher-paying jobs and higher-quality jobs, which resulted in higher income, and therefore higher tax revenues. The benefit-cost analysis results indicated that the cost of the intervention (approximately $300 per person) was rapidly offset by these increased tax revenues (Vinokur, van Ryn, Gramlich, and Price, 1991). Other analyses indicated that women in general and people with less education, who were at higher levels of disadvantage, benefited more from the JOBS intervention (Vinokur et al., 1992). Additional analyses indicated that the JOBS intervention was most successful with those people who were at highest risk for subsequent episodes of depressive symptoms.

The primary limitation of the JOBS project is that it was explicitly designed for and has been tested only on job losers in the context of the unemployment insurance offices. It is unclear whether the JOBS intervention can have similar impacts on other groups of unemployed persons who are not recent job losers, such as persons reentering the job market after long periods of time or for the first time or discouraged workers who are no longer seeking employment. A second limitation arises from the attempts to disseminate the intervention on a broad scale to assess how easily it can be adopted by other social service systems. It remains unclear whether it can be delivered with integrity in less well controlled circumstances.

A detailed intervention manual for the JOBS program is available. A more extensive replication of the research evaluating the impact of the JOBS program is currently under way, and a training manual for replicating the JOBS intervention and copies of research reports are also available.

Programs Aimed at Preventing Depressive Disorders Among Adults at Risk Because of Poverty and Minority Status

Depressive disorders, referred to here as depression, are a major health problem (see Chapters 5 and 6). Not only is depression one of the most common of the serious mental disorders, but, partly because of stigma and partly because of lack of knowledge regarding its symptoms and the availability of effective treatments, most persons who have the disorder do not receive treatment. This is especially true for certain ethnic minorities and those in poverty. How to reach and support these populations in effective ways represents a major challenge for prevention research and practice. Two pioneering efforts in this area are described below.

The prevalence of clinical depression is between 9 and 14 percent in the general population. Shapiro and colleagues indicated that only 20 percent of individuals meeting criteria for major depression get treatment from mental health specialists (Shapiro, Skinner, Kessler, Von Korff, German, Tischler et al., 1984). This major underutilization of services is even worse for certain groups, such as Hispanics. For example, in the UCLA Epidemiologic Catchment Area (ECA) sample, only 11 percent of Mexican Americans meeting diagnostic criteria for DSM-III disorders had sought mental health services, compared with 22 percent of similarly diagnosed non-Hispanic whites at the same site (Hough, Landsverk, Karno, Burnam, Timbers, Escobar, and Regier, 1987). Not only do certain minority groups underutilize services much more than others, but they also show higher levels of stressful life events and higher levels of depressive symptoms (Roberts, 1987).

Two of the earliest randomized trials investigating prevention of depression in adults included minorities as major segments of their samples. The *San Francisco Depression Prevention Research Project* focused on public sector primary health care facilities as an ideal site for identifying individuals at risk for depression (Muñoz, Ying, Armas, Chan, and Gurza, 1987). Shapiro et al. (1984) found that although only 20 percent of depressed individuals sought mental health care, 75 percent sought other types of health care. Thus the prevalence of depression in primary care populations is much higher than in the general population. It made sense, then, that persons who were at risk for depression would also seek help there. Given their medical and economic problems, some proportion of those seeking help would be nonsymptomatic but at risk, and others symptomatic but not yet over the threshold into a clinical episode of depression. This randomized controlled preventive trial screened primary care low-income medical patients, the majority of whom were members of ethnic minority groups, identified those who already met criteria for major depression or other mental disorders, and referred them for treatment. Those who did not meet DIS/DSM-III criteria, were not receiving mental health treatment, had been enrolled in the primary care clinic for at least six months, and spoke either English or Spanish were invited to participate in the randomized trial of this selective intervention.

The intervention consisted of a course in cognitive behavioral methods to gain greater control of mood. Doctoral-level psychologists were the instructors, and they followed a protocol (Muñoz and Ying, 1993a). A Spanish-language version was also used. Topics focused on (1) the nature of depression and social learning theory; (2) self-control approaches; (3) how thoughts, activities, and interpersonal interactions affect mood; and (4) how to identify and change those behaviors. The course was conducted in a small-group format with no more than 10 participants per group. The class intervention consisted of eight weekly two-hour sessions.

To date, this is the only randomized controlled prevention trial intended to test whether an intervention could prevent new clinical episodes of major depression. The impact of the prevention project was evaluated in a randomized trial comparing experimental and control group members at 6- and 12-month follow-up periods. Participants in the experimental group had significantly fewer depressive symptoms at both time points. At 12-month follow-up, 4 of the 72 control participants and 2 of the 67 experimental participants met DIS/DSM-III criteria for major depression. The low incidence did not allow sufficient statistical power to test whether the rate of new cases was significantly reduced.

Participants assigned to the experimental group showed the intended changes in the cognitions and behaviors hypothesized to be risk factors for depressive symptoms. Compared with the control group, those assigned to receive the depression prevention course became less pessimistic, had more positive (self-rewarding) and fewer negative (self-punishing) thoughts, and engaged in more pleasant and social activities at one or more follow-up assessment periods. In addition, reductions in negative thoughts and increases in levels of pleasant activity were shown to lead to reductions in depressive symptoms.

Prevention of depression might have additional benefits in terms of reducing utilization of unnecessary medical services. The Depression Prevention Research Project did not find significant differences in medical service utilization between the experimental and the control groups. Further analyses revealed that patients with higher levels of somatization had a greater number of medical visits as stressful life events increased than did nonsomatizers (Miranda and Pérez-Stable, 1993). This suggests that attempts to reduce medical service costs ought to focus on teaching somatizers to cope better with stress. Like most studies of depression, this project relied heavily on self-report data, and outcomes could be made more powerful by adding other sources of data, particularly on the relationship between mood changes and other domains of functioning, such as work or interpersonal relationships. A manual is available for this intervention (Muñoz, 1993a).

Vega and colleagues identified low-income immigrant women of Mexican heritage at consistently high risk for distress and depressive symptomatology (Vega, Valle, and Kolody, in press; Vega and Murphy, 1990; Vega, Valle, Kolody, and Hough, 1987). Ethnographic research identified natural support systems as critical to the well-being of this group. Specifically, the profile of risk that emerged involved both household and extrahousehold factors. Women in the target group typically were experiencing increased burdens and diminished resources, low control, and a sense of personal powerlessness because of chronic economic and social marginality. Their living conditions in families with husbands having unsteady employment or physical handicaps, and the responsibility of caring for large families, placed these women under substantial stress. In addition, most spoke only Spanish, and their social roles were limited to housekeeping.

Counterbalancing protective factors could be mobilized, however. Vega et al. (in press) indicated that emotional and material support, including resource redistribution, transportation, and translation assistance, are all key forms of social support in scarce supply for this population.

Projecto Bienestar was aimed at reaching women who were at high risk for depression but currently had mild or no depressive symptomatology (Vega and Murphy, 1990; Vega, Valle, Kolody, and Hough, 1987). The rationale for the selective intervention (Roskin, 1982) argued that attempts to modify the environment by providing opportunities to strengthen individual capacities for coping with critical developmental tasks and unanticipated stressful circumstances could have preventive effects regarding the onset of depression.

Two types of interventions were provided. The first replicated the cultural style of natural helpers (*Servidoras*) found in low-income communities of Southern California and was a one-to-one intervention carried out by these helpers in the community. These natural helpers were trained and supervised by project staff. The second intervention (*Merienda educativa*) was a peer group intervention organized and led by a *Servidora*. Each type of intervention consisted of 12 contacts, but actual exposure varied depending on the group.

Projecto Bienestar was evaluated in a randomized trial comparing the one-on-one and group interventions with a control group over the course of one year. In general, the *Merienda* group intervention showed significant effects that were nonlinear. The one-on-one intervention showed no effects. The results for the group intervention indicated no significant differences between women with low and high baseline levels of symptoms of depression and those in the control group. On the other hand, for women in the middle range of depression scores, the group intervention had clear positive effects, suggesting that there are strong and complex interactions between baseline depression levels and the effect of the preventive intervention. Nevertheless, for women whose baseline depression scores are at midlevel, the group intervention appears to be effective in preventing subsequent depressive symptoms.

The complexity of the findings suggests that this intervention should be tailored carefully, through screening or other means, to particular subpopulations of the general population in question. In addition, these results suggest that further analyses may reveal interesting and informative relationships between baseline depressive symptoms and preventive interventions.

Program Aimed at Supporting Adult Children Providing Care for Ill Parents

The stressful role of caregiving has been reported to have negative effects on physical (Golodetz, Evans, Heinritz, and Gibson, 1969), social (Cantor, 1983), and psychological well-being (Lawton and Maddox, 1985; Klein et al., 1977; Busse, 1976). Toseland (1990) has reviewed evidence suggesting that various supportive interventions for children of parents needing caregiving can have protective effects against the stresses associated with caregiving for chronic disorders. A variety of research suggests that both peer-led and professional-led support groups may be of value in reducing the stressors associated with chronic caregiving. The target group for these interventions consisted of the adult daughters and daughters-in-law who were the primary caregivers for their parents.

In Toseland, Rossiter, and Labrecque's (1989) preventive intervention, *Peer- and Professionally-Led Groups to Support Family Caregivers*, groups of caregivers met for a total of eight weekly two-hour sessions. Both peer and professional leaders relied heavily on supportive interventions, including ventilation of stressful experiences, expressions of support, and understanding and affirmation of members' ability to cope.

The professional-led sessions followed a two-part protocol including education and discussion as well as problem-solving training. Topics in the education and discussion section included introduction to the support group, caregiver emotions, care receivers' reaction to illness, taking care of oneself, communication between caregivers and care receivers, community resources, medical needs, pharmacology, nursing home placement processes, and managing within the home. A problem solving component involved a six-step model including (1) identifying the problem, (2) anticipating its consequences, (3) identifying its antecedents, (4) generating alternative solutions, (5) evaluating the solutions, and (6) carrying out a plan. Peer-led sessions were less structured and used a self-help approach that emphasized mutual support, the sharing of common concerns, and free exchange of information.

The interventions were evaluated in a three-group randomized trial: (1) peer-led sessions, (2) professional-led sessions, and (3) control group. Both peer- and professional-led experimental groups produced increases in psychological well-being compared with the control condition. Participants in the experimental conditions also reported statistically significant differences with controls in their levels of psychiatric symptoms on the global severity index and the positive symptom index (Toseland, 1990). In addition, results favored the experimental groups in the areas of somatization, obsessive-compulsiveness, and phobic anxiety. Furthermore, participants in the experimental groups differed significantly from those in the control group in social support and in social support network size. Both peer-and professional-led experimental groups also showed higher levels of knowledge of community resources. The patterns of improvement did reflect, to some degree, the nature of the intervention. Peer-led groups spent more time socializing and sharing personal experiences and experienced higher levels of informal social support, whereas professional-led groups tended to focus more on highly structured skills and knowledge.

Follow-up after one year (Toseland, 1990) showed that both peer-led and professional-led experimental groups were more effective than the control group in helping caregivers of frail, older persons reduce the stress of pressing problems, increase formal and informal social supports, and make more personal changes in their caregiving role. The experimental groups also reported higher levels of interpersonal competence, but the initial differences in mental health symptoms were not observed one year later, indicating that improvements in coping and competence may not be enough to prevent psychiatric symptoms.

Toseland (1990) and colleagues suggested several possibilities for improving the effectiveness of interventions for caregivers. For example, for those already experiencing debilitating psychiatric symptoms, psychotherapeutically oriented treatment interventions may be more appropriate. On the other hand, short-term improvements in social support could be sustained for caregivers without serious psychiatric symptoms if preventive interventions were incorporated by either extending weekly group sessions or making periodic booster sessions available. Local chapters of the Alzheimer's Disease and Related Disorders Association could sponsor such groups.

Findings and Leads

• The Caregivers Support Program and the JOBS project both found that the interventions were most successful with people who were at highest risk. Projecto Bienestar was most effective, however, with women with midlevel depressive symptom scores. Interventions should be carefully tailored to groups in which they will have the most impact.

• A practical implication of the findings on the JOBS project is that a preventive intervention that both reduces mental health problems and is cost-effective could be implemented at a relatively low cost. In addition, the benefit-cost analyses suggest that the intervention could pay for itself in higher levels of tax revenues in a relatively short period, clearly under one year.

• As a general intervention for those at risk for depressive symptoms, the San Francisco Depression Prevention Project shows the key role of thoughts and activities, thus reinforcing a broad range of research on the relationship between cognitions, behaviors, and mood. The project demonstrates that randomized controlled trials with low-income, public sector primary care populations are feasible, these trials may include non-English-speaking persons, the prevalence of depressive symptoms is very high, and preventive interventions can reduce depressive symptoms. The next step is to carry out a randomized controlled trial with sufficient statistical power (see Muñoz, 1993b, Table 1) to adequately test whether onset of first episode of major depressive disorder can be prevented. Once a clinical episode has occurred, the probability of relapse is very high (see Chapter 5). Therefore research programs should concentrate on the prevention of the first episode.

• The Perceived Personal Control Preventive Intervention Model (Caplan, 1977) is potentially applicable to a wide range of community institutions, including the general hospital. This model could be adapted to a variety of developmental transitions in which the enhancement of coping skills and personal control is important.

• The Caregiver Support Program has been shown to increase coping resources and reduce stress-related symptoms in social service workers. Modifications in the Caregiver Support Program might include providing training to all members of work teams and developing organizational-level reward structures for successfully implementing the program concepts and skills.

• When outcome data are limited to self-report measures, the full impact of the preventive program may not be known. Adding other sources of outcome data, such as from standardized tests or from family members or teachers of the participant, can increase the validity of the findings.

INTERVENTIONS FOR THE ELDERLY

Old age brings important changes in the social and biological life of the individual, including its own developmental tasks, risk factors, and a need for compensating protective factors. In older persons, work diminishes as a major source of stress and satisfaction, and new challenges emerge. Offspring leave the family, and for some older people the role of grandparent emerges. Retirement becomes a milestone for persons who earned their living outside the home. Perhaps most important, illness in oneself or in one's family or the death of a spouse or other loved ones may produce major life changes for the aging individual.

Developmental challenges that emerge in this period include caring for others, particularly a spouse, coping with severe and incapacitating illness in oneself or in loved ones, as well as coping with loss and death. In addition, maintaining meaningful roles and finding new social roles that give life meaning constitute an important but often ignored developmental task.

Accordingly, risk factors for the elderly include relationship loss and bereavement, chronic illness and caregiver burden, social isolation, and loss of meaningful social roles. On the other hand, protective factors include social support in a wide variety of forms—family, peers, informal relationships, more formal support groups, responsive health and social services such as respite care, and opportunities for new productive social roles.

The prevention programs reviewed in this section address (1) caregiver burden, an important potential risk factor for the elderly and (2) loss of a loved one or spouse, a risk factor that is almost inevitable for the elderly.

Evidence from a Quasi-Experimental Study: Relieving Caregiver Burden

Elderly caregivers of profoundly disabled elderly spouses and parents face major stressful burdens. Demographic trends make it clear that this burden will increase dramatically as we enter the twenty-first century. (For further discussion of caregiver burden, see the sections on Alzheimer's disease in Chapters 5 and 6.)

Caregivers are more likely than others to experience problems in the areas of social participation and psychological distress. Furthermore, the relationship between the patient and the caregiver, living arrangements, the caregiver's perceived adequacy of social support, and the caregiver's gender are related to the probability of experiencing lower levels of well-being. As George and Gwyther (1988) observed, "there are no data suggesting that the stresses of caregiving place one at risk for psychiatric disorder as defined by conventional diagnostic criteria. Nonetheless, our research results suggest that caregivers are a group at risk for substantial psychological distress" (p. 317).

No randomized controlled trial data are available; most studies in this area have used quasi-experimental design. The *Duke University Family Support Program* (George and Gwyther, 1988; Gwyther and Brooks, 1983) is described here as an illustration of the work that currently exists. It is a quasi-experimental design in a longitudinal survey context. The program consisted of community support groups for the family caregivers and memory-impaired older adults. Three basic functions of support groups were identified: (1) Persons sharing a common problem frequently report the need for more information. Support groups are a potentially useful mechanism for information transfer and exchange. (2) In addition, support groups provide neutral support based on the fact that persons have experienced a specific problem and feel psychologically isolated. They can share experiences, coping strategies, and perhaps a sense of mutual understanding and validation. (3) Finally, support groups in some cases perform an advocacy function, mobilizing community support for their problem, and/or educating the community. This advocacy role can, itself, present therapeutic opportunities by augmenting the range of choices for self-efficacy.

Each family support program group had co-facilitators consisting of one family caregiver and one professional service provider, who provided access to local agencies with physical and material resources as well as professional expertise. In addition, the development of one-to-one networks was specifically recommended by the family support program, consisting of dyadic relationships between caregivers with common interests.

In evaluating the intervention, George and Gwyther (1988) explicitly focused only on risk factors; they did not measure psychological well-being as an outcome of their intervention. They focused specifically on knowledge of Alzheimer's disease and related disorders, knowledge of available community-based services, use of the services, and feelings of being misunderstood and/or lonely. In addition, the study examined membership in the support group versus no membership.

The intervention had a strong effect on knowledge of Alzheimer's disease and knowledge of community services, but little effect on use of community services. Nevertheless, it also had strong effects on reduction of feelings of loneliness and feelings that no one understands the caregiver's situation. Longitudinal analyses of results substantially confirmed these initial cross-sectional findings with few exceptions. Future studies would benefit from more rigorous methodological design and inclusion of psychological measures of outcomes. A manual for this program is available (Gwyther and Brooks, 1983). In North Carolina, the manual has been supplemented by training sessions for the support group leaders, called support group facilitators.

Other forms of assistance are also needed to ease caregiver burden. Respite care is the service that caregivers desire most but is least available. Respite care involves temporary relief from the responsibility of caregiving and can be delivered as an in-home, day center, or institutional service for periods of time ranging from a few hours to a few days.

Programs Aimed at Enhancement of Coping with Widowhood and Bereavement

Bereavement is a life event that deserves serious attention in understanding the mental health of persons of all ages (IOM, 1984). Widowhood and bereavement will affect increasingly large groups of the elderly in the coming years. Widows and widowers experience grief, including feelings of sadness, despair, anger, and guilt. They also experience feelings of profound disruption as well as the role loss associated with losing a spouse. After the immediate needs following the death of a spouse have been met, including funeral arrangements, legal arrangements, immediate social service arrangements, and the initial support from loved ones, the widow or widower is often left alone and is expected by others to recover rapidly. This period of transition, from six weeks to two months after the death, appears to be more difficult than the period immediately following the death.

Many bereaved people will live many more years after their loss, and some are at risk for a variety of problems. Bereavement has been studied extensively as a risk factor, and Marris's (1958) and Parkes's (1965) early epidemiological work suggests that bereavement reactions can increase the risk of depression. Epidemiological research also indicates that conjugal bereavement is associated with higher risk for elevated levels of physical deterioration and death (Lieberman and Videka-Sherman, 1986). In addition, widows and widowers are more likely than single or married peers to be socially isolated, to live in poverty, to be emotionally troubled, and to have fewer meaningful social activities (IOM, 1984).

Protective factors for the bereaved include emotional and social support, higher levels of social engagement and interaction, formation of meaningful new social roles, as well as the opportunity in mutual-help groups for the catharsis and interaction that can lead to personal insight.

Widow-to-Widow: A Mutual Help Program for the Widowed, developed by Silverman (1988) as a service program, involves recruiting widowed aides who have some perspective on their own grief and who are in a position to reach out to other widowed persons in their transition state. Widowed helpers were recruited by word of mouth and through local community action programs. Identification of the newly widowed was done through funeral directors, who became involved in Widow-to-Widow programs as sponsors and served on advisory boards. Outreach typically began with a first contact two months after the death. Initial contact was by mail, and the initial social visits later evolved into group discussions.

Vachon and colleagues evaluated the Widow-to-Widow program in a research trial in Toronto (Vachon, Sheldon, Lancee, Lyall, Roger, and Freeman, 1982, 1980; Vachon, 1979). They randomly assigned 162 newly widowed women to control and experimental groups. The intervention consisted of one-to-one support by another widow, practical help in locating community resources, and small group meetings. The intervention was not limited to any predefined duration or phase of bereavement.

Widows who participated in the program were more apt to have begun new relationships and activities and did so more quickly. They also experienced fewer depressive symptoms on a psychiatric screening instrument than women in the control group. This was particularly true for women who experienced high stress immediately after the death of their spouse. Over the two years of the randomized trial, most women recovered with or without help; however, those receiving the intervention recovered more quickly (Vachon et al., 1980).

The Widow-to-Widow program focused almost exclusively on widowed women. Presumably, such a mutual support program could also be useful for widowed men. Randomized trials of this form of support would provide information about the range of impact of the program and about subgroups at higher risk who could be more likely to benefit from the intervention, but few have been conducted.

The Widow-to-Widow program model seems already to have been widely disseminated through such organizations as the American Association of Retired Persons (AARP). Careful trials to assess which program models would be particularly well suited for dissemination, which individuals would be most likely to benefit, and whether depressive disorders are prevented would be important next steps in the development of these programs.

Evidence from a Quasi-Experimental Study: Mutual-Help Groups for Widowed Persons

THEOS, a national network of self-help groups that aid widowed persons, was the vehicle used to reach widows and widowers in a preventive program addressing issues of bereavement (Lieberman and Videka-Sherman, 1986). The research design, which was complex but quasi-experimental, compared participants in the mutual-help program (experimental group) to a probability sample of widowed persons in a longitudinal data set (comparison group). The experimental group showed improved mental health status over a one-year period, whereas the control group showed deterioration on all mental health measures except depression.

In addition, experimental group members who made strong social linkages in THEOS showed more positive changes on six of the eight mental health measures (depression, anxiety, somatic symptoms, well-being, self-esteem, and mastery) than those who attended meetings but did not develop other social linkages within THEOS.

These results were checked by examining whether high-participation experimental group members were different in other important ways, including having special aptitudes and skills that would account for the establishment of their new social linkages. No important differences were found, with the possible exception that low meeting attenders had somewhat lower need-for-affiliation scores. In short, a variety of risk factors associated with social isolation appeared to have been reduced by participation in THEOS mutual-help intervention, and a number of measures of precursor symptoms of mental disorders showed improvement in comparison with a control group.

Lieberman and Videka-Sherman (1986) pointed out that their analyses strongly suggest that the mere passage of time could not account for the positive changes observed in the high-participation experimental members. Nor did improvements in mental health scores appear to be simply the result of attendance. Instead, a particular type of high-intensity mutual support involvement appeared to be the active mechanism of the intervention.

Findings and Leads

- The Widow-to-Widow program was most successful with those women who experienced high stress immediately after the death of their spouse. This result suggests increased targeting of this high-risk group. Trials are needed to determine whether depressive disorders can be prevented.
- A variety of naturally occurring mutual-help groups could be rigorously evaluated to assess their preventive potential, particularly when the mutual-help groups are aimed at aiding persons in coping with major life transitions, losses, illnesses, or stigmatizing experiences.

A NEW GENERATION OF DEVELOPMENTAL STUDIES

Recently, a new generation of preventive intervention research studies have been designed and supported by federal, state, and private sources. These studies have adhered to high methodological standards and hold great promise for identifying causality and malleability of individual and combined risk factors, demonstrating efficacy and effectiveness of single- or multiple-component interventions, and assessing not only reduction of risk factors but also reduction of incidence of mental disorders. Because this work is still in progress, the programs are not reviewed here, but the project titles and investigators are included in the reference list. Some of the research to note over the next decade will come from investigators such as D. Cicchetti, whose work focuses on preventing developmental problems in children with depressed mothers; B. Egeland, whose work is with children of high-risk mothers; D. Olds, who is replicating the Prenatal/Early Infancy Project in Memphis with a different high-risk sample; J. Coie and N. Guerra, whose prevention demonstration projects to prevent conduct disorder point the way for combining research methodologies with service programs; T. Field, whose work with high-risk mothers and their babies is showing psychological and physiological benefits from the therapeutic use of touch; W. Beardslee, whose aim is to prevent depression in children and adolescents who have been exposed to parental depression; J. Reid and C. Webster-Stratton, who in separate indicated prevention programs are pushing the boundaries with children who have precursor symptoms of conduct disorder through the application of techniques that have proved successful in treatment settings; and G. Clarke, whose school-based interventions are yielding the first data on prevention of major depressive disorders among adolescents at high risk for depression.

MAJOR FINDINGS AND PROMISING LEADS

• Although their numbers are relatively small, some excellent illustrations of preventive interventions are available. These illustrations point the way toward further work by highlighting successes as well as problems. The design of new prevention programs should consider such illustrations and adapt methodologies and strategies for intervention accordingly.

• There are data that clearly show that preventive interventions can reduce risk factors that are associated with the onset of many mental disorders. However, as yet, there is no evidence that preventive interventions reduce the incidence of mental disorders. Risk reduction findings are encouraging about the eventual prevention of the initial onset of some disorders, such as major depressive disorder and alcohol abuse.

• The criteria presented here for the assessment of prevention programs that have been completed and published can be a guide for researchers, practitioners, and policymakers as they make critical decisions for this field.

• Although there are numerous prevention service programs throughout the life span, most prevention research programs are targeted to the needs of infants, preschoolers, elementary-age children, and adolescents. There is a nationwide and unfortunate lack of prevention research programs targeted to the needs of adults, especially the elderly.

• Although there are excellent reasons to target an intervention for a specific age or stage of life, and for a particular disorder or problem, there is usually no single intervention at a single point in time that accomplishes comprehensive goals of prevention for a lifetime. The ultimate goal to achieve optimal prevention should be to build the principles of prevention into the ordinary activities of everyday life and into community structures to enhance development over the entire life span. This would include promoting consensual community values and norms.

• Attention should be given to the potential risks of short-term interventions that are beneficial but are then curtailed or terminated.

• Many prevention programs clearly demonstrate that education, physical health care, employment, and mental health care are not separable. Improvements in one area can affect other areas. A logical extension of this finding is support for collaboration among the agencies and institutions in these domains.

• Risk factors can occur in single or multiple domains, such as home, school, peer group, neighborhood, or work site. When risk factors occur in multiple domains, interventions are required in all of them. Prevention programs from infancy to adolescence have clearly demonstrated the feasibility of multidomain interventions.

• Risk factors can also occur across generations in the same family. The Prenatal/Early Infancy Project has clearly shown that positive outcomes can be secured for both infants and their mothers from a single comprehensive interaction. Prevention programs should take advantage of opportunities to reduce risks, assess outcomes, and compare benefits and costs for members of different generations within a household, such as adult children serving as caregivers for disabled parents.

• Many prevention research programs have similar methodological complications: difficulty in adhering to a strict randomized controlled trial design; high attrition of participants; lack of documentation of fidelity in delivering the intervention; lack of multiple measures of outcomes from multiple sources; and insufficient long-term follow-up, which can prevent the collection of outcome data on incidence of multiple disorders.

• Some prevention programs get scaled up into field trials or quickly become translated into service programs. Others that have positive outcomes and seem to be equally well designed, however, do not. One factor that contributes to the difference is marketing, such as encouraging a school or an agency to use a new program.

• Social competence enhancement has been shown to be a successful intervention with young children. Social competence programs have extended the basic social competence curriculum of Shure and Spivack to address stressors and interpersonal challenges of different developmental periods. Social competence interventions should probably be included in risk reduction interventions seeking to strengthen resilience in populations at risk for early behavior problems. Again, however, it is important to note that to date, the long-term preventive effects of such interventions on the incidence of most mental disorders is unknown and follow-up studies are needed.

• Prevention research suggests the importance of using interventions beginning in the preschool and elementary age periods to create normative consensual behavior regarding substance use and bullying. With such early intervention, those at risk might be hypothesized to be more committed to the normative standards of the larger community and to be less likely to violate widely shared community standards for behavior.

• The combined evidence suggests that some proportion of conduct disorder may be preventable. Developmentally adjusted interventions in early childhood, during the elementary grades, and in adolescence have been tested and have, in isolated experiments and with some confirmatory data from quasi-experimental studies, shown modest but statistically significant effects in preventing later delinquent behaviors and related indicators of conduct disorder during adolescence. Few of these preventive interventions have used diagnostic criteria to ascertain effects on the incidence of the disorder. Nevertheless, there is promise in several components, including early childhood education, parent training, enhancement of social and academic competence, and school curricula promoting consensual norms antithetical to risk behavior for disorder, such as substance use.

• Interventions that have been highly successful at certain developmental stages, such as home visiting with families with infants and preschoolers, might also be useful at other stages of the life span, such as with the elderly, who may be homebound, and single parents or dual-career parents who cannot work another scheduled event into their lives.

• Service programs can provide good leads regarding intervention, community context, and exchange of ideas. Such programs can also be brought into the preventive intervention research cycle and tested for their effectiveness in reducing psychological symptoms and mental disorders. For example, Healthy Start in Hawaii and Homebuilders provide excellent ideas.

• The combined evidence suggests that a number of programs have successfully focused on prevention of depressive symptoms in adults and the elderly, but data on the prevention of the first episode of major depressive disorder are not yet available, in part because of inadequate sample sizes in preventive trials.

• In general, research on preventive interventions that emphasize an ecological perspective has been neglected. As yet, there are no communitywide prevention research programs that target multiple age groups and attempt to change community norms. Such research has special issues, such as difficulty in randomization. However, for some problems, it may be necessary to foster new consensual values and norms in neighborhoods and communities. Beginning work in the areas of substance abuse and alcohol prevention and in Olweus's program to reduce bullying shows promise.

• Even though biological risk factors have a significant role in the onset of mental disorders, there are few prevention programs other than prenatal care and childhood immunizations that address these factors. As knowledge grows in this area over the next decade, growth in the number of programs addressing these factors is expected.

• Changes in laws and pricing have affected the availability of alcohol and appear to be successful in the prevention of alcohol use. There are also some data to suggest that peer-led didactic curricula can reduce and prevent alcohol use.

• Many prevention research programs are most successful with the individuals within the sample who are at highest risk, but there are many exceptions. Much remains to be learned about tailoring interventions to groups in which they will have the most impact. Consideration will need to be given to benefit-cost issues as well as the potential harmful effects of screening and labeling individuals as being at risk.

REFERENCES

Alexander, J. F.; Parsons, B. V. (1980) Functional Family Therapy. Monterey, CA: Brooks/Cole Publishing.

Alexander, J. F.; Parsons, B. V. (1973) Short-term behavioral intervention with delinquent families: Impact on family process and recidivism. Journal of Abnormal Psychology; 18: 219–225.

Alpert-Gillis, L. J.; Pedro-Carroll, J. L.; Cowen, E. L. (1989) The Children of Divorce Intervention Program: Development, implementation, and evaluation of a program for young urban children. Journal of Counseling and Clinical Psychology; 57: 583–589.

Andrews, S. R.; Blumenthal, J. B.; Johnson, D. L.; Kahn, A. J.; Ferguson, C. J.; Lasater, T. M.; Malone, P. E.; Wallace, D. B. (1982) The skills of mothering: A study of Parent-Child Development Centers. Monographs of the Society for Research in Child Development, 47; 6, Serial No. 198.

Baumrind, D. (1983) Why adolescents take chances—and why they don't. Paper presented at the National Institute for Child Health and Human Development, Bethesda, MD.

Beardslee, W. R. (Judge Baker Children's Center, Boston, MA). "Prevention for Families with Affective Disorder." National Institute of Mental Health Grant No. RO1 MH48696.

Beardslee, W. R.; Hoke, L.; Wheelock, I.; Rothberg, P. C.; van de Velde, P.; Swatling, S. (1992) Preventive intervention for families with parental affective disorders: Initial findings. American Journal of Psychiatry; 149(10): 1335–1340.

Beardslee, W. R. (1990) Development of a clinician-based preventive intervention for families with affective disorders. Journal of Preventive Psychiatry and Allied Disciplines; 4: 39–61.

Beardslee, W. R.; Salt, P.; Porterfield, K.; Rothberg, P. C.; van de Velde, P.; Swatling, S.; Hoke, L.; Moilanen, D. L.; Wheelock, I. (1993) Comparison of preventive interventions for families with parental affective disorder. Journal of the American Academy of Child and Adolescent Psychiatry; 32(2): 254–263.

Berkman, L. F. (1984) Assessing the physical health effects of social networks and social support. Annual Review of Public Health; 5: 413–432.

Berrueta-Clement, J. R.; Schweinhart, L. J.; Barnett, W. S.; Epstein, A. S.; Weikart, D. P. (1984) Changed Lives: The Effects of the Perry Preschool Program on Youths Through Age 19 (High/Scope Educational Research Foundation, Monograph 8). Ypsilanti, MI: High/Scope Press.

Bierman, K. L. (1986) Process of change during social skills training with preadolescents and its relation to treatment outcomes. Child Development; 57: 230–240.

Bloom, B. L. (1985) University of Colorado Separation and Divorce Program: A program manual. Washington, DC: Government Printing Office; DHHS Pub. No. (ADM) 88–1556.

Bloom, B. L.; Asher, S. J.; White, S. W. (1978) Marital disruption as a stressor: A review and analysis. Psychological Bulletin; 85: 867–894.

Bloom, B. L.; Hodges, W. F. (1988) The Colorado Separation and Divorce Program: A preventive intervention program for newly separated persons. In: R. H. Price, E. L. Cowen, R. P. Lorion, and J. Ramos-McKay, Eds. Fourteen Ounces of Prevention: A Casebook for Practitioners. Washington, DC: American Psychological Association.

Bloom, B. L.; Hodges, W. F.; Caldwell, R. A. (1982) A preventive program for the newly separated: Initial evaluation. American Journal of Community Psychology; 10(3): 251–264.

Bloom, B. L.; Hodges, W. F.; Kern, M. B.; McFaddin, S. C. (1985) A preventive intervention program for the newly separated. American Journal of Orthopsychiatry; 55: 9–26.

Botvin, G. J.; Baker, E.; Filazzola, A. D.; Botvin, E. M. (1990a) A cognitive-behavioral approach to substance abuse prevention: One-year follow-up. Addictive Behaviors; 15: 47–63.

Botvin, G. J.; Baker, E.; Tortu, S.; Botvin, E. M. (1990b) Preventing adolescent drug abuse through a multimodal cognitive-behavioral approach: Results of a 3-year study. Journal of Consulting and Clinical Psychology; 58: 437–446.

Bronfenbrenner, U. (1979) The Ecology of Human Development: Experiments by Nature and Design. Cambridge, MA: Harvard University Press.

Brophy, J.; Good, T. L. (1986) Teacher behavior and student achievement. In: M. C. Wittrock, Ed. Handbook of Research on Training. 3rd ed. New York, NY: Macmillan Press; 328–375.

Bry, B. H. (1982) Reducing the incidence of adolescent problems through preventive intervention: One- and five-year follow-up. American Journal of Community Psychology; 10: 265–276.

Busse, E. W. (1976) Hypochondriasis in the elderly: A reaction to stress. Journal of American Geriatrics Society; 24: 145–149.

Cantor, M. (1983) Strain among caregivers: A study of experience in the U.S. The Gerontologist; 23: 556–561.

Caplan, G. (1977) Support systems and community mental health. Paper presented at a seminar at Harvard University: Boston, MA.

Caplan, G.; Killilean, M. (1976) Support Systems and Mutual Help: Multidisciplinary Explorations. New York, NY: Grune & Stratton.

Caplan, M.; Weissberg, R. P.; Grober, J. S.; Sivo, P. J.; Grady, K.; Jacoby, C. (1992) Social competence promotion with inner-city and suburban young adolescents: Effects on social adjustment and alcohol use. Journal of Consulting and Clinical Psychology; 60: 56–63.

Caplan, R. D.; Vinokur, A. D.; Price, R. H.; van Ryn, M. (1989) Job seeking, reemployment and mental health: A randomized field experiment in coping with job loss. Journal of Applied Psychology; 74(5): 759–769.

Carnegie Council on Adolescent Development. (1989) Turning Points: Preparing American Youth for the 21st Century. Washington, DC: Carnegie Corporation.

Carnine, D.; Carnine, L.; Karp, J.; Weissberg, P. (1988) Kindergarten for economically disadvantaged children: The direct instruction component. In: C. Warger, Ed. A Resource Guide to Public School Early Childhood Programs. Alexandria, VA: Association for Supervision and Curriculum Development; 73–78.

Cauce, A. M.; Comer, J. P.; Schwartz, D. (1987) Long-term effects of a systems-oriented school prevention program. American Journal of Orthopsychiatry; 57: 127–131.

CDC (Centers for Disease Control). (1992) Early childhood vaccination levels among urban children—Connecticut 1990 and 1991. Mortality & Morbidity Weekly Report; 40: 888–891.

CDC (Centers for Disease Control). (1991) Measles vaccination among selected groups of pre-school children—United States. Mortality & Morbidity Weekly Report; 40: 36–39.

CDC (Centers for Disease Control). (1990) 1989 Update: Measles outbreak, Chicago, 1989. Mortality & Morbidity Weekly Report; 39(319): 325–326.

Center for the Study of Social Policy with The Annie E. Casey Foundation. (1992) Kids Count Data Book. Washington, DC: Center for the Study of Social Policy.

Cicchetti, D. (University of Rochester, Rochester, NY). "Preventive Intervention for Toddlers of Depressed Mothers." National Institute of Mental Health Grant No. RO1 MH45027.

Clarke, G. (Oregon Health Sciences University, Eugene, OR). "School Based Prevention of Adolescent Depression." National Institute of Mental Health Grant No. RO3 MH48118–02.

Cohen, J. (1988) Statistical Power Analysis for the Behavioral Sciences. 2nd ed. Hillsdale, NJ: Lawrence Erlbaum Associates.

Cohen, N. W. (1977) Minimizing emotional sequelae of caesarean childbirth. Birth and Family Journal; 4: 114–119.

Cohen, S.; Wills, T. A. (1985) Stress, social support, and the buffering hypothesis. Psychological Bulletin; 98: 310–357.

Coie, J. (Duke University, Durham, NC). "Multi-Site Prevention of Conduct Disorder." National Institute of Mental Health Grant No. RO1 MH48043.

Coie, J.; Krehbiel, G. (1984) Effects of academic tutoring on the social status of low-achieving, socially rejected children. Child Development; 55: 1465–1478.

Coie, J.; Hawkins, J. D.; Ramsey, S.; Watt, N. (1991) Prevention research: Conceptual model of strategies and procedures. Paper presented at the National Prevention Conference, June 1991, Washington, DC.

Comer, J. P. (1988) Educating poor minority children. Scientific American; 259(5): 42–48.

Comer, J. P. (1985) The Yale-New Haven Primary Prevention Project: A follow-up study. Journal of the American Academy of Child and Adolescent Psychiatry; 24(2): 154–160.

Cook, P. J.; Tauchen, G. (1984) The effect of minimum drinking age legislation on youthful auto fatalities, 1970–1977. Journal of Legal Studies; 13: 169–190.

Cook, P. J.; Tauchen, G. (1982) The effect of liquor taxes on heavy drinking. Bell Journal of Economics; 13: 379–390.

Cutts, F. T.; Zell, E. R.; Mason, D.; Bernier, R. H.; Dini, E. F.; Orenstein, W. A. (1992) Monitoring progress toward U.S. preschool immunization goals. Journal of the American Medical Association; 267: 1952–1955.

DHHS (Department of Health and Human Services). (1991) Healthy People 2000: National Health Promotion and Disease Prevention Objectives. Washington, DC: Government Printing Office; DHHS Pub. No. (PHS) 91–50212.

Donovan, B. (1977) The Caesarean Birth Experience: A Practical, Comprehensive and Reassuring Guide for Parents and Professionals. Boston, MA: Beacon Press.

Dumas, J. D. (1989) Treating antisocial behavior in children: Child and family approaches. Clinical Psychology Review; 1: 197–222.

Egeland, B. (University of Minnesota, Minneapolis, MN). "An Evaluation of STEEP: A Program for High-Risk Mothers." National Institute of Mental Health Grant No. RO1 MH41879.

Elias, M. J.; Gara, M.; Schuyler, T.; Brandon-Muller, L. R.; Sayette, M. A. (1991) The promotion of social competence: Longitudinal study of a preventive school-based program. American Journal of Orthopsychiatry; 61: 409–417.

Elias, M. J.; Gara, M.; Ubrlaca, M.; Rothbaum, P. A.; Clabby, J. F.; Schuyler, T. (1986) Impact of a preventive social problem intervention on children's coping with middle-school stressors. American Journal of Community Psychology; 14: 259–275.

Ellickson, P. L.; Bell, R. M. (1990) Drug prevention in junior high: A multi-site longitudinal test. Science; 247: 1299–1305.

Elliott, D. S.; Huizinga, D.; Menard, S. (1989) Multiple Problem Youth: Delinquency, Substance Use and Mental Health Problems. New York, NY: Springer-Verlag.

Emshoff, J. G. (1990) A preventive intervention with children of alcoholics. Prevention in Human Services; 7(1): 225–254.

Farrington, D. P.; Loeber, R.; Elliott, D. S.; Hawkins, J. D.; Kandel, D. B.; Klein, M. W.; McCord, J.; Rowe, D. C.; Tremblay, R. E. (1990) Advancing knowledge about the onset of delinquency and crime. In: B. B. Lahey and A. E. Kazdin, Eds. Advances in Clinical Child Psychology. Vol. 13. New York, NY: Plenum Press; 283–342.

Feldman, L. H. (1991a) Assessing the effectiveness of family preservation services in New Jersey within an ecological context. New Jersey Division of Youth and Family Services: Bureau of Research, Evaluation and Quality Assurance.

Feldman, L. H. (1991b) Evaluating the impact of intensive family preservation services in New Jersey. In: D. E. Biegel and K. Wells, Eds. Family Preservation Services: Research and Evaluation. Newbury Park, CA: Sage Publications; 47–71.

Felner, R. D.; Adan, A. M. (1988) The School Transitional Environment Project: An Ecological Intervention and Evaluation. In: R. Price, E. L. Cowen, R. P. Lorion, and J. Ramos-McKay, Eds. Fourteen Ounces of Prevention: A Casebook for Practitioners. Washington, DC: American Psychological Association; 111–122.

Felner, R. D.; Ginter, M.; Primavera, J. (1982) Primary prevention during school transitions: Social support and environmental structure. American Journal of Community Psychology; 10: 277–290.

Field, T. (University of Miami, Miami, FL). "Preventing Depression in Infants of Depressed Mothers." National Institute of Mental Health Grant No. R37 MH46586.

Field, T. M.; Schanberg, S. M.; Scafidi, F.; Bauer, C. R.; Vega-Lahr, N.; Garcia, R.; Nystrom, J.; Kuhn, C. M. (1986) Tactile/kinesthetic stimulation effects on preterm neonates. Pediatrics; 77(5): 654–658.

Field, T. M.; Widmayer, S. M.; Stringer, S.; Ignatoff, E. (1980) Teenage, lower-class, black mothers and their preterm infants: An intervention and developmental follow-up. Child Development; 51(2): 426–436.

Fraser, M. W.; Hawkins, J. D.; Howard, M. O. (1988) Parent training for delinquency prevention. Child and Youth Services; 11: 93–125.

George, L. K.; Gwyther, L. P. (1988) Support group for caregivers of memory-impaired elderly: Easing caregiver burden. In: L. A. Bond and B. M. Wagner, Eds. Families in Transition: Primary Prevention Programs That Work. Newbury Park, CA: Sage Publications; 309–331.

Golodetz, A.; Evans, R.; Heinritz, G.; Gibson, C. (1969) The care of chronic illness: The responsor role. Medical Care; 7: 385–394.

Gordus, J. P. (1984) Coping with unemployment: I. The trainers' guide. Industrial Development Division, Institute of Science and Technology, The University of Michigan. Unpublished paper.

Gottfredson, D. C. (1988) An evaluation of an organization development approach to reducing school disorder. Evaluation Review; 11: 739–763.

Gottfredson, D. C. (1986) An empirical test of school-based environmental and individual interventions to reduce the risk of delinquent behavior. Criminology; 24: 705–731.

Gottfredson, D. C.; Gottfredson, G. D. (1992) Theory-guided investigation: Three field experiments. In: J. McCord and R. E. Tremblay, Eds. Preventing Antisocial Behavior: Interventions from Birth Through Adolescence. New York, NY: Guilford Press; 311–329.

Gottfredson, D. C.; Karweit, N. L.; Gottfredson, G. D. (1989) Reducing Disorderly Behavior in Middle Schools. Baltimore, MD: Center for Research on Elementary and Middle Schools.

Gottfredson, G. D. (1984) A theory-ridden approach to program evaluation. American Psychologist; 39: 1101–1112.

Gottman, J. G.; Markman, H. J.; Notarius, C. I. (1977) The topography of marital conflict: A sequential analysis of verbal and nonverbal behavior. Journal of Marriage and the Family; 46: 461–478.

Grych, J. H.; Fincham, F. D. (1992) Interventions for children of divorce: Toward greater integration of research and action. Psychological Bulletin; 111: 434–454.

Guerra, N. (University of Illinois at Chicago). "Preventing the Emergence of Anti-Social Behavior in High-Risk Children." National Institute of Mental Health Grant No. R18 MH48034.

Gwynn, C.; Brantley, H. (1987) Effects of a divorce group intervention for elementary school children. Psychology in the Schools; 24: 161–164.

Gwyther, L. P.; Brooks, B. (1983) Mobilizing networks of mutual support: How to develop Alzheimer caregivers' support groups. Durham, NC: Duke University Center of the Study of Aging and Human Development.

Hamburg, D. A. (1992) Today's Children: Creating a Future for a Generation in Crisis. New York, NY: Times Books.

Hansen, W. B. (1992) School-based substance abuse prevention: A review of the state of the art in curriculum, 1980–1990. Health Education Research; 7: 403–430.

Hansen, W. B.; Graham, J. W. (1991) Preventing alcohol, marijuana, and cigarette use among adolescents: Peer pressure resistance training versus establishing conservative norms. Preventive Medicine; 20: 414–430.

Hansen, W. B.; Johnson, C. A.; Flay, B. R.; Graham, J. W.; Sobel, J. (1988) Affective and social influence approaches to the prevention of multiple substance abuse among seventh grade students: Results from Project SMART. Preventive Medicine; 17: 135–154.

Hausman, A. J.; Spivak, H.; Prothrow-Stith, D.; Roeber, J. (1992) Patterns of teen exposure to a community-based violence prevention project. Journal of Adolescent Health; 13: 668–675.

Hawkins, J. D.; Catalano, R. F. (1992) Communities That Care: Action for Drug Abuse Prevention. San Francisco, CA: Jossey-Bass Publications.

Hawkins, J. D.; Catalano, R. F.; Jones, G.; Fine, D. (1987) Delinquency prevention through parent training: Results and issues from work in progress. In: J. Wilson and G. Loury, Eds. Children to Citizens: Families, Schools, and Delinquency Prevention. Vol. 3. New York, NY: Springer-Verlag; 186–204.

Hawkins, J. D.; Catalano, R. F.; Miller, J. R. (1992) Risk and protective factors for alcohol and other drug problems in adolescence and early adulthood: Implications for substance abuse prevention. Psychological Bulletin; 112(1): 64–105.

Hawkins, J. D.; Catalano, R. F.; Morrison, D. M.; O'Donnell, J.; Abbott, R. D.; Day, L. E. (1992) The Seattle Social Development Project: Effects of the first four years on protective factors and problem behaviors. In: J. McCord and R. Tremblay, Eds. The Prevention of Antisocial Behavior in Children. New York, NY: Guilford Press.

Hawkins, J. D.; Doueck, H. J.; Lishner, D. M. (1988) Changing teaching practices in mainstream classrooms to improve bonding and behavior of low achievers. American Educational Research Journal; 25: 31–50.

Hawkins, J. D.; Lam, T. (1987) Teacher practices, social development, and delinquency. In: J. D. Burchard and S. N. Burchard, Eds. Prevention of Delinquent Behavior. Newbury Park, CA: Sage Publications; 241–274.

Heaney, C. A. (1992) Enhancing social support at the workplace: Assessing the effects of the Caregiver Support Program. Health Education Quarterly; 18(4): 477–494.

Hinman, A. R. (1988) Public health considerations. In: S. A. Plotkin and E. A. Mortimer Jr., Eds. Vaccines. Philadelphia, PA: W. B. Saunders; 587–611.

Hinman, A. R.; Koplan, J. R. (1985) Pertussis and pertussis vaccine: Further analysis of benefits, risks and costs. Developmental Biology Standards; 61: 429–437.

Hohmann, M.; Banet, B.; Weikart, D. P. (1979) Young Children in Action: A Manual for Preschool Educators. Ypsilanti, MI: High/Scope.

Holder, H. D.; Blose, J. O. (1987) Impact of changes in distilled spirits availability on apparent consumption: A time series analysis of liquor-by-the-drink. British Journal of Addiction; 82: 623–631.

Horacek, H. J.; Ramey, C. T.; Campbell, F. A.; Hoffman, K. P.; Fletcher, R. H. (1987) Predicting school failure and assessing early intervention with high-risk children. Journal of the American Academy of Child and Adolescent Psychiatry; 26: 758–763.

Hough, R. L.; Landsverk, J. A.; Karno, M.; Burnam, M. A.; Timbers, D. M.; Escobar, J. I.; Regier, D. A. (1987) Utilization of health and mental health services by Los Angeles Mexican Americans and non-Hispanic whites. Archives of General Psychiatry; 44: 702–709.

House, J. S. (1981) Work Stress and Social Support. Reading, MA: Addison-Wesley.

Infant Health and Development Program. (1990) Enhancing the outcomes of low birth-weight premature infants: A multi-site randomized trial. Journal of the American Medical Association; 263: 3035–3042.

IOM (Institute of Medicine). (1988) Prenatal Care: Reaching Mothers, Reaching Infants. Washington, DC: National Academy Press.

IOM (Institute of Medicine). (1985) Preventing Low Birthweight. Washington, DC: National Academy Press.

IOM (Institute of Medicine). (1984) Bereavement: Reactions, Consequences and Care. Washington, DC: National Academy Press.

Israel, B. I.; Rounds, K. A. (1987) Social networks and social support: A synthesis for health educators. Advances in Health Education and Promotion; 2: 311–351.

Jessor, R. (1993) Successful adolescent development among youth in high-risk settings. American Psychologist; 48(2): 117–126.

Jessor, R.; Jessor, S. L. (1977) Problem Behavior and Psychosocial Development: A Longitudinal Study of Youth. New York, NY: Academic Press.

Johnson, C. A.; Pentz, M. A.; Weber, M. D.; Dwyer, J. H.; Baer, N. A.; MacKinnon, D. P.; Hansen, W. B.; Flay, B. R. (1989) Relative effectiveness of comprehensive community programming for drug abuse prevention with high-risk and low-risk adolescents. Journal of Consulting and Clinical Psychology; 58: 447–456.

Johnson, D. L. (1991) Primary prevention of behavior problems in young children: The Houston Parent-Child Development Center. In: R. Price, E. L. Cowen, R. P. Lorion, and J. Ramos-McKay, Eds. Fourteen Ounces of Prevention: A Casebook for Practitioners. Washington, DC: American Psychological Association; 44–52.

Johnson, D. L. (1990) The Houston Parent-Child Development Center Project: Disseminating a viable program for enhancing at-risk families. Prevention in Human Services; 7: 89–108.

Johnson, D. L.; Walker, T. (1987) Primary prevention of behavior problems in Mexican-American children. American Journal of Community Psychology; 15: 375–385.

Joksch, H. C. (1988) The impact of severe penalties on drinking and driving. Washington, DC: AAA Foundation for Traffic Safety.

Jones, M. B.; Offord, D. R. (1989) Reduction of antisocial behavior in poor children by nonschool skill development. Journal of Child Psychology and Psychiatry and Allied Disciplines; 30: 737–750.

Kalter, N.; Pickar, J.; Lesowitz, M. (1984) School-based developmental facilitation groups for children of divorce: A preventive intervention. American Journal of Orthopsychiatry; 54: 613–623.

Kandel, D. B.; Yamaguchi, K.; Chen, K. (1992) Stages of progression in drug involvement from adolescence to adulthood: Further evidence for the gateway theory. Journal of Studies on Alcohol; 53: 447–457.

Kazdin, A. E. (1990) Prevention of conduct disorder. Paper presented to the National Conference on Prevention Research, National Institute of Mental Health, Bethesda, MD.

Kazdin, A. E. (1987) Treatment of antisocial behavior in children: Current status and future directions. Psychological Bulletin; 102: 187–203.

Kellam, S. G.; Branch, J. D.; Agrawal, K. C.; Ensminger, M. E. (1975) Mental Health and Going to School. Chicago, IL: University of Chicago Press.

Kellam, S. G.; Rebok, G. W. (1992) Building developmental and etiological theory through epidemiologically based preventive intervention trials. In: J. McCord and R. E. Tremblay, Eds. Preventing Antisocial Behavior: Interventions from Birth Through Adolescence. New York, NY: Guilford Press; 162–195.

Kendell, R. E.; Rennie, D.; Clark, J. D.; Dean, C. (1981) The social and obstetric correlates of psychiatric admission in the puerperium. Psychological Medicine; 11: 341–351.

Kessler, R. C.; House, J. S.; Turner, J. B. (1987) Unemployment and health in a community sample. Journal of Health and Social Behavior; 28: 51–59.

Kessler, R. C.; Turner, J. B.; House, J. S. (1988) Effects of unemployment on health in a community survey: Main, modifying, and mediating effects. Journal of Social Issues; 44(4): 69–85.

Kinney, J. M.; Madsen, B.; Fleming, T.; Haapala, D. A. (1977) Homebuilders: Keeping families together. Journal of Consulting and Clinical Psychology; 45: 667–673.

Klein, N. C.; Alexander, J. F.; Parsons, B. V. (1977) Impact of family systems intervention on recidivism and sibling delinquency: A model of primary prevention and program evaluation. Journal of Consulting and Clinical Psychology; 45: 469–474.

Klepp, K. I.; Halper, A.; Perry, C. L. (1986) The efficacy of peer leaders in drug abuse prevention. Journal of School Health; 56(9): 407–411.

Kraemer, H. C. (1992) Reporting the size of effects in research studies to facilitate assessment of practical or clinical significance. Psychoneuroendocrinology; 17(6): 527–536.

Kraemer, H. C.; Fendt, K. H. (1990) Random assignment in clinical trials: Issues in planning (Infant Health and Development Program). Journal of Clinical Epidemiology; 43: 1157–1167.

Kreig, T. L. (1982) Is raising the legal drinking age warranted? The Police Chief; 32–34.

Lally, J. R.; Mangione, P. L.; Honig, A. S. (1988) The Syracuse University Family Development Research Program: Long-range impact on an early intervention with low-income children and their families. In: D. Powell, Ed. Advances in Applied Developmental Psychology: Parent Education as Early Childhood Intervention, Vol. 3. Norwood, NJ: Ablex Publishing.

Lally, J. R.; Mangione, P. L.; Honig, A. S.; Wittner, D. S. (1988) More pride, less delinquency: Findings from the ten-year follow-up study of the Syracuse University Family Development Research Program. Zero to Three; 8(4): 13–18.

Lawton, M. P.; Maddox, G. L. (1985) Annual Review of Gerontology and Geriatrics. New York, NY: Springer.

Levenstein, P. (1992) The Mother-Child Home Program: Research methodology and the real world. In: J. McCord and R. E. Tremblay, Eds. Preventing Antisocial Behavior: Interventions from Birth Through Adolescence. New York, NY: Guilford Press; 43–66.

Levy, D.; Sheflin, N. (1985) The demand for alcoholic beverages: An aggregate time-series analysis. Journal of Public Policy and Marketing; 4: 47–54.

Lieberman, M. A.; Videka-Sherman, L. (1986) The impact of self-help groups on the mental health of widows and widowers. American Journal of Orthopsychiatry; 56(3): 435–449.

Lochman, J. E. (1992) Cognitive-behavioral intervention with aggressive boys: Three-year follow-up and preventive effects. Journal of Consulting and Clinical Psychology; 60: 426–432.

Lochman, J. E.; Coie, J. D.; Underwood, M. K.; Terry, R. (in press) Effectiveness of a social relations intervention program for aggressive and nonaggressive rejected children. Journal of Consulting and Clinical Psychology.

Lochman, J. E.; Curry, J. F. (1986) Effects of social problem-solving training and self-instruction training with aggressive boys. Journal of Clinical Child Psychology; 15: 159–164.

McAlister, A. L. (1983) Social-psychological approaches. In: T. J. Glynn, C. G. Leukefeld, and J. P. Ludford, Eds. Preventing Adolescent Drug Abuse: Intervention Strategies. NIDA Research Monograph No. 47; Washington, DC: Government Printing Office; 36–50.

McAlister, A. L.; Perry, C.; Killen, J.; Slinkard, L. A.; Maccoby, N. (1980) Pilot study of smoking, alcohol, and drug abuse prevention. American Journal of Public Health; 70: 719–721.

McMahon, R. J.; Wells, K. C. (1989) Conduct disorders. In: E. J. Mach and R. A. Barkley, Eds. Treatment of Childhood Disorders. New York, NY: Guilford Press; 73–132.

Madden, J.; O'Hara, J.; Levenstein, P. (1984) Home again: Effects of the Mother-Child Home Program on mother and child. Child Development; 55: 636–647.

Markman, H. J. (1984) The longitudinal study of couples' interactions: Implications for understanding and predicting the development of marital distress. K. Hahlweg and N. Jacobson, Eds. Marital Interactions: Analysis and Modification. New York, NY: Guilford Press; 253–281.

Markman, H. J. (1981) Prediction of marital distress: A 5-year follow-up. Journal of Consulting and Clinical Psychology; 49(5): 760–762.

Markman, H. J. (1979) Application of a behavioral model of marriage in predicting relationship satisfaction of couples planning marriage. Journal of Consulting and Clinical Psychology; 47(4): 743–749.

Markman, H. J.; Renick, M. J.; Floyd, F.; Stanley, S. M.; Clements, M. (1993) Preventing marital distress through effective communication and conflict management: A 4- and 5-year follow-up. Journal of Consulting and Clinical Psychology; 61(1): 70–77.

Marris, P. (1958) Widows and Their Families. London, England: Routledge and Kegan Paul.

Miranda, J.; Pérez-Stable, E. J. (1993) The effects of preventive intervention on the use of medical services. In: R. F. Muñoz and Y. W. Ying, Eds. The Prevention of Depression: Research and Practice. Baltimore, MD: Johns Hopkins University Press.

Mulford, H. A.; Ledolter, J.; Fitzgerald, J. L. (1992) Alcohol availability and consumption: Iowa sales data revisited. Journal of Studies on Alcohol; 53: 487–494.

Muñoz, R. F. (1993a) The depression prevention course. In: R. F. Muñoz and Y. W. Ying, Eds. The Prevention of Depression: Research and Practice. Baltimore, MD: Johns Hopkins University Press.

Muñoz, R. F. (1993b) The prevention of depression: Current research and practice. Applied and Preventive Psychology; 2: 21–33.

Muñoz, R. F.; Ying, Y. W. (1993) The Prevention of Depression: Research and Practice. Baltimore, MD: Johns Hopkins University Press.

Muñoz, R. F.; Ying, Y.; Armas, R.; Chan, F.; Gurza, R. (1987) The San Francisco depression prevention research project: A randomized trial with medical outpatients. In: R. F. Muñoz, Ed. Depression Prevention: Research Directions. Washington, DC: Hemisphere Press; 199–215.

Murray, D. M.; Johnson, C. A.; Luepker, R. V.; Mittelmark, M. B. (1984) The prevention of cigarette smoking in children: A comparison of four strategies. Journal of Applied Social Psychology; 14: 274–288.

National Vaccine Advisory Committee. (1991) The measles epidemic: The problems, barriers, and recommendations. Journal of the American Medical Association; 266: 1547–1552.

Olds, D. (University of Colorado, Denver, CO). "Study of Home Visitation for Mothers and Children." Maternal and Child Health Bureau Grant No. MCJ-360579.

Olds, D. L.; Henderson, C. R.; Tatelbaum, R.; Chamberlin, R. (1988) Improving the life-course development of socially disadvantaged mothers: A randomized trial of nurse home visitation. American Journal of Public Health; 78(11): 1436–1444.

Olds, D. L.; Henderson, C.; Tatelbaum, R.; Chamberlin, R. (1986) Preventing child abuse and neglect: A randomized trial of nurse home visitation. Pediatrics; 78(1): 65–78.

Olds, D. L.; Kitzman, H. (1990) Can home visitation improve the health of women and children at environmental risk? Pediatrics; 86(1): 108–116.

Olweus, D. (1991) Bully/victim problems among schoolchildren: Basic facts and effects of an intervention program. In: K. Rubin and D. Pepler, Eds. The Development and Treatment of Childhood Aggression. Hillsdale, NJ: Lawrence Erlbaum Associates.

O'Malley, P. M.; Wagenaar, A. C. (1991) Effects of minimum drinking age laws on alcohol use, related behaviors and traffic crash involvement among American youth: 1976–1987. Journal of Studies on Alcohol; 52: 478–491.

Parkes, C. M. (1965) Bereavement and mental illness: Part 2. A classification of bereavement reactions. British Journal of Medical Psychology; 33: 14–15.

Patterson, G. R.; Reid, J. B.; Jones, R. R.; Conger, R. E. (1975) Families with Aggressive Children, Vol. I. Eugene, OR: Castalia.

Pedro-Carroll, J. L.; Cowen, E. L. (1985) The Children of Divorce Intervention Program: An investigation of the efficacy of a school-based prevention program. Journal of Counseling and Clinical Psychology; 53: 603–611.

Pedro-Carroll, J. L.; Cowen, E. L.; Hightower, A. D.; Guare, J. C. (1986) Preventive intervention with latency-aged children of divorce: A replication study. American Journal of Community Psychology; 14: 277–289.

Penning, M.; Barnes, G. E. (1982) Adolescent marijuana use review. International Journal of the Addictions; 17: 749–791.

Pentz, M. A.; Dwyer, J. H.; MacKinnon, D. P.; Flay, B.; Hansen, W. B.; Wang, E. Y. I.; Johnson, C. A. (1989) A multicommunity trial for primary prevention of adolescent drug abuse. Journal of the American Medical Association; 261: 3259–3266.

Perry, C. L. (1986) Community-wide health promotion and drug abuse prevention. Journal of the School of Health; 56: 359–363.

Perry, C. L.; Grant, M.; Ernberg, G.; Florenzano, R. U.; Langdon, M. C.; Myeni, A. D.; Waahlberg, R.; Berg, S.; Andersson, K.; Fisher, K. J.; Blaze-Temple, D.; Cross, D.; Saunders, B.; Jacobs, D. R.; Schmid, T. (1989) WHO Collaborative Study on Alcohol Education and Young People: Outcomes of a four-country pilot study. The International Journal of the Addictions; 24: 1145–1171.

Peter, G. (1992) Childhood immunizations. New England Journal of Medicine; 327(25): 1794–1800.

Petersen, A. C.; Compas, B. E.; Brooks-Gunn, J.; Stemmler, M.; Ey, S.; Grant, K. E. (1993) Depression in adolescence. American Psychologist; 48: 155–168.

Plotkin, S. A.; Mortimer, E. A. (1988) Vaccines. Philadelphia, PA: Harcourt Brace Jovanovich, Inc.; 302.

Price, R. H.; van Ryn, M.; Vinokur, A. (1992) Impact of a preventive job search intervention on the likelihood of depression among the unemployed. Journal of Health and Social Behavior; 33: 158–167.

Reid, J. (Oregon Social Learning Center, Eugene, OR). "Oregon Prevention Research Center." National Institute of Mental Health Grant No. P50 MH46690.

Renick, M. J.; Blumberg, S. L.; Markman, H. J. (1992) The Prevention and Relationship Enhancement Program (PREP): An empirically based preventive intervention program for couples. Family Relations; 41: 141–147.

Rickel, A. U.; Allen, L. (1987) Preventing Maladjustment from Infancy through Adolescence. Newbury Park, CA: Sage Publications.

Roberts, R. E. (1987) Epidemiological issues in measuring preventive effects. In: R. F. Muñoz, Ed. Depression Prevention: Research Directions. Washington, DC: Hemisphere Press; 45–75.

Robins, L. N. (1980) The natural history of drug abuse. Acta Psychiatrica Scandinavica; 62(Suppl. 284): 7–20.

Robins, L. N.; Przybeck, T. R. (1985) Age of onset of drug use as a factor in drug and other disorders. In: C. L. Jones and R. J. Battjes, Eds. Etiology of Drug Abuse: Implications for Prevention. NIDA Research Monograph No. 56. Washington, DC: Government Printing Office; DHHS Pub. No. ADM 85–1335: 178–192.

Rose, S. A.; Feldman, J. F.; Rose, S. L.; Wallace, I. F.; McCarton, C. (1992) Behavior problems at 3 and 6 years: Prevalence and continuity in full-terms and preterms. Development and Psychopathology; 4: 361–374.

Rosenberg, M. L.; Mercy, J. A. (1991) Assaultive violence. In: M. L. Rosenberg and M. A. Fenley, Eds. Violence in America: A Public Health Approach. New York, NY: Oxford University Press; 14–50.

Roskin, M. (1982) Coping with life changes: A preventive social work approach. American Journal of Community Psychology; 10: 331–340.

Ross, J. G.; Saavedra, P. J.; Shur, G. H.; Winters, F.; Felner, R. D. (1992) After-school program for primary grade latchkey students on precursors of substance abuse. Journal of Community Psychology; Office of Substance Abuse Prevention Special Issue: 22–38.

Rotheram, M. J. (1982) Social skill training with underachievers, disruptive, and exceptional children. Psychology in the Schools; 19: 532–539.

Rotheram, M. J.; Armstrong, M.; Booraem, C. (1982) Assertiveness training in fourth and fifth grade children. American Journal of Community Psychology; 10(5): 567–582.

Saffer, H.; Grossman, M. (1987) Beer taxes, the legal drinking age, and youth motor vehicle fatalities. Journal of Legal Studies; 16: 351–374.

Sameroff, A. J.; Chandler, M. J. (1975) Reproductive risk and the continuum of caretaking casualty. In: F. D. Horowitz, M. Hetherington, and S. Scarr-Salopatek, Eds. Review of Child Development Research. Vol. 4. Chicago, IL: University of Chicago Press; 187–244.

Sandler, I. N.; West, S. G.; Baca, L.; Pillow, D. R.; Gersten, J. C.; Rogosch, F.; Virdin, L.; Beals, J.; Reynolds, K. D.; Kallgren, C.; Tein, J. Y.; Kreige, G.; Cole, E.; Ramirez, R. (1992) Linking empirically-based theory and evaluation: The Family Bereavement Program. American Journal of Community Psychology; 20(4): 491–523.

Schinke, S. P.; Botvin, G. J.; Orlandi, M. A. (1991) Substance Abuse in Children and Adolescents: Evaluation and Intervention. Newbury Park, CA: Sage Publications.

Schinke, S. P.; Orlandi, M. A.; Cole, K. C. (1992) Boys and Girls clubs in public housing developments: Prevention services for youths at risk. Journal of Community Psychology; 118–128.

Schweinhart, L. J. (1987) Can preschool programs help prevent delinquency? In: J. Q. Wilson and G. C. Loury, Eds. From Children to Citizens: Families, Schools, and Delinquency Prevention. New York, NY: Springer-Verlag; 13–53.

Schweinhart, L. J.; Weikart, D. P. (1992) High/Scope Perry Preschool Program outcomes. In: J. McCord and R. E. Tremblay, Eds. Preventing Antisocial Behavior: Interventions from Birth Through Adolescence. New York, NY: Guilford Press; 67–86.

Shapiro, S.; Skinner, E. A.; Kessler, L. G.; Von Korff, M.; German, P. S.; Tischler, G. L.; Leaf, P. J.; Benham, L.; Cottler, L.; Regier, D. A. (1984) Utilization of health and mental health services: Three epidemiological catchment area sites. Archives of General Psychiatry; 41: 971–978.

Shure, M. B.; Spivack, G. (1988) Interpersonal cognitive problem solving. In: R. H. Price, E. L. Cowen, R. P. Lorion, and J. Ramos-McKay, Eds. Fourteen Ounces of Prevention: A Casebook for Practitioners. Washington, DC: American Psychological Association; 69–82.

Shure, M. B.; Spivack, G. (1982) Interpersonal problem-solving in young children: A cognitive approach to prevention. American Journal of Community Psychology; 10: 341–356.

Shure, M. D.; Spivack, G. (1980) Interpersonal problem solving as a mediator of behavioral adjustment in preschool and kindergarten children. Journal of Applied Developmental Psychology; 1: 29–44.

Silverman, P. R. (1988) Widow-to-widow: A mutual help program for the widowed. In: R. Price, E. Cowen, R. P. Lorion, and J. Ramos-McKay, Eds. Fourteen Ounces of Prevention: A Casebook for Practitioners. Washington, DC: American Psychological Association; 175–186.

Slavin, R. E.; Madden, N. A.; Karweit, N. L.; Livermon, B. J.; Dolan, L. (1990) Success for All: First year outcomes of a comprehensive plan for reforming urban education. American Educational Research Journal; 27: 255–278.

Spivack, G.; Shure, M. B. (1974) Social Adjustment of Young Children. San Francisco, CA: Jossey-Bass Publications.

Springer, F.; Phillips, J.; Phillips, L.; Cannady, L. P.; Derst-Harris, E. (1992) CODA: A creative therapy program for children in families affected by abuse of alcohol or other drugs. Journal of Community Psychology; OSAP Special Issue: 55–74.

Stolberg, A. L.; Garrison, K. M. (1985) Evaluating a primary prevention program for children of divorce. American Journal of Community Psychology; 13: 111–124.

Strayhorn, J. M.; Weidman, C. S. (1991) Follow-up one year after parent-child interaction training: Effects on behavior of preschool children. Journal of the American Academy of Child and Adolescent Psychiatry; 30: 138–143.

Stuart, R. B. (1974) Teaching facts about drugs: Pushing or preventing? Journal of Educational Psychology; 66: 189–201.

Sullivan, L. W. (1991) The prevention of violence: A top HHS priority. Public Health Reports; 106: 268–269.

Tadmor, C. S. (1988) The Perceived Personal Control preventive intervention for a caesarean birth population. In: R. H. Price, E. L. Cowen, R. P. Lorion, and J. Ramos-McKay. Fourteen Ounces of Prevention: A Casebook for Practitioners. Washington, DC: American Psychological Association; 141–152.

Tadmor, C. S.; Brandes, J. M. (1984) The perceived personal control crisis intervention model in the prevention of emotional dysfunction for a high risk population of caesarean birth. The Journal of Primary Prevention; 6: 244–255.

Tadmor, C. S.; Brandes, J. M.; Hofman, J. E. (1988) Preventive intervention for a caesarean birth population. Journal of Preventive Psychiatry; 3(4):

Thoits, P. (1986) Social support as coping assistance. Journal of Consulting and Clinical Psychology; 54: 416–423.

Toseland, R. W. (1990) Long-term effectiveness of peer-led and professionally-led support groups for caregivers. Social Service Review; 64: 308–327.

Toseland, R. W.; Rossiter, C. M.; Labrecque, M. S. (1989) The effectiveness of peer-led and professionally-led groups to support family caregivers. The Gerontologist; 29(4): 465–471.

Tremblay, R. E.; McCord, J.; Bioleau, H.; Charlebois, P. I.; Gagnon, C.; LeBlanc, M.; Larivee, S. (1991) Can disruptive boys be helped to become competent? Psychiatry; 54: 148–161.

Tremblay, R. E.; Vitaro, F.; Bertrand, L.; LeBlanc, M.; Beauchesne, H.; Boileau, H.; David, L. (1992) Parent and child training to prevent early onset of delinquency: The Montreal Longitudinal-Experimental Study. In: J. McCord and R. Tremblay, Eds. Preventing Antisocial Behavior: Interventions from Birth Through Adolescence. New York, NY: Guilford Press; 117–138.

U.S. Advisory Board on Child Abuse and Neglect. (1990) Child Abuse and Neglect: Critical

First Steps in Response to a National Emergency. Washington, DC: Government Printing Office.

USPHS (U.S. Public Health Service) Expert Panel on the Content of Prenatal Care. (1989) Caring for Our Future: The Content of Prenatal Care. Report of the Public Health Service Expert Panel on the Content of Prenatal Care. Washington, DC: Department of Health and Human Services.

Vachon, M. L. S. (1979) Identity change over the first two years of bereavement: Social relationships and social support in widowhood. York University, Toronto, Canada: Unpublished doctoral dissertation.

Vachon, M. L. S.; Sheldon, A. R.; Lancee, W. J.; Lyall, W. A. L.; Roger, J.; Freeman, S. J. J. (1982) Correlates of enduring distress patterns following bereavement: Social network, life situations and personality. Psychological Medicine; 12: 783–788.

Vachon, M. L. S.; Sheldon, A. R.; Lancee, W. J.; Lyall, W. A. L.; Roger, J.; Freeman, S. J. J. (1980) A controlled study of self-help intervention for widows. American Journal of Psychiatry; 137: 1380–1384.

Vega, W. A.; Murphy, J. (1990) Projecto Bienestar: An example of a community-based intervention. In: Culture and the Restructuring of Community Mental Health: Contributions in Psychology. Series No. 16; Westport, CT: Greenwood Press; 103–122.

Vega, W. A.; Valle, R.; Kolody, B. (submitted for publication) Preventing depression in the Hispanic community: An outcome evaluation of Projecto Bienestar.

Vega, W. A.; Valle, R.; Kolody, B.; Hough, R. (1987) The Hispanic social network prevention intervention study: A community-based randomized trial. In: R. F. Muñoz, Ed. Depression Prevention: Research Directions. Washington, DC: Hemisphere Publishing; 217–231.

Vinokur, A. D.; Schul, Y.; Price, R. H. (1992) Demographic assets and psychological resources in the reemployment process: Who benefits from the JOBS intervention for the unemployed? Michigan Prevention Research Center Working Paper, Institute for Social Research, University of Michigan.

Vinokur, A. D.; van Ryn, M.; Gramlich, E. M.; Price, R. H. (1991) Long-term follow-up and benefit/cost analysis of the JOBS Project. Journal of Applied Psychology; 76(2): 213–219.

Wagenaar, A. C.; Holder, H. D. (1991) A change from public to private sale of wine: Results from natural experiments in Iowa and West Virginia. Journal of Studies on Alcohol; 52: 162–173.

Weaver, S. C.; Tennant, F. S. (1973) Effectiveness of drug education programs for secondary school students. American Journal of Psychiatry; 130: 812–814.

Webster-Stratton, C. (University of Washington, Seattle, WA). "Preventing Conduct Disorders in Head Start Children." Administration for Children and Families Grant No. 93–600 (90CD0949/01) and "Parent Training Models for Anti-social Children." Institute for Nursing (National Center for Nursing Research) Grant No. NR 01 075–09.

Weikart, D. P.; Schweinhart, L. J.; Larner, M. B. (1986) A report on the High/Scope preschool curriculum comparison study: Consequences of three preschool curriculum models through age 15. Early Childhood Research Quarterly; 1: 15–45.

Weissberg, R. P.; Caplan, M. Z.; Sivo, P. J. (1989) A new conceptual framework for establishing school-based competence promotion programs. In: L. A. Bond and B. E. Compas, Eds. Primary Prevention and Promotion in the Schools: Primary Prevention of Psychopathology, Vol. 12. Newbury Park, CA: Sage Publications: 255–296.

White, C. C.; Koplan, J. P.; Orenstein, W. A. (1985) Benefits, risks, and costs of immunization for measles, mumps, and rubella. American Journal of Public Health; 75(7): 739–744.

8

Treatment Research and Prevention Research: A Collaborative Frontier

Prevention and treatment are part of a continuum of interventions aimed at reducing the incidence and prevalence of mental disorders, but they have different targets and purposes (see Chapter 2). Treatment interventions attempt to alleviate or eliminate an episode or delay recurrence of a mental disorder among identified patients who have met the full criteria for diagnosis. Preventive interventions are aimed at preventing or at least delaying the onset of a mental disorder among persons who have not yet met these criteria and therefore are not yet classified as patients. One heuristic reason to view treatment and prevention on a continuum derives from the potential value of extrapolating knowledge gained from one area of intervention research and applying it to the other.

Treatment intervention research and preventive intervention research are similar in several respects. They share a knowledge base, and the core sciences that support prevention and treatment have been instrumental in the advancement of both fields. Using the best available scientific methods, researchers in both fields increasingly are evaluating the efficacy and effectiveness of interventions, thus providing more information for community practitioners. Also, both treatment and prevention research continue to try to recruit competent scientists to their respective fields in the face of inadequately funded training programs (see Chapter 12).

Commissioned papers for this chapter were prepared by J. Asarnow and R. Koegel and by S. Glynn, K. Mueser, and J. Herbert, and are available as indicated in Appendix D.

Effective psychosocial and pharmacological treatments are now available for many of the mental disorders in DSM-III-R (Kaplan and Sadock, 1989; Karasu, 1989; Dobson and Shaw, 1988; see also Chapter 5). When these treatment interventions are used, they can substantially reduce the morbidity, chronicity, and disability of mental disorders. One justification for mining the principles grounded in treatment intervention research to learn lessons for designing, conducting, and analyzing preventive intervention research programs is that preventive interventions and treatment interventions are often based on similar multifactorial causal models. Therefore it is possible that if a particular treatment intervention is effective for treating an already developed mental disorder, the same or a similar intervention may be effective in preventing the disorder in individuals who are at high risk. Moreover, even if the preventive intervention fails to prevent the onset of the disorder, it may delay onset or may lessen the severity of the disorder. Many treatment interventions aimed at enhancing protective factors, such as literacy and academic and social skills, are generic and not specific to any one mental disorder, and they are good in and of themselves. They may also provide beneficial effects when used in preventive intervention research programs, regardless of how critical they may be in actually preventing a mental disorder.

In this discussion, as in the rest of this report, the terms *intervention program* and *intervention trial* are carefully delineated. The intervention program is the activity or activities provided to the targeted population. Its design includes considerations regarding the timing, duration, and environment of those activities, as well as the interveners involved. The intervention trial is the research component designed with experimental and methodological protocols to analyze and validate the success of the intervention program. *Intervention research program* is the inclusive term for the program plus the trial.

Principles and lessons that can be shared between treatment intervention research and preventive intervention research are listed and described in this chapter. The list is illustrative, rather than exhaustive, and the principles and lessons fall into several categories according to the main concept to which they apply. The categories applicable to the design of intervention programs include risk and protective factors and etiological chains; co-morbidity of disorders; progressive course of maladaptive behavior; individual differences; multimodal interventions; timing, duration, and environment of interventions; and the effects of interventions on family members. Principles and lessons applicable to research methodology, ethical and cultural concerns, and dissemination are also presented. The suggestions in this chapter regarding translations from treatment to prevention are made with cautious optimism and the realization that only a growing body of empirical trials of preventive interventions can validate the applicability of these considerations.

INTERVENTION PROGRAM DESIGN

Risk and Protective Factors and Etiological Chains

Treatment interventions have been developed from knowledge of risk and protective factors that influence the course and outcome of mental disorders; likewise, preventive interventions have been developed from knowledge based on risk and protective factors that affect the onset of mental disorders. Some of these risk and protective factors are undoubtedly the same for treatment and prevention, and some are undoubtedly different. Research on the factors thought to be associated with onset of disorders—and thus of particular interest in prevention—and on how and where they fit within causal models is still at an early stage (see Chapter 6). Nevertheless, treatment research involving risk and protective factors affecting the course of disorders can provide additional insight. For example, many treatment studies have shown that when language, communication, and social skills are improved—giving individuals more functional control in their environments—disruptive, aggressive, self-injurious, and stigmatizing behaviors can be greatly reduced (Liberman, 1988). This consideration may have utility in prevention of stress-induced onset of disorders whose precursors include information-processing deficits.

As described in Chapter 2, risk factors that function as precursor signs and symptoms of a disorder can be used in indicated preventive interventions to target individuals at high risk for onset. Currently, whether those risk factors were part of the prodrome of the disorder can be known only in retrospect, after onset. Identification of prodromal phases could facilitate use of a treatment intervention to push the boundaries from treatment into an indicated prevention, which, because of its proximity to treatment on the intervention spectrum for mental disorders (see Figure 2.1), is where lessons from treatment are likely to be most applicable.

In the course of schizophrenia, for example, delay in treating the early stages of the disorder leads to maladaptive coping strategies by families and patients, the appearance of negative symptoms, refractoriness to drug therapy, social withdrawal, and greater chronicity. A treatment demonstration project in England by Falloon and colleagues documented a decrease in the prevalence of chronic schizophrenia when early detection and treatment intervention were provided by mental health teams working closely with general practitioners to reduce the duration and intensity of the disorder (Falloon, Shanahan, LaPorta, and Krekorian, 1990). Falloon reported reductions in chronic schizophrenia following an intervention that focused on individuals showing early stages of schizophrenia. Key features of this treatment intervention were (1) the identification of individuals hypothesized to be at risk to move further down the pathway to a chronic schizophrenic disorder, at a point relatively close to the disorder onset; (2) the use of proven, multimodal interventions, including both pharmacological and psychosocial components; and (3) integration of the treatment program within the primary health care and family systems (Falloon, 1992). Thus one prospect for a preventive intervention research program for schizophrenia might be to offer education on the early warning signs of psychosis in middle and high schools and colleges to students, parents, and teachers, as well as through the mass media, so that early identification of precursor signs and symptoms with a high likelihood of leading to the onset of disorder would lead to early indicated prevention, including psychosocial interventions for the individual and his or her family. However, the prevalence of schizophrenia is only 1 percent, and there are considerable dangers in the effects of labeling false positives, so the initiation of such a program would have to be considered very carefully.

Another example of using treatment interventions to push the boundaries from treatment into indicated preventive intervention is in the area of depression. DeRubeis, Hollon, and colleagues have reviewed evidence from studies that have followed up patients who were treated for depression (Hollon, DeRubeis, and Seligman, 1992; DeRubeis, Evans, Hollon, Garvey, Grove, and Tuason, 1990). Overall, the relapse rates for patients who received cognitive therapy were considerably lower than for those who received pharmacotherapy. Thus cognitive preventive interventions might help avert a first episode of depression, especially in individuals with precursor symptoms.

With the development of reliable and sensitive means of detecting prodromal phases of a disorder, the current public education programs on recognition and treatment of depressive and anxiety disorders, sponsored by the National Institute of Mental Health (NIMH) (e.g., NIMH Panic Disorder Campaign (NIMH, 1991)) could be expanded to include identification and preventive intervention of early precursors associated with these and other mental disorders. Information regarding the early precursors of panic and agoraphobia (such as an initial, transient panic experience) could be provided to the public through radio, television, and newspaper "health messages." Such an educational campaign might result in early identification and indicated preventive interventions, such as cognitive-behavioral approaches for the individual and his or her family, before the full syndrome develops. A research trial could be developed to determine the efficacy of such an approach.

Co-morbidity of Disorders

There is a high rate of co-morbidity in mental disorders. Half of persons with mental disorders have more than one diagnosis (Wolf, Schubert, Patterson, Grande, Brocco, and Pendleton, 1988). Furthermore, three out of four individuals with substance abuse disorders are also diagnosed with another mental disorder (Ross, Glaser, and Germanson, 1988). Data from the Epidemiologic Catchment Area study show that approximately half of mental disorders in the United States occur in persons with a history of some other mental disorder (Robins, Locke, and Regier, 1990).

Treatment research has found that one disorder (the primary disorder) usually occurs at an earlier stage than the other disorder(s) (typically described as secondary). For example, co-morbidity between anxiety disorders and substance use disorders has been found in a number of clinical studies (Roy, DeJong, Lamparski, Adinoff, George, Moore et al., 1991; Chambless, Cherney, Caputo, and Rheinstein, 1987), with phobias almost always preceding substance abuse (Christie, Burke, Regier, Rae, Boyd, and Locke, 1988; Hesselbrock, Meyer, and Keener, 1985; Weiss and Rosenberg, 1985). Klein (1980) suggests that co-morbidity between primary phobia and secondary substance abuse is traditionally attributed to anxiety, which leads to the use of alcohol and drugs as a form of self-medication. This interpretation has been supported by reports that the majority of patients with phobias consciously use drugs and alcohol to manage their fears (Bibb and Chambless, 1986). Other examples of a primary disorder leading to a secondary one include cocaine, marijuana, and amphetamine abuse triggering schizophrenia, panic disorder predating agoraphobia, and dysthymia being followed by major depression.

This evidence on co-morbidity of mental disorders suggests several rationales for preventive intervention research (Kessler and Price, in press). First, when one disorder causes or leads to a second, prevention of the first disorder is a plausible preventive strategy for the second. Preventing the onset of an initial primary disorder could, in principle, reduce the number of lifetime cases of other mental disorders and the substantial impairment, disability, and handicap associated with them.

Thus preventive interventions aimed at preventing the initial primary disorder should include outcome measures that assess effects on the incidence of multiple disorders. Second, when precursor signs and symptoms of a primary disorder are identified, preventive interventions should focus not only on the prevention of the primary disorder but also on the other likely co-morbid disorders that could develop. For example, a program to prevent anxiety symptoms from developing into a phobia should be accompanied by preventive strategies to decrease the potential for substance abuse. This might be done by weakening or eliminating causal pathways from the first set of precursor symptoms of the primary disorder to a likely set of precursors for a second disorder that could develop. Third, possible causal mechanisms linking two or more disorders provide a special opportunity for both prevention and etiological research. Interventions aimed at common causes may reduce the incidence of two or more co-morbid states. Finally, individuals who are at high risk for a mental disorder because of their having a primary physical disorder may benefit from preventive interventions. For example, individuals recovering from a myocardial infarction or coronary artery graft surgery—one half of whom can be expected to develop a depressive disorder—would be prime candidates for preventive interventions, especially if they have had precursor symptoms of depression (Brown, Munford, and Munford, 1993).

Progressive Course of Maladaptive Behavior

Treatment research has documented strong associations between children with dysthymic disorder, a persistent depressive condition, and the subsequent development of major depression (Kovacs, Feinberg, Crouse-Novak, Paulauskas, and Finkelstein, 1984a; Kovacs, Feinberg, Crouse-Novak, Paulauskas, Pollock, and Finkelstein, 1984b). Likewise, the early appearance of low levels of disruptive behaviors, such as inattention to classroom or home rules, in young children can progress to full-blown oppositional, conduct, or antisocial disorders that develop at a later age (Koegel, Camarata, and Koegel, 1992; Loeber, Brinhaupt, and Green, 1990). In a similar manner, patterns of seeking attention and social validation and avoiding challenging or anxiety-provoking situations in childhood may establish behavioral trends that can escalate to a mental disorder at a later stage in life. Thus it would appear that preventive intervention research would need to separate normative from abnormal developmental patterns of behavior and focus on eliminating or reducing those elements in the social environment that reinforce abnormal modes of coping and adaptation.

Individual Differences

Treatment in most areas of medicine has been guided by an appreciation of the special needs and responses of the individual patient. In treatment research the focus is often on which type of treatment is best for individual patients with specific mental disorders. Contributing to individual differences are the underlying gene-environment risk patterns and the role they play in etiology and the availability of social and other environmental resources.

One type of treatment intervention design that recognizes the importance of individual differences is the modular approach, which offers discrete elements of the intervention incrementally, in a hierarchy beginning with interventions that are least costly and intrusive to the subject population, depending on each individual's needs and responses (Liberman, Mueser, and Glynn, 1988; Liberman, 1981; Lazarus, 1974). For example, a wide range of modules have been developed for individuals with chronic mental disorders. The modules help teach skills in conversation, money management, home finding and maintenance, and medication self-management. Each identified skill area has specific, targeted behaviors for training (Liberman, 1988).

The modular approach has three primary advantages for treatment. First, it permits considerable latitude in designing a program to fit the specific needs of a given individual, while ensuring that some core elements are consistently applied to all. This approach depends on defining which subgroups will respond to which interventions. An eclectic approach can be developed, using modules that draw from cognitive, social, behavioral, and pharmacological domains.

Second, the modular approach can achieve greater efficiency in cost-effectiveness through providing only as much intervention as is needed and desired. Some targeted individuals may require many months or even years of intervention, whereas others may show the desired change in risk factors with a minimal, brief intervention.

Third, the modular approach fits well with a competence-based approach to intervention. Because many intervention programs aim to enhance skills that confer protection against risk factors—both enduring psychobiological vulnerabilities in the individual and stressful life events—monitoring the acquisition of skills in the targeted population can reveal the point at which incremental, modular intervention has achieved its objective in any one individual. In a like manner, preventive interventions that are flexible and tailored to individual needs may yield better results than a preventive intervention that attempts to change all targeted participants in much the same way with much the same type, intensity, and duration of intervention. Preventive interventions should take cognizance of individual differences in the degree to which participants are "at risk," possess personal or environmental protective factors, and display readiness for intervention.

Multimodal Interventions

The complexity of mental disorders has led to the use of multimodal treatment interventions including pharmacological and psychosocial-behavioral approaches. These combined approaches have tended to be more effective than either alone (Kaplan and Sadock, 1989; Karasu, 1989). Such combined biopsychosocial interventions also may be more effective than unidimensional interventions in prevention trials.

Before considering the use of pharmacological agents in prevention, the benefit-risk ratio of such a strategy must be carefully weighed. There are several reasons to limit the use of pharmacological agents in prevention programs that have children and adolescents as participants. First, the efficacy of drug therapy for many mental disorders in children is not well documented. Second, the adverse side effects of psychoactive drugs, especially on physical and mental development, may be greater for youths than for adults. Third, the potential for stigmatization may be greater when medications are used.

Some medications have proved effective in alleviating symptoms of some mental disorders and in forestalling relapse. Therefore it may be reasonable—but only with adults, not with children—to study the potential of these psychotropic drugs for preventing or delaying the onset of a disorder if administered to individuals who have precursor signs and symptoms and are at extremely high risk for the disorder. However, this is an extremely controversial issue. Even with adults, benefit-risk ratios for medication strategies must be carefully weighed. Medications with serious and frequent side effects would probably exceed a threshold considered acceptable. In indicated preventive interventions, knowing that an individual is entering a high-risk period for the development of a mental disorder might justify the administration of a psychotropic medication known to be effective with the disorder of concern. The amount of medication could be titrated downward to a subclinical, yet potentially effective, preventive dose in individuals who have shown precursor signs or symptoms of the disorder. Thus judicious administration of antidepressant and antipsychotic medications might find a place in the prevention of depressive and schizophrenic disorders among individuals at extremely high risk for developing these illnesses. This pharmacological preemptive strategy has been used to treat toxic, drug-induced psychoses in individuals thought to be at risk for schizophrenic disorder (Machiyama, 1992). Similarly, rapid treatment of serious panic symptoms with pharmacotherapy and cognitive behavior therapy might prove effective in preempting the development of agoraphobia.

Timing, Duration, and Environment of Interventions

The timing of interventions may be critical to success. For example, parent training with parents of conduct disordered children has been shown to be effective in producing clinically significant behavior changes in children up to age 12½ (Dishion and Patterson, 1992). However, that research has also shown that parents of older children are more likely than parents of younger children to drop out of the intervention before completion. The importance of intervening during sensitive periods, before precursor problem behaviors become rigidly set, is highlighted by the disappointing results of intensive and long-term residential social learning therapy for predelinquent boys. Even though there were efficacious results while the youth were living under close supervision (Phillips, Phillips, and Fixsen, 1971), long-term follow-up studies failed to document a significant effect of the social learning therapy on emergence of delinquency and other antisocial personality traits. It has been suggested that aggression crystallizes around age 8 and that preventive interventions should start before then (McCord and Tremblay, 1992). Both sets of findings suggest that providing parent training in early childhood is likely to be more successful in reducing the prevalence of child conduct problems than is delaying intervention until middle or late childhood, when oppositional and aggressive behavior patterns have stabilized (Loeber and Dishion, 1983).

Duration of interventions may also be critical. The achievement of prevention of mental disorders based on short-term interventions is unlikely to be successful. The literature on treatment intervention research repeatedly shows that the impact of a time-limited treatment tends to be diluted and lost over time because of subsequent intervening biopsychosocial events, natural living environments, and other transactions between individuals and their social settings (Forehand, 1992). Ideally, to sustain the progress derived from the initial intervention, prevention programs need a developmental perspective, with an integrated and comprehensive series of age-specific interventions timed to enhance and sustain healthy adaptation and skills and prevent dysfunction at multiple points over the life course. Successful interventions will need to have a sustained source of funding.

To achieve durable and generalizable effects from preventive interventions, the use of long-term strategies with the continuous or intermittent infusion of elements of the prevention program will need to be carefully considered. These may include the use of "booster" programs or the involvement of natural helpers (such as parents, caregivers, teachers, and peers) to ensure that the individual's social environment will continue to reinforce and strengthen the targeted protective factors. Many effective psychosocial and behavioral treatments have employed natural helpers instead of professional therapists to deliver the interventions (Stein, 1992; Falloon, 1988; Tharp and Wetzel, 1979). Involving natural helpers bearing close relationships with the targeted high-risk individuals may be fruitful in the delivery of preventive interventions as well, especially because these often take place in naturalistic, nonclinical community settings.

With regard to the site of the intervention, Webster-Stratton's (1992) findings from treatment research suggested that low-income, young, single mothers of infants and toddlers were the least likely group to profit from a video-assisted intervention program administered in a clinical setting. These young mothers, constrained by lack of mobility and babysitters, might have responded better to treatment delivered through home visits. In another example of the importance of choice of site, soldiers who have experienced "combat fatigue" or stress syndromes have been treated with combined pharmacological and exposure-in-vivo approaches as close to their front-line positions as possible, rather than in far-off hospitals (Rahe, in press), with the aim of returning the soldiers to duty as quickly as possible. Preventive intervention programs also may have different levels of participation and effectiveness depending on where they are delivered.

Treatment research has illustrated that behaviors and skills transfer to novel environments and demonstrate durability if programming for generalization is a part of the intervention (Liberman, McCann, and Wallace, 1976). Generalization requires specifically linking the intervention in one setting to other situations involving peers, family, school, and work. Generalization techniques include

• gradually "fading" the intervention (such as gradually reducing social reinforcement from the teacher for appropriate social behavior from almost continuous to very intermittent);
• using in vivo interventions (such as teaching the child at risk for conduct disorder to verbally negotiate conflict situations with peers on the playground);
• making the interventions relevant to the participant's natural

environment (such as, while coaching unemployed persons at risk for depression on job interviewing skills, making sure that the person role playing the employer accurately represents a coldly rejecting interviewer as well as a congenial interviewer, or having a person at risk for alcoholism use drink-refusal skills in a variety of environments, such as restaurants, bars, and homes, and in response to overtures from bartenders, peers, family members, and strangers);

- overlearning (such as requiring repetition when teaching discriminations or skills); and

- self-instruction and self-management (Eckman, Wirshing, Liberman, Marder, Johnston-Cronk, Mintz, and Zimmerman, 1992; Dobson, 1987).

Other strategies to increase durability include the use of "booster" programs. Pharmacotherapists have documented and accepted the need for "maintenance" drug treatment for chronic and recurrent mental disorders. However, a double standard applies in clinicians' thinking about continuing an indefinite psychosocial treatment for a chronic mental disorder. If the pharmacological treatment is withdrawn and the patient relapses, the treatment is viewed as efficacious; on the other hand, if the psychosocial treatment is withdrawn and the patient relapses, this is considered evidence that the treatment is ineffective. The importance of prolonged, maintenance, and booster treatments for serious and chronic mental disorders has recently received greater recognition, and it is likely that preventive interventions will also increasingly be designed with these attributes.

Intervention Effects on Family Members

Interventions with one family member have been shown to have salutary effects on other family members. For example, treatment delivered to patients with diagnosed mental disorders not only helps to reduce relapse and improve the functional status for the patients directly served, but also reduces the emotional burden, dysphoria, and risks of mental disorder for family members and other caregivers deriving from the untreated mental disorder of the patient (Falloon, 1992; Harris and Bruey, 1988; Zarit, 1988; Falloon, Boyd, McGill, Razani, Moss, Gilderman, and Simpson, 1985). For example, treatment or maintenance interventions for a depressed mother might reduce the emotional risks for her child. Similarly, preventive interventions with a parent, sibling, or child might also reduce risks for other family members, but unless these potential positive "side effects" are anticipated, opportunities to measure them will be lost.

METHODOLOGICAL RESEARCH ISSUES

Treatment research has advanced in the past decade through the use of rigorous, controlled clinical trial methodology (Karasu, 1990). Trials have been carefully designed, conducted, and analyzed. The research has been hypothesis-driven, including a focus on the role of risk and protective factors in the onset and course of the disorder (Liberman, 1986). When treatment trials have concluded, patients have been followed up to determine the full effects of the intervention.

Treatment fidelity has been improved through the use of operationalized therapy manuals (Liberman, 1993). Until treatment research progressed to the point where therapy manuals became prerequisites for NIMH funding, it was impossible to compare the results of studies of psychotherapy conducted by different investigators, therapists, and academic centers. With the advent of these manuals, therapists could ensure fidelity of the subsequent replication and cooperative and collaborative multisite studies (Wallace, Liberman, MacKain, Blackwell, and Eckman, 1992).

Many of these same research principles are being applied to prevention trials. Preventive intervention research should be hypothesis-driven, with specification of the linkages and intervening mechanisms through which the interventions are expected to affect identified risk and protective factors and mediate delay or prevention of disorders. Participants in prevention trials should be followed up for long enough periods to determine the full effects of the intervention on the diagnosable disorder(s). Fidelity can be increased through the use of well-specified and replicable written manuals that clearly spell out what aspects of the intervention can be adapted to meet the needs of different cultural, socioeconomic, and age groups.

ETHICAL AND CULTURAL CONSIDERATIONS

In the design of an intervention program, and of the research methodology necessary to test its efficacy and effectiveness, caution is needed to guard against unintended negative effects. A pillar of ethics in delivery of health care is "do no harm." Unfortunately, treatment research has resulted in examples of untoward iatrogenic effects from both pharmacological and psychosocial interventions (Flanagan and Liberman, 1982; Gutheil and Appelbaum, 1982). The mechanisms of action and long-term effects and side effects of many of our pharmacological and psychosocial treatments remain to be clarified. This is particularly true during childhood, when many biological, psychological, and social systems are developing rapidly. Similarly, as mentioned earlier, applying diagnostic labels at an early age, although sometimes helpful, can stigmatize a child or adolescent, resulting in detrimental school and peer interactions that, in themselves, may produce psychological disorders (Dodge, 1983). Treatment research has shown many times that diagnostic classifications and treatment techniques must be modified and adapted to meet the special needs of culturally diverse population groups (Mezzich, Kleinman, Fabrega, Good, Johnson-Lowell, Lin et al., 1992). Failure of prevention researchers to address these needs can increase the risks of inadvertent adverse effects of preventive interventions or lack of positive effects.

Even emotionally supportive interventions have been found to produce mixed effects. The Cambridge-Somerville project, initiated in 1935, was designed to prevent delinquency, alcoholism, and mental illness by intervening with an experimental group composed of a sample of "troubled" and average boys in working-class neighborhoods. In retrospect, it is not clear whether this project would today be classified as a treatment or an indicated preventive intervention. Nevertheless, the lesson it provides remains of concern today. These boys were matched to a control group, with five years of biweekly visits by social workers for counseling and assistance with family problems (McCord, 1992). The experimental group also received tutoring, access to social and community programs, and medical and psychiatric attention. A 30-year follow-up found that almost twice as many individuals in the experimental group as in the control group had adverse outcomes, including criminal behavior, alcoholism, and serious mental disorder (McCord, 1992). These negative effects of the well-meaning intervention may have been the result of the labeling of youths who received the clinical intervention, leading to a self-fulfilling prophecy of "mental illness" or "deviance." Alternatively, there may have been inadvertent social reinforcement of early signs of deviance by the professional human service workers over the five years of intervention.

Adverse effects of universal preventive interventions that are issued through the mass media or school-based programs also may occur. For example, it is possible that some educational campaigns designed to reduce substance abuse, smoking, or hazardous sexual behavior could actually produce higher levels of these behaviors than were found in control groups. In particular, media-based campaigns may backfire when targeted to individuals who are at high risk for disorders.

DISSEMINATION ISSUES

Experiences from efforts to disseminate findings from efficacious treatment research programs to practitioners can enhance the prospects for successful adoption of innovative prevention methods. In treatment research, traditional dissemination methods, such as journal articles and conferences, have had serious limitations because so few professionals are able to translate this information into clinical practice (Backer, Liberman, and Kuehnel, 1986; Norris and Larsen, 1976; Garvey and Griffith, 1971; Havelock, 1969). Factors that have appeared to promote the use of clinical treatment innovations by practitioners include interpersonal contacts between potential adopters and those knowledgeable about the innovation, outside consultation on the adoption process, organizational support for innovation, persistent championship by agency staff, and effectiveness and adaptability of the innovation (Corrigan, MacKain, and Liberman, 1993; Backer et al., 1986). These lessons learned by treatment researchers certainly could be applied to the goal of more effective methods of dissemination and widespread public utilization of the results of prevention research.

FINDINGS AND LEADS

• When precursor signs and symptoms of an initial primary disorder are identified, preventive interventions should focus not only on the prevention of the primary disorder but also on the other likely co-morbid disorders that could develop. Outcome measures should be used to assess intervention effects on the incidence of multiple disorders.

• With the development of reliable and sensitive means of detecting prodromal phases of a disorder, treatment intervention techniques can be used in indicated preventive interventions for individuals at high risk for developing a disorder.

• Preventive interventions should be tailored to take cognizance of individual differences in the degree to which participants are "at risk," possess personal or environmental protective factors, and display readiness for intervention.

• Preventive interventions should aim to achieve durable and generalizable effects. Long-term strategies may include the use of "booster" sessions and the involvement of natural helpers from the individual's social environment.

• Preventive interventions with one individual can have salutary effects on other family members. Benefit-cost and cost-effectiveness analyses would do well to consider these other outcomes.

• Preventive intervention programs can have powerful effects. It is imperative, therefore, to be alert to inadvertent adverse outcomes.

• The usefulness of viewing treatment and prevention as part of a spectrum of interventions for mental disorders, instead of in opposition to each other, is apparent. Many principles that have emerged from research in one area can be borrowed, fully formed, for use in the other. Over the next decade, the cutting edge for progress will lie in the development of mutual respect, equal opportunity, and pragmatic collaboration among the scientists and advocates in the prevention and treatment fields.

REFERENCES

Backer, T. E.; Liberman, R. P.; Kuehnel, T. S. (1986) Dissemination and adoption of innovative psychosocial intervention. Journal of Consulting and Clinical Psychology; 54: 111–118.

Bibb, J. L.; Chambless, D. L. (1986) Alcohol use and abuse among diagnosed agoraphobics. Behavior Research Therapy; 24: 49–58.

Brown, M. A.; Munford, A. M.; Munford, P. R. (1993) Behavior therapy of psychological distress in patients after myocardial infarction or coronary bypass. Journal of Cardiopulmonary Rehabilitation; 13: 201–210.

Chambless, D. L.; Cherney, J.; Caputo, G. D.; Rheinstein, B. J. (1987) Anxiety disorders and alcoholism. Journal of Anxiety Disorders; 1: 24–40.

Christie, K. A.; Burke, J. D., Jr.; Regier, D. A.; Rae, D. S.; Boyd, J. H.; Locke, B. Z. (1988) Epidemiologic evidence for early onset of mental disorders and higher risk of drug-use in young adults. American Journal of Psychiatry; 145: 971–975.

Corrigan, P. W.; MacKain, S. J.; Liberman, R. P. (1993) Skills training modules: A strategy for dissemination and utilization of a rehabilitation innovation. In: J. Rothman and E. Thomas, Eds. Intervention Research. Chicago, IL: The Haworth Press.

DeRubeis, R. J.; Evans, M. D.; Hollon, S. D.; Garvey, M. J.; Grove, W. M.; Tuason, V. B. (1990) How does cognitive therapy work? Cognitive change and symptom change in cognitive therapy and pharmacotherapy for depression. Journal of Consulting and Clinical Psychology; 58(6): 862–869.

Dishion, T. J.; Patterson, G. R. (1992) Age effects in parent training. Behavior Therapy; 23: 719–729.

Dobson, K. S. (1987) Handbook of Cognitive Behavioral Therapies. New York, NY: Guilford Press.

Dobson, K. S.; Shaw, B. F. (1988) The use of treatment manuals in cognitive therapy: Experience and issues. Journal of Consulting and Clinical Psychology; 56(5): 673–680.

Dodge, K. A. (1983) Behavioral antecedents of peer social status. Child Development; 54: 1386–1399.

Eckman, T. A.; Wirshing, W.; Liberman, R. P.; Marder, S. R.; Johnston-Cronk, K.; Mintz, J.; Zimmerman, K. (1992) Techniques for training schizophrenic patients in illness self-management: A controlled trial. American Journal of Psychiatry; 149: 1549–1555.

Falloon, I. R. (1992) Early intervention for first episodes of schizophrenia: A preliminary exploration. Psychiatry; 55(1): 1–3.

Falloon, I. R. H., Ed. (1988) Handbook of Behavioral Family Therapy. New York, NY: Guilford Press.

Falloon, I. R. H.; Boyd, J. L.; McGill, C. W.; Razani, J.; Moss, H. B.; Gilderman, A. M.; Simpson, G. M. (1985) Family management in the prevention of morbidity of schizophrenia. Archives of General Psychiatry; 42: 887–896.

Falloon, I. R. H.; Shanahan, W.; LaPorta, M.; Krekorian, H. A. R. (1990) Integrated family, general practice and mental health care in the management of schizophrenia. Journal of the Royal Society of Medicine; 83: 225–228.

Flanagan, S.; Liberman, R. P. (1982) Ethical issues in the practice of behavior therapy. In: M. Rosenbaum, Ed. Ethics and Values in Psychotherapy. New York, NY: Free Press.

Forehand, R. (1992) Parental divorce and adolescent maladjustment: Scientific inquiry vs. public information. Behavior Research and Therapy; 30(4): 319–327.

Garvey, W. D.; Griffith, B. C. (1971) Scientific communication: Its role in the conduct of research and creation of knowledge. American Psychologist; 26: 349–362.

Gutheil, T. G.; Appelbaum, P. S. (1982) Clinical Handbook of Psychiatry and the Law. New York, NY: McGraw Hill.

Harris, S. L.; Bruey, C. T. (1988) Families of the developmentally disabled. In: I. R. H. Falloon, Ed. Handbook of Behavioral Family Therapy. New York, NY: Guilford Press.

Havelock, R. G. (1969) Planning for innovation through dissemination and utilization of knowledge. Ann Arbor, MI: University of Michigan, Center for Research on Utilization of Scientific Knowledge, Institute for Social Research.

Hesselbrock, M. N.; Meyer, R. E.; Keener, J. J. (1985) Psychopathology in hospitalized alcoholics. Archives of General Psychiatry; 42: 1050–1055.

Hollon, S. D.; DeRubeis, R. J.; Seligman, M. E. P. (1992) Cognitive therapy and the prevention of depression. Applied and Preventive Psychology; 1: 89–95.

Kaplan, H.; Sadock, B. J., Eds. (1989) Comprehensive Textbook of Psychiatry. Baltimore, MD: Williams & Wilkins.

Karasu, T. B. (1990) Toward a clinical model of psychotherapy for depression, II: An integrative and selective treatment approach. American Journal of Psychiatry; 147(3): 269–278.

Karasu, T. B. (1989) New frontiers in psychotherapy. Journal of Clinical Psychiatry; 50(4): 148.

Kessler, R. C.; Price, R. H. (in press) Primary prevention of secondary disorders: A proposal and an agenda. American Journal of Community Psychology.

Klein, D. (1980) Anxiety reconceptualized. Comprehensive Psychiatry; 21: 411–427.

Koegel, R. L.; Camarata, S. M.; Koegel, L. K. (1992) Aggression and non-compliance: Behavior modification through naturalistic language remediation. In: J. L. Matson, Ed. Autism in Children and Adults: Etiology, Assessment and Intervention. Sycamore, IL: Sycamore Press.

Kovacs, M.; Feinberg, T. L.; Crouse-Novak, M. A.; Paulauskas, S. L.; Finkelstein, R. (1984a) Depressive disorders in childhood. I. A longitudinal prospective study of characteristics and recovery. Archives of General Psychiatry; 41(3): 229–237.

Kovacs, M.; Feinberg, T. L.; Crouse-Novak, M. A.; Paulauskas, S. L.; Pollock, M.; Finkelstein, R. (1984b) Depressive disorders in children. II. A longitudinal study of the risk factors for a subsequent major depression. Archives of General Psychiatry; 41(7): 643–649.

Lazarus, A. A. (1974) Multimodal behavior therapy. In: C. M. Franks and G. T. Wilson, Eds. Annual Review of Behavior Therapy. New York, NY: Brunner/Mazel.

Liberman, R. P. (1993) Innovations in skills training for the seriously mentally ill. Innovations and Research; 2: 43–60.

Liberman, R. P. (1988) Psychiatric Rehabilitation of Chronic Mental Patients. Washington, DC: American Psychiatric Press.

Liberman, R. P. (1986) Coping and competence as protective factors in the vulnerability-stress model of schizophrenia. In: M. J. Goldstein, I. Hand, and K. Hahlweg, Eds. Treatment of Schizophrenia. Berlin, West Germany: Springer-Verlag; 201–216.

Liberman, R. P. (1981) Individualizing treatment strategies in depression. In: Behavior Therapy for Depression: Present Status and Future Directions. New York, NY: Academic Press.

Liberman, R. P.; McCann, M.; Wallace, C. J. (1976) Generalization of behavior therapy with psychotics. British Journal of Psychiatry; 129: 490–496.

Liberman, R. P.; Mueser, K. T.; Glynn, S. (1988) Modular strategies in behavioral family therapy. In: I. R. H. Falloon, Ed. Handbook of Behavioral Family Therapy. New York, NY: Guilford Press.

Loeber, R.; Brinhaupt, V. P.; Green, S. M. (1990) Attention deficits, impulsivity, and hyperactivity with or without conduct problems: Relationships to delinquency and unique contextual factors. In: R. J. McMahon and R. Peters, Eds. Behavior Disorders of Adolescence. Research, Intervention and Policy in Clinical and School Settings. New York, NY: Plenum Press.

Loeber, R. T.; Dishion, T. (1983) Early predictors of male delinquency: A review. Psychological Bulletin; 93: 68–99.

Machiyama, Y. (1992) Chronic methamphetamine intoxication model of schizophrenia. Schizophrenia Bulletin; 18: 107–113.

McCord, J. (1992) The Cambridge-Somerville Study: A pioneering longitudinal-experimental study of delinquency prevention. In: J. McCord and R. E. Tremblay, Eds. Preventing Antisocial Behavior: Interventions from Birth Through Adolescence. New York, NY: Guilford Press; 196–208.

McCord, J.; Tremblay, R. E. Eds. (1992) Preventing Antisocial Behavior: Interventions from Birth Through Adolescence. New York, NY: Guilford Press.

Mezzich, J. E.; Kleinman, A.; Fabrega, H.; Good, B.; Johnson-Powell, G.; Lin, K-M.; Manson, S.; Parron, D. (1992) Cultural Proposals for DSM-IV. Submitted to the DSM-IV Task Force by the Steering Committee, NIMH-Sponsored Group on Culture and Diagnosis.

NIMH (National Institute of Mental Health). (1991) Panic Disorder. Department of Health and Human Services (Public Health Service). Washington, DC: Government Printing Office; DHHS Pub. No. (ADM) 92–1869.

Norris, E. L.; Larsen, J. K. (1976) Critical issues in mental health service delivery: What are the priorities? Hospital and Community Psychiatry; 27: 561–566.

Phillips, E. L.; Phillips, E. A.; Fixsen, D. L. (1971) Achievement place: Modification of the behaviors of pre-delinquent boys within a token economy. Journal of Applied Behavior Analysis; 4: 45–59.

Rahe, R. H. (in press) Combat stress and post-traumatic stress disorders. In: R. P. Liberman and J. Yager, Eds. Stress in Psychiatric Disorders. New York, NY: Springer.

Robins, L. N.; Locke, B. Z.; Regier, D. A. (1990) An overview of psychiatric disorders in America. In: L. N. Robins and D. A. Regier, Eds. Psychiatric Disorders in America. New York, NY: Free Press; 328–366.

Ross, H. E.; Glaser, F. B.; Germanson, T. (1988) The prevalence of psychiatric disorders in patients with alcohol and other drug problems. Archives of General Psychiatry; 45: 1023–1031.

Roy, A.; DeJong, J.; Lamparski, D.; Adinoff, B.; George, T.; Moore, V.; Garnett, D.; Kerich, M.; Linnoila, M. (1991) Mental disorders among alcoholics: Relationship to age of onset and cerebrospinal fluid neuropeptides. Archives of General Psychiatry; 48: 423–427.

Stein, L. I., Ed. (1992) Innovative Community Mental Health Programs: New Directions for Mental Health Services, No. 56. San Francisco, CA: Jossey-Bass Publications.

Tharp, R.; Wetzel, S. (1979) Behavior Modification in the Natural Environment. New York, NY: Academic Press.

Wallace, C. J.; Liberman, R. P.; MacKain, S. J.; Blackwell, G.; Eckman, T. A. (1992) Effectiveness and replicability of modules for teaching social and instrumental skills to the severely mentally ill. American Journal of Psychiatry; 149: 654–658.

Webster-Stratton, C. (1992) Individually administered videotape parent training: "Who benefits?" Cognitive Therapy and Research; 16: 31–35.

Weiss, K. J.; Rosenberg, D. J. (1985) Prevalence of anxiety disorder among alcoholics. Journal of Clinical Psychiatry; 46: 3–5.

Wolf, A. W.; Schubert, D. S. P.; Patterson, M. B.; Grande, T. P.; Brocco, K. J.; Pendleton, L. (1988) Associations among major psychiatric diagnoses. Journal of Consulting and Clinical Psychology; 56: 292–294.

Zarit, S. H. (1988) Senile dementia. In: I. R. H. Falloon, Ed. Handbook of Behavioral Family Therapy. New York, NY: Guilford Press.

9

Mental Health Promotion

To this point in the report, the emphasis has been on decreasing risk factors and increasing protective factors with the ultimate goal of reducing numbers of new cases of mental disorders. But "health" is not simply the absence of disease. Indeed, recent reports (Mechanic, 1991, 1986) indicate that people have a much broader concept of health that includes successful physical and psychosocial functioning and encompasses spiritual growth. For example, answers to the common question, "In general, would you say your health is excellent, good, fair, poor, or bad?" actually encompass comprehensive and integrated concepts of health. The responses to such subjective assessments of health status not only tend to be given within a holistic frame of reference that may not sharply distinguish between physical and psychological aspects of the respondent's health (Eastwood, 1975), but also go beyond the presence or absence of disease. They tend to incorporate appraisals that relate to the development and sustenance of the concept of self—including individual competence, activity, and self-efficacy (Mechanic and Hansell, 1987).

The importance of this more complex view of health, for programmatic as well as theoretical purposes, is underscored by a strong link between the subjective assessment of health status and many health measures, including mortality (Idler, 1992; Ware, 1986). Specifically,

---

This chapter is based in part on a commissioned paper by N. Dinges, available as indicated in Appendix D.

several studies that have controlled for other risk factors have observed large differences in mortality over significant follow-up periods between those individuals who rated their subjective health status as excellent and those who rated it as poor (Idler and Kasl, 1991; Idler and Angel, 1990; Kaplan and Camacho, 1983; Mossey and Shapiro, 1982). If such assessments can predict something as basic as survival, then future preventive intervention efforts cannot afford to ignore the multidimensional nature of health, especially in terms that move beyond an exclusive concern with disease models and an artificial dichotomy between physical and psychological health.

With this expanded concept of health in mind, the present chapter embarks on a different line of inquiry from that pursued earlier in the report. Here the focus on pathology and the attendant risk-oriented approaches to preventive intervention momentarily is set aside, and the discussion turns instead to the state of the art of research and intervention specific to promoting mental health. As explained in Chapter 2, mental health promotion activities are offered to individuals, groups, or large populations to enhance competence, self-esteem, and a sense of well-being rather than to intervene to prevent psychological or social problems or mental disorders.

In many respects, the goals of decreasing risk and increasing protection in the disease-oriented model and the goals of promoting mental health are not mutually exclusive, either in practice or in outcome. There is also overlap in the techniques used to achieve these goals. For example, cognitive and behavioral interventions frequently are employed to prevent depression by reducing anger, regulating anxiety, and increasing positive cognitions (Lewinsohn, Hoberman, and Clarke, 1989; Muñoz, Ying, Armas, Chan, and Gurza, 1987). Likewise, the same cognitive and behavioral techniques may characterize attempts to enhance personal harmony and well-being (Walsh, 1992; da Silva, 1990). Consequently, it sometimes may be difficult to distinguish the pursuit of prevention from the pursuit of promotion; moreover, achieving one can result in the other. However, there are enormous differences, conceptually and philosophically, between these two goal orientations that must be recognized. Such differences have far-reaching implications for how people talk about these endeavors, why they participate in them, what they expect to gain, and the manner and extent to which they are willing to support them.

Mental health promotion represents the logical extension of the intervention spectrum depicted in Figure 2.1, yet it remains separate, outside of the illness model. It encompasses matters of individual as well as collective well-being and optimal states of wellness (Chopra,

1991; Stokols, 1991; Travis and Ryan, 1988; Ardell, 1986). Substantial resources—public as well as private—are currently being expended in the attempt to promote mental health. The expenditures are almost certainly large, perhaps similar in extent to the prevention research and service programs reviewed elsewhere in this report, but there has been no accounting. Programs, many of which are cited below, exist in schools, health service organizations, businesses, industries, and municipal governments. Other, perhaps not so apparent, examples can be found in religion, recreation, and physical exercise, all of which can be used to enhance mental well-being. The enthusiasm of commitment to such activities is infectious; personal testimony in regard to success abounds. Yet careful, rigorous examination of the efficacy, let alone the effectiveness, of these activities and of their associated costs and benefits has not yet been conducted. Thus the development of a scientific body of knowledge in regard to mental health promotive interventions represents a truly pioneering labor. Toward this end, the committee offers a review of the field as a foundation on which to build and raises a number of questions as a blueprint for progress.

CONCEPTUAL UNDERPINNINGS

Chapter 1 describes several of the problems involved in identifying, defining, and classifying mental disorders. There is, unfortunately, even less clarity about and little common nomenclature for discussing mental health and well-being. The reasons for this discrepancy are intriguing and include socioeconomic (Starr, 1980) as well as cultural (Kleinman, 1988; Manson, Tatum, and Dinges, 1982) factors. Although deserving fuller study, such analysis is beyond the immediate purview of this chapter. However, scholars have attempted to define this domain.

One of the major theoretical forerunners of the contemporary literature on psychological well-being is found in work on the dimensions of positive mental health and the related concept of happiness (Bradburn, 1969; Jahoda, 1958). The initial writings focused on the individual traits that were thought to define the mentally healthy person (Heath, 1977; Jahoda, 1958), which evolved from enumeration of core characteristics to more complex schemas that attempted to describe similarities in the dimensions that characterize well-functioning individuals, families, groups, and organizations (Adler, 1982). The original concepts of positive mental health and psychological well-being have further evolved to include the closely related constructs of competence, self-efficacy, and individual empowerment (Bandura, 1992, 1991; Sternberg and Kolligian, 1990; Swift and Levin, 1987). A recurrent element of such schemas has been the concept of self-esteem and its variants. Although this concept is prominently associated with the psychology of the self, other disciplines have also examined its role in their attempts to explain a wide range of human activities that are relevant to mental health promotion.

Goldschmidt (1974) asserted that humans are preprogrammed to be essentially concerned with the maintenance and furtherance of a positive self-image, reinforcing other theorists who previously had pointed out that the concept of self lies at the very center of humankind's symbolic system. Thus "normal" individuals in "normal" communities act to enhance the quality of the symbolic self, even though the actions required for this purpose may vary considerably from culture to culture. The most pertinent point about this theoretical position is that the social institutions of a given culture must provide means to maintain and promote the self-symbols of its members at the same time that these institutions must ensure their own basic survival. Taken by itself, the concept of "culture" is inadequate because it lacks a theory of motivation to account for cultural behavior. The concept of the self-image, when combined with cultural behavior, provides just such a motivating concept.

The importance of self-esteem maintenance and enhancement has achieved a broad disciplinary acceptance as a unifying concept, helping explain behaviors intended to attain psychological well-being. This desire to sustain self-esteem may partly explain why humans perceive it as a threat to be defined as an object (Kelman, 1975), and thus this motive may be the source of efforts in contemporary empowerment movements. Obviously, such movements owe much to the self-actualization principles of the past decades of humanistic psychology. Contemporary theorists have expanded these earlier views to a conceptual framework of self-esteem as a cultural construction (Solomon, Greenberg, and Pyszczynski, 1991). However conceived, there is little doubt that self-esteem has attained considerable importance in the thinking that informs mental health promotion efforts (Mecca, Smelser, and Vasconcellos, 1989).

Although the motives of self-esteem and mastery have been at the forefront of these developments, other concepts have appeared and received fleeting attention, only to disappear for lack of sufficient empirical verification or perhaps for lack of theoretical credibility. For example, the notion of trauma/stress conversion—which refers to the transformation of a painful, distressing, or shocking experience into one that induces strength and resiliency (Finkel and Jacobsen, 1977; Finkel, 1975, 1974)—enjoyed a brief exposure before being overwhelmed by the apparently more theoretically compelling complexities described in the literature on the stress-coping process. The idea that successfully coping with an objectively traumatic event could lead to personality strengths continues to have some appeal and is included in some models of the stress-coping process (IOM, 1982; see also the commissioned paper by Glynn, Mueser, and Herbert, available as indicated in Appendix D). But the potential for positive outcomes has been overlooked while attention has focused on negative effects (Zautra and Sandler, 1983).

Even less well received, if not actively scorned by many mental health professionals, have been proponents of the "transformative" health movement (Walsh, 1992; Grof and Grof, 1989; Tart, 1989, 1975; Wilber, Engler, and Brown, 1986; Walsh and Shapiro, 1983; Ferguson, 1980; Walsh and Vaughan, 1980), who have written extensively from a humanistic and "transpersonal" psychology perspective. This movement emphasizes the holistic nature of the human condition and sees it as inextricably rooted in social context. Its proponents argue that, by systematically focusing attention on the interplay of spiritual, physical, and psychological dimensions of everyday life experience, individuals can recast their sense of self, to the benefit of themselves and others.

Other theoretical contributions have focused on less sweeping, but nonetheless important, aspects of what seems to be an unlimited human need to think well of oneself by whatever means are available. The New Age forms that this need sometimes takes today can mask the perennial essential human striving that underlies it. Whether mundane or transcendent in purpose, the concept of self-esteem remains at the core of cultural behavior and manifests itself according to prevailing norms of the day. Contemporary forms of mental health promotion are thus now beginning to converge with spiritually oriented, transpersonal wellness movements (Murphy, 1992; McGuire, 1988).

Societies and their respective cultures vary in their ability to provide institutionalized means for preserving and enhancing the self-images and cultural identities of their members. Several theorists have pointed to the inherent interdependence of humans in finding an effective, socially adaptive fit between social structure and environmental demands. For example, Mechanic (1974) assessed the literature on personal coping abilities. He concluded that adaptation is widely perceived as being dependent on the ability of individuals to develop personal mastery over their environment. In Mechanic's view, this position was contradicted by the evidence for the interdependence of people in finding group solutions to socioenvironmental problems.

This perspective has been more recently elaborated by Antonovsky (1987, 1979) in positing the concept of "salutogenesis." (It is perhaps an indication of the dominating conceptual framework of pathogenesis that new terms have to be coined to describe a presumably qualitatively different health status on the positive end of the spectrum.) Antonovsky's salutogenic orientation grew out of his own background in traditional public health, but it came to be focused on the origins of and sustaining conditions for health rather than the etiology of illness. He proposed the concept of "generalized resistance resources" as the basis of health and included among such resources any phenomenon that was effective in combating a wide variety of stressors. Although such resources are easy to identify in the abstract (e.g., social supports, money, and ego strength), Antonovsky sought to specify the common elements of the dynamic process by which such resources promoted healthy functioning. He posited a "sense of coherence" as the organizing concept, defined as

a global orientation that expresses the extent to which one has a pervasive, enduring, though dynamic, feeling of confidence that one's internal and external environments are predictable and that there is a high probability that things will work out as well as can reasonably be expected. (Antonovsky, 1979, p. xiii)

Antonovsky's subsequent work has extended the model to examine the empirical support for and the heuristic value of adopting the salutogenic perspective (Antonovsky, 1987). It is consistent with notions of communal coping (David, 1979) that come from quite different theoretical and empirical origins. Likewise, there are clear parallels to the moral or behavioral codes that serve as the central themes for organizing life in other segments of our society. Consider, for example, the concept of *sa' a naghai bik'e hozhq*, or simply *hozhq*, in the Navajo world view:

Kluckhohn (1968) identified *hozhq* as the central idea in Navajo religious thinking. But it is not something that occurs only in ritual song and prayer, it is referred to frequently in everyday speech. A Navajo uses this concept to express his happiness, his health, the beauty of his land, and the harmony of his relations with others. It is used in reminding people to be careful and deliberate, and when he says good-bye to someone leaving, he will say *hozhqqgo naninaa doo* "may you walk or go about according to *hozhq*." (Witherspoon, 1977, p. 47)

Sa' a naghai bik'e hozhq encompasses the notions of connectedness, reciprocity, balance, and completeness that underlie contextually oriented views of human health and well-being (Stokols, 1987; Farella, 1984; Moos, 1979; Sandner, 1979). As a subsequent section of this chapter suggests, many contemporary mental health promotion activities in the United States can be construed as expressions of attempts to achieve a "sense of coherence," irrespective of the conceptual schema that informs the particular approach.

HEALTH PROMOTION PROGRAMS

The concepts described above have guided the development of the content, process, and outcome criteria of the various mental health promotion programs. The committee has chosen from among these programs some examples that illustrate the range and diversity of these activities on the contemporary scene, but has made no attempt to evaluate these programs according to any more stringent criteria.

The best current, single source of mental health promotion literature is contained in the annotated bibliography prepared by Trickett, Dahiyat, and Selby (in press). However, the mental health promotion literature constitutes a minute portion of the entire bibliography, only 22 of 1,326 references, and Trickett's definition of mental health promotion was not especially clear. He focused on articles "dealing with mental health education as a preventive strategy . . . and preventive interventions intended to promote varied aspects of mental and physical health" (Trickett et al., in press). About half of the 22 articles focused on preventing illnesses. This is itself a statement about the relative attention that has been given to mental health promotion.

The mental health promotion examples cited by Trickett range from those that focus on the acquisition of health-enhancing habits (Albino, 1984) to specific intervention programs in child and maternal health (Groves, Leeson, and Slovine, 1989; Peters, 1988; Bronstein, 1984; Chamberlain, 1984). These include efforts across the developmental life span (Re, Noble, and Howard, 1990) targeting issues specific not only to youth but also to older adults (Leventhal, Prohaska, and Hirschman, 1985; Gioiella, 1983). A large portion of the literature reviewed by Trickett and his colleagues reveals that, regardless of focus, social resources are a critical element in most promotive endeavors (Kulbok, 1985), especially insofar as natural support groups can form the basis for promoting desirable behaviors and empowering individuals (Albino and Tedesco, 1987; Mechanic, 1985).

Supporting and strengthening family functioning is, of course, a focal issue in many mental health promotion efforts (Duffy, 1988; Bowman, 1983), which reinforces earlier views of the critical role of the family in providing the foundation for healthy child, adolescent, and adult functioning (David, 1979). However, echoing Bradburn's earlier empirical research on the structure of individual well-being, Dunst, Trivette, and Thompson (1991) found that the prevention of poor outcomes could not be equated with the strengthening of family functioning, and that the absence of individual problems did not necessarily indicate the presence of positive family functioning.

The work of Spivack and Shure (1974; Shure and Spivack, 1978) on interpersonal, cognitive problem-solving deserves to be included among mental health promotion efforts, especially since it has gained relatively broad acceptance in school-based efforts to promote self-esteem and prosocial behavior (Groves et al., 1989). This program, "I Can Problem Solve: An Interpersonal Cognitive Problem-Solving Program," is included as an illustrative preventive intervention research program in Chapter 7 and is an example of how the same program may serve both preventive and promotive functions. The recent studies of resilient youth (Wyman, Cowen, Work, and Parker, 1991; Parker, Cowen, Work, and Wyman, 1990; Work, Cowen, Parker, and Wyman, 1990; Cowen and Work, 1988) also serve as examples of mental health promotion, as do the various studies of resilience and invulnerability (Beardslee, 1989; Garmezy, 1985; Werner and Smith, 1982).

Still other examples of mental health promotion present a more complex array of human activities from which to draw and a considerably greater challenge in terms of categorization. Because these are not typically oriented to scientific validation, it can be difficult to trace a clear line from their theoretical underpinnings to the methods used and the outcome criteria by which results might be judged. Just as Kleinman (1984) described the heterogeneity of indigenous systems of healing, so too can the myriad of human activities that may be motivated by mental health promotion efforts be seen as local forms of expression in a wide range of contexts.

One of the best places to look for examples of such mental health promotion efforts is among the diverse settings that provide some form of nonprofessional "healing," a term that is becoming widely embraced as a metaphor for less stigmatized, more participatory, holistic, and positively oriented approaches to addressing the (dis-)order of the human condition. It commonly is assumed that such practices are sought by those desperately grasping for a solution to a terminal illness after having exhausted the resources of professional biomedicine or by those lacking the motivation or discipline to comply with a medically prescribed regimen. This, however, is a misconception (Eisenberg, Kessler, Foster, Norlock, Calkins, and Delbanco, 1993). McGuire found that although a few adherents had participated in ritual healing practices as a last resort, most were attracted by a larger system of beliefs of which health-illness concerns were only a part. "For most adherents, therefore, the use of alternative healing typically involves a totally different definition of medical reality, an alternative etiology of illness, and a specific theory of health, deviance, and healing power" (McGuire, 1988, p. 5).

Equally important, McGuire's research did not support the rather common misconception that alternative healing practices and the systems of belief that informed such practices were characteristic of rural, poorly educated, lower-class persons, or that such practices had waned with increasing social mobility. Rather, her study demonstrated that alternative healing had considerable appeal to well-educated, economically secure, middle- and upper-middle-class residents of suburban communities.

A similar conclusion probably can be drawn with respect to the consumers of contemporary mental health promotion activities. Indeed, the "meaning-making" functions—that is, the communication of a structure for perceiving and assigning significance to people, places, and events—of participation in these practices may have many mental-health-promoting effects. This is perhaps what Antonovsky (1987, 1979) had in mind when he referred to the ability to maintain high levels of health by translating difficult, complex bombardment by environmental stimuli into a meaningful whole that provides a sense of coherence. Such concepts clearly go beyond those contained in the models of competence, positive mental health, and self-efficacy reviewed above.

Mental health promotion activities are common throughout many cultures. Among Native Americans, for example, the sweat lodge ritual can be and often is used by relatively well-functioning persons. The cultural practice in this case involves the sweat lodge purification ritual (*Inipi Onikare*), which is regarded as a "serious and sacred occasion in which spiritual insights, personal growth, and physical and emotional healing may take place. The purpose of purification is experienced on numerous levels of awareness, including the physical, psychological, social, and spiritual" (Wilson, 1988, p. 44). Many symbolic aspects of the physical construction of the sweat lodge and the various objects are part of the ritual (Brown, 1971). Of more direct relevance here are the psychological effects attributed to the ritual process, which includes a physically close circular arrangement of participants to increase unity and bonding, individual prayers involving self-disclosure of personal concerns and needs, as well as the needs and concerns of others, and the "opening" of the Four Doors through a cycle of prayers (actual opening of the sweat lodge door with change in heat and light conditions), which is controlled by the medicine person, who works to lead the group to

see more fully the symbolic nature of the ritual as a paradigm of life's central struggles. The juxtaposition of darkness and light may then take on deeper symbolic values as the paradigms of life versus death; insight versus ignorance;

growth versus stagnation; hope versus despair; relief versus suffering; renewal versus stasis; connection versus separation; communality versus aloneness, and will versus resignation. (Wilson, 1988, p. 54)

Wilson provides an explanation of the psychobiological aspects of altered states of consciousness that have commonly been observed and measured during the ritual and of the shifts in hemispheric dominance of the brain that are part of the altered states of consciousness commonly produced by ritual participation. Other aspects of the ritual are designed to promote a sense of the continuity of the community and the continuity of the individual in the culture. The conclusion of the ritual is typically accompanied by a number of positive psychological outcomes, including a sense of emotional release and a feeling of renewal and inner strength. Clearly, for many people, participation in the church and related religious activities serves similar purposes and offers comparable benefits. These benefits have been particularly well-documented for African-Americans (Neighbors, 1990; Dressler, 1987, 1985; Maypole and Anderson, 1987; Neighbors, Jackson, Bowman, and Gurin, 1983).

Another example of a contemporary form of mental health promotion can be found in groups combining Eastern meditation practices such as Zen, transcendental meditation, and yoga, and tenets of the human potential movement that have gained increasing popularity in many parts of the country. According to McGuire (1988), Eastern meditation practices in the United States trace their historical roots to the latter part of the nineteenth century but did not receive much public recognition until they were popularized through press coverage beginning in the 1960s and 1970s. Their increasing popularity was brought about in part by the growth of the self-realization goals of the human potential movement, whose adherents subsequently turned to Eastern spirituality for their longer-term development. McGuire noted as well that many Eastern spiritual forms have attracted not only the stereotypical countercultural youth but also middle-aged, established, and educated persons. Because the membership of Eastern meditation groups and the human potential movement appears to overlap considerably, McGuire treats them as one in her systematic examination of their core elements.

Ideal concepts of health and wellness are a prominent element of such groups, which emphasize balance among physical, psychological, and spiritual levels of the individual, as well as energy, flexibility, and self-awareness (Goleman and Epstein, 1983). They emphasize a holistic view of these elements in interaction and use such concepts in both literal and metaphorical ways to refer to both physical and spiritual well-being. Thus they emphasize a life-style characterized by balance in all spheres of life, seeking moderation and avoiding excess as a means of achieving a state of optimal balance. Life-style choices are a prominent feature of the means by which the desired state of well-being can be attained. These choices extend to larger social, environmental, political, and economic issues in an attempt to address real causes and not just the symptoms of imbalanced states.

The source of health, as well as of overall well-being, is conceived of as a universal life force that is more spiritual than mechanistic. This force provides the basic energy required for states of physical and spiritual well-being, and many of the practices of the groups are oriented to adjusting such energies into a harmonious flow. Eclecticism characterizes the choice of healing and health practices in both individual and group form. Meditation, massage, yoga, and dance therapy might be among the simultaneous or serial choices of health-oriented practices to bring about purification or promote balance and personal growth.

The element of flexibility as a criterion of well-being is fundamental for judging the beneficial outcomes of the belief system and life-style choices of adherents to Eastern meditation and the human potential movement. Practice, technique, beliefs, and methods of managing one's life are not given eternal validity but are rather viewed as appropriate for a particular time, place, and problem that at some point no longer applies. Thus the impermanence of both physical and psychological substance are considered the natural state, and self-awareness and self-responsibility are key requirements of general well-being. A generalized faith in the expectation that usefulness of whatever practice one is employing also characterizes this approach. Hence, being part of the "flow" without fully understanding or being able to control it is considered an important corollary of the generalized expectation of beneficial outcomes.

There are striking parallels between the beliefs and practices of Eastern meditation and human potential adherents derived from non-Western cultures and those articulated in the more formalized conceptual framework of generalized resistance resources and sense of coherence proposed by Antonovsky (1987, 1979). In Csikszentmihalyi's (1990) examination of the psychology of optimal experience, he depicted both as related to "flow" as the organizing concept.

The reemergence of such concepts, which appear to have long histories and broad cross-cultural recognition, leads to the issue of the rediscovery of fundamental aspects of psychological well-being that can inform mental health promotion. A common misconception is that such belief systems espouse some unattainable utopian ideal of mental health that has little relation to everyday existence. To the contrary, such belief systems are oriented to understanding how human beings manage to find positive meaning and identity-sustaining experiences as they go about coping with life's adversities (da Silva, 1990). Over 20 years ago, Bradburn (1969) empirically demonstrated in studies with humans that a subjective sense of psychological well-being consisted of a balance of positive and negative emotions, not just positive ones.

Most of the intervention strategies discussed to this point have been individually rather than collectively oriented in design and implementation. There is, in addition, an emerging emphasis on linking individual-focused, small-group/organizational, and community approaches to mental health promotion (Fawcett, Paine, Francisco, and Vliet, 1993; Hawkins and Catalano, 1992; Weiss, 1991; Braithwaite and Lythcott, 1989; Winett, King, and Altman, 1989; Green and Raeburn, 1988; McLeroy, Bibeau, Steckler, and Glanz, 1988; Green, 1986). This perspective assumes that the healthfulness of a situation and the well-being of its participants are influenced by the diverse interplay among biological, psychological, and social factors. It also assumes that the effectiveness of any health promotion activity can be enhanced through the coordination of individual and group action at different levels: family members who attempt to improve their health practices, corporate managers who shape organizational health policies, and public health officials who supervise community health services (Green and Kreuter, 1990; Winett et al., 1989; Pelletier, 1984). This particular perspective has encouraged promotive policies and community interventions at municipal, regional, national, and even international levels.

For instance, *Toward a State of Esteem* (California Department of Education, 1990), a legislatively mandated review, outlines a comprehensive plan for engineering massive increases in self-esteem and personal as well as social responsibility. Such change is advocated across private and public sectors, targeted simultaneously at individuals, families, schools, neighborhoods, business, and government, through a wide variety of means. Examples include nurturing and family life programs for teenage parents (Family Development Resources, Inc., Adolescent Family Life Programs), as well as specialized training for foster care and institutional staff to promote personal and social responsibility among their wards (Sacramento County Foster Parent Training Program). Other examples are in-service and credentialing requirements for educators that emphasize self-esteem enhancement skills (Action Education, Annual California Self-Esteem Conference), real-life skills curricula (College Readiness Program, Partnership Academy Program), and parent-school collaboration in education (Project Self-Esteem, New Parents as Teachers Project). Still other examples include community partnerships in after-school projects that promote constructive, prosocial experiences and serve as alternatives to activities that may place youth at risk of delinquency and violence (Urban Youth Lock-In, Stop-Gap Theatre); peer-support groups that foster learning, self-confidence, and motivation among welfare recipients (GAIN, GOALS Program); and strategies that positively reinforce employee responsibility in the work place (New Ways to Work). A basic theme is simultaneous, coordinated action across these different domains.

Recent examples of intercity and cross-national cooperation in mental health promotion include the World Health Organization's (WHO) Healthy Cities Project (World Health Organization, 1988, 1986, 1984; Ashton, Grey, Barnard, 1986; Hancock and Duhl, 1985). Recognizing that healthy cities continually create and improve physical and social environments conducive to their residents' well-being, WHO orchestrates, through technical assistance and resource materials, the development and implementation of citywide health plans. Healthy Cities Indiana (Flynn and Rider, 1991) represents the U.S. counterpart, in which Indiana University, the state public health association, six Indiana cities, and the W.K. Kellogg Foundation have combined their efforts to bring about planned change to improve community life. Other communities are rapidly adopting similar plans, such as the Healthy Communities Initiative, a cooperative venture between the National Civic League and the U.S. Public Health Service. Specific examples include the Kansas Initiative, involving the Wesley Foundation and an array of citizen as well as institutional participants (Fawcett et al., 1993), and the Colorado Healthy Communities Initiative, which employs community and agency coalitions, supported by the Colorado Trust. As is evident, these endeavors frequently engender significant investment by private as well as public sponsors. The Municipal Foreign Policy Movement has provided a similar forum for intercity development of legislation in health promotion and environmental protection (Agran, 1989; Shuman, 1986). Regardless of the particular form such enterprises take, all value citizen action in, mutual investment toward, and shared responsibility for promoting health, well-being, and positive life-styles.

GAPS IN OUR KNOWLEDGE

The current level of knowledge about the mental health promotion activities that are occurring in this country is sparse. Gaps in knowledge include a wide variety of topics that could be addressed in a research agenda.

A useful body of theory exists as one component in the knowledge base for mental health promotion activities. Several lines of inquiry might prove especially fruitful in expanding our understanding. What is the motivation for psychological well-being, and what are the conditions under which it emerges? How many dimensions are necessary for a complete accounting of the variations in psychological well-being? Do the different forms of alternative mental health promotion noted above reflect significant needs that have not been met by other mental health interventions? Do promotion efforts arise from attempts to counteract the social stigma that frequently accompanies the onset of disease in an individual? Does the pursuit of wellness, holism, empowerment, and a sense of coherence reflect the need for buffers against the social loss involved in the illness experience (Kleinman, 1984)? Perhaps our attention has been so focused on psychopathology that we have missed the significance of the tremendous grass-roots efforts that are being expended in the pursuit of psychological well-being.

McGuire's (1988) analysis of the new individualism involved in urban ritual healing suggests that conventional, institutional forms of healing may be losing their effectiveness in providing means for maintaining and furthering self-esteem. Did conventional healing ever provide sufficient avenues for pursuit of the positive self-symbol, or were such avenues limited to the fortunate few? Perhaps mental health practitioners and researchers have failed to understand that lay definitions of psychological well-being are at variance with professional views, just as medical practitioners have long operated with different explanatory models of physical disease from those of their patients (Kleinman, 1980). Perhaps it is time to consider how the psychological, biosocial, cultural, and spiritual dimensions intersect in contemporary definitions of psychological well-being and mental health promotion.

Cultural variations in mental health promotion activities and the ways in which specific cultural practices might inform mental health promotion might prove to be particularly significant areas of inquiry. Do alternative forms of mental health promotion serve different sectors of society or subcultures of the mass culture? What determines a person's choice of mental health promotion resources, and how does being placed in a devalued social role affect such choices (as may occur with subcultural group members)? Has the multicultural nature of our society been a significant factor in the emergence of diverse modes of mental health promotion?

A closely related issue concerns the extent of simultaneous use of different methods of mental health promotion. Options from conventional and alternative systems are sometimes presented as polar choices requiring allegiance to one or the other orientation. But individuals often choose more than one option, as in participation in workplace wellness programs during the week and ritual healing practices on the weekend. Individuals' simultaneous use of different methods may be an expression of their self-determination and may reflect goal-oriented striving to incorporate new sources of information to promote self-esteem.

The types, forms, scope, frequency, and location of mental health promotion activities are poorly understood. How many people participate in mental health promotion activities? Of what kind? What are their sociodemographic characteristics, particularly with respect to subcultural variation and geographic location? Where are mental health promotion activities occurring, and where else could they be implemented? Schools and work sites are obviously prime locations, but perhaps there are many other venues the potential of which has been underestimated, such as churches, neighborhoods, and cities. How are these activities organized, and who uses them? Much contemporary mental health promotion activity appears to emanate from religious and spiritual beliefs that historically have not been available for empirical study in the United States. Can such activities now be studied?

A critical issue concerns how to determine the actual outcomes of participation in different potential mental health promotion activities. What criteria are to be used in evaluating the outcomes of these activities? This question goes directly to the issue of the impacts of conventional and alternative forms of mental health promotion. Is one or the other superior in outcomes for specific groups of individuals? Is a combination of involvements more effective for long-term psychological well-being? If alternative methods yield promotive benefits, how do they produce such effects? Do they achieve outcomes different from or similar to those of more conventional methods? Not much is known about the harm some mental health promotion activities might cause. What potential adverse effects are there? Are particular forms of mental health promotion likely to cause harm? Are specific groups of individuals more at risk?

We simply do not understand the full range of the phenomena involved in mental health promotion and certainly lack the evidence to reject alternative sources as useless. Kleinman (1984) suggested that no policies be advanced that might control nonprofessional indigenous healers in the United States until research could demonstrate if such activities were beneficial or counterproductive to the nation's health. An analogous position probably is advisable with respect to the complexities involved in the measurement of the myriad forms of potential mental health promotion activities engaged in by the U.S. public.

Mechanic (1991) has taken a similar position with regard to research on the sources of health and disease, which vary widely in a given community. Referring to researching the idea of health in broad terms, he comments: "Definition and measurement is central to the challenge, but to allow the easily measurable to guide our definitions of what is important and our research efforts would be exceedingly foolish" (p. 32).

A related issue concerns the criteria by which costs and benefits are calculated. The social and economic costs and benefits of conventional mental health promotion activities figure prominently in any research agenda. Are alternative mental health promotion efforts more socially acceptable and cost-effective than those provided through conventional means? If workplace wellness programs can demonstrate positive cost-effectiveness, may there be equal or greater benefits involved for those who participate in alternative mental health promotion, or some combination of the two?

People in our society are deeply committed to health promotion pursuits, expending enormous resources to attain happiness and dignity. Success often has been equivocal, certainly uneven, and the ideas of mental health promotion are to some extent culture-bound. Nonetheless, this endeavor—the promotion of mental health and well-being—will continue. Hence it behooves us to proceed thoughtfully and with care on a research agenda regarding these activities.

FINDINGS AND LEADS

• Health, wellness, zest, resilience, self-efficacy, empowerment, order, balance, harmony, integrity, energy, flexibility, a sense of coherence: each represents some facet of an underlying human experience that is desirable, satisfying, perhaps even necessary. In the quest to understand and ultimately attempt to prevent suffering, it is important to not lose sight of another, equally powerful imperative, that is, the need to nurture positive regard for one's self and the world around us. There appear to be many ways of accomplishing this goal of promotion of mental health; clearly, each entails more than seeking freedom from disease or ailment.

• Research on mental health promotion, defined as distinct from enhancement of protective factors within an illness model, may be a difficult concept for some to accept. In part, this may reflect a tension between expressing an openness to new ways of thinking about mental health on the one hand, and attempting to be scientifically rigorous and skeptical on the other. An analogous tension in the physical illness field was partially resolved in 1992 when the National Institutes of Health established an Office of Unconventional Medical Practices—later renamed the Office of Alternative Medicine—and began systematically to explore such interventions. The decision to use federal support to determine the effectiveness of unconventional medical practices was controversial and momentous. It was an acknowledgment of the wide application of such practices and an openness to their potential usefulness.

- Traditional mind-body dichotomies are alternative ways of understanding the same phenomenon. The concept of health promotion has begun to integrate these perspectives.
- In Chapter 7, a small, but growing body of scientific evidence could be cited in regard to the efficacy of interventions for decreasing risk factors and enhancing protective factors with an ultimate goal of preventing mental disorders. No comparable corpus of knowledge is available with respect to mental health promotion. The current level of understanding about the potential contribution of conventional and alternative approaches to the goals of mental health promotion is sparse.
- Current public and private expenditures to promote mental health are substantial. They are perhaps similar to the amounts spent on prevention research and service programs reviewed elsewhere in this report. Because we know little about the outcomes from promotion activities, it would be useful to assess them scientifically. A research agenda could begin by cataloging mental health promotion activities across the life course and crafting outcome criteria that could be used in rigorous evaluations down the road.
- Enthusiasm for the health promotion movement should not interfere with a willingness to evaluate potential harm from such activities. For example, although mental health promotion activities do not use an illness model, persons with severe mental disorders may seek out such activities, viewing them as alternatives to standard treatment. Ethical issues such as this will be paramount in any attempts to bring methodological rigor to the mental health promotion field.

REFERENCES

Adler, P. T. (1982) An analysis of the concept of competence in individuals and social systems. Community Mental Health Journal; 18(2): 34–45.

Agran, L. (1989) Mayor as global leader. Paper presented at Macalester College Mayors' Forum. St. Paul, MN.

Albino, J. E. (1984) Prevention by acquiring health-enhancing habits. In: M. C. Roberts and L. Peterson, Eds. Prevention of Problems in Childhood: Psychological Research and Applications. New York, NY: John Wiley and Sons; 200–231.

Albino, J. E.; Tedesco, L. A. (1987) Public health and community wellness. Prevention in Human Services; 5(2): 207–239.

Antonovsky, A. (1987) Unraveling the Mystery of Health: How People Manage Stress and Stay Well. San Francisco, CA: Jossey-Bass Publications.

Antonovsky, A. (1979) Health, Stress and Coping. San Francisco, CA: Jossey-Bass Publications.

Ardell, D. B. (1986) High-Level Wellness: An Alternative to Doctors, Drugs and Disease. Berkeley, CA: Ten Speed Press.

Ashton, J.; Grey, P.; Barnard, K. (1986) Healthy Cities: WHO's new public health initiative. Health Promotion; 1: 319–324.

Bandura, A. (1992) Self-efficacy mechanism in psychobiologic functioning. R. Schwarzer, Ed. Self-efficacy: Thought Control of Action. Philadelphia, PA: Hemisphere Publishing Corporation.

Bandura, A. (1991) Self-efficacy in physiological activation and health-promoting behavior. In: J. Madden, IV, Ed. Neurobiology of Learning, Emotion and Affect. New York, NY: Raven Press; 229–269.

Beardslee, W. R. (1989) The role of self-understanding in resilient individuals: The development of a perspective. American Journal of Orthopsychiatry; 59(2): 266–278.

Bowman, T. W. (1983) Promoting family wellness. In: D. R. Mace, Ed. Prevention in Family Services: Approaches to Family Wellness. Newbury Park, CA: Sage Publications; 39–48.

Bradburn, N. M. (1969) The Structure of Psychological Well-Being. Chicago, IL: Aldine.

Braithwaite, R. L.; Lythcott, N. (1989) Community empowerment as a strategy for health promotion for black and other minority populations. Journal of the American Medical Association; 261: 282–283.

Bronstein, P. (1984) Promoting healthy emotional development in children. Journal of Primary Prevention; 5(2): 92–110.

Brown, J. E. (1971) The Sacred Pipe: Black Elk's Account of the Seven Rites of the Oglala Sioux. Baltimore, MD: Penguin Books.

California Department of Education. (1990) Toward a State of Esteem. Sacramento, CA: Office of State Printing.

Chamberlin, R. W. (1984) Strategies for disease prevention and health promotion in maternal and child health. Journal of Public Health Policy; 5(2): 185–197.

Chopra, D. (1991) Perfect Health: The Complete Mind/Body Guide. New York, NY: Harmony Books.

Cowen, E. L.; Work, W. C. (1988) Resilient children, psychological wellness, and primary prevention. American Journal of Community Psychology; 16(4): 591–607.

Csikszentmihalyi, M. (1990) Flow: The Psychology of Optimal Experience. New York, NY: Harper Collins Publications.

da Silva, P. (1990) Self-management strategies in early Buddhism: A behavioral perspective. In: J. Crook and D. Fontana, Eds. Space in Mind: East-West Psychology and Contemporary Buddhism. Rockport, MA: Element Books; 123–132.

David, H. P. (1979) Healthy family functioning: Cross-cultural perspectives. In: P. Ahmed and G. Coehlo, Eds. Toward a New Definition of Health: Psychosocial Dimensions. New York, NY: Plenum Press; 251–320.

Dressler, W. (1987) The stress process in a southern black community: Implications for prevention research. Human Organization; 46: 211–220.

Dressler, W. (1985) Extended family relationships, social support and mental health in a southern black community. Journal of Health and Social Behavior; 26: 39–48.

Duffy, M. E. (1988) Health promotion in the family: Current findings and directives for nursing research. Journal of Advanced Nursing; 13(1): 109–117.

Dunst, C. J.; Trivette, C. M.; Thompson, R. B. (1991) Supporting and strengthening family functioning: Toward a congruence between principles and practice. Prevention in Human Services; 9(1): 19–43.

Eastwood, M. R. (1975) The Relationship Between Physical and Mental Illness. Toronto, Ontario, Canada: University of Toronto Press.

Eisenberg, D. M.; Kessler, R. C.; Foster, C.; Norlock, F. E.; Calkins, D. R.; Delbanco, T. L. (1993) Unconventional medicine in the United States. The New England Journal of Medicine; 328(4): 246–252.

Farella, J. R. (1984) The Main Stalk: A Synthesis of Navajo Philosophy. Tucson, AZ: University of Arizona Press.

Fawcett, S. B.; Paine, A. L.; Francisco, V. T.; Vliet, M. (1993) Promoting health through community development. In: D. Glenwick and L. A. Jason, Eds. Promoting Health and Mental Health in Children, Youth, and Families. New York, NY: Springer.

Ferguson, M. (1980) The Aquarian Conspiracy: Personal and Social Transformation in the 1980's. Los Angeles, CA: Jeremy P. Tarcher.

Finkel, N. J. (1975) Strens, traumas, and trauma resolution. American Journal of Community Psychology; 3: 172–178.

Finkel, N. J. (1974) Stress and traumas: An attempt at categorization. American Journal of Community Psychology; 2: 265–273.

Finkel, N. J.; Jacobsen, C. A. (1977) Significant life experiences in an adult sample. American Journal of Community Psychology; 5: 165–177.

Flynn, B.; Rider, M. S. (1991) Healthy Cities Indiana: Mainstreaming community health in the United States. American Journal of Public Health; 81: 510–511.

Garmezy, N. (1985) Stress resistant children: The search for protective factors. In: J. E. Stevenson, Ed. Recent Research in Developmental Psychopathology. Oxford, England: Pergamon Press; 213–233.

Gioiella, E. C. (1983) Healthy aging through knowledge and self-care. Prevention in Human Services; 3(1): 39–51.

Goldschmidt, W. (1974) Ethology, ecology, and ethnological realities. In: G. V. Coelho, D. A. Hamburg, and J. E. Adams, Eds. Coping and Adaptation. New York, NY: Basic Books; 13–31.

Goleman, D.; Epstein, M. (1983) Meditation and well-being: An Eastern model of psychological health. In: R. Walsh and D. H. Shapiro, Eds. Beyond Health and Normality: Explorations of Exceptional Well-Being. New York, NY: Van Nostrand Reinhold; 229–253.

Green, L. W. (1986) The theory of participation: A qualitative analysis of its own expression in national and international health policies. Advances in Health Education and Promotion; 1: 211–236.

Green, L. W.; Kreuter, M. W. (1990) Health promotion as a public health strategy for the 1990's. Annual Review of Public Health; 11: 319–334.

Green, L. W.; Raeburn, J. M. (1988) Health promotion: What is it? What will it become? Health Promotion; 3: 151–159.

Grof, S.; Grof, C., Eds. (1989) Spiritual Emergency: When Personal Transformation Becomes a Crisis. Los Angeles, CA: Jeremy P. Tarcher.

Groves, D. R.; Leeson, L. L.; Slovine, T. M. (1989) Choices for positive living: A private/public partnership program to promote mental fitness and self-esteem in adults and children. Prevention in Human Services; 6(2): 59–66.

Hancock, T.; Duhl, L. (1985) Healthy Cities: Promoting health in the urban context. A background paper for the Healthy Cities symposium. Copenhagen, Denmark: World Health Organization.

Hawkins, J. D.; Catalano, R. F., Eds. (1992) Communities That Care. San Francisco, CA: Jossey-Bass Publications.

Heath, D. H. (1977) Maturity and Competence: A Transcultural View. New York, NY: Gardner Press.

IOM (Institute of Medicine). (1982) Stress and Human Health: Analysis and Implications of Research. New York, NY: Springer.

Idler, E. L. (1992) Self assessed health and mortality: A review of studies. In: S. Maes, H. Leventhal, and M. Johnston, Eds. International Review of Health Psychology. New York, NY: John Wiley and Sons.

Idler, E. L.; Angel, R. J. (1990) Self-rated health and mortality in the NHANES-I Epidemiologic Follow-Up Study. American Journal of Public Health; 80: 446–452.

Idler, E. L.; Kasl, S. V. (1991) Health perceptions and survival: Do global evaluations of health status predict mortality? Journal of Gerontology: Social Sciences; 46: 555–565.

Jahoda, M. (1958) Current Concepts of Positive Mental Health. New York, NY: Basic Books.

Kaplan, G. A.; Camacho, T. (1983) Perceived health and mortality: A nine-year follow-up of the Human Population Laboratory cohort. American Journal of Epidemiology; 117: 292–304.

Kelman, S. (1975) The social nature of the definition problem in health. International Journal of Health Services; 5(4): 626–642.

Kleinman, A. (1988) Rethinking Psychiatry. New York, NY: Academic Press.

Kleinman, A. (1984) Indigenous systems of healing: Questions for professional, popular, and folk care. In: J. W. Salmon, Ed. Alternative Medicines: Popular and Policy Perspectives. New York, NY: Tavistock Publications; 138–164.

Kleinman, A. (1980) Patients and Healers in the Context of Culture: An Exploration of the Borderland Between Anthropology, Medicine and Psychiatry. Berkeley, CA: University of California Press.

Kluckhohn, C. (1968) The philosophy of Navajo Indians. In: M. H. Fried, Ed. Readings in Anthropology. 2nd ed. New York, NY: Crowell.

Kulbok, P. P. (1985) Social resources, health resources, and preventive health behavior: Patterns and predictions. Public Health Nursing; 2(2): 67–81.

Leventhal, H.; Prohaska, T. R.; Hirschman, R. S. (1985) Preventive health behavior across the life span. In: J. C. Rosen and L. J. Solomon, Eds. Prevention in Health Psychology. Hanover, NH: University Press of New England.

Lewinsohn, P. M.; Hoberman, H. M.; Clarke, G. N. (1989) The coping with depression course: Review and future directions. Canadian Journal of Behavioral Sciences; 21(4): 470–493.

Manson, S. M.; Tatum, E.; Dinges, N. G. (1982) Prevention research among American Indian and Alaska Native communities: Charting future courses for theory and practice in mental health. In: S. M. Manson, Ed. New Directions in Prevention Among American Indian and Alaska Native Communities. Portland, OR: Oregon Health Sciences University; 15–64.

McGuire, M. B. (1988) Ritual healing in suburban America. New Brunswick, NJ: Rutgers University Press.

McLeroy, K. R.; Bibeau, D.; Steckler, A.; Glanz, K. (1988) An ecological perspective on health promotion programs. Health Education Quarterly; 15: 351–378.

Maypole, D.; Anderson, R. (1987) Culture-specific substance abuse prevention for blacks. Community Mental Health Journal; 23: 135–139.

Mecca, A. M.; Smelser, N. J.; Vasconcellos, J. (1989) The social importance of self-esteem. Berkeley, CA: University of California Press.

Mechanic, D. (1991) Researching the idea of health. In: P. E. Bebbington, Ed. Social Psychiatry: Theory, Methodology, and Practice. New Brunswick, NJ: Transaction Publishers; 23–34.

Mechanic, D. (1986) The role of social factors in health and well-being: The biopsychosocial model from a social perspective. Integrative Psychiatry; 4: 2–11.

Mechanic, D. (1985) Health and behavior: Perceptions on risk prevention. In: J. C. Rosen and L. J. Solomon, Eds. Prevention in Health Psychology. Hanover, NH: University Press of New England; 6–17.

Mechanic, D. (1974) Social structure and personal adaption: Some neglected dimensions. In: G. V. Coehlo, D. A. Hamburg, and J. E. Adams, Eds. Coping and Adaptation. New York, NY: Basic Books; 32–46.

Mechanic, D.; Hansell, S. (1987) Adolescent competence, psychological well-being and self-assessed physical health. Journal of Health and Social Behavior; 28: 364–374.

Moos, R. H. (1979) Social ecological perspectives on health. In: G. C. Stone, F. Cohen, and N. E. Adler, Eds. Health Psychology: A Handbook. San Francisco, CA: Jossey-Bass Publications; 523–547.

Mossey, J. M.; Shapiro, E. (1982) Self-rated health: A predictor of mortality among the elderly. American Journal of Public Health; 72: 115–135.

Muñoz, R. F.; Ying, Y. W.; Armas, R.; Chan, F.; Gurza, R. (1987) The San Francisco Depression Prevention Research Project: A randomized trial with medical outpatients. In: R. F. Muñoz, Ed. Depression Prevention: Research Directions. Washington, DC: Hemisphere Press; 199–215.

Murphy, M. (1992) The Future of the Body: Explorations into the Further Evolution of Human Nature. Los Angeles, CA: Jeremy P. Tarcher.

Neighbors, H. W. (1990) The prevention of psychopathology in African Americans: An epidemiologic perspective. Community Mental Health Journal; 26(2): 167–179.

Neighbors, H. W.; Jackson, J.; Bowman, P.; Gurin, G. (1983) Stress, coping and black mental health: Preliminary findings from a national study. Prevention in Human Services; 2: 4–29.

Parker, G. R.; Cowen, E. L.; Work, W. C.; Wyman, P. A. (1990) Test correlates of stress resilience among urban school children. The Journal of Primary Prevention; 11(1): 19–36.

Pelletier, K. R. (1984) Healthy People in Unhealthy Places: Stress and Fitness at Work. New York, NY: Dell Publishing Company.

Peters, R. D. (1988) Mental health promotion in children and adolescents: An emerging role for psychology. Canadian Journal of Behavioral Sciences; 20(4): 389–401.

Re, A.; Noble, B. N.; Howard, G. (1990) Techniques for promoting a healthier society: Thoughts on prevention planning and needs assessment. Journal of Primary Prevention; 10(3): 207–221.

Sandner, D. (1979) Navajo Symbols of Healing: A Jungian Exploration of Ritual, Image and Medicine. Rochester, VT: Healing Arts Press.

Shuman, M. H. (1986) Dateline main street: Local foreign policies. Foreign Policy; 65: 154–174.

Shure, M. B.; Spivack, G. (1978) Problem-solving techniques in childrearing. San Francisco. CA: Jossey-Bass Publications.

Solomon, S.; Greenberg, J.; Pyszczynski, T. (1991) A terror management theory of social behavior: The psychological functions of self-esteem and cultural worldviews. Advances in Experimental Social Psychology; 24: 93–159.

Spivack, G.; Shure, M. B. (1974) Social Adjustment of Young Children: A Cognitive Approach to Solving Real-Life Problems. San Francisco, CA: Jossey-Bass Publications.

Starr, P. (1980) The Social Transformation of American Medicine. Cambridge, MA: Harvard University Press.

Sternberg, R. J.; Kolligan, J., Jr. (1990) Competence Considered. New Haven, CT: Yale University Press.

Stokols, D. (1991) Establishing and maintaining healthy environments: Toward a social ecology of health promotion. Wellness Lecture Series. Berkeley, CA: University of California Press.

Stokols, D. (1987) Conceptual strategies of environmental psychology. In: D. Stokols and I. Altman, Eds. Handbook of Environmental Psychology. New York, NY: John Wiley and Sons.

Swift, C.; Levin, G. (1987) Empowerment: An emerging mental health technology. Journal of Primary Prevention; 8: 71–94.

Tart, C. (1989) Open Mind, Discriminating Mind: Reflections on Human Possibilities. San Francisco, CA: Harper & Row.

Tart, C. (1975) Transpersonal Psychologies. New York, NY: Harper & Row.

Travis, J. W.; Ryan, R. S. (1988) The Wellness Workbook. Berkeley, CA: Ten Speed Press.

Trickett, E. J.; Dahiyat, C.; Selby, P. (in press) Primary Prevention in Mental Health: An Annotated Bibliography. Rockville, MD: Department of Health and Human Services.

Walsh, R. (1992) The search for synthesis: Transpersonal psychology and the meeting of East and West, psychology and religion, personal and transpersonal. Journal of Humanistic Psychology; 32(1): 19–45.

Walsh, R.; Shapiro, D. H. (1983) Beyond health and normality: Explorations of exceptional well-being. New York, NY: Van Nostrand Reinhold.

Walsh, R.; Vaughan, F. (1980) Beyond Ego: Transpersonal Dimensions in Psychology. Los Angeles, CA: Jeremy P. Tarcher.

Ware, J. E., Jr. (1986) The assessment of health status. In: L. H. Aiken and D. Mechanic, Eds. Applications of Social Science to Clinical Medicine and Social Policy. New Brunswick, NJ: Rutgers University Press; 204–228.

Weiss, S. M. (1991) Health at work. In: S. M. Weiss, J. E. Fielding, and A. Baum, Eds. Perspectives in Behavioral Medicine: Health at Work. Hillside, NJ: Lawrence Erlbaum Associates; 1–10.

Werner, E. E.; Smith, R. S. (1982) Vulnerable, But Invincible: A Longitudinal Study of Resilient Children and Youth. New York, NY: McGraw-Hill.

Wilber, K.; Engler, J.; Brown, D. P. (1986) Transformations of Consciousness. Boston, MA: Shambhala Publications.

Wilson, J. (1988) Culture and trauma: The sacred pipe revisited. In: J. Wilson, Z. Harel, and B. Kahana, Eds. Human Adaptation to Extreme Stress: From Holocaust to Vietnam. New York, NY: Plenum Press; 38–71.

Winett, R. A.; King, A. C.; Altman, D. G. (1989) Health Psychology and Public Health: An Integrative Approach. New York, NY: Pergamon Press.

Witherspoon, G. (1977) Language and Art in the Navajo Universe. Ann Arbor, MI: University of Michigan Press.

Work, W. C.; Cowen, E. L.; Parker, G. C.; Wyman, P. A. (1990) Stress resilient children in an urban setting. Journal of Primary Prevention; 11(1): 3–18.

World Health Organization. (1988) WHO Healthy Cities Project: An update. Geneva, Switzerland: WHO.

World Health Organization. (1986) The Ottawa charter for health promotion. Health Promotion; 1: *ii-v*.

World Health Organization. (1984) Health promotion: A discussion document on the concept and principles. Health Promotion; 1: 73–76.

Wuthnow, R. (1976) The Consciousness Reformation. Berkeley, CA: University of California Press.

Wyman, P. A.; Cowen, E. L.; Work, W. C.; Parker, G. R. (1991) Developmental and family milieu correlates of resilience in urban children who have experienced major life stress. American Journal of Community Psychology; 19(3): 405–426.

Zautra, A.; Sandler, I. (1983) Life event needs assessment: Two models for measuring preventable mental health problems. Prevention in Human Services; 2(4): 35–58.

AN AGENDA FOR THE
NEXT DECADE

10

Designing, Conducting, and Analyzing Programs Within the Preventive Intervention Research Cycle

S uccessful science benefits from cumulative progress, and the field of prevention of mental disorders is no exception. The previous chapters have detailed the progress to this point, including the diverse lessons that can be taken from other areas in health research. It is apparent from the review in Chapter 7 that an encouraging number of well-designed research programs on the reduction of risk factors associated with the onset of mental disorders do exist. The task over the next decade will be to enlarge that body of work into a prevention science by instituting rigorous standards for designing, conducting, and analyzing future preventive intervention research programs. By adhering to such standards, prevention can achieve the credibility and validity necessary for its interventions to reduce the incidence of mental disorders.

Only rigorous standards can lead to an enrichment or expansion of the knowledge base essential for prevention efforts. Outcomes from trials built on such standards can serve to refine hypotheses and concepts related to risk and protective factors. The model building and hypothesis testing inherent in prevention research can elucidate pathways taken by individuals as they move toward or away from the onset of a mental disorder, as well as intervening mechanisms and brain-behavior-environment interactions that result in mental disorders or avert their occurrence, even in individuals at very high risk. In addition,

Commissioned papers for this chapter were prepared by H. Kraemer and K. Kraemer and by S. Fawcett and colleagues and are available as indicated in Appendix D.

empirical validation of preventive interventions can usefully inform and broaden clinical practice. Epidemiological evidence, for example, can suggest causal factors that can best be tested in a preventive intervention research trial, which may, in turn, suggest molecular or behavioral mechanisms for further study.

THE PREVENTIVE INTERVENTION RESEARCH CYCLE

Just as the development of prevention into a science requires a series of rigorously designed research programs for its collective progress, so an individual research program requires a series of carefully planned and implemented steps for its success. Figure 10.1 presents the committee's concept of how these steps build upon another in the preventive intervention research cycle. The process proceeds in much the same sequence as it has in the report to this point. The first step is to identify and define operationally and reliably the mental disorder(s) or problem. The second step is to consider relevant information from the core biological and behavioral sciences and from research on the treatment of mental disorders, and to review risk and protective factors associated with the onset of the disorder(s) or problem, as well as prior physical and mental disorder prevention intervention research. The investigator then embarks on designing and testing the preventive intervention, by conducting rigorous pilot studies and confirmatory and replication trials (the third step) and extending the initial positive findings in large-scale field trials (the fourth step). If the trials are successful, the researcher facilitates the dissemination and adoption of the program into community service settings (the fifth step). Most of the research programs presented as illustrations in Chapter 7 are at the third step.

Although the review processes that constitute the first and second steps in Figure 10.1 are considered to be part of the preventive intervention research cycle, the original studies in these areas, with the exception of the previous studies on the prevention of mental disorders or problems, are not. For the individual researcher, it is the activities in the third and fourth steps that constitute preventive intervention research per se. Likewise, it is not the community service program and its evaluation but the facilitation by the investigator of the program's widespread dissemination and adoption (the fifth step) that is part of the research cycle. The knowledge exchange processes that operate between the researcher and the community at this step are discussed in more detail in Chapter 11. (In this report, the term *community* refers not just to a community as a whole, but also to an element within a community, such as a school, health care clinic, advocacy group, or neighborhood.)

The final steps in the cycle, represented by the feedback loop, are to review the results of any subsequent epidemiological studies to determine if the prevention program actually resulted in reductions in incidence of the targeted problem or disorder(s) and to respond to community representatives regarding their research interests and suggestions for further work.

Each step in the cycle is outlined below. Sections later in the chapter present a host of issues relevant primarily to the research activities in steps three and four—including methodological issues pertaining to experimental design, sampling, measurement, and statistics and analysis, as well as documentation issues. Cultural, ethical, and economic issues that require attention throughout the cycle are also presented.

In this discussion the terms *preventive intervention program* and *preventive intervention trial* are carefully delineated. The preventive intervention program is the activity or activities that are provided to the target population (e.g., home visitation with mothers and their infants or a substance use resistance training curriculum delivered to school children by their teacher). The preventive intervention trial is the research component designed with experimental protocols to evaluate and validate the success of the intervention program. *Preventive intervention research program* is the inclusive term for the program plus the trials.

Identification of the Problem or Disorder(s) and Review of Information Concerning Its Extent

The first step in the preventive intervention research cycle is to identify the disorder, cluster of disorders, or problem that is to be the target of the intervention. Knowledge regarding the diagnostic criteria and course of the disorder, as well as its incidence and prevalence, can be helpful in determining whether a preventive intervention for a particular disorder is warranted. Problems that are appropriate targets for intervention can include those such as child maltreatment that are serious social problems in their own right but are also risk factors associated with the onset of mental disorders. At this step in the research cycle, the investigator also considers the personal, social, and economic costs associated with the suffering and disability resulting from the problem or disorder.

Further, because prevention research almost always touches the community in some way, even at its earliest stages, a partnership in project planning between the researcher and the community is highly desirable. Questions to ask at this point include: Is the particular problem or disorder a matter of concern within the social unit—

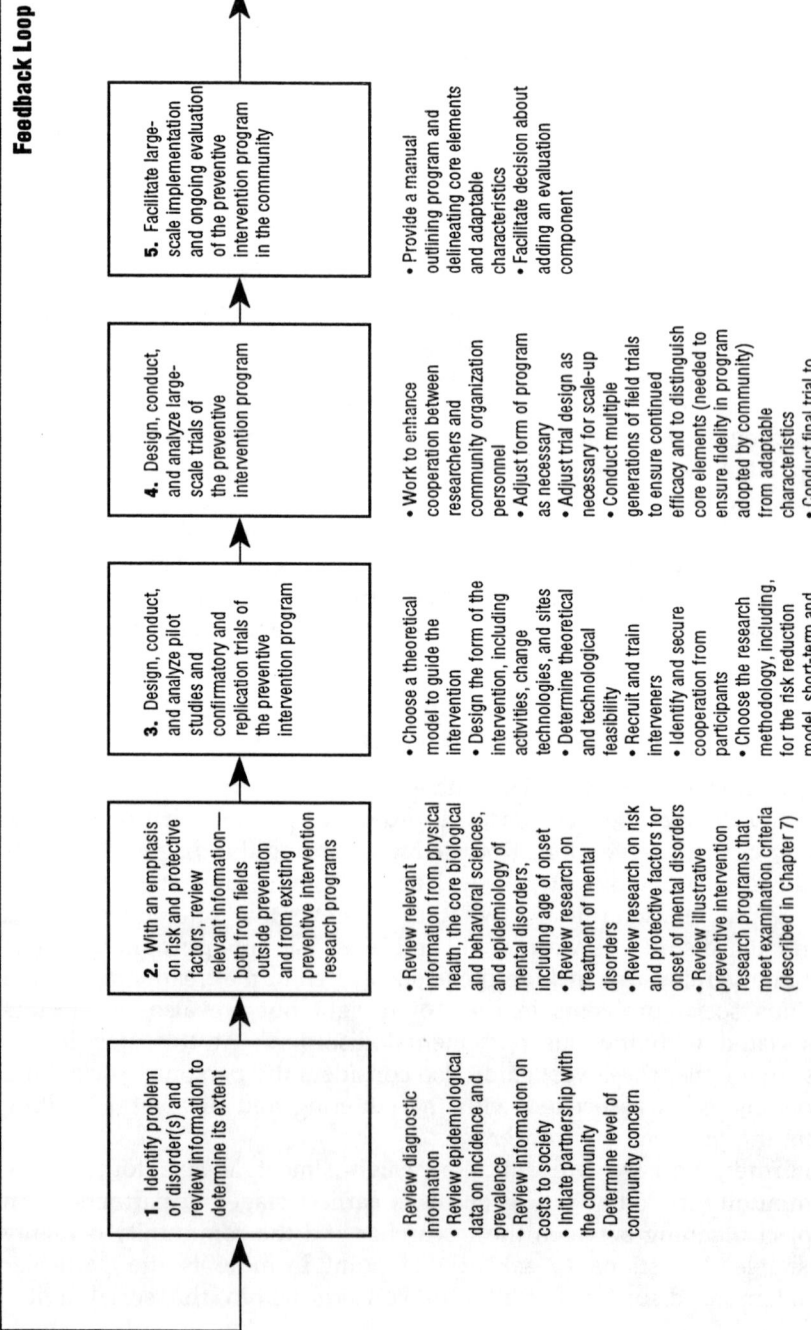

Feedback Loop

1. Identify problem or disorder(s) and review information to determine its extent

- Review diagnostic information
- Review epidemiological data on incidence and prevalence
- Review information on costs to society
- Initiate partnership with the community
- Determine level of community concern

2. With an emphasis on risk and protective factors, review relevant information—both from fields outside prevention and from existing preventive intervention research programs

- Review relevant information from physical health, the core biological and behavioral sciences, and epidemiology of mental disorders, including age of onset
- Review research on treatment of mental disorders
- Review research on risk and protective factors for onset of mental disorders
- Review illustrative preventive intervention research programs that meet examination criteria (described in Chapter 7)

3. Design, conduct, and analyze pilot studies and confirmatory and replication trials of the preventive intervention program

- Choose a theoretical model to guide the intervention
- Design the form of the intervention, including activities, change technologies, and sites
- Determine theoretical and technological feasibility
- Recruit and train interveners
- Identify and secure cooperation from participants
- Choose the research methodology, including, for the risk reduction model, short-term and intermediate outcome measures to determine

4. Design, conduct, and analyze large-scale trials of the preventive intervention program

- Work to enhance cooperation between researchers and community organization personnel
- Adjust form of program as necessary
- Adjust trial design as necessary for scale-up
- Conduct multiple generations of field trials to distinguish efficacy and to distinguish core elements (needed to ensure fidelity in program adopted by community) from adaptable characteristics
- Conduct final trial to determine effectiveness
- Document thoroughly

5. Facilitate large-scale implementation and ongoing evaluation of the preventive intervention program in the community

- Provide a manual outlining program and delineating core elements and adaptable characteristics
- Facilitate decision about adding an evaluation component

malleability of theorized
risk and protective factors
and long-term outcome
measures to determine
effects on incidence of
problem or disorder(s)
• Determine efficacy in
pilot studies and
confirmatory and
replication trials
• Document thoroughly

FIGURE 10.1 The preventive intervention research cycle. Preventive intervention research is represented in boxes three and four. Note that although information from many different fields in health research, represented in the first and second boxes, is necessary to the cycle depicted here, it is the review of this information, rather than the original studies, that is considered to be part of the preventive intervention research cycle. Likewise, for the fifth box, it is the facilitation by the investigator of the shift from research project to community service program with ongoing evaluation, rather than the service program itself, that is part of the preventive intervention research cycle. Although only one feedback loop is represented here, the exchange of knowledge among researchers and between researchers and community practitioners occurs throughout the cycle. The feedback loop demonstrates both the continuity of the cycle and the necessity to incorporate many different types of feedback into each step, including community responses, additions to the knowledge base, and ultimate effects of programs on incidence and prevalence of disorders. Cross-cutting issues regarding methodology, documentation, and cultural, ethical, and economic concerns are treated in the text.

community, school, neighborhood, mental health service agency—where the research would be carried out? Would the community be responsive to the development of a research program to address such concerns? Giving the community a voice in defining the problem and in formulating the research program and procedures can be done in many ways, such as by having a representative from the community, perhaps a delegate from a service agency, participate with the research team on an ongoing basis (Kelly, Dassoff, Levin, Schreckengost, and Altman, 1988; Weiss, 1984; Snowden, Muñoz, and Kelley, 1979; see also the commissioned paper by Fawcett, Paine, Francisco, Richter, and Lewis, and commentaries by Gallimore and Rothman, available as indicated in Appendix D.)

Review of Risk and Protective Factors and Relevant Information from the Knowledge Base

Information regarding the concept of risk reduction and how it can be applied in research programs on the prevention of mental disorders can be obtained from a review of prevention programs in physical health (see Chapter 3). Knowing specifics about the predisposing biopsychosocial risk factors and environmental and personal protective factors that converge and interact to determine the onset of any mental disorder is critical for decisions that are made about the nature and targets of any preventive intervention strategy. To acquire this knowledge, the investigator can access a panoply of research disciplines, including molecular biology; behavioral, population, and molecular genetics; gene-environment interactions; neuroscience; developmental, experimental, and social psychology; sociology; behavior analysis; cognitive science; developmental psychopathology; and population and developmental epidemiology (see Chapters 4 and 5). The investigator next examines what is known regarding the relevant risk and protective factors affecting the onset of the disorder(s) or problem(s) of interest (see Chapter 6). This review provides information that will be useful later in choosing a theoretical model that specifies the mechanism or processes through which these factors have effects. In addition, the review can reveal information on sociodemographic or biological characteristics that may be helpful in targeting a population at risk, as well as identify modifiable risk or protective factors as potential targets for preventive intervention. A review of the relevant publications on prior preventive intervention research programs (see Chapter 7) is another essential step to take before designing the research program. Finally, some of the most important information about protective factors has come from research on the treatment of mental disorders (see Chapter 8). Treatments to strengthen the social support network and social competence of an individual afflicted with a mental disorder, for example, have consistently been shown to improve that person's outcome. This points toward preventive interventions to reinforce these protective factors and thereby diminish the likelihood of stress-induced initial onset of illness.

Pilot Studies and Confirmatory and Replication Trials

Once the pertinent information has been reviewed, the investigator can begin the process of designing, conducting, and analyzing the research program. Initially, a small-scale, rigorously designed pilot study is done in a carefully controlled setting, often within a community institution, to test methods and procedures. A pilot study is exploratory in nature, and many alterations in design are made. Then the investigator applies the methods and procedures that appear to be successful to a larger population in a confirmatory trial to determine the efficacy of the research program, efficacy being "the extent to which a specific intervention, procedure, regimen, or service produces a beneficial result under ideal conditions" (Last, 1988). If a research program proposes to change risk or protective factors and does so, but the targeted factors are not causal, then the program will lack efficacy, failing to prevent the mental disorder even if it succeeds in altering the risk factor. Thus a well-controlled confirmatory trial can provide relevant data to confirm or deny the causal roles of hypothesized risk and protective factors. Finally, if the results from the confirmatory trial are encouraging, the same methods and procedures are applied in a replication trial to ensure continued efficacy. The Prenatal/ Early Infancy Project (Olds, Henderson, Tatelbaum, and Chamberlin, 1988, 1986), discussed in Chapter 7, is an example of a research program that is now being replicated in a new location.

At this third step in the cycle, the investigator faces a number of decisions. The first of these is the choice of a theoretical model to guide the preventive intervention program. With this model in place, the form of the intervention program itself can be designed. The features of the program—including such things as intervention techniques and site— are chosen here, although they may be adjusted somewhat in step four, when the program is applied in a large-scale field trial. Intervention program design issues are distinct from the methodological issues involved in designing the research component of the program, a task that is encountered both in this step and in step four and thus is discussed as a cross-cutting issue later in this chapter. When the design work is done, the processes of recruiting and training interveners and identifying and securing the cooperation of appropriate participants can begin. Then the studies or trials are conducted. Thorough documentation of all these choices and the reasons for them is essential to subsequent analysis, both in this step and in step four. This is discussed as a cross-cutting issue below.

Choosing a Theoretical Model to Guide the Intervention Program

To prevent the targeted disorder or problem, the investigator chooses a theoretical model based on the available body of knowledge that addresses one or more of the following factors:

- The presence of risk factors and absence of sufficient protective factors correlated with the disorder that may be both causal and malleable, that is, can be altered through intervention.
- The mechanisms that link the presence of risk factors and the absence of protective factors to the initial onset of symptoms (which may involve gene-environment interactions).
- The triggers that activate these mechanisms (including stressful life events, physical illness, and developmental changes).
- The processes that mediate the triggering event and the onset of symptoms.
- The processes that occur once symptoms have developed. Ideally, these processes can be attenuated through indicated preventive interventions before they cross the threshold criteria for diagnosis of the disorder.

The choice of a theoretical model stems not only from formulations of risk and protective factors, mechanisms, triggers, and processes, but also from analysis of interventions. Whether a particular theoretical approach can guide prevention strategies depends on the data supporting it. Practically, most current evidence is limited to assessment of risk and protective factors, although there is considerable speculation regarding mechanisms and triggers. Therefore, for now, basing preventive interventions on the risk reduction model, that is, on theories involving the reduction of risk factors and/or enhancement of protective factors, is the most productive strategy. This may ultimately lead to studies on incidence of disorders. No matter which theoretical model is used, the ultimate goal of reducing the incidence of mental disorders is the same.

Designing the Form of the Intervention Program

The intervention program is made up of (1) the activity or activities that are provided to the targeted population, such as an educational curriculum, supportive counseling, and child care, at a planned frequency and for a set amount of time; (2) the psychological, biobehavioral, educational, organizational, or social techniques and procedures—sometimes called *change technologies*—used; and (3) the site in which the intervention takes place.

Theoretical and technological factors are closely intertwined and affect the choice of the intervention activities and change technologies. For example, educational interventions require teaching techniques known to work. Specific teaching techniques may work well with certain groups but not with others. If the instructors are not able to teach the participants the skills that are thought to decrease the probability of the disorder or problem, the theory cannot be tested, nor the intervention implemented. Interventions may thus have to be redesigned for different groups to address how they learn; language, educational level, cultural background, rural versus urban setting, and generational cohort will need to be considered. In addition to learning theory, intervention activities and change technologies may draw heavily on operations research, social psychology, behavioral modification technology, and a variety of other fields. They may include the use of biological-pharmacological, educational, or skills-building programs, environmental change strategies, new social policies, and regulations or laws.

A variety of questions are typically addressed at this stage in the prevention research process, such as: Is this intervention acceptable and feasible for the targeted population? Has consideration been given to ethical concerns, cultural factors, and linguistic differences? Have issues of access been addressed, including potential barriers in the host institution or community and dissemination of information regarding the availability of the intervention? In addition, questions about intervention intensity (that is, the frequency and length of intervener-participant contacts), the feasibility of administering the intervention to a group instead of individuals, and the use of special technologies such as video tapes, computer-aided learning, and specialized medical techniques are addressed at this stage.

Preventive interventions, in general, should be short enough to be practical, yet intensive and long-lasting enough to be effective. Obviously, it is best if they are not too costly, but the more relevant issue is whether the potential benefits justify the cost. With the possible exception of certain structural interventions, such as helping a participant secure a job, brief interventions usually cannot be expected to have long-term effects in preventing major disorders. Attempts to change behavior or instill certain skills and to sustain these changes over time require intensity of effort, not only from investigators, but also from participants.

Finally, it is useful to obtain information regarding how well the program and its component parts have been received. Feedback to the prevention researcher in this stage can come from the participants in the studies and trials as well as from community leaders (Krueger, 1988; Manoff, 1985).

Recruiting and Training Interveners

The choice of the interveners can be crucial to the success of the preventive intervention program. Sometimes the interveners are professionals; often they are not. Frequently, they have a natural relationship with the participant—such as being a teacher, parent, doctor, or neighbor (see Chapter 7). Careful selection, provision of initial training and ongoing supervision, payment of a salary, a reasonable workload, and involvement, as appropriate, with the interdisciplinary research team, help ensure high quality and low attrition of interveners.

Identifying and Securing Cooperation from Appropriate Participants

The researcher next decides for whom the intervention is appropriate. In general, the less expensive and the less likely to have any unintended adverse side effects the intervention is, the more widely it can be implemented (universal). As the intervention becomes more expensive, and as it becomes more potent, it becomes increasingly important for ethical as well as economic reasons to focus its implementation to reach the population most at risk (selective, then indicated). (See Chapter 2 for a discussion of population groups.) However, this is not to say that universal interventions are inexpensive to deliver. An intervention with even a low cost per participant becomes a large expense when delivered to thousands of participants. However, these delivery costs may be more than offset by the savings realized when disorders are prevented, especially if an entire lifetime of disability and expensive treatment can be avoided.

One crucial element in identifying appropriate participants is the current understanding of the nature of the problem or disorder (reviewed in steps one and two of the research cycle), in part because individuals who already have the disorder in question must be excluded from the preventive intervention and individuals who are at especially high risk should be included. For most mental disorders, genetic predispositions have only a probabilistic influence on the manifestation of the illness. The onset of a disorder often depends on the nature of the interaction between genetic predisposition and environment. Therefore, if genes related to mental disorders are eventually identified, individuals with these genes may be particularly appropriate participants in prevention trials for indicated interventions.

Another crucial element is information about who in the population is at risk for the disorder or problem. This information comes not only from risk studies but also from treatment research (reviewed in step two). For example, a high incidence of a particular disorder within a population group identified by age, gender, or culture provides clues about whom to target. Finally, a knowledge of the developmental periods of risk and the ages of onset (from epidemiological studies reviewed in step two) is also valuable for decisions regarding when to intervene.

The investigator next develops a plan to successfully engage the targeted participants. These participants, by definition, do not have a problem that they are necessarily motivated to cure or relieve. There is no way of ascertaining whether any one individual in an at-risk group will develop the disorder if the intervention is not received. Therefore potential participants may not be willing to participate. Influential members of the community can often help by providing access to the targeted group and gaining their cooperation. The investigator can then inform the potential participants not only about any risks involved, but also about how the intervention may be useful to them. Incentives for participation, such as payment for interviews, video tapes of children, printed educational materials, and free transportation, are often presented at this time.

Noncompliance and attrition are major issues in prevention research programs. The intervention potentially can have its largest effects on participants who are receptive to its aims, participate in all intervention sessions, follow through on requests, and continue with the program until it is completed. But participants who do not comply may be those at the highest risk. Efforts to promote compliance are essential to well-designed interventions. One way to sustain participation is to shape the intervention so it is sensitive to the local culture and customs of the targeted group. For example, it is useful to uncover the targeted population's daily routine—including their daily tasks, their values and goals, and their culturally prescribed rules, norms, and scripts—as well as the motives, feelings, and meanings they may associate with the intervention (Gallimore, Goldenberg, and Weisner, in press; O'Donnell and Tharp, 1990). Making participation easy by crafting interventions congruent with these elements, and relevant to people's lives, will increase participation.

Large-Scale Field Trials

Large-scale field trials offer an opportunity to expand preventive intervention programs found to be efficacious in initial confirmatory and replication trials to large-scale field conditions. Here also, the benefits and costs of the intervention can be more realistically assessed. These trials help to assess the generality of the efficacy of the program with different personnel, participants, settings, cultures, and conditions. A large amount of research in the field of social innovation and organizational change has addressed these questions. Such trials may require involvement with community service agencies or organizations of various kinds, including social service agencies, mental health clinics, primary health care clinics, schools, and day care centers—all here referred to for convenience as organizations—and will definitely require the involvement of many more interveners. Therefore the investigator, although still theoretically in charge, can lose some control over the fidelity of the implementation unless considerable attention is paid to the details regarding the delivery of the intervention and the recording of data.

Experience tells us that research in naturalistic settings can be beset with complications and failure (Hiltz, 1974). The changes in personnel at this point are often the crucial element. Poor communication and operational tensions between researchers and the organization's personnel are common (Hood, 1990). These problems can lead to certain unwelcome results: personnel may fail to follow through in filling out forms or keeping records, may slow down the work, may provide false or misleading information, may circumvent established procedures, and may even sabotage or move to terminate the project (Hiltz, 1974). Furthermore, researchers are not ordinarily trained to deal with the interorganizational and interpersonal complexities of large-scale field trials.

Projects involving collaborative work between researchers in universities and institutes, on the one hand, and organizational personnel, on the other, can be brought into focus through the lens of interorganizational theory. Hasenfeld and Furman (in press) have specifically suggested the use of the following principles to facilitate these research relationships:

- the problem and purpose should be manifest for both parties from the start,
- the benefits for each party and the reasons for participating should be clear, and
- the expectations and costs should be explicit.

In addition, a more satisfactory exchange may occur at this step if a community representative was involved earlier. Such a process helps to protect the community interests and engenders commitment for participation in the field trials. Rossi (1977) pointed out, in addition, that results of projects are unpredictable and often equivocal and can result in disappointment or bitterness within the community organization. Organizational personnel typically are skeptical at the beginning, but once work is in progress they may develop high and unrealistic expectations about results, especially when their investment of time and effort is substantial. Taking time initially to jointly establish feasible objectives for both entities can minimize this kind of dissonance.

The researcher can enhance the prospects for a cooperative relationship by selecting a compatible organization whose concerns and activities are conducive to those involved in empirical study (Alkin, 1985). Good matches can be found in organizations that

- are open to innovation,
- have been involved in research before,
- train students,
- use information and research regularly in decision making,
- encourage staff to take courses (providing released time or tuition support), and
- include a number of staff who teach or have taught courses.

Personnel are then given information on research objectives and methods. Training sessions can include orientation meetings, workshops, special seminars, and informal discussions.

Interorganizational collaboration is also a consideration in the selection of the investigator's own staff. Shadish, Cook, and Leviton (1991) have proposed a set of attributes to look for in recruiting such individuals, including the ability to function in complex, uncertain and ambiguous situations, a programmatic leaning, negotiation and communication skills, flexibility, and the ability to respond rapidly to requests.

Additional guidelines to aid in the shaping of productive interorganizational exchange can be derived from the experiences of a team of intervention researchers with extensive experience (Schilling, Schinke, Kirkham, Meltzer, and Norelius, 1988). They advise that researchers

- approach and orient the organization at least six months in advance,
- invite suggestions from the organization on research objectives and procedures,
- gear operations, if possible, to tangibly benefit the organization's program,

- make procedures compatible with organizational processes,
- specify costs to the organization openly and clearly,
- indicate personnel time demands, client risk, and potential liability,
- provide ongoing recognition to personnel for effort and accomplishments,
- provide ongoing feedback through progress reports, and
- help implement intervention products in the organizational setting.

Even for the most carefully designed preventive intervention, a single randomized field trial is not likely to result in an innovation prototype ready for large-scale implementation in the community. Furthermore, critical research questions concerning such issues as the plausibility of causal hypotheses regarding the role of risk or protective factors and the assessment of subsequent rates of disorder may require multiple generations of preventive trials. Both multiple generations and multiple sites may be required to determine the "active ingredients" in the intervention, that is, to distinguish the core elements, which must be included to ensure fidelity when a program is adopted by a community, from the less essential features, or adaptable characteristics (see Chapter 11 for further discussion of this critical issue).

After efficacy has been established in large-scale field trials, a final trial is needed to determine the program's effectiveness (as distinct from its efficacy), that is, "the extent to which a specific intervention, procedure, regimen, or service, *when deployed in the field*, [emphasis added] does what it is intended to do for a defined population" (Last, 1988). For this trial the investigator turns the carefully tuned intervention program over to the organization that hopes to run it, but leaves the research component in place. This stage in the research cycle is frequently not achieved, but the Centers for Disease Control and Prevention is currently planning to test the Infant Health and Development Program (see Chapter 7 and program abstract, available as indicated in Appendix D) for effectiveness in field trials. Convincing documentation of the program's effectiveness (its efficacy already having been established) would be likely to lead to widespread dissemination of the program.

Facilitation of Large-Scale Implementation of the Preventive Intervention Program in the Community

When researchers and community organizations work together at all stages of the program, they can avoid the problem of "manifest" but not "true" adoption of an innovative preventive intervention. Rappaport, Seidman, and Davidson (1979) have shown what can happen when a community "adopts" an intervention program shown by research to be efficacious and effective, but modified by community organizations in a manner that produces unexpected negative consequences for the recipients. This need not happen, but ensuring a positive large-scale implementation effort requires considerable knowledge and attentiveness to the concepts of core elements and adaptable characteristics. At this step, the investigator can provide a manual describing the program to guide implementation. The investigator can also facilitate a decision by the organization to include an ongoing evaluation component in the program. (See Chapter 11 for a description of other ways to facilitate the exchange of knowledge between investigator and community organization.)

METHODOLOGICAL ISSUES

It is essential to delineate explicitly the goals at the outset of designing the research component of a preventive intervention research program. For example, is the goal to reduce an occupational, social, educational, family, or personal risk factor—such as child abuse, marital stress, unemployment, or aggressive behavior? Is it also to enhance protective factors? Is the goal to intervene with mechanisms, triggers, and processes related to the onset of disorder? In addition to these goals, the ultimate goal of preventing or delaying the development of a full-blown mental disorder(s) should be explicitly stated even though at this stage that may not be the goal of the preventive intervention itself.

The goals influence the types of research methodology that will be used, as well as the answers to methodological questions encountered in steps three and four of the preventive intervention research cycle. Questions concerning the structure and duration of the trial and follow-up period, sampling, measurement, and statistics and analysis are considered here, including: What are the characteristics of the population to be used in sampling? How large should the sample be? What are the methods to be used to produce and measure changes in the targeted risk and protective factors in the population? What are the methods to be used to measure changes over time in the incidence of the targeted disorder(s) or problem?

Structure and Duration of the Trial and Follow-up Period

Structure of the Trial

The randomized controlled trial, in which members of a population are randomly allocated into experimental and control groups, usually is the preferred experimental design in research studies, and it provides the most rigorous means for hypothesis testing available in preventive intervention trials as well. Random assignment helps to ensure that the participants' responses are unbiased estimates of what the average responses would have been if all members of the population could have been assigned to one of the two groups. Frequently, when trials are designed, there are conceptual or hypothesis-driven reasons to include more than one intervention for evaluation. Hence a particular prevention trial may have more than one experimental group, and therefore random assignment is made to multiple groups.

Randomized control groups are particularly important in selective and indicated prevention trials, especially if the targeted groups have been chosen carefully enough to ensure that they are at very high risk. In such trials the interventions are working against the probabilities associated with the "natural" course of the pathological process. If this course is increasingly negative, the results of the intervention can appear to be an increase in problems that did not exist before the intervention. On the other hand, some problems are self-limiting, and positive results may be due to the passage of time rather than the intervention. A finding of lower incidence of disorder in the experimental group as compared to higher incidence in the control group is the best way of documenting the effect of a preventive intervention.

Although randomized controlled trials remain the optimal design for preventive intervention trials, quasi-experimental time series designs can sometimes permit investigators to capitalize on policy or regulatory changes and conduct natural experiments in the real world, as, for example, with the Intervention Campaign Against Bully-Victim Problems (Olweus, 1991) reviewed in Chapter 7. Campbell (1991) has described a number of policy-oriented interventions that can be analyzed by using interrupted time series and regression, discontinuity analyses.

The logic of the interrupted time series analysis is relatively straightforward. The independent variable, in this case the preventive intervention, is expected to produce a change in the group under observation. The intervention "interrupts" a series of baseline observations at a specified point. If the intervention does indeed have an effect, the time series preceding it should differ from the time series subsequent to it. In a treatment study, for example, Liberman and Eckman (1981) used an interrupted time series design to assess the impact of two brief inpatient interventions on suicide ideation and attempts. Both treatments markedly reduced suicide attempts when two years following intervention were compared with two years prior to hospitalization. Such simple quasi-experimental time series designs cannot rule out alternative explanations for a change in the variable of interest. Thus it is more desirable to use controlled, experimental forms of time series, such as multiple baseline, multiple schedule, reversal, withdrawal, and multi-element designs (Barlow and Hersen, 1973) or to combine time series with nonequivalent control group designs, as Cook and Campbell (1979) suggest.

Obviously, one cannot have as much confidence in the results of quasi-experimental designs as true experiments. Therefore quasi-experimental designs should be used only when it is not possible to randomize. An important problem with nonequivalent control group designs is that researchers simply may not be able to create control groups that are similar enough to the experimental group.

Several other problems severely restrict the conclusions that can be drawn equally from both true experiments and quasi-experiments. Consider, for example, instances in which, despite efforts by the research team, participants in a control group know that they are not receiving the desired intervention. The control group, as an "underdog," may be motivated to reduce or reverse the expected effect of the intervention (Cook and Campbell, 1979), the so-called "John Henry effect." On the other hand, members of a control group may be demoralized in knowing that they are not receiving the desired intervention, and there may be a decrement in their performance. Because control groups are often intact groups that may interact with one another, such as students in a particular classroom or residents of a particular block or neighborhood, their proximity increases the likelihood that they will act in concert or develop similar perceptions of the experiment.

Duration of the Trial and Follow-up

The length of the intervention as described above—short enough to be practical and yet long enough to be effective—governs the length of the preventive intervention trial as well. In addition, because a decrease in the incidence of a disorder is the major long-term goal, participants should be followed longitudinally in prospective designs. Therefore follow-up periods can be quite lengthy, but this is a complex issue. The longer the duration of follow-up, the greater the power—that is, the statistical capacity to be able to demonstrate a significant result—may be to detect the efficacy of the program in showing short-term as well as long-term positive effects. This is not, however, necessarily so. If multiple factors are involved in the onset of a disorder, lengthy follow-up provides more opportunity for uncontrolled factors to influence outcome.

Long time frames also may be necessary in order to get beyond the age of risk of onset. Preventive intervention trials cannot prove that a particular disorder has been permanently prevented; they can only provide evidence that the onset of the disorder has been delayed for as long as the trial proceeds. A participant still free of the targeted disorder at the end of the trial's follow-up period may have the onset of the disorder one day later, unless the trial has followed the participant completely through the age at risk. For many mental disorders, however, risk of onset continues through the life span.

The longer the trial and follow-up, however, the greater the cost and difficulty, and the longer the delay in obtaining answers to the research questions. Consideration of cost, of course, plays a crucial part in the setting of the follow-up time. Funding sources are understandably reluctant to fund research programs that will take 10 to 20 years to produce results. But the current practice of short-term support is especially limiting in regard to research on prevention of mental disorders.

Lengthy follow-up periods that delay the reporting of results have disadvantages in terms of scientific practice as well. As time goes on, the importance attached to certain research questions changes. Also changing are the methods of measurement, diagnostic criteria, and other issues that must be taken into consideration. Therefore a balance must be found between the gain in power and precision resulting from long-term follow-up and the loss in relevance and quality of content or substance that may be incurred. This also suggests that data should be kept on symptoms and behaviors because the definition of disorders is subject to change.

The practical limitations placed on the duration of a preventive intervention trial and follow-up in part can be dealt with by timing the implementation carefully. Selecting participants who are moving into their period of highest risk for the onset of the disorder, a period of critical developmental challenge and maturation, or a period of high responsiveness to protective effects, permits detection of effects that are sufficiently large and immediate.

Sampling

The choice of the sample from the targeted population has methodological repercussions. The major problem in using selective and indicated preventive interventions is the identification of the high-risk group. Obviously, it is critical that the definition of high risk be a valid one. The sensitivity and specificity of screening tests are used in the determination of risk status. Sensitivity is the proportion of truly diseased persons in the screened populations who are identified as diseased by the screening test. Specificity is the proportion of truly nondiseased persons who are so identified by the screening test. Sensitivity and specificity of identification criteria tend to "see-saw"; that is, the cost of having high specificity is usually low sensitivity. It is possible to develop criteria with high sensitivity, but the result will be a far looser definition of what constitutes high risk.

It is useful to obtain samples that span the full range of gender and culture among individuals at risk. Since passage of the National Institutes of Health Revitalization Act of 1993, such representative samples are legally required. A trial of a preventive intervention that excludes women produces results that do not necessarily generalize to women; one that excludes minorities may yield results that do not necessarily generalize to minorities. The principle is clear: If one excludes any group from a trial, the results of that trial cannot be assumed to generalize to that group. For this reason, in implementing indicated interventions in which there are stringent inclusion and exclusion criteria, the effects of these restrictions on the generalizability of the results of the trial to the population at large must be carefully considered. In locations that include large segments of non-English-speaking individuals, studies must include assessment and interventions in the appropriate language (Muñoz and Ying, 1993; Maccoby and Alexander, 1979).

The use of a universal population presents methodological problems of a different sort. Such a population is typically diverse and may include participants who are not receptive to the program for a variety of reasons. The heterogeneity, combined with the low incidence rates of the disorder likely in such a population, creates a situation in which very large sample sizes are necessary to detect any indication of efficacy or effectiveness. Because the effects may seem quite small, the clinical or policy significance of the prevention program may be underestimated. Uniform implementation of both intervention and measurement protocols in universal interventions across entire communities may be difficult. Such problems reduce statistical power, either by increasing the heterogeneity of response or decreasing the reliability of the response measures.

For a trial using a universal population, the investigator can plan secondary analyses to focus on those subgroups likely to be most at risk and most receptive to the intervention, in order to generate results comparable to those that would be obtained with the selective or indicated populations. Thus the investigator can have both generalizability of results and the possibility of specific a priori subgroup analyses of special interest. The costs and difficulties of such studies are, however, often substantial.

Another method for analyzing subgroups is stratification, that is, the separation of a sample into several subsamples, sometimes along a continuum, according to specified criteria such as age or level of education. Stratification can be useful when factors measurable at baseline, that is, at the beginning of the intervention, are believed to correlate strongly with onset of the disorder or problem. In such a situation, greater power can be achieved when samples are stratified before randomization (thus creating subsamples) and participants from the subsamples are randomized to the intervention and control groups.

If there are certain subgroups of the population of special interest, naturalistic sampling will likely yield too small a sample size to draw definitive conclusions that can be generalized to each subgroup separately. To answer questions about subgroups adequately, the investigator should ensure that there is adequate power through oversampling of these groups. Alternatively, it is often desirable to design a separate trial for each subgroup with a sample size adequate to answer the questions.

Measurement

Although the processes of focusing attention on the questions that require answers, selecting the appropriate measures (and thus excluding the rest), deciding when and how often to measure, choosing the best measurement techniques or instruments, and taking steps to ensure the reliability and validity of the selected measures are perhaps the most tedious and difficult parts of a trial, these are also among the most essential procedures in determining its success or failure.

What to Measure

Careful selection of primary outcome measures is essential to the success of a preventive intervention trial. These are usually the measures of changes in the theorized mediating variables, including risk and protective factors, that are assumed to be responsible for the reduction in risk. They may be psychological outcomes such as measures of precursor signs or symptoms, social outcomes such as reduction of poverty, or biological outcomes such as reduction of the incidence of low birthweight. Finally, in the prevention of mental disorders, it is particularly desirable for programs explicitly to include measures of the incidence of mental disorders. One benefit of including incidence measures is that they may reveal that a risk factor that was found to be malleable was not causal, thus contributing to the knowledge base about etiology.

Evidence of risk reduction is used as the primary outcome measure, that is, the measure used most often to document the results of the trial, in part because it is available first. For example, in the Perry Preschool Program, a selective preventive intervention with preschoolers that was intended to increase their intellectual and social development (see Chapter 7), the long-term results, including measures of such factors as how long the children stayed in school, took many years to be documented. However, short-term measures of behavioral problems, such as lower rates of aggression, lying, and stealing, served as early evidence of the success of the intervention. Documentation of the changes in risk and protective factors for the child could have been extended for a more complete picture of mediating variables. Although disorder incidence measures were not included in the Perry Preschool Program, it is one of the few research programs to have included long-term outcome measures of any sort.

Measures of process are also appropriate. Because prevention programs typically have many components, it can be difficult to determine which one accounts for the success of the intervention. However, it may be possible to examine, on a more exploratory level, the impact of the different components by gathering data that are descriptors of process. Measures of process are selected to reflect certain characteristics of the participants, program, activities, change technologies, and so on, and of the interaction of these, that might help to generate hypotheses as to why and how the program might work. For example, what is it that the intervener actually said and did during home visits, or how do teachers respond to participants' aggressive outbursts at school? This set of measures can include consideration of risks, costs, inconvenience, and dosage effects. Measures that reflect different theoretical models can be chosen to elucidate most salient elements of the intervention.

Measures of compliance are another type of process measure. Participants at the outset of a preventive intervention trial may simply refuse to participate. If they agree to participate, they may not comply, in whole or in part, with the procedures and activities of the prevention program. It is useful to document the extent of compliance of individual participants throughout the trial. If the program does not prove to be efficacious, it is important to gain insights as to why participants did not comply, as a basis for consideration in the design of future prevention efforts.

A primary goal of a trial is efficacy, but process measures may provide information that can be useful in improving the design of a subsequent prevention effort. Furthermore, such data provide documentation of the fidelity of the program, that is, the extent to which the components of the program as designed were actually delivered and received by the participants.

When and How Often to Measure

Random assignment does not yield groups that are identical on all baseline variables. Therefore an extensive collection of baseline information, including targeting variables, is necessary. Without this, the investigator's ability to draw firm conclusions about what would have happened in the experimental group in the absence of the intervention is compromised. The baseline information is also needed to determine eligibility for the program, to ensure that the elements in the prevention program are not already in place in the participants' environment before the experiment, to describe the population to which the results might be expected to generalize, to document the success of the randomization procedures, and, in secondary analysis, to detect those subgroups for which there is differential outcome. If there are dropouts or missing data, baseline information is also necessary to investigate the possibilities of resulting sampling bias. Figure 10.2 shows the points on the time line for the trial and follow-up at which the baseline and other measures are taken.

After the baseline assessment, the greater the frequency of observation, the more precise the measurement of onset and course. Outcome measures on each participant should be taken frequently enough to determine the timing of short-term effects. Long-term outcome measures taken at follow-up to determine incidence should be continued past the mean age of onset for the disorder. Frequent follow-up can bind the participants more closely to the program and promote receptivity and compliance. However, too great a frequency of observation (particularly when the assessments are difficult, long, tiresome, stressful, or invasive) may annoy the participants and produce the opposite effect. The quality of information (validity and reliability) may suffer; dropouts may increase. Clearly, some balance must be achieved.

Which Measuring Techniques and Instruments to Use

The selection of outcome measures for use at baseline, over the short term, and during follow-up includes consideration of the relative value

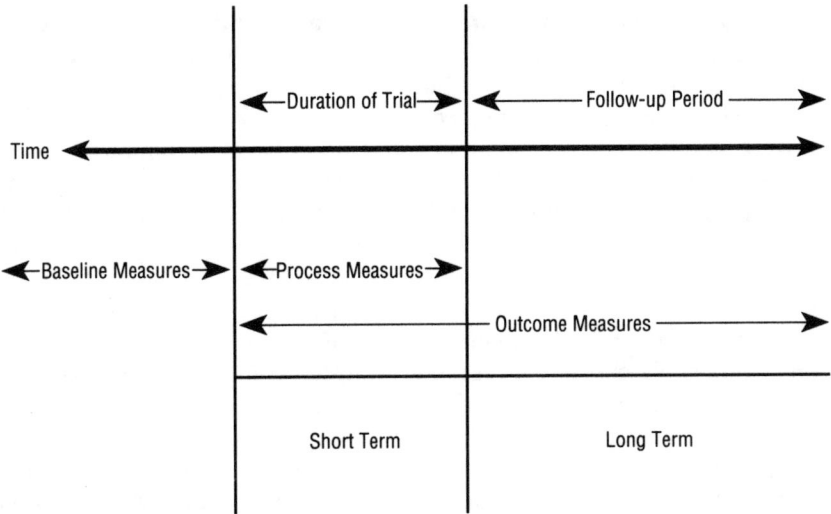

FIGURE 10.2 Measurement points along the time line for the intervention trial and follow-up period. The total length of time varies according to disorder targeted (to get past mean age of onset) and how closely the program is tied to age of highest risk.

and use of continuous (that is, a scaled or dimensional response) measures and the more usual categorical (that is, a number of nonhierarchial responses) measures. Almost always, a variable can be measured with either technique, but the yield is different. When they are appropriate, continuous measures can increase statistical power, but the crucial issue in deciding on the outcome measures in a trial of a prevention program is that of selecting the most valid and reliable measures available.

The most likely strategy to detect effects and to be cost-effective includes both categorical and continuous measures. For example, the intervention may produce a modest reduction in the incidence of new cases that meet the designated diagnostic criteria for a particular disorder or in the existence of specific risk factors (categorical measures), but may produce a very great reduction or attenuation in the severity and duration of risk factors, including precursor symptoms (continuous measures). Also, even if the intervention failed to prevent the onset of a disorder, it might reduce the severity, duration, or disability of the disorder (continuous measures). An example from infectious disease may illuminate this point. If an antibiotic taken prophylactically to prevent traveler's diarrhea produced only a modest reduction in the frequency or incidence of a threshold for diagnosing the enteritis (e.g., presence of bacteria in stool with at least one episode of diarrhea with or without abdominal discomfort), but produced a very large reduction in the severity of the diarrhea (i.e., reduced frequency and amount of loose stools as well as reduced frequency and severity of abdominal discomfort), then the verdict of that prevention trial might be that the antibiotic was indeed useful in prophylaxis. A similar argument could be made for the effectiveness of fluoridated water in preventing the number and severity of caries; the effectiveness of a cognitive behavior therapy preventive intervention on the depth, duration, and disability of major depressions; and the effectiveness of family- and school-based educational and skills training programs with children at risk for conduct disorder on the incidence and severity of subsequent delinquency, substance abuse, and antisocial behavior.

Whether the chosen measures are categorical or continuous, they should display high internal consistency and construct validity based on earlier psychometric analyses and research as well as high reliability with different assessors. With the advent of the DSM-III and DSM-III-R, certain comprehensive diagnostic instruments that can elicit all the signs and symptoms of mental disorders have come into general use and provide a means for improving the reliability and replicability of diagnosis. Diagnostic interviews such as the Diagnostic Interview Schedule (DIS), the Present State Examination, the Schedules for Clinical Assessment in Neuropsychiatry (SCAN), and the Structured Clinical Interview for DSM-III-R (SCID) (all of which can provide continuous and categorical measures) can improve the detection of symptoms. They also lead to operational criteria for improving the accuracy of rating the presence or absence of symptoms or disorders. When diagnosticians are trained in the use of these structured instruments, they become more consistent, systematic, and precise—thereby enhancing the reliability, validity, and power of the preventive intervention trial. In addition, the work groups responsible for producing DSM-IV and ICD-10 have purposely interacted in their development of diagnostic criteria, and these classification systems are coming closer together.

How Many Measures and Instruments to Use

Measures should be carefully chosen and relatively independent. Every variable measured yields both signal and noise. Multiple noisy measures (unreliable measures) of the same signal used separately add no signal to the system, only noise. The signal is merely repeated along with the noise. For this reason, in any set of highly correlated measures, the investigator should either select the best and delete the rest or combine them into one measure. This strategy not only reduces the number of analyses, thus diminishing the risk of false positive results, but also diminishes the risk of false negative results, because combining multiple measures of the same signal frequently results in "tuning out" much of the noise and thus "tuning in" the signal, resulting in a combined measure that is more reliable.

Having many measurements and diagnostic assessments may compromise the quality control of the measurements. When there are only a few crucial measurements on which the success of a trial depends, the investigator can spend a great deal of time and effort to select the best instruments, provide adequate training and orientation to the assessors, and institute adequate quality control procedures. But if hundreds of variables are collected, expedient measures of limited validity become a temptation, and the consistency and care in assessing each variable may be compromised. The fatigue of both participants and assessors can further impair the quality of measurements. What is sometimes called a "rich" data set that contains a large number of variables may, on closer inspection, be rich only in noise, not in signal.

Very large data sets require more staff effort to maintain and analyze. A large number of variables will not be helpful if key variables that will reflect the hypotheses are inadequately measured. Investment in quality control of key variables that includes error checking, detection, and correction procedures is critical to achieve a valid result.

How to Ensure Reliability and Validity of Measures

Reliability "refers to the degree to which the results obtained by a measurement procedure can be replicated," and *validity* "is an expression of the degree to which a measurement measures what it purports to measure" (Last, 1988). Seldom do diagnostic procedures in any area of medicine have a reliability coefficient above 80 percent. Many diagnostic procedures in common use have reliability coefficients between 40 and 60 percent. The issue of reliability of diagnosis in psychiatry has certainly received far more attention than has reliability of diagnosis in most other fields of medicine. But the principle remains: unreliability tends to attenuate power, necessitating larger sample sizes (Kraemer, 1979); therefore, it is especially important to develop reliable methods.

A common error made in addressing the issue of validity is to collect many poor measurements in the hope that these will somehow make up for the absence of one highly valid measure. But multiple poor measurements that do not accurately assess the construct of interest can lead to false positive or false negative results. To add to the confusion, multiple outcome measures can produce contradictory findings, making it impossible to draw any conclusions at all. In addition, lack of sensitivity to cultural variations in meaning can confound the validity of measurement; for example, among the Navajo the concept of "home" includes the extended family, whereas in the mainstream culture it is restricted to the nuclear family. If a measure includes only nuclear family members, it will miss an essential part of Navajo life and therefore be less valid.

To ensure validity, outcome measures ideally should be assessed "blind" to the group to which the participants have been assigned. Measurement and assessment procedures that include any subjective component may be affected by the assessor's knowledge of group membership. Thus a certain response pattern, when observed in a participant known to be in the experimental group, may be assessed differently from the same response pattern observed in a participant known to be in the control group. This phenomenon introduces measurement bias and compromises the validity of the results. A quality control check on raters' blindness can be done by administering a questionnaire to raters at several times during the prevention trial, asking them to make guesses about the assignment of the participants.

As is the case in many randomized controlled trials, however, it is simply not possible to blind all assessors to the group membership of the participants. When the measure is based on self-report, it is often not possible to blind the participants to their own group membership. This situation places a premium on measures that are objective. It also makes the implementation of training and orientation procedures for assessors, and quality control procedures such as periodic reliability testing of the assessors over the course of the study, more vital to the validity of trials of prevention strategies than might otherwise pertain.

Adherence to the measurement protocols of the research program, for both experimental and control groups, adds to validity and reliability. Requirements for such adherence to protocol are often viewed as a rigidity that runs counter to good clinical care, and maintaining these protocols is difficult over the course of a long-term study. Such requirements are often seen as a challenge to the morale and commitment of the researchers, particularly to those who are also clinicians. Special efforts must be made both to inform all research colleagues of the necessity for such adherence and the consequences of deviations from protocol in terms of the validity and power of the results, and to ensure the enthusiastic participation and commitment of all participants to the goals of the study.

Statistics and Analysis

Strategies for Data Analysis

Randomized controlled trials in which participants are followed longitudinally inevitably entail collection of a great deal of data, no matter how parsimonious the investigator has been in choosing and pruning the type and frequency of measures and instruments. Many statistical methods for analyzing these data exist. For categorical data, the most familiar of these methods are logistic regression, log-linear modeling, and discriminant analysis.

For continuous measures, methods for the analysis of repeated measures are required. Considerable interest has been generated recently by the use of random effects regression models as alternatives to repeated measures analysis of variance and covariance or MANOVA designs (Gibbons, Hedeker, Elkin, Waternaux, Kraemer, Greenhouse et al., in press; Laird and Ware, 1982). In this methodology a separate curve is fit to each participant's response data, using a few clinically interpretable parameters to define the mathematical model for the curve. Unlike the more familiar repeated measures analysis of variance designs, these methods are relatively tolerant of missing data, irregular follow-up, and dropout. Moreover, because these approaches use scaled response data, they can be more powerful than approaches using binary indicators of disorder applied in the same context.

Latent structural equation modeling is a statistical tool for examining the relationships among multiple variables. This statistical methodology is available to clinical researchers as part of major software statistical packages. It permits simultaneous testing of complex multivariate hypotheses and may have considerable promise as a tool for exploratory data analysis. However, its utility in formal statistical hypothesis testing is less clear, because the validity of the statistical tests depends on the correctness of strong assumptions about multivariate distributions and on the existence of a clear theoretical model (i.e., Fergusson, Harwood, and Lloyd, 1991).

As more data regarding age of onset are gathered, the preferred analytic strategy for comparing incidence rates across groups is likely to be survival analysis. Survival analysis is a flexible and powerful statistical method for analyzing incidence of illness when time to onset is known. Like the more familiar contingency table methods based on counts of numbers of participants who have onset of the disorder during some follow-up interval, survival analysis can be used to compare the risk of becoming ill in two or more groups. Indeed, because survival analysis depicts incidence across the whole follow-up period, it provides a more detailed picture of outcome. Both parametric and nonparametric approaches are widely available, the former being more powerful when the distributional assumptions are valid, and the latter being less restrictive and more familiar. Survival analysis is typically more powerful than simple counts of incidence during a specified period, particularly when base rates are low. The methodology adjusts for participants who are lost to follow-up. As with regression analysis, covariates can be analyzed, including both main effects and interactions.

The probability of a participant's surviving through a period of risk without developing a disorder may change as the duration of the intervention and follow-up increases. This changing probability is called the survival function. For example, the longer a participant proceeds through the period of risk for a disorder, the lower the probability for developing the disorder. Statistical methods of survival analysis are being used in treatment trials and epidemiological studies of onset and natural history (Elandt-Johnson and Johnson, 1980).

Typically, there are individual differences in the susceptibility among participants in any group—based on risk and protective factors—and these differences are reflected in different survival function shapes. Some participants may be essentially immune to the disorder, and, at the other extreme, some may already be experiencing the precursor signs or symptoms of the disorder at the initiation of the trial. Survival function curves begin at 100 percent and either decrease or plateau as participants succumb to the disorder. Thus it is possible to identify individual differences among participants, as well as to detect differences in effects of the experimental and control conditions.

Groups of participants with high survival curves (i.e., close to the 100 percent level of survival) are "low risk," and those with low survival curves are "high risk," but these are relative terms, with no precise definition. Participants selected from the general population are likely to be "low risk," and participants selected because they have risk factors such as a family history of the disorder are likely to be "high risk" in terms of *lifetime* risk. In the real world, an individual participant's survival curve is a hypothetical construct that cannot actually be seen. However, the *average* survival curve for any group of participants can be estimated and provides information about delay of onset in that group. For example, Figure 10.3 presents three survival curves using new data from the Five Cities Program of Cardiovascular Risk Prevention (see Chapter 3 and the commissioned paper by Kraemer and Kraemer, available as indicated in Appendix D). These survival curves demonstrate the reported onset of smoking in three male birth cohorts: A: (1901

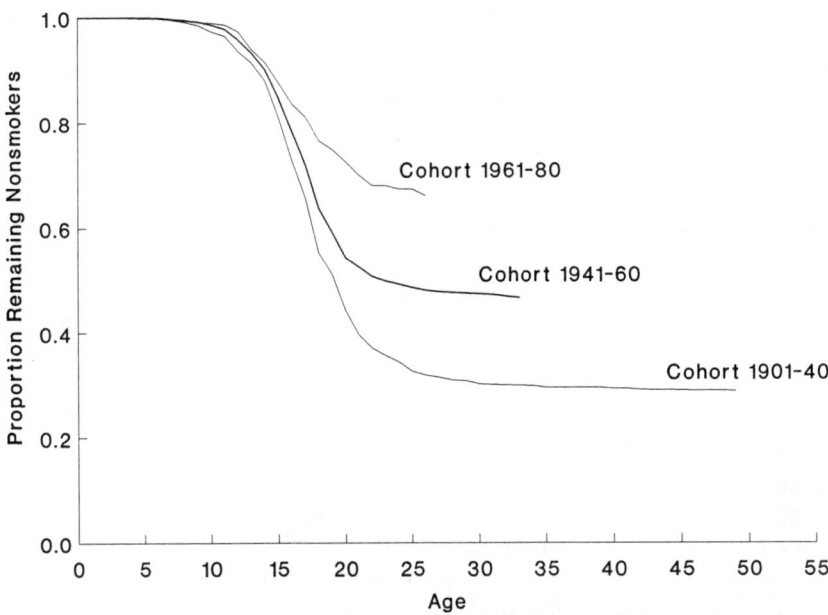

FIGURE 10.3 Survival function estimates. Using data from the Five Cities Program of Cardiovascular Risk Prevention, three survival curves demonstrate the stages in the distribution of onset of smoking in three male birth cohorts: A: (1901 to 1940); B: (1941 to 1960); and C: (1961 to 1980).

to 1940); B: (1941 to 1960); and C: (1961 to 1980). The last cohort was born after the publicity and widespread education following the Surgeon General's recommendation against smoking for health reasons. The change in the distribution of onset of smoking is clear. The onset of smoking came later, particularly in cohort C, and the lifetime prevalence (indicated by the plateau value) of smoking decreased in the later cohorts, leaving more nonsmoking "survivors" and a higher plateau value.

For a given group, the point in time at which its curve reaches the 50 percent point is the median survival time or median onset time. Thus the median age of onset of smoking for cohort A was about 20 years, and for cohort B, about 22 years. For cohort C, the median time is not less than 25 years (at which point 65 percent have survived without smoking), and there may be no median age of onset overall, for fewer than 50 percent may have the onset of smoking during their lifetime.

An interesting aspect of survival analysis is the hazard function, which is the probability of becoming ill at each point in time. Analyses of changes in risk over time may be particularly sensitive indicators of a program's efficacy and effectiveness. The hope is that the intervention program might begin to exert an effect at its inception and gradually build to its full effect as it is fully implemented with desired impacts on the participants' risk and protective factors. The hazard function curve quantifies the probability per unit time that a participant who has survived up to a particular time will have the onset of the disorder in the very short ensuing time interval.

By restricting consideration to those who have survived up to a particular point in time, the investigator can control for factors before that point that have already exerted their effects. By restricting the consideration of the hazard function curve to a short time period, factors that exert their influence on onset of disorder during that time interval only can be identified. Whereas the survival function curve must be either constant or decreasing downward from its initial 100 percent level, the hazard function curve can take any shape at all. It may be flat, it may increase as it does for disorders associated with aging, or it may decrease as it does for disorders primarily associated with infancy. Depending on the natural history and risk periods for the disorder, hazard curves may grow, recede, or have one or several peaks.

Whereas survival and hazard functions can illuminate the changes in incidence of mental disorders among participants in a prevention program, impacts of the program on the severity of the disorders that do develop among participants for whom the prevention program failed, such as the degree of impairment or disability, relapse pattern, or duration of episodes, require the use of prevalence assessments to highlight the differences between the experimental and control groups.

Currently, however, it may not be practical or feasible to obtain valid measures of time to onset for survival analysis. For an insidiously developing disorder, such as schizophrenia, the time to onset may be difficult to ascertain and, at least from the point of view of analyzing a prevention research program, relatively unimportant. If survival methods cannot be used, random effects regression models permit the best use of incomplete follow-up data for participants and help avoid some of the problems of sample bias associated with low retention rates during a trial. However, such problems do not disappear; every missing data point or dropout from the study costs some degree of power.

The Unit of Analysis and Statistical Power Consideration

When interventions are delivered to groups rather than to individuals, the appropriate unit of analysis is the group. Because there are typically far fewer groups than there are individual participants, use of the group as the unit of analysis may appear to result in a major sacrifice in power. However, power is not totally determined by the degrees of freedom, that is, the number of independent comparisons that can be made between the members of a sample. Power is more strongly affected by the size of the effect. Therefore groups can be used as the unit of analysis, and "two-stage" statistical models can be used for that purpose (Gibbons et al., in press).

The number of individuals or groups necessary to detect clinically significant effects with sufficient power is dependent on the design of the trial. The number may vary from two cities per group to tens of thousands of individuals, so choices made in sampling (such as whether entire communities or individuals are being studied), as well as choices made in measurement (such as whether categorical or continuous measures are used), can have an effect on the power achieved.

Power calculations should precede the initiation of a preventive intervention trial to determine the requisite sample size (Muñoz, 1993). For example, for a universal preventive intervention trial targeting the general population with a short follow-up period to measure the onset of a disorder that has a low baseline frequency and unreliable diagnosis, having one million participants may not yield adequate power to detect statistically significant effects. On the other hand, for a trial of a potent selective preventive intervention sampling a relatively high risk population and using frequent, repeated measurements that are valid and reliable, with a long follow-up period and good retention of subjects, a sample size of 50 per group might be adequate. It is important to keep in mind that false positives will always be more frequent with small samples than with large ones. The issue, then, is not only how many participants to use, but also how to design the trial to get the greatest power within the limits of the trial's feasibility. Once issues of feasibility and likelihood of effects being found are determined, standard power calculations (Cohen, 1988) can be used to determine the number of participants that are needed.

DOCUMENTATION ISSUES

For the committee's examination of preventive intervention research programs, it compiled a list of criteria, which appear in Chapter 7, to be used in identifying research programs of particular merit. In documenting research programs in the future, the investigator may find these guidelines useful. But an even higher standard will be desirable in the next decade of preventive intervention research. For example, efforts will need to be made to assess costs and benefits in a realistic way (see the section on economic issues below).

When the research program has been completed, the design, sampling, measurement, and analytic decisions should be specified in the peer-reviewed literature and manuals in sufficient detail that they can be replicated by others. The background and rationale are also relevant. When the results have been analyzed, the statistical methods used should be reported in such a way that the proper inferences can be made about the effectiveness of the prevention program. Descriptive statistics can be used to describe the groups at baseline and to demonstrate the randomization of the groups. If the sample was stratified, descriptive data can be presented for each stratum.

Some details should be presented about how many participants were recruited, how many screened, how many passed and failed that screening (and why), how many consented (and why refusals occurred), how many of those who consented were actually randomized (and why some were omitted), and, of those randomized, how many entered their assigned groups (and why others did not). Of those who entered the randomized groups, how many completed the follow-up (and why did others not)? Of those who dropped out of the experimental and control groups, how long did they last in the protocol? What baseline factors were associated with dropout, and were they the same in the experimental as in the control group? How many of those in the experimental and control groups complied with the protocol (and why did others not)? In short, any information on the sample pertinent to sampling bias, measurement bias, or any other type of bias should be presented so that readers can judge how convincing the results are. A flowchart format can sometimes present these data clearly and efficiently.

There should be brief descriptions of the protocols for recruitment, retention, experimental and control delivery, and of measurement. Documentation of the quality of measurement (reliability or validity) is always valuable in aiding judgments of the results.

The estimated survival curves or hazard curves (or both), in addition to simple summary statements of statistical significance, are valuable in assessing the size and hence the clinical or policy importance of statistically significant results. They are also essential in assessing whether nonsignificant results are the result of low power and thus worth further pursuit or the result of ineffective preventive intervention and thus not worth further consideration. If the secondary results prove informative, these might be documented with separate survival or hazard curves for subgroups found substantially different in response or for subgroups substantially different in terms of process (such as compliant versus noncompliant subjects).

ISSUES OF CULTURE, ETHNICITY, AND RACE

As discussed earlier in this chapter, the success of preventive interventions—whether at the level of the individual, family, community, or nation—depends heavily on the contexts in which they are delivered. Clearly, anticipating the social and cultural elements of these contexts and accounting for such elements in terms of content, format, staffing, and implementation are critical to subsequent outcomes. Given the cultural diversity that characterizes this country, no discussion of the current and future status of preventive intervention research is complete without systematic attention to culture, ethnicity, and race (Muñoz, Chan, and Armas, 1986).*

Throughout the preventive intervention research cycle, investigators must be sensitive to the attitudes, values, beliefs, and practices of the cultural groups with whom they are working, as matters of good science and therapeutic leverage, as well as professional ethics (Kavanagh and Kennedy, 1992; Locke, 1992; Vega, 1992; Galanti, 1991). However, they must strive for more, namely, a set of skills and a perspective that have become commonly known as *cultural competence* (Isaacs and Benjamin, 1991; Cross, Bazron, Dennis, and Isaacs, 1989; Lefley, 1982).

Sensitivity and competence can be conceptualized as existing along a continuum (Orlandi, 1992). Cultural sensitivity is the awareness of a body of important information relevant to the population(s) of interest, which should inform the entire research process, from defining the sampling frame, through negotiating access, to actual intervention and dissemination of results. Such sensitivity can be, and typically is, learned through formal, didactic means and by familiarity with the rapidly growing literatures. It is a necessary but insufficient condition for cultural competence.

Competence is achieved through personal experience, either closely supervised practice or actual immersion in the field, which leads to the

---

*This section is based, in part, on discussions at a one-day meeting, convened by the Institute of Medicine, that focused on preventive intervention research issues related to special populations. (See Appendix C for participants at this meeting.)

acquisition and mastery of the skills needed to fit intervention to context. Being competent involves employing the means by which to improve the probability that this fit will occur, that the prospective participants will embrace it, that the gains will be truly useful and valued, and that their diffusion to other potential beneficiaries will be maximized.

The evidence is increasingly clear in regard to the link between cultural competence and the success (or failure) of preventive intervention research and programming (Orlandi, 1992; Neighbors, Bashshur, Price, Selig, Donabedian, and Shannon, 1991; Manson, 1982). Thus some have argued for extensive retooling of graduate curricula in the social, behavioral, and health sciences to emphasize such skills (Bolek, Debro, and Trimble, 1992). Though crucial to the evolution of sound preventive intervention research over the long haul, an immediate emphasis should be to encourage investigators to obtain first-hand experience and to collaborate closely with other professionals, perhaps themselves members of the communities of interest. Those who accept this challenge will undergo a process of discovery, gaining insight into the equivalents between their own cultural framework (professional as well as personal in origin) and that of the people with whom they work. Ultimately, cultural competence specific to prevention will emerge through the conduct of preventive interventions themselves, critical reflection on what does and does not work, and constructive exchanges intended to capitalize on success and reduce the likelihood of future failure.

The committee identified a number of points throughout the preventive intervention research cycle at which issues of cultural competence become especially salient and must be addressed. Several examples illustrate the nature and frequency of such occurrences:

• Forging relationships between researchers and community. Prevention research, typically conceptualized within and springing from academic settings, needs to be married with indigenous efforts, particularly those mounted by leaders of the communities of interest. The notion of prevention strikes a resonant chord in most ethnic minority communities. Considerable activity already is under way that is consonant with the intrinsic goals of prevention and with the quest for more knowledge about how best to achieve these goals. Sometimes those community leaders may themselves function as senior investigators. More often, they broker interactions between researchers and participant communities, facilitating the accommodations required to blend their separate strengths and resources. In order for this process to work, traditional power relationships must be transformed. Mutual respect, appropriate responsibility, equity in decision making, and shared commitment to negotiating differences are central to that transformation. Lacking these conditions, the ensuing power differential can become a major barrier to the research process.

• Identifying risks, mechanisms, triggers, and processes. Attempts to understand risk and protective factors, triggers, and processes regarding the onset of a disorder or problem should allow for the possibility of alternative explanation and circumstances among cultural groups (Neighbors, 1990). For example, risk factors can be unique to a specific population. Consider Levy and Kunitz's (1987) inquiry into suicide among the Hopi. They observed that rates of suicide are high not only among Hopi in "progressive villages" and off-reservation border-towns, but also in traditional villages. Specifically, Hopis at increased risk for suicide include the children of parents who entered into traditionally disapproved marriages, such as across tribes, mesas, and even clans of disparate social status. The labeling of parents as "deviant" in this regard stigmatizes their children, thereby engendering a distinct series of stressors. Typical inquiries about marital status would not have arrived at this discovery, missing an important, systematic risk for suicide and related mental health problems.

• Employing relevant theoretical frameworks. Choosing theory to guide the intervention entails more than attending to the presumed links between cause and effect. It also must accommodate the relationship between what participants will (or are expected to) learn and those things valued by them. Different groups of people have different attributional styles, even different assumptions about consequences and costs. Numerous illustrations of the kinds of problems that can be caused by these differences can be found in Paul's (1955) book *Health, Culture, and Community: Case Studies of Public Reactions to Health Programs*. The best is the description by Wellin (1955) of what it took to mount a successful health intervention program in Peru. The problem was dysentery and typhoid; the solution was for people to boil their own water. The difficulty, however, was that the Peruvian community in question lacked an understanding of germ theory. Moreover, the interveners never anticipated that obtaining wood to fuel the fires necessary to boil water was difficult and costly. Analogous examples, both more current and closer to home, include similar disjunctions between conventional intervention models and health beliefs about hypertension among African-Americans (Dressler, 1987), intravenous drug use and HIV infection among African-Americans and Hispanics (Page, Chitwood, Smith, Kane, and McBride, 1990; Singer, Flores,

Davison, Burke, Castillo, Scanlon, and Rivera, 1990), and alcohol abuse among Native Americans (Thurman, Jones-Saumty, and Parsons, 1990; Walker, Walker, and Kivlahan, 1988).

- Preparing the content, format, and delivery of preventive interventions. Individuals and groups are adapted to ethnocultural niches, defined in familial, social, political, and economic terms. To ignore the historical and evolving nature of these niches is to court failure, if not disaster, for prevention research. There is ample documentation that unintended negative effects can accrue from cultural insensitivity and incompetence (McCord, 1978). Thus considerable effort should be expended to inform intervention efforts along these lines. Pilot work and pretesting ought to accompany all attempts to transfer prevention technology across cultural boundaries. In this regard, ethnography stands out among the available methods (Trotter, Rolf, Quintero, Alexander, and Baldwin, in press; Gilbert, 1990; Montagne, 1988). For example, anthropological field work with Native Hawaiian children revealed that peer assistance was important in children's daily activities, that learning occurred most often in "child-constructed" contexts, and that children were seldom individually directed and monitored by adults (Gallimore et al., in press). These observations shaped a remedial school program, aimed at improving the educational attainment of Native Hawaiians, that encouraged peer teaching in independent learning centers in which groups of three to seven children studied together. This design of the educational environment resulted in higher frequencies of on-task behavior, peer assistance, and work completion in contrast to other classroom designs (Tharp and Gallimore, 1988). Hence the infusion of local knowledge permits social validation of intervention goals and procedures, enhances compatibility with valued ends, and increases participation.

- Adopting appropriate narrative structures and discourse. What people are willing to discuss, how they talk about it, and with whom they share certain matters vary in important ways across ethnic minority and cultural groups (Kleinman, 1988, 1980). For example, there often is a great deal of discomfort in Hispanic families with respect to sexual issues (Marin and Marin, 1991). Thus an AIDS prevention program intended to reach Hispanics must recognize that discomfort talking about sexual behaviors is normative and approach the topic carefully or risk losing audience participation. How individuals refer to and discuss a given disorder or problem also can differ markedly by ethnicity and culture. "Down in the dumps," "feeling blue," and "feeling low"— idioms, metaphors, and labels commonly used in white, middle-class America to refer to depression—do not have the same currency among

Asian-Americans (Kinzie, Manson, Do, Nguyen, Bui, and Than, 1982) or Native Americans (Manson, 1993; Manson, Shore, and Bloom, 1985). Likewise, there are differences across ethnic groups in regard to the choice of person in whom to confide specific thoughts or feelings. African-Americans are much less open to discussing issues of shame and anger stemming from racial discrimination with persons whom they perceive as unlikely to have shared similar experiences and who are thus, presumably, less empathic (Neighbors et al., 1992; Jones and Matsumoto, 1982; Jones, 1978). For slightly different reasons, many Native Americans will not volunteer their beliefs about witchcraft as the cause of mental health problems, in part because such matters typically are kept secret from outsiders and, when disclosed, often meet with disdain or ridicule (Manson et al., 1985).

● Tapping critical decision-making processes. The means by which decisions are processed and the locus of responsibility for decision making can be quite different from one ethnic or cultural group to another. For example, nearly one third of Native American tribes explicitly invest a great deal of authority in women, largely as a function of the matrilineal structure of their social organization. Indeed, in some of these tribes, at the time of marriage, men will relocate from their parental homes to those of their wives and their wives' mothers. Decisions, then, that bear directly on the economics of the household, the allocation of family time and resources, and other life-style matters typically are more the responsibility of the women, of both generations, than the men. Though their role has been slightly eroded, family councils among Hmong refugees, who relocated to the United States after fleeing from Vietnam, remain central to conflict resolution and mediation of domestic disputes (Norton and Manson, 1993; Bloom, Kinzie, and Manson, 1985). Imagine the probability of success of preventive interventions that ignore, or even run counter to, such decision-making processes.

● Determining points of intervention leverage. Just as it shapes decision-making processes, social structure also influences access to people and defines points of leverage for subsequent intervention. A home visiting model for prevention, akin to that employed by Olds (see Chapter 7), would need, for example, among the Navajo, to take into account seasonal household migration and concomitant shifts in care-giving responsibilities (Dinges, 1982). At winter residences, maternal grandmothers, who produce many of the crafts for market, assume a central role in childrearing as a consequence of their sedentary activities. By contrast, during summer months, and being free from school, older female siblings are responsible for caring for younger children at the large, extended family camps located deep in the foothills, close to traditional grazing lands. Not only does the configuration of the family, and the corresponding roles, change, but so do developmental tasks for young children. *Projecto Bienestar*, as described by Vega and colleagues (see Chapter 7), which focused on Mexican-American women at high risk of depression, paid close attention to similar elements of household composition and residential patterns, facilitating access to these individuals and enhancing their participation in the intervention.

• Recognizing social networks and natural helpers. *Projecto Bienestar* (Vega, Valle, and Kolody, submitted for publication; Vega and Murphy, 1990; Vega, Valle, Kolody, and Hough, 1987) also underscores the importance of the resources and strengths that exist in all communities, but which are accorded special prominence in ethnic minority groups. As noted in Chapter 7, natural helpers (*Servidoras*) were employed to deliver the intervention. This approach was congruent with the local social ecology, reduced the social distance that often separates participant from intervener, minimized errors due to cultural incompetence, and increased the likelihood that intervention skills and knowledge would be dispersed beyond the intended audience and continue to be delivered past the funding of the program. This same lesson is evident in reports of prevention programming among Southeast Asian refugees (Bliatout, Rath, Do, Kham One, Bliatout, and Lee, 1985; Le Xuan and Bui, 1985; Lum, 1985; True, 1985), Asian-Americans and Pacific Islanders (Murase, Egawa, and Tashima, 1985), other Hispanic populations (Szapocznik and Kurtine, 1993; Bestman, 1986), and Native Americans (Manson and Brenneman, in press; DHHS, 1990).

• Seeking fidelity of implementation. Many factors impinge on the fidelity with which an intervention is delivered, as it moves from highly controlled tests of efficacy to effectiveness and from application in one community to another. An investigator struggling with this issue asks (or is asked): Does what has been done or must be done in order to deliver the intervention compromise its integrity, and, thus, its comparability to the original model? Service providers are seldom concerned with such questions; their mandate is to "make it work" in terms of the clients' best interests. No simple answers emerge for the researcher. Clearly, the researcher has license to use the cultural equivalents of the settings, units of intervention, key constructs, attributional processes, means of instruction, and reinforcement strategies that were used in the original model. But he or she then must carefully document the nature of these equivalences, how they were determined, and what forms they take subsequently in the intervention. In many instances, the adaptations will pose little threat to fidelity. For example, supplementing written curricula with audio-taped versions for literacy-limited older Native American participants in a cognitive-behavioral intervention to prevent depression (Manson and Brenneman, in press) represents a minor deviation from the "Coping with Depression Course" developed by Lewinsohn, Clarke, and Hoberman (1989). Delivering the course through the continuing adult education division of tribally controlled colleges (Gallagher and Thompson, 1983) is another minor adaptation of the intervention. However, reworking the language of the intervention by substituting local idioms and metaphors for depression and drawing analogies between progressive relaxation techniques and indigenous forms of meditation carry the adapted intervention another step away from the original model. Here again, extensive documentation of effectiveness is essential.

• Replicating interventions across diverse and changing populations. The cross-cultural literature on prevention illustrates the great diversity among and within ethnic minorities. For example, some Asian-Americans have lived in the United States for four to five generations, although most, over 50 percent, have been here for fewer than 10 years. Among these individuals, then, language, including English fluency, varies significantly. Indeed, according to the 1990 census (U.S. Census Bureau, 1990), from 24 to 76 percent of the various Asian-American groups do not speak English "very well." A dozen or more distinct groups of Asian-Americans—Japanese, Chinese, Koreans, Vietnamese, Cambodians, and Hmong to name but a few—make up this special population, speaking more than 75 different languages. Similar diversity is evident among African-Americans, Hispanics, Native Americans, and Native Alaskans. Given such variability, interventions cannot be assumed to transfer easily across these lines, any more so than their original extension from the population for whom they were first designed.

Many investigators find the challenge of accommodating diversity of this nature and magnitude almost too daunting to consider. But the quest for cultural competence in this field carries with it an excitement. It promises to enrich the developing science of prevention and yield fulfillment from having successfully bridged differences thought unspannable.

ETHICAL ISSUES

All types of scientific research face challenges in ensuring that their activities adhere to fundamental standards of integrity. Many of these complex issues are reviewed in *Responsible Science: Ensuring the Integrity of the Research Process* (NAS, 1992). Policy recommendations were made to help scientists, research institutions, and government agencies protect the scientific process and minimize scientific misconduct, defined as "fabrication, falsification, or plagiarism in proposing, performing, or reporting research" (NAS, 1992, p. 27). This broad range of issues is applicable to prevention research, but the more narrow concern in this section is the ethical issues regarding the participants in preventive intervention research programs.*

Three factors combine to complicate the ethical issues involved in research on the prevention of mental disorders. First, the various disciplines and techniques that are being integrated into prevention research programs each carry their own complex ethical issues. Second, prevention research programs conducted in communities often require commitments, promises, and risks not encountered in basic research. Third, in many cultures mental disorders carry a special stigma.

The development of a specific ethical code for prevention research is premature and perhaps not even desirable. What is needed, however, is a sensitivity on the part of the individual investigator, and of the research community in general, regarding the importance of ethical issues throughout the preventive intervention research cycle. Investigators individually and as a field must recognize these issues in changing circumstances and respond responsibly—with appropriate questions, skills, and decisions. The development of this competence begins with formal training in basic principles but then requires a continuing process of self-education to instill the habit of ethical accountability.

We can begin to think about ethical issues regarding participants in research on the prevention of mental disorders by drawing on considerations from ethics in other areas of clinical research. Several professional associations and the federal government have developed guidelines that apply to research with human subjects. The federal government has a formal policy for the protection of human subjects in all research projects (DHHS, 1991); therefore this policy automatically applies to participants in preventive intervention research projects. Institutional Review Boards (IRBs) at the researcher's home institution must follow certain requirements for approval of research. These requirements include assurances that

---

*This section is based, in part, on discussions at a one-day meeting, convened by the Institute of Medicine, that focused on ethical considerations in preventive intervention research. (See Appendix C for participants at this meeting.)

- risks to subjects are minimized,
- risks to subjects are reasonable in relation to anticipated benefits,
- selection of subjects is equitable,
- informed consent is sought,
- informed consent is appropriately documented,
- data collection is monitored to ensure the safety of subjects, and
- adequate provisions are made to protect the privacy of subjects

and to maintain the confidentiality of data.

Additional requirements of the IRBs are made to ensure the rights and welfare of subjects who are likely to "be vulnerable to coercion or undue influence," such as children, pregnant women, and economically or educationally disadvantaged persons—all potential targets for preventive interventions (DHHS, 1991, p. 6).

In addition to being bound by the values and standards that guard scientific integrity and by the IRB policies, preventive intervention research programs must address numerous specific ethical issues regarding participants. Pope (1990) has suggested several general guidelines for investigators to routinely consider:

- Do no harm. It is true that for some individuals, families, and communities, under some circumstances, being involved in prevention programs may have harmful proximal or distal consequences (Lorion, 1987). Pope stressed that focusing on the supposed welfare of the many cannot justify the harm that may come to the few. The importance of this issue is heightened by the fact that preventive interventions, by their very nature, involve people who are deemed "at risk" yet may not ever exhibit the disorder or behavior in question. But what standards of evidence are to be used in determining who is "at risk," especially in view of the fact that the importance of specific risk factors is not always well known.

Withholding a preventive intervention that is thought to be efficacious, as can happen in a randomized controlled trial design, may also be thought of as constituting inhumane treatment. This is not a problem early in the research cycle, when the investigator has little scientific evidence for believing that a particular prevention program does what it is intended to do, that is, reduce risks and maybe even lower incidence. Also, the preventive intervention is not like treatment, which is an attempt to deal with a current mental disorder that needs attention. However, the ethical dilemma of a randomized controlled trial design becomes more compelling at the stage of large-scale field trials, when the documentation of evidence from confirmatory and replication trials is encouraging (Muñoz and Ying, 1993). One way of dealing with this dilemma is to have field trials in whole communities or neighborhoods, with control groups being entirely from communities where there is no access to the prevention program (CBASSE, 1993; Seitz, 1987; Cook and Campbell, 1979). Another way of dealing with this problem is to offer the intervention to the waiting list control group after the study has been completed if the results favor the experimental intervention.

Systematic methods must be developed for identifying the possible harm that may occur as a result of a particular intervention or failure to act. Although the methods used to identify possible harm will differ according to the population being targeted, the strategies of intervention being considered, and the problems being addressed, Pope has identified several crucial questions to be considered. First, what are the possibilities for direct harm to people participating in the intervention or to those indirectly affected, such as families, peers, or neighbors? This includes emotional, developmental, physical, interpersonal, educational, economic, and a host of other potential damages. Second, to what degree can delayed damages be anticipated? Because it is hoped that preventive interventions will produce positive long-term effects, it is reasonable to assume that harmful consequences also may be passed along, perhaps even to future generations. Third, if a community is the focus of an intervention, in what way might it be disrupted? Will its natural leadership and social cohesiveness be disturbed? If the group of prevention researchers differs significantly from the community in terms of such factors as social class, race, religion, or politics, what will be the effect on the community? What is informed consent for a community? Fourth, what effects that might be considered harmful could occur in the context of the community's relationship with the larger society? For example, in a project intended to minimize the incidence of serious depression, anxiety, and impulsive behavior in an economically disadvantaged neighborhood, it could be argued that some of these conditions are natural responses to severe poverty. Helping residents learn to adapt to desperate conditions might merely serve as a subtle, perhaps unintended, form of social control that could hinder the community's ability to identify the true source of its suffering and take effective action (Pope, 1990). And finally, what are the possibilities that effective prevention of one outcome will make another outcome worse?

• Practice with competence. In the early stages of a developing field, new approaches and techniques are frequently formulated, applied with enthusiasm, and then discarded when they prove unproductive. However, prevention is moving beyond this point and now possesses a growing body of knowledge and a set of skills that are prerequisites to action. Researchers can accomplish much by carefully analyzing a proposed intervention to identify the information and areas of expertise likely to be necessary for the competent planning, initiation, management, and evaluation of that project. Because prevention programs focus on individuals, families, and communities—involving economic, political, psychological, social, educational, religious, and other diverse aspects—an interdisciplinary team approach may be a necessity, with each member bringing complementary sets of competences. Without such interweaving of disciplines, important social or scientific facets may go unexamined, possibly leading to unexpected harmful results.

• Do not exploit. Researchers are often in a position of power relative to the program's participants, and there are numerous ways this power may be abused. In conducting an intervention effort in an economically disadvantaged neighborhood, for example, researchers may spend many hours establishing relationships with community members, in the process learning "secrets" that would not be apparent to outsiders. If the "life stories" of the residents are used inappropriately—perhaps for professional advancement, with little regard for the impact on those who revealed the information in a bond of trust—both the scientific and the personal damages may be considerable (Pope, 1990). It is critical, then, that researchers be clear about their own contextual constraints before making promises to communities (Trickett and Levin, 1990). Time constraints, economic resources, planning for the research program's termination—all of these issues carry ethical implications for how an intervention program is presented and whether or not it is conducted in good faith.

• Treat participants with respect and dignity. At heart, all ethical principles flow from respect for the human dignity of others. Pope maintained that "scrupulous attention must be paid those aspects of our education and training, of our institutional structures, of the language and content of our theories, research, and interventions which tend to diminish the degree to which we can appreciate, hold as fundamentally important, and respond appropriately to the full human dignity of others. When the people who are affected by our primary prevention strategies become primarily known as 'research subjects,' 'populations-at-risk,' . . . case studies, etc., we may lose sight of the fact that they are all full human beings struggling with life just as we are" (Pope, 1990, p. 57). In addition, individual characteristics such as race, ethnicity, gender, social class, sexual orientation, and age determine, to a larger extent than is commonly acknowledged, how interventions are conceived and implemented. The ethical ramifications of how this information is used need to be considered for each intervention.

• Protect confidentiality. Preventive interventions often involve collection of extremely sensitive and potentially damaging information, such as narcotic use, frequently from large numbers of people. Researchers must identify the sorts of information that are or ought to be treated as confidential. This process includes, but is not limited to, checking carefully any legislation or case law that might govern confidentiality of such things as school records, membership lists of civil or religious organizations, and personal information obtained through interviews. The next step is to ensure that all parties involved or likely to be affected by the intervention clearly understand the boundaries between what is and is not confidential. In addition, the researchers must develop effective mechanisms for handling documents to safeguard their privacy and must develop procedures (including training procedures) to guard against accidental disclosure of confidential information through casual conversation or other means outside the scientific process.

Confidentiality poses especially difficult ethical concerns when researchers discover illegal activity such as evidence of violence, including child maltreatment, which under various state laws may have to be reported to the appropriate social welfare or law enforcement authorities. This combination of circumstances raises serious questions for those who consider as inviolable the trust and confidentiality between researcher and participant (Sieber, 1993). Should the researcher stop and warn a participant who starts to mention abuse? Should the researcher take what is reported and follow the law or seek ethical or legal loopholes to avoid the law? Should the researcher actively seek and report evidence of abuse and neglect? How much professional discretion should the researcher exercise in deciding what degree of abuse requires reporting, in relation to the likely outcome of reporting for the researcher, the project, the institutions involved, the person suspected of committing the abuse, and the person being abused?

Researchers involved in socially sensitive studies can obtain certificates of confidentiality that may preempt state reporting requirements and court subpoenas. They are available from the Department of Health and Human Services and the Department of Justice. Through continued examination of issues of confidentiality, on which opinions now vary considerably, researchers may identify ways to better ensure the efficacy and effectiveness of preventive intervention research programs while exercising responsibility for the welfare of victims and rehabilitation of perpetrators of violence.

• Obtain informed consent. An individual's right to understand a proposed intervention and to freely give or refuse consent to participate stands as a cornerstone of research with human subjects. Weithorn

(1987) has reviewed the ethical issues and federal regulations pertaining to informed consent for prevention. Research with children presents special problems. Children may be more susceptible to harmful consequences, such as stigma and labeling, of research participation; they also may be limited in their ability to provide informed consent because of their immature psychological functioning, limited understanding, and their dependent status as minors. Researchers should not confuse the ability of a child to understand procedures when explained with the more complex and mature cognitive task of making the comparative and contingent risk assessment judgments that are required in informed consent.

The ethical dilemmas that arise regarding informed consent often focus on questions of when and from whom to obtain consent, and what types of information to disclose in the consent process. For example, investigators are required to disclose to prospective participants the purposes and procedures involved in the research, possible risks or discomforts, expected benefits to the participants or others, and appropriate alternatives that might be beneficial. Federal laws, however, allow for less than complete disclosure under certain circumstances, although the boundaries are not always clearly defined. Weithorn presented some of the difficulties for a hypothetical study designed to prevent psychopathology in the children of schizophrenics. What should parents and children be told about the reasons for their inclusion in the project? A completely open disclosure would inform them, for example, that some percentage of the children of schizophrenics are likely to develop serious psychological disorders based on their membership in this risk group (Weithorn, 1987). But many investigators fear that such full disclosure would be harmful to the families, causing additional psychological trauma. Moreover, labeling of the group as "at risk" could possibly alter the behavior and expectations of family members and others, placing the child at further risk for the development of problems. A similar, and perhaps even more traumatic, disclosure would be the identification of a person found to be at risk of a mental disorder because of possession of a certain gene, a possibility in the not-too-distant future.

Weithorn (1987) concluded that prevention researchers should regard the federal regulations covering informed consent as an important guide, but view them as the minimum adequate standards and not as a substitute for careful reference to the moral principles that underlie them.

The principles of informed consent are especially difficult to apply when a universal preventive intervention involves an entire community. For example, a minority member in the community may oppose the project, yet nonetheless may be subjected to its indirect effects. Methods of recognizing and weighing the rights of these individuals are needed.

• Promote equity and justice. At a minimum, preventive interventions must not directly affirm or contribute to inequality or injustice. But a truly ethical approach must go beyond the minimum, to active promotion of equity and justice (Pope, 1990). As with the other ethical areas, there are no simple answers concerning how to enhance the general social well-being. Keeping this goal clearly in mind, however, will help ensure that ethical dilemmas are not ignored or discounted, and that researchers and institutions explicitly attend to them.

To identify and attempt to resolve the various ethical issues destined to arise in preventive interventions, researchers will often be best served by joining with the members of the community—the providers of data and the targets of interventions (Trickett and Levin, 1990). As Conner (1990) has pointed out, ethical issues often involve trade-offs among competing sets of values that may or may not be shared between researchers and community members. He concludes that clients should play a central role in planning, implementing, and evaluating prevention programs.

Rather than simply moving into a community and implementing large-scale prevention programs, researchers might announce their plans and then formally listen to the community's response—including the response from broader constituencies than the program's direct participants—before proceeding (Pope, 1990). In a prevention program for children, for example, Trickett and Levin (1990) note that parents might assume a variety of roles that could increase the sensitivity of researchers to potential ethical issues and provide a forum for their resolution. Also, involving administrators in the planning of a school intervention program may lead to a commitment for continuing the program beyond its externally funded demonstration phase—itself an ethical issue.

Although there is consensus about the importance of ethics in prevention research on mental disorders, ethical accountability in this area has not yet received the emphasis it deserves. This remains a developing field, in need of increasing numbers of individuals and organizations possessing heightened sensitivity to ethical concerns and new skills for designing and conducting ethically appropriate intervention programs. Raising these ethical issues is not to suggest that initiation of preventive interventions should await unanimity on the goals and methods (Lorion, 1987). Rather, careful identification and analysis of these issues can be useful in broadening scientific perspective and in increasing awareness of the potential range and impact of unintended consequences.

ECONOMIC ISSUES

The allocation of available resources to activities aimed at reducing the burden of mental problems in our society requires some capacity to estimate the benefits and costs of our efforts. Analysis of costs and benefits can help inform decision makers about which kinds of interventions for mental disorders hold the most promise for yielding net benefits. The basic goal is to reach a decision on whether a particular intervention program is worth undertaking or whether an existing program should be discontinued, expanded, or reduced in scope.

Analysis of benefits and costs seeks systematically to identify and measure all the benefits and costs of a program (Muñoz and Ying, 1993). Obviously, if benefits exceed costs, then society profits from having the program available. On the other hand, if costs exceed benefits, a decision to allocate scarce resources to other purposes would seem warranted. There are two main methods for doing such an analysis. In cost-benefit analysis, costs and benefits are expressed in dollars. This process is adequate and straightforward for some measures, but it means that dollar amounts have to be assigned to all important outcomes. Assigning dollar amounts is difficult or nearly impossible for some measures, such as life and health. Cost-effectiveness analysis, on the other hand, avoids some of the above controversy by using two categories of outcome measures—dollars and health outcomes. Health outcomes can be presented, for example, in "years of healthy life gained."

The assumption is often made that preventive efforts are cost-effective. Some programs provide evidence that this may be true, but much more confirmation is desirable. The following useful framework is adapted from work by Russell (1986) for analyzing the cost-effectiveness of potential preventive efforts:

- Population and risk. The aggregate or net cost of an intervention depends on the size of the targeted population relative to the number of persons in the population who would be likely to develop the negative outcomes without the intervention. Even interventions that are relatively inexpensive per person may be quite costly in the aggregate if the target population is large and the number of persons in the population at risk is small. The more specific the definition of risk groups, the more likely the intervention will be cost-effective, other factors being equal.
- Cost and frequency of administration of the intervention. Preven-

tive interventions vary greatly in their cost. School curriculum innovations, for example, may be relatively inexpensive. Schools can replace ongoing programming with much more effective curricula at relatively little new cost in time or effort. On the other hand, intensive personal interventions using expensive professional personnel can be quite costly per person served. The cost of the intervention depends also on start-up costs, the size of the sample, and the required frequency of contacts with participants; as observed in Chapter 7, many preventive interventions require multiple contacts over an extended period of time. Thus the cost of an intervention is a product of its initial cost and the frequency of administration.

• Potency of the intervention. Interventions vary in the power of their effects. The efficiency of an intervention—as measured by the proportion of those at risk affected and the size of the effect—should be taken into account in evaluations of cost-effectiveness.

• Uncertainty of risk. For many problems and disorders the causal status of associated risk factors, and therefore the benefits from interventions targeted toward reducing those risk factors, remain uncertain, as do possible adverse events. When the risk of developing the disorder or problem is low and uncertain, thought must be given to the costs associated with exposing large populations to interventions that offer no advantages to most and possible adverse effects to some.

• Time. Another relevant consideration is the temporal proximity of the result of the intervention to its administration. Benefits are much greater for interventions that bring quick and persisting results than for those with delayed results or results that lessen over time.

Once the preventive intervention moves into the community for the large-scale field trials, as well as on into the service realm, the costs and benefits may fall on different segments of society. The service agency or organization may be willing to share part of the cost. To the extent that a service agency assumes the cost for a preventive intervention, the cost-effectiveness of the intervention should be measured against the cost-effectiveness of other potential services. Alternatively, the preventive intervention may be carried as a public service announcement or administered by a community volunteer agency. Even though there may not be direct costs for the health sector or service agencies, these interventions would still entail costs in that they compete for alternative uses of the resources.

Many potential preventive intervention research programs are consistent with the policy priorities for school districts, and the classroom and teacher resources required to conduct them could be achieved at relatively low cost. On the other hand, if the program requires the hiring and training of a new cadre of mental health worker—or even the retraining of existing personnel—the costs of the program could be so great as to compromise its viability.

The cost of prevention programs stems not only from the monetary cost of the intervention, but also from the potential costs involved for those receiving the service. This response cost or burden includes the participant's having to travel to a specific location, pay for travel or time lost for other activities, and undergo uncomfortable or time-consuming procedures, as well as the overall amount of effort involved in receiving the intervention. Perceived response cost may vary across sociocultural groups, even if monetary costs remain the same. For example, accepting "free" babysitting services while receiving a preventive intervention may be unacceptable to those cultural groups for whom sharing the childrearing responsibility is considered unwise or dangerous.

Prevention programs should not be funded by withdrawing resources from needed, and usually underfunded, treatment services (see Chapter 2 for definitions). Even though preventive interventions may have a significant impact in terms of increased socialization and reduced psychopathology, cognitive impairment, and psychosocial dysfunction, they are unlikely to result in an immediate reduction in the need for treatment interventions. In part, this is because those currently being treated are a small proportion of those suffering from a disorder.

Cost-benefit and cost-effectiveness analyses appear only infrequently in the treatment literature (Cardin, McGill, and Falloon, 1985; Weisbrod, Test, and Stein, 1980; Paul and Lentz, 1977) and are almost nonexistent in the prevention literature. As requests for these analyses increase over the next decade, there are several important points that policymakers and prevention researchers should consider (Gramlich, 1984). For example, benefits from prevention programs may increase over time. Short-term evaluations may show small or nonexistent benefits, but benefits may accrue as children are engaged over time in less crime, depend less on welfare, or begin to reap the benefits of higher levels of educational achievement. In addition, a well-designed and sensitive benefit-cost analysis can identify gainers and losers in society. Net social benefits may be received by participants in the program themselves, taxpayers, and potential victims of crime. Evaluation can show who gains and who loses as well as how big the overall gain or loss actually is.

One example of a pioneering benefit-cost analysis of a prevention program is that done for the Perry Preschool Program, a selective preventive intervention (Berrueta-Clement, Schweinhart, Barnett, Epstein, and Weikart, 1984). (See Chapter 7 for a description of the program.) The investigators documented the costs of high-quality pre-school education and the benefits resulting from positive program outcomes. Results suggested that the total net benefit to preschool participants themselves was approximately $5,000. On the other hand, the total net benefit to taxpayers and potential crime victims was estimated at around $23,000 for one year of preschool by the time the program recipients reached 19 years of age. As the authors observed, "changes in economic success, self-sufficiency, and social responsibility can be predicted quantitatively from observed effects at age 19" (Berru-eta-Clement et al., 1984, p. 89).

Another example of a benefit-cost analysis of a preventive program is that done for the JOBS Project for the Unemployed, a selective preventive intervention aimed at helping the recently unemployed find new employment (Vinokur, van Ryn, Gramlich, and Price, 1991). (See Chapter 7.) Results from a 2½-year follow-up of participants in a randomized field experiment that included a jobs program aimed at increasing reemployment and preventing poor mental health outcomes showed the continued beneficial effects of the intervention on monthly earnings, quality of reemployment, and episodes of employer and job changes. Results of a benefit-cost analysis demonstrated large net benefits of the intervention not only to the participants, but also to federal and state governments, based on increased tax revenues produced by reemployed workers in the randomized trial. Not only did the benefits of the program exceed all costs within less than two years, but, because the wage differences appeared to persist, the benefits were expected to continue to accumulate over many years. According to the researchers' estimates, by the time experimental group participants reach age 60, they can be expected to have accrued $48,151 more benefit per person than their counterparts in the control groups, assuming they continue to be employed.

CONCLUSION

If the research standards and methodology outlined here are system-atically and rigorously applied within the preventive intervention research cycle and the guidelines on cultural, ethical, and economic issues are carefully considered at each step, prevention research will yield progressively more powerful results over the next decade. The ensuing development of prevention into a science will provide a firm base of knowledge for policymakers. This knowledge will inform their decisions on the allocation of available resources toward the ultimate goal of realizing the opportunities presented by the science for the alleviation of the personal and societal suffering and burdens associated with mental disorders.

REFERENCES

Alkin, M. C. (1985) A Guide for Evaluation Decision Makers. Beverly Hills, CA: Sage Publications.

Barlow, D. H.; Hersen, M. (1973) Single-case experimental designs: Uses in applied clinical research. Archives of General Psychiatry; 29(3): 319–325.

Berrueta-Clement, J. R.; Schweinhart, L. J.; Barnett, W. S.; Epstein, A. S.; Weikart, D. P. (1984) Changed Lives: The Effects of the Perry Preschool Program on Youths Through Age 19 (High/Scope Educational Research Foundation, Monograph 8).Ypsilanti, MI: High/Scope Press.

Bestman, E. (1986) Cross-cultural approaches to service delivery to ethnic minorities: The Miami Model. In: M. Miranda and H. Kitano, Eds. Mental Health Research and Practice in Minority Communities: Development of Culturally Sensitive Training Programs. Rockville, MD: National Institute of Mental Health; DHHS Pub. No. (ADM) 86–1466: 199–226.

Bliatout, B. T.; Rath, B.; Do, V. T.; Kham One, K.; Bliatout, H. Y.; Lee, D. T. (1985) Mental health and prevention activities targeted to Southeast Asian refugees. In: T. C. Owan, Ed. Southeast Asian Mental Health: Treatment, Prevention, Services, Training, and Research. Washington, DC: National Institute of Mental Health; DHHS Pub. No. (ADM) 85–1399: 183–207.

Bloom, J. D.; Kinzie, J. D.; Manson, S. M. (1985) Halfway around the world to prison: Vietnamese in Oregon's criminal justice system. International Journal of Medicine and Law; 4: 563–572.

Bolek, C. S.; Debro, J.; Trimble, J. E. (1992) Overview of selected federal efforts to encourage minority drug abuse research and researchers. Drugs and Society; 6(3/4): 345–375.

Campbell, D. T. (1991) Methods for the experimenting society. Evaluation Practice; 12(3): 223–260.

Cardin, V. A.; McGill, C. W.; Falloon, I. R. H. (1985) An economic analysis: Costs, benefits and effectiveness. In: I. R. H. Falloon, Ed. Family Management of Schizophrenia. Baltimore, MD: Johns Hopkins University Press; 115–123.

CBASSE (Commission on Behavioral and Social Sciences and Education). (1993) Understanding Child Abuse and Neglect. Panel on Research on Child Abuse and Neglect, National Research Council. Washington, DC: National Academy Press.

Cohen, J. (1988) Statistical Power Analysis for the Behavioral Sciences (2nd ed.). Hillsdale, NJ: Lawrence Erlbaum Associates.

Conner, R. F. (1990) Ethical issues in evaluating the effectiveness of primary prevention programs. In: E. J. Trickett and G. B. Levin, Eds. Ethical Implications of Primary Prevention. New York, NY: The Haworth Press.

Cook, T. D.; Campbell, D. T. (1979) Quasi-Experimentation: Design and Analysis Issues for Field Settings. Chicago, IL: Rand McNally.

Cross, T. L.; Bazron, B. J.; Dennis, K. W.; Isaacs, M. R. (1989) Toward a Culturally Competent System of Care: Vol. I. Washington, DC: Georgetown University Child Development Center.

DHHS (Department of Health and Human Services). (1991) National Institutes of Health.

Office for Protection from Research Risks. Code of Federal Regulations: Part 46— Protection of Human Subjects. Washington, DC: Government Printing Office.

DHHS (Department of Health and Human Services). (1990) Breaking new ground for American Indian and Alaska Native youth at risk: Program summaries. Rockville, MD: Office for Substance Abuse Prevention; (OSAP Technical Report 3); DHHS Pub. No. (ADM) 90–1705.

Dinges, N. G. (1982) Mental health promotion with Navajo families. In: S. M. Manson, Ed. New Directions in Prevention Among American Indian and Alaska Native Communities. Portland, OR: Oregon Health Sciences University; 119–143.

Dressler, W. (1987) The stress process in a Southern black community: Implications for prevention research. Human Organization; 46: 211–220.

Elandt-Johnson, R. C.; Johnson, N. L., Eds. (1980) Survival Models and Data Analysis. New York, NY: John Wiley and Sons.

Fergusson, D. M.; Harwood, L. J.; Lloyd, M. (1991) Confirmatory factor models of attention deficit and conduct disorder. Journal of Child Psychology and Psychiatry; 32(2): 257–274.

Galanti, G. (1991) Caring for Patients from Different Cultures. Philadelphia, PA: University of Pennsylvania Press.

Gallagher, D.; Thompson, L. W. (1983) Cognitive therapy for depression in the elderly: A promising model for treatment and research. In: L. D. Breslau and M. R. Haug, Eds. Depression and Aging: Causes, Care, and Consequences. New York, NY: Springer Publishing Company.

Gallimore, R.; Goldenberg, C. N.; Weisner, T. S. (in press) The social construction and subjective reality of activity settings: Implications for community psychology. American Journal of Community Psychology; 21.

Gibbons, R. D.; Hedeker, D.; Elkin, I.; Waternaux, C.; Kraemer, H. C.; Greenhouse, J. B.; Shea, M. T.; Imber, S. D.; Sotosky, S. M.; Watkins, J. T. (in press) Some conceptual and statistical issues in analysis of longitudinal psychiatric data. Archives of General Psychiatry.

Gilbert, J. (1990) Ethnographic research strategies in the cross-cultural substance use and abuse field. The International Journal of the Addictions; 25(2A): 123–148.

Gramlich, E. M. (1984) Commentary on Changed Lives. In: J. R Barreuta-Clement, L. J. Schweinhart, W. S. Barnett, A. S. Epstein, and D. P. Weikart, Eds. Changed Lives: The Effects of the Perry Preschool Program on Use Through Age 19. Ypsilanti, MI: Monographs of the High Scope Educational Research Foundation; 8: 200–203.

Hasenfeld, Y.; Furman, W. M. (in press) Intervention research as an interorganizational exchange. In: J. Rothman and E. J. Thomas, Eds. Intervention Research: Design and Development for Human Services. Binghamton, NY: The Haworth Press.

Hiltz, S. R. (1974) Evaluating a pilot social service project for widows: A chronicle of research problems. Journal of Sociology and Social Welfare; 2(4): 217–224.

Hood, P. D. (1990) How can studies of information consumers be used to improve the education communication system? Knowledge in Society; 3(2): 8–25.

The Infant Health and Development Program. (1990) Enhancing the outcomes of low birth weight, premature infants: A multisite randomized trial. Journal of the American Medical Association; 263(22): 3035–3042.

Issacs, M. R.; Benjamin, M. P. (1991) Toward a Culturally Competent System of Care: Vol. II. Washington, DC: Georgetown University Child Development Center.

Jones, E. (1978) Effects of race on psychotherapy process and outcome: An exploratory investigation. Psychotherapy: Theory, Research, and Practice; 15: 226–236.

Jones, E.; Matsumoto, D. (1982) Psychotherapy with the underserved: Recent developments. In: L. Snowden, Ed. Reaching the Underserved: Mental Health Needs of Neglected Populations. Beverly Hills, CA: Sage Publications.

Kavanagh, K. H.; Kennedy, P. H. (1992) Promoting Cultural Diversity: Strategies for Health Care Professionals. Newbury Park, CA: Sage Publications.

Kelly, J. G.; Dassoff, N.; Levin, I.; Schreckengost, S. P.; Altman, B. E. (1988) A Guide to Conducting Prevention Research in a Community: First Steps. New York, NY: The Haworth Press.

Kinzie, J. D.; Manson, S. M.; Do, T. V.; Nguyen, T. T.; Bui, A.; Than, N. P. (1982) Development and validation of a Vietnamese-language depression rating scale. American Journal of Psychiatry; 139(10): 1276–1281.

Kleinman, A. (1988) The Illness Narratives. New York, NY: Basic Books.

Kleinman, A. (1980) Patients and Healers in the Context of Culture. Berkeley, CA: University of California Press.

Kraemer, H. C. (1979) Ramifications of a population model for kappa as a coefficient of reliability. Psychometrika; 44: 461–472.

Krueger, R. A. (1988) Focus Groups: A Practical Guide for Applied Research. Newbury Park, CA: Sage Publications.

Laird, N. M.; Ware, J. H. (1982) Random effects models for longitudinal data. Biometrics; 38: 963–974.

Last, J. M. (1988) A Dictionary of Epidemiology. New York, NY: Oxford University Press.

Le Xuan, K.; Bui, D. D. (1985) Southeast Asian mutual assistance associations: An approach for community development. In: T. C. Owan, Ed. Southeast Asian Mental Health: Treatment, Prevention, Services, Training, and Research. Rockville, MD: National Institute of Mental Health; DHHS Pub. No. (ADM) 85–1399: 209–224.

Lefley, H. P. (1982) Cross-cultural training for mental health personnel. Final Report. Miami, FL: University of Miami School of Medicine; NIMH Training Grant No. 5-T24-MH15249.

Levy, J. E.; Kunitz, S. J. (1987) A suicide prevention program for Hopi youth. Social Science and Medicine; 25(8): 931–940.

Lewinsohn, P. M.; Clarke, G. N.; Hoberman, H. H. (1989) The Coping with Depression Course: Review and future directions. Canadian Journal of Behavioral Science; 21(4): 470–493.

Liberman, R. P.; Eckman, T. (1981) Behavior therapy vs insight-oriented therapy for repeated suicide attempters. Archives of General Psychiatry; 38(10): 1126–1130.

Locke, D. C. (1992) Increasing Multicultural Understanding: A Comprehensive Model. Newbury Park, CA: Sage Publications.

Lorion, R. P. (1987) The other side of the coin: The potential for negative consequences of preventive interventions. In: Preventing Mental Disorders: A Research Perspective. National Institutes of Health. Washington, DC: DHHS Pub. No. (ADM) 87–1492.

Lum, R. G. (1985) A community-based mental health service to Southeast Asian refugees. In: T. C. Owan, Ed. Southeast Asian Mental Health: Treatment, Prevention, Services, Training, and Research. Rockville, MD: National Institute of Mental Health; DHHS Pub. No. (ADM) 85–1399: 283–306.

Maccoby, N.; Alexander, J. (1979) Reducing heart disease risk using the mass media: Comparing the effect on three communities. In: R. F. Muñoz, L. R. Snowden, and J. G. Kelly, Eds. Social and Psychological Research in Community Settings. San Francisco, CA: Jossey-Bass Publications.

Manoff, R. K. (1985) Social Marketing: New Imperative for Public Health. New York, NY: Random House.

Manson, S. M. (1993) Culture and depression: Discovering variations in the experience of illness. In: W. J. Lonner and R. S. Malpass, Eds. Psychology and Culture. Needham, MA: Allyn and Bacon.

Manson, S. M. (1982) New Directions in Prevention Among American Indian and Alaska Native Communities. Portland. OR: Oregon Health Sciences University Foundation.

Manson, S. M.; Brenneman, D. (in press) Chronic disease among older American Indians: Preventing depression and related problems of coping. In: D. Padgett, Ed. Handbook on Ethnicity, Aging, and Mental Health. Westport, CT: Greenwood Press.

Manson, S. M.; Shore, J. H.; Bloom, J. D. (1985) The depressive experience in American Indian communities: A challenge for psychiatric theory and diagnosis. In: A. Kleinman and B. Good, Eds. Culture and Depression. Berkeley, CA: University of California Press; 331–368.

Marin, G.; Marin, B. (1991) Research with Hispanic Populations. Beverly Hills, CA: Sage Publications.

McCord, J. E. (1978) A thirty-year follow-up of treatment effects. American Psychologist; 33(3): 284–289.

Montagne, M. (1988) The metaphorical nature of drugs and drug taking. Social Science and Medicine; 26(4): 417–424.

Muñoz, R. F. (1993) The prevention of depression: Current research and practice. Applied and Preventive Psychology; 2: 21–33.

Muñoz, R. F.; Chan, F.; Armas, R. (1986) Primary prevention: Cross-cultural perspectives. In: J. T. Barter and S. W. Talbott, Eds. Primary Prevention in Psychiatry: State of the Art. Washington, DC: American Psychiatric Press.

Muñoz, R. F.; Ying, Y. W. (1993) The Prevention of Depression: Research and Practice. Baltimore, MD: Johns Hopkins University Press.

Murase, K.; Egawa, J.; Tashima, N. (1985) Alternative mental health services models in Asian/Pacific communities. In: T. C. Owan, Ed. Southeast Asian Mental Health: Treatment, Prevention, Services, Training, and Research. Rockville, MD: National Institute of Mental Health; DHHS Pub. No. (ADM) 85–1399: 225–227.

NAS (National Academy of Sciences). (1992) Responsible Science: Ensuring the Integrity of the Research Process. Washington, DC: National Academy Press.

Neighbors, H. W. (1990) The prevention of psychopathology in African Americans: An epidemiologic perspective. Community Mental Health Journal; 26(2): 167–179.

Neighbors, H. W.; Bashshur, R.; Price, R.; Selig, S.; Donabedian, A.; Shannon, G. (1992) Ethnic minority health service delivery: A review of the literature. Research in Community and Mental Health; 7: 55–71.

Norton, I. M.; Manson, S. M. (1993) An association between domestic violence and depression among Southeast Asian refugee women. Journal of Nervous and Mental Disease; 180(11): 729–730.

O'Donnell, C. R.; Tharp, R. G. (1990) Community intervention guided by theoretical development. In: A. S. Bellack, M. Hersen, and A. E. Kazdin, Eds. International Handbook of Behavior Modification and Therapy. 2nd ed. New York, NY: Plenum Press; 251–266.

Olds, D. L.; Henderson, C. R.; Tatelbaum, R.; Chamberlin, R. (1988) Improving the life-course development of socially disadvantaged mothers: A randomized trial of nurse home visitation. American Journal of Public Health; 78(11): 1436–1445.

Olds, D. L.; Henderson, C. R.; Tatelbaum, R.; Chamberlin, R. (1986) Improving the delivery of prenatal care and outcomes of pregnancy: A randomized trial of nurse home visitation. Pediatrics; 77(1): 16–28.

Olweus, D. (1991) Bully/victim problems among schoolchildren: Basic facts and effects of an intervention program. In: K. Rubin and D. Pepler, Eds. The Development and Treatment of Childhood Aggression. Hillsdale, NJ: Lawrence Erlbaum Associates.

Orlandi, M. A. (1992) Defining cultural competence: An organizing framework. In: M. A. Orlandi, Ed. Cultural Competence for Evaluators. Washington, DC: Office of Substance Abuse Prevention; DHHS Pub. No. (ADM) 92–1884.

Page, J. B.; Chitwood, D. D.; Smith, P. C.; Kane, N.; McBride, D. C. (1990) Intravenous drug use and HIV infection in Miami. Medical Anthropology Quarterly; 4(1): 56–71.

Paul, B. P. (1955) Health, Culture and Community: Case Studies of Public Reactions to Health Programs. New York, NY: Sage Publications.

Paul, G. L.; Lentz, R. (1977) Psychosocial Treatment of Chronic Mental Patients. Cambridge, MA: Harvard University Press.

Pope, K. S. (1990) Identifying and implementing ethical standards for primary prevention. In: E. J. Trickett and G. B. Levin, Eds. Ethical Issues of Primary Prevention. New York, NY: The Haworth Press.

Rappaport, J.; Seidman, E.; Davidson, W. S. (1979) Demonstration research and manifest versus true adoption: The natural history of a research project to divert adolescents from the legal system. In: R. F. Muñoz, L. R. Snowden, and J. G. Kelly, Eds. Social and Psychological Research in Community Settings. San Francisco, CA: Jossey-Bass Publications; 101–144.

Rossi, P. H. (1977) Boobytraps and pitfalls in evaluation of social actions programs. In: F. G. Caro, Ed. Readings in Evaluation Research. 2nd ed. New York, NY: Sage Publications.

Russell, L. B. (1986) Is Prevention Better than Cure? Washington, DC: The Brookings Institution.

Schilling, R. F.; Schinke, S. P.; Kirkham, M. A.; Meltzer, N. J.; Norelius, K. L. (1988) Social work research in social service agencies: Issues and guidelines. Journal of Social Service Research; 11(4): 75–87.

Seitz, V. (1987) Outcome evaluation of family support programs: Research design alternatives to true experiments. In: S. L. Kagan, D. Powell, B. Weissbound, and E. Zigler, Eds. America's Family Support Programs: Perspectives and Prospects. New Haven, CT: Yale University Press.

Shadish, W. R., Jr.; Cook, T. D.; Leviton, L. C. (1991) Foundation of Program Evaluation. Newbury Park, CA: Sage Publications.

Sieber, J. (1993) Issues Presented by Mandatory Reporting Requirements. Paper commissioned by the CBASSE Panel on Child Abuse and Neglect, National Research Council. Washington, DC.

Singer, M.; Flores, C.; Davison, L.; Burke, G.; Castillo, Z.; Scanlon, K.; Rivera, M. (1990) SIDA: The economic, social, and cultural context of AIDS among Latinos. Medical Anthropology Quarterly; 4(1): 72–114.

Snowden, L. R.; Muñoz, R. F.; Kelly, J. G. (1979) The process of implementing community-based research. In: R. F. Muñoz, L. R. Snowden, and J. G. Kelly, Eds. Social and Psychological Research in Community Settings. San Francisco, CA: Jossey-Bass Publications; 14–29.

Szapocznik, J.; Kurtine, W. M. (1993) Family psychology and cultural diversity. American Psychologist; 48(4): 400–407.

Tharp, R. G.; Gallimore, R. (1988) Rousing Minds to Life: Teaching, Learning, and Schooling in Social Context. Cambridge, MA: Cambridge University Press.

Thurman, P. J.; Jones-Saumty, D.; Parsons, O. A. (1990) Locus of control and drinking behavior in American Indian alcoholics and non-alcoholics. American Indian and Alaska Native Mental Health Research; 4(1): 31–39.

Trickett, E. J.; Levin, G. B. (1990) Paradigms for Prevention: Providing a Context for Confronting Ethical Issues. New York, NY: The Haworth Press.

Trotter, R. T., II; Rolf, J.; Quintero, G. A.; Alexander, C.; Baldwin, I. (in press) Cultural models of drug abuse and AIDS on the Navajo Reservation: Navajo youth at risk. Medical Anthropology Quarterly.

True, R. H. (1985) An Indochinese mental health service model in San Francisco. In: T. C. Owan, Ed. Southeast Asian Mental Health: Treatment, Prevention, Services, Training, and Research. Rockville, MD: National Institute of Mental Health; DHHS Pub. No. (ADM) 85–1399: 329–342.

U.S. Census Bureau. (1990) Census of Population. Unpublished tabulations.

Vega, W. A. (1992) Theoretical and pragmatic implications of cultural diversity for community research. American Journal of Community Psychology; 20(3): 375–391.

Vega, W. A.; Murphy, J. (1990) Projecto Bienestar: An example of a community-based intervention. In: W. A. Vega and J. W. Murphy, Eds. Culture and the Restructuring of Community Mental Health. Westport, CT: Greenwood Press; 103–122.

Vega, W. A.; Valle, R.; Kolody, B. (submitted for publication) Preventing depression in the Hispanic community: An outcome evaluation of Projecto Bienestar.

Vega, W. A.; Valle, R.; Kolody, B.; Hough, R. (1987) The Hispanic social network prevention intervention study: A community-based randomized trial. In: R. Muñoz, Ed. Depression Prevention: Research Directions. Washington, DC: Hemisphere Publishing.

Vinokur, A.D.; van Ryn, M.; Gramlich, E. M.; Price, R. (1991) Long-term follow-up and benefit-cost analysis of the Jobs Program: A preventive intervention for the unemployed. Journal of Applied Psychology; 76(2): 213–219.

Walker, P. S.; Walker, R. D.; Kivlahan, D. (1988) Alcoholism, alcohol abuse, and health in American Indians and Alaska Natives. In: S. M. Manson and N. G. Dinges, Eds. Behavioral Health Issues Among American Indians and Alaska Natives: Explorations on the Frontiers of the Biobehavioral Sciences. Denver, CO: University of Colorado Health Sciences Center.

Weisbrod, B. A.; Test, M. A.; Stein, L. I. (1980) Alternative to mental hospital treatment: III. Economic benefit-cost analysis. Archives of General Psychiatry; 37: 400–405.

Weiss, C. H. (1984) Increasing the likelihood of influencing decisions. In: L. Rutman, Ed. Evaluation Research Methods: A Basic Guide. Beverly Hills, CA: Sage Publications: 159–190.

Weithorn, L. A. (1987) Informed consent for prevention research involving children: Legal and ethical issues. In: Preventing Mental Disorders: A Research Perspective. Washington, DC: National Institute of Mental Health. DHHS Pub. No. (ADM) 87–1492.

Wellin, E. (1955) Water boiling in a Peruvian town. In: B. P. Paul, Ed. Health, Culture and Community. New York, NY: Russell Sage Foundation; 71–103.

11

The Knowledge Exchange Process: From Research into Practice

The success of the preventive intervention research cycle, described in Chapter 10, for a given research program lies only partly in how well it works to expand the knowledge base for prevention. The cycle's ultimate merit—and the justification for the expenditure of large amounts of research monies—lies in how effectively that knowledge can be exchanged among researchers, community practitioners, and policymakers to successfully implement the program in real-life settings and ultimately, with widespread application, to reduce the incidence of mental disorders.

This chapter focuses on the process of exchanging knowledge. The term *knowledge exchange* has been chosen for this process because it implies two-way communication, including the feedbacks represented by the loop in Figure 10.1. The term *dissemination* is used when only a one-way flow of information is implied, for example, from researchers to other researchers through publication of a journal article. Therefore, although the role the researchers play, as described in Chapter 10, is critical to the success of knowledge exchange, it is only one part of a more complicated process. The community's role is equally important, not only in how it implements the program and provides feedback, but also in how it goes about gathering the needed information. Policymakers at federal, state, and local levels also have a critical role to play in gathering information to use in setting priorities for research and in supporting standards of excellence.

Researchers and community practitioners come to the knowledge exchange table with very different perspectives and value systems. Most researchers, by nature, are cautious. They appreciate the complexity of etiology and the diverse pathways in the occurrence of mental disorders and usually are skeptical about unidimensional interventions, which may not generalize across populations diverse in age and culture. They have high standards for the quality of the evidence they believe is needed before practice recommendations can be made. This circumspect approach contributes to slowness in publication of evidence. For example, pilot studies and early field trials often are not published because the researchers believe that doing so might be "premature."

Although community practitioners, along with representatives from community organizations, may understand the reasons for caution, they are faced on a daily basis with the need for preventive services, and they often are frustrated by what they perceive as the unwillingness of the researchers to provide direction. The bottom line for practitioners, who often must answer to policymakers in state legislatures and local councils, is straightforward: What works? How long does it take? How much will it cost?

When these questions cannot be answered from the results of completed field trials within the research cycle, or when practitioners have creative ideas for new interventions, they proceed to create their own prevention programs. Currently, this is being done at the federal, state, and local levels of government and by private foundations. Such programs are primarily "service" in nature, although some, including demonstration projects, have evaluation components attached to them. The result is that large expenditures are being made without knowing the effectiveness of these services.

THE ROLE OF THE COMMUNITY

The role of the community—defined here as policymakers, community practitioners, and representatives of host organizations—is complicated and time-consuming. Part of this complexity is due to the very nature of "community," which can rarely be regarded as a unitary whole. Rather, it is a heterogeneous group of individuals, institutions, and special interest groups, among whom it can be difficult to achieve consensus. The role of the community includes the following functions: defining the problem and assessing the needs, ensuring the readiness of the host organization, selecting a model program, balancing fidelity and adaptability while implementing the program, evaluating the program's effectiveness, and providing feedback to the researchers. Attention to this process is necessary for programmatic planning at federal, state, and local levels of government and with private foundations.

Defining the Problem and Assessing the Needs

When community leaders, pressed by the urgency of local needs, must decide whether to initiate a service program for a particular mental disorder or problem, many factors will influence their decision. These include the degree of community concern about a specific problem, such as substance abuse, compared with concern over other priorities, such as education and police protection; the scarcity of resources for health care, especially mental health care; the availability of an effective model; the safety and cultural relevance of the model; and the availability of local interveners to deliver the program.

The community must define for itself what needs and problems it has and what it wants to accomplish. Initially, a community may be more interested in treatment and maintenance programs than preventive interventions. The timing for the introduction of a prevention program must be right for a community; a program foisted onto a community, even by a local practitioner rather than a researcher, is unlikely to succeed.

Ensuring the Readiness of the Host Organization

If the host organization, such as a service agency, school, church, or city council, has had success in reaching out into its geographic community previously, has developed referral sources, and is respected within its community, it will have a better chance of success. Also, if the bureaucratic structure within the organization has some flexibility regarding its structures for communication, coordination, decision making, and role definition, it will be more able to adapt and implement a prevention program (Price and Lorion, 1989).

Selecting a Model Program

The questions that the community and the host organization will focus on in selecting a particular model program include: Does the program address the needs and problems identified by the community? Is the program really ready for distribution? Has it demonstrated its efficacy and effectiveness? What aspects of the program would have to be adapted to fit the needs of this particular community, such as cultural issues? How much does the program cost, and how long must it continue to achieve positive effects? Is technical assistance available from someone who understands this particular program, such as someone from the original research team?

Criteria to Use in Examining Programs

For a community searching for a model, practicality is paramount. An ideal model that has proved its efficacy and effectiveness through confirmatory, replication, and large-scale field trials is as yet, owing to the status of current prevention research, unlikely to be available. Nevertheless, communities can be guided by the quality of evidence that is available from various prevention programs, some that have been tested in trials and others that have not. The following guidelines regarding a hierarchy of evidence have been adapted from work by the Canadian Task Force on the Periodic Health Examination and the U.S. Preventive Service Task Force (Battista and Fletcher, 1988; Spitzer, 1979).

Grade I: Evidence obtained from multiple randomized controlled trials (confirmatory and replication trials and large-scale field trials).

Grade II: Evidence obtained from multiple randomized controlled trials (confirmatory and replication trials but no large-scale field trial).

Grade III: Evidence obtained from at least one properly randomized controlled trial.

Grade IV: Evidence obtained from well-designed controlled trials without randomization.

Grade V: Evidence obtained from well-designed cohort or case-control studies, preferably more than one.

Grade VI: Evidence obtained from multiple time series studies with or without the intervention. Dramatic results in uncontrolled experiments (such as the results of the introduction of penicillin in the 1940s) could constitute this type of evidence.

Grade VII: Evidence suggested by respected authorities, based on clinical experience, descriptive studies, prior service delivery programs, or reports by expert committees.

A community can use the criteria listed in Chapter 7 to assess the quality of preventive intervention research programs. It can also use the forward-looking methodologies presented in Chapter 10 to guide its selection of a program. By making opinion subordinate to evidence and by searching for the highest level of evidence available, the community, in its program selection, increases the likelihood that its efforts will be successful.

Information Sources to Use in Examining Programs

Throughout the preventive intervention research cycle, there can be information and data ready to be exchanged with community practitioners and policymakers for general use. There are five main routes by which research findings are commonly disseminated: academic journals and books, manuals, clearinghouses, professional conferences, and direct working relationships between researchers and communities to facilitate implementation of the prevention programs. When a research program is being reviewed by a community, published papers and manuals should be obtained from libraries, clearinghouses, or the researchers themselves.

The committee reviewed the amount of knowledge dissemination currently available for examination by community practitioners and policymakers, as well as by other researchers. A description of this review process and the findings follows.

Research Publications. Peer-reviewed journal publication is the usual method of dissemination in all scientific fields, but it does entail a time lag between establishment of the data, the acceptance of the paper, and the distribution of the journal. In addition, many of these journals can be difficult for nonresearchers to locate.

The first step in the committee's review was to determine how large the prevention literature related to mental disorders was; then it could determine what portion of this was based on research. The following sources of information were used:

- MEDLINE searches.
- Computer Retrieval of Information on Scientific Projects (CRISP) files from 1988 through 1992 on research grants that identified prevention of mental disorder, alcoholism, or drug addiction as one of the main areas of emphasis. These files included grants from all three of the former ADAMHA research institutes—National Institute of Mental Health (NIMH), National Institute of Drug Abuse (NIDA), and National Institute of Alcoholism and Alcohol Abuse (NIAAA)—as well as other National Institutes of Health research institutes and the former Office of Substance Abuse Prevention (OSAP).
- Lists of research grants from the Prevention Research Branches of NIMH, NIDA, and NIAAA.
- Personal inquiries to NIMH Preventive Intervention Research Center (PIRC) directors as well as researchers of numerous "illustrative programs" identified by the research institutes, service agencies, private foundations, and many other sources.

- An annotated bibliography prepared under contract for NIMH. In 1991, NIMH contracted to compile an annotated bibliography of published work in the field of primary prevention in mental health (Trickett, Dahiyat, and Selby, in press). This compendium was a follow-up of an earlier bibliography that covered materials on primary prevention in mental health through early 1983 (Buckner, Trickett, and Corse, 1985). Because the field of prevention continues to have multiple definitions of its scope and boundaries, the editors' decisions as to what to include in both bibliographies were, by necessity, arbitrary. The second bibliography focused on published materials from later 1983 through mid-1991. It emphasized primary prevention, but where the boundaries between primary and secondary prevention were not clear, publications were included. A broad definition of primary prevention was used, including the concept of risk, prevention of specific disorders, enhancement of specific competences, empowerment, early intervention, and biosocial approaches to development. Although the main emphasis was on preventive interventions, articles were included if they had direct implications for preventive interventions or provided a conceptual perspective that was "heuristically rich." The data bases used for the search included PsycINFO, MEDLINE, SOCIOFILE, ERIC, and AIDS at the National Library of Medicine. The search also included journals that were identified as specifically representing the field, volumes emanating from primary prevention conferences, and information derived directly from NIMH Prevention Research Branch (PRB) researchers and the NIMH Panel on Biosocial Approaches.

In summary, the editors noted that, compared with the 1985 annotated bibliography, the second bibliography reflected how "the boundaries of primary prevention are stretching both in a biosocial direction on the one hand, and in an empowerment direction on the other" (Trickett et al., in press).

The committee analyzed the second bibliography and treated it as a main source for locating literature on prevention. Although it was not an all-encompassing source of available and/or relevant literature, and did not use the definitions of prevention and prevention research that the committee adopted (see Chapter 2), it was the most complete annotated bibliography dealing with prevention of mental disorders available.

The committee's findings are as follows. The bibliography has 1,326 entries, with 1,990 authors. These entries include journal articles, books, chapters, and monographs. For the committee's purposes, 109 of these entries were excluded from analysis because they centered on AIDS, a topic outside the committee's purview. Of the remaining references, 808 were journal articles, which included theoretical papers; findings from risk studies; descriptions of methodologies; descriptions of prevention programs, some with evaluation components; results from quasi-experimental research studies; and findings from approximately 25 preventive intervention research programs that, according to the abstracts, had used randomized controlled trial designs. These 808 articles were published in 224 journals. (This wide array of journals publishing prevention articles related to mental disorders from 1983 to 1991, compiled by using only the NIMH prevention bibliography as the source, can be found in Appendix E.) More than half of these 224 journals published only one prevention article. Many prestigious academic journals have published few or no prevention papers related to mental disorders. Notably absent from representation in the bibliography or publishing only one article were journals such as *The New England Journal of Medicine, Nature, Lancet, British Journal of Medicine,* and *Science.*

Table 11.1 lists the journals that have published the most prevention articles. The editors of the bibliography identified *Prevention in Human Services* and the *Journal of Primary Prevention* as the two journals that specifically represent this field, and indeed they may be because they have the most publications, 92 and 82, respectively, accounting for approximately 22 percent of the 808 journal articles. Unfortunately, these journals are not readily accessible, nor is their existence common knowledge. During the committee's work, the *Journal of Primary Prevention* was not easy to locate, even in the academic libraries in the Washington, D.C., area. It is not indexed in MEDLINE, nor is it available at the National Library of Medicine (NLM) or the NIH library. *Prevention in Human Services* is indexed and can be found at the NLM but not at the NIH library. The limited library circulation of these two journals make them essentially unavailable except by individual subscription.

During the course of its work, the committee compiled approximately 2,000 references. This data base, quite different from the NIMH prevention bibliography, is available as part of the background materials (available as indicated in Appendix D).

The committee next wanted to determine, in general, how many publications had been made available from funded research programs related to prevention of mental disorders. To do this, a cross-referencing of research projects and published work was done for one representative funding agency. The committee used NIMH as the example and cross-referenced NIMH-funded principal investigators with the bibliography prepared for NIMH. This check did not necessarily reveal that the investigators had published findings from NIMH-supported research,

TABLE 11.1   Journals Cited Most Often in NIMH Prevention
Bibliography, 1983 to 1991

	Number of Articles
Prevention in Human Services	92
Journal of Primary Prevention	82
American Journal of Community Psychology	49
Journal of Preventive Psychiatry and Allied Disciplines	25
Journal of Drug Education	24
Personnel and Guidance Journal	23
American Journal of Orthopsychiatry	19
American Psychologist	18
Child Abuse and Neglect: The International Journal	18
Journal of Consulting and Clinical Psychology	18
Journal of School Health	15
Journal of Community Psychology	13
Community Mental Health Journal	10
Infant Mental Health Journal	10
School Psychology Review	10
Journal of the American Academy of Child and Adolescent Psychiatry	8
International Journal of the Addictions	7
Public Health Reports	7
Social Science and Medicine	7
Acta Psychiatrica Scandinavica	6
American Journal of Psychiatry	6
Health Psychology	6
Journal of Behavioral Medicine	6
Journal of Drug Issues	6
Journal of Studies on Alcohol	6

only that they had written and published material on prevention. Of the 112 grantees funded by the NIMH PRB from FY 1985 through FY 1991, 43 had entries in the bibliography. The entries totaled 168, but one researcher accounted for 28 of these. Many NIMH PRB researchers, including those whose projects are completed, have never published their findings in peer-reviewed academic journals; others have written book chapters that contain some data.

At the request of the committee, each NIMH PIRC director prepared a list of publications generated directly from support of the PIRCs. Table 11.2 shows the number and type of publications from the six centers and the number of years the centers have been funded (one center is no longer in existence). These publications were mostly in the areas of theory, methodology, and risk, but some included data from preventive intervention research trials. The publication rates generated from the

TABLE 11.2 Publications from NIMH Preventive Intervention Research Centers (as of August 1993)

	Years in Operation	Type of Publication						
		Peer-Reviewed Journal Articles*	Books*	Chapters*	Research Manuals	Bibliographies	Manuscripts Submitted	Total
Prevention Research Center, Hahnemann University	(1983–1987)	2	0	3	1	0	0	6
Michigan Prevention Research Center, University of Michigan	(1983–present)	26	0	17	17	4	5	69
Preventive Intervention Research Center for Child Health, Albert Einstein College of Medicine, Montefiore Medical Center	(1983–present)	53	2	37	0	1	10	103
Prevention Research Center, Department of Mental Hygiene, The Johns Hopkins School of Hygiene and Public Health	(1984–present)	12	1	8	3	0	5	29
Program for Prevention Research, Arizona State University	(1984–present)	53	2	15	8	0	12	90
Oregon Social Learning Center, University of Oregon	(1990–present)	5	0	1	0	0	0	6

* Published or in press.

PIRCs have been uneven. It is recognized that many preventive interventions require a long follow-up period to assess the effects of the programs and investigators are reluctant to publish findings prematurely. However, if the theory, methods, and results are not published in a timely fashion, communities and practitioners have little access to this information and cannot use it in designing their local programs.

Manuals. The advantage of manuals is that they can include details of the prevention intervention method that journals may not be interested in but which are crucial in the replication of a program by other researchers and in the adoption of the program by a community. However, preparation of manuals is very time-consuming; it is difficult to get funding for their printing and distribution; and they receive little recognition by academic departments when reviewing researchers' careers for promotion and tenure. The bibliography did not contain any entries for manuals. However, several of the researchers funded by the NIMH PRB, including those working within the PIRCs, have produced manuals. (See the abstracts in the background materials, available as indicated in Appendix D, for examples of programs that have manuals.)

Clearinghouses. There is no federal clearinghouse for published information on prevention of mental disorders. Table 11.3 lists several clearinghouses with materials relevant to prevention of mental disorders. The Center for Substance Abuse Prevention (CSAP, formerly OSAP) has one of the world's largest clearinghouses in its topic area, but little of its information deals with findings from rigorous preventive intervention research programs. The National Center on Child Abuse and Neglect (NCCAN) has a clearinghouse on child maltreatment literature, but only a small part of it is relevant to prevention. The National Prevention Coalition (NPC), a private, nonprofit organization affiliated with the National Mental Health Association, has the only clearinghouse that includes a concentrated focus on preventive intervention programs, and some of this material is research based. NPC currently has a grant from the Pew Foundation to provide program information to communities, but it does not have the capability to provide ongoing assistance on highly technical issues.

National Conferences. NIMH, NIDA, CSAP, and NIAAA hold national conferences focused on prevention, and others such as NCCAN have national conferences with some attention to prevention issues, but the crossover between agencies in each other's meetings is still rather

TABLE 11.3   Clearinghouses That Provide Information Related to the Prevention of Mental Disorders

---

CSAP National Resource Center for the Prevention of Perinatal Abuse of Alcohol and Other Drugs
Center for Substance Abuse Prevention
Substance Abuse and Mental Health Services Administration
U.S. Department of Health and Human Services
Lewin-VHI
9302 Lee Highway
Suite 310
Fairfax, VA 22031
703-218-5600

Clearinghouse on Child Abuse and Neglect Information
National Center on Child Abuse and Neglect
U.S. Department of Health and Human Services
P.O. Box 1182
Washington, DC 20013-1182
1–800-FYI-3366

Mental Health Policy Resource Center
1730 Rhode Island Avenue, NW
Suite 308
Washington, DC 20036
202-775-8826

National Clearinghouse for Alcohol and Drug Information
Center for Substance Abuse Prevention
Substance Abuse and Mental Health Services Administration
U.S. Department of Health and Human Services
P.O. Box 2345
Rockville, MD 20847-2345
301-468-2600

National Committee to Prevent Child Abuse
332 South Michigan Avenue
Suite 1600
Chicago, IL 60604
312-663-3520

National Criminal Justice Reference Service
National Institute of Justice Clearinghouse
Department of Justice
1600 Research Blvd
Dept. F
Rockville, MD 20850
1-800-851-3420

(continued)

TABLE 11.3   *(Continued)*

National Maternal and Child Health Clearinghouse
Maternal and Child Health Bureau
U.S. Department of Health and Human Services
8201 Greensboro Drive, Suite 600
McLean, VA 22102
703-821-8955

National Mental Health Association
National Prevention Coalition
1021 Prince Street
Alexandria, VA 22314-2971
703-684-7722

National Prevention Evaluation Research Collection
Center for Substance Abuse Prevention
Substance Abuse and Mental Health Services Administration
U.S. Department of Health and Human Services
Aspen Systems Corporation
1600 Research Blvd
MS-1C
Rockville, MD 20850
301-251-5180

National Resource Center on Worksite Health Promotion
777 North Capitol Street, NE
Suite 800
Washington, DC 20002
202-408-9320

ODPHP National Health Information Center
Office of Disease Prevention and Health Promotion
U.S. Department of Health and Human Services
P.O. Box 1133
Washington, DC 20013-1133
1-800-336-4797

Ontario Prevention Clearinghouse
The Ministry of Community and Social Services
415 Yonge Street
Suite 1200
Toronto, Ontario M5B 2E7
Canada
416-408-2121

Resource Center on Substance Abuse Prevention and Disability
1331 F Street, NW
Suite 800
Washington, DC 20077-1514
202-783-2900

limited. There is, however, an increasing awareness of the need for more cross-fertilization of ideas and exchange of research data.

Working Directly with Researchers. After reviewing information sources regarding prevention programs, a community may choose to seek direct consultation with prevention researchers, especially those who have conducted the program the community is interested in adopting. Currently, however, there is no formal federally funded mechanism for researchers to work directly with communities to develop preventive interventions for mental disorders. Sometimes this interaction does take place on an ad hoc basis. The NIMH PRB has recognized the need to include plans for knowledge exchange in continuation grant applications of the PIRCs. SAMHSA's Center for Mental Health Services has indicated an interest in being a link between prevention researchers and communities. However, its current Prevention and Program Development Branch was not mandated in the ADAMHA reorganization, so its continued existence is not ensured, nor does it currently have its own funding. Prevention resources have been limited to discretionary management funds from the director's office. The Centers for Disease Control and Prevention (CDC) works directly with communities through an extensive network of state public health departments on issues such as violence and suicide and has recently made a commitment to the scaling-up of the Infant Health and Development Program (see Chapters 7 and 10). The Department of Health and Human Services' Office of Disease Prevention and Health Promotion has disseminated some information on prevention of mental disorders but concentrates its efforts on physical disorders. At the state level, mental health departments or authorities are a possible mechanism for researchers to work directly with communities, but few states have made a significant commitment to prevention of mental disorders (Goldston, 1991).

Balancing Fidelity and Adaptability While Implementing the Program

Maintaining *fidelity* means that a program seeks to maintain the original tested model as closely as possible, whereas allowing *adaptability* means that a program is permitted to have leeway and is encouraged to use innovations wherever necessary to adjust to local circumstances. As mentioned in Chapter 10, Price and Lorion (1989) have proposed that the appropriate resolution of the fidelity versus adaptability dilemma requires distinguishing between the *core elements* of the intervention and the *adaptable characteristics* that can be adjusted to local circumstances.

BOX 11.1

Case Study: Replication of the Prenatal/Early Infancy Project

"The Prenatal/Early Infancy Project in Elmira, New York, demonstrated impacts on birthweight, maternal health, reduction in child abuse, and improved maternal education or employment status when it was an experimental research program, but when the local health department took it over, the program was altered. As a demonstration project, the program had multiple sources of funding, including HHS, The Robert Wood Johnson Foundation, and the W. T. Grant Foundation. When the six-year grant funding ended in 1983, the local health department absorbed the program, while changing its definition and extent of services, target population, and caseload per home visitor. As a result of these changes, all of the original home visitors left within a few months. One director of county services told us that the program was no longer achieving the same reductions in low birthweight as the original project.

"The program's absence of final evaluation data in 1983, reduced financial support, and location within the local health department all contributed to the changes. Some of these changes resulted from a reluctance to invest substantially in a program whose benefits had not yet been fully demonstrated at that time. But a difference in philosophy also prompted the change in program focus. Local officials told us there was not unanimous agreement with the research program's broad health and social service orientation and intensity. They also did not agree with limiting services to the target population of first-time mothers—particularly low-income, unmarried teen mothers—even though these women were among the ones who benefited most from the experimental program. Local officials believed that some minimum level of home-visiting services should be provided to a larger group of pregnant women, which may be diluting the overall impact of the formerly targeted, high-intensity services." (GAO, 1990).

Unfortunately, researchers have rarely described their prevention programs in these terms. Sometimes it may be possible in retrospect to distinguish between what is core technology and what is not. When these elements are not specified, it is left to the community practitioners to decide, not always with the best results. The accompanying case study (see Box 11.1) shows what can happen to a preventive intervention program when fidelity is not maintained. (See Chapter 7 for a description of the original program.)

Evaluating the Program's Effectiveness

Because the transfer of programs from research to community settings always necessitates some adaptation, if for no other reason than that new personnel are involved, the success of the program should never be taken for granted. The true test of a prevention program is not the efficacy and effectiveness in the research setting but the effectiveness in the real-life setting with the community in charge of the program. To determine that effectiveness, a program evaluation is done after the program has been completed. Ideally, evaluation is also done at multiple points along the way while the preventive services are being delivered. To increase objectivity, at least some of the program evaluators should be external to the program delivery process. The program evaluators must be involved from the beginning of the program's implementation in the community so they understand what the core elements and adaptable characteristics are. Ideally, such an evaluation not only critiques the prevention program but also provides feedback about the effects of the program on the needs and problems originally identified by the community.

Quality assurance and quality control are a major concern, especially as prevention programs are "reinvented." These programs evolve and change in response to adaptations required by real-life exigencies. Thus quality assurance issues must be included in the documentation and evaluation of prevention programs that are installed in community settings. For example, it is essential that the goals and interventions are explicitly stated in written form; that documentation of the provision or delivery of the preventive interventions in the community fits the description of the interventions in the prevention program manual and provides a paper trail to audit the program's quality; and that all documentation be readily available for review.

Evaluation of a prevention program will ensure its quality if (1) there are frequent audits of the fidelity of the interventions to their program design; (2) there are in-person reviews of the program by senior-level personnel; (3) staff are held accountable for the quality of the preventive interventions; (4) the program designers and agency leadership are held accountable for achieving desired outcomes; and (5) opportunities exist for frequent reviews by all personnel to resolve problems, suggest changes, modify program design, and provide mutual support.

Providing Feedback to the Researchers

Researchers need to receive feedback from the community about their programs—the successes, the problems, and the creative solutions developed at the local level. It is also critical that they hear about current community needs so that when research priorities are set, these needs can be taken into consideration. The community can also raise ethical issues, including selection of targeted populations, consideration of the values and interests of diverse cultures, and potential negative effects. (See the commissioned paper by Fawcett and colleagues, and the commentaries by Rothman and Gallimore, in the background materials, available as indicated in Appendix D.)

STRATEGIES FOR OVERCOMING BARRIERS TO THE KNOWLEDGE EXCHANGE PROCESS

There are many barriers to the knowledge exchange process. Barriers to the adoption of innovative and effective prevention programs include those related to the prevention programs themselves; to the practitioners, clinicians, educators, and administrators involved in the service delivery; and to the host organizations.

Barriers in the Prevention Program

One of the challenges to innovators in the prevention field will be to "package" their programs in such a way as to make them easy to disseminate and "user-friendly." User-friendliness can be increased by encouraging second- and third-generation users of the program to reinvent the program to better fit the constraints and opportunities in the local jurisdiction. Giving those responsible for implementing a prevention program permission to adapt the program components to fit local conditions—as long as the adaptations do not jeopardize the fidelity of the key, effective core elements of the program—increases the likelihood that the program will be accepted by the community.

Another element that can increase user-friendliness is "packaging." For widespread adoption of a prevention program to occur, the program needs to be packaged in a format that enables potential adopters or users to readily acquire the skills required for faithful utilization. Such packaging includes print materials with high degrees of specificity and operational description, audiovisual demonstrations of the methods in action, and well-designed workshops and training programs.

Barriers Related to the Practitioner, Clinician, Educator, or Administrator

Many attitudinal obstacles to the use of prevention programs can arise in a wide diversity of audiences. For example, prevention programs are sometimes viewed by clinicians and others in the mental health enterprise as foreign to their traditional mandate to "treat the sick." Skepticism and nihilism toward shifting resources to prevention are often expressed. Moreover, innovations in prevention programs that are complex, demanding, extended in time, and linked to a team for implementation can encounter problems in fidelity of delivery (Yeaton and Sechrest, 1981).

One of the keys to unlocking any potential opposition to engaging in preventive interventions is to provide relevant training to practitioners, educators, and other human service workers, equipping them with new knowledge, attitudes, and competences that will enable them to use the prevention programs with confidence. Thus, training the host of professional and paraprofessional interveners for prevention programs is a major requirement in elevating the status of prevention in mental health. One prerequisite for productive training or retraining of clinicians is to have trainers and consultants available who possess clinical credibility and administrative savvy and are readily recognized and respected by organization staff and managers alike. Teaching techniques—employing such methods as setting educational objectives, modeling or demonstrating the new skills to be learned, behavioral rehearsal with active coaching, and positive feedback for performance of the requisite skills (Kuehnel and Flanagan, 1984)—need to be used so that new competences can be successfully acquired and used.

Overcoming resistance among clinicians can also be achieved by a process of consultation and technical assistance similar in nature to that discussed in Chapter 10 at the point in the research cycle when trials are moved into the community. In the service arena the process before implementation of the prevention program includes (1) the identification of a relevant need in the target organization and among the organization's staff; (2) a feasibility assessment related to personal and organizational readiness for adoption of the prevention program; (3) the development of consensus for adoption of the prevention program; (4) the broadening of job descriptions and performance appraisals to include competences related to preventive interventions; and (5) the development of an implementation strategy.

Barriers Within the Host Organization

To overcome bureaucratic and other inertia within the institutions that will be the legitimate purveyors of prevention programs, a sine qua non is to have the active support of the host organization—from top management to local unit chiefs and team leaders. Support must be translated into oral and written endorsements of prevention as a priority within the organization's mission statement and long-term goals; concordance with the philosophy and basic assumptions of prevention; and allocation of resources (including time, staff, space, and equipment), as enunciated in annual reports and statements of goals, that matches the priorities and support needs of the prevention program.

Also vital for successful implementation of prevention programming is the presence, within the organization, of an advocate of prevention who is a credible formal or informal leader in the organization. This person coordinates the initial efforts to introduce an innovative prevention program, consults with the experts who are disseminating the program, communicates with top management as well as with line-level staff to solve problems related to implementation, and offers training and encouragement to those applying the prevention program.

Staff roles must be defined by the functions explicitly described by the prevention program, and conflicts involving overlapping roles and disciplinary differences—as can arise on an interdisciplinary team— should be openly discussed and resolved. Resolution of staff conflicts can be facilitated by reconciling job descriptions with the competences needed for delivering the prevention program.

IMPROVING COMMUNITY ACCESS TO RESEARCH KNOWLEDGE

As described above, several existing federal and state institutions— such as SAMHSA's CSAP and CMHS, the Office of Disease Prevention and Health Promotion, the Centers for Disease Control and Prevention, and state mental health departments—are currently serving as brokers to communities of information provided by prevention researchers on intervention programs related to mental disorders. However, these efforts have been scattered, without mandate, and "catch-as-catch-can." Perhaps the utilization of prevention programs in mental health can take cues from successful experiences in technology transfer found in other areas of our society. For example, in agriculture, field agents of a state university's extension services work hand-in-hand with farmers to help them adopt new seeds, fertilizers, pesticides, equipment, and planting and harvesting techniques. Another example comes from the pharmaceutical industry, where "detail" sales representatives visit physicians in their offices and hospitals to provide information on new drugs and facilitate their adoption.

Any national research agenda for prevention of mental disorders will have to include the development of mechanisms for promoting the proper utilization and application of prevention technologies that have been validated in confirmatory, replication, and large-scale field trials. One model that could be considered is the concept of research knowl-

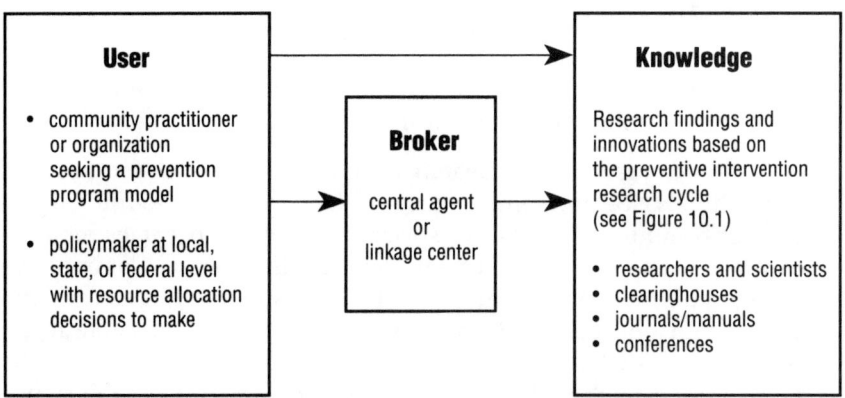

FIGURE 11.1 The process by which practitioners and policymakers access knowledge based on prevention research. Length of arrow indicates relative ease of access.

edge exchange centers, adapted from work by Liberman and Phipps (1987), which could be established regionally or nationally to serve as the broker, linkage center, or central agent between prevention researchers and scientists on the one hand, and practitioners, educators, administrators, and policymakers on the other. Figure 11.1 depicts a model that shows how such a center could provide this link.

Among the training and consulting roles that such a center would fill are (1) identifying new prevention programs from the scientific literature, clearinghouses, and conferences and from ongoing communication and liaison with innovators in the prevention field; (2) reviewing the quality of evidence regarding efficacy and effectiveness provided from the programs; (3) assisting "user communities" to choose and adapt prevention programs to fit their local constraints and resources and to ensure fidelity to the core characteristics of the program; (4) facilitating communities' evaluation of their prevention programs; and (5) using the feedback gained from working with the communities to assist researchers in refining and improving their prevention innovations so they can be ever more effective, efficient, and practical.

Of course, the community could go directly to the researchers and data sources themselves, but access to knowledge about effective preventive intervention research programs may be easier through a linkage center or broker. The amount and quality of interpersonal contacts between the linkage center or broker and the recipient organization may be critical to the successful adoption of the preventive program by the community.

CONCLUSION

The committee's examination of the knowledge exchange process uncovered a number of points worthy of special attention:

• When a prevention research program is adopted for use as a community service program, issues of fidelity are paramount. Consideration of community needs and special populations becomes moot if a program is changed so much that it no longer is effective. Communities must be informed about the hazards of assuming that a program effective with one population will necessarily be generalizable to another.

• Increased methodological rigor must be applied to the design of preventive intervention research programs over the next decade. This is likely to lead to more articles being published in high-quality journals.

• Many research findings relevant to the prevention of mental disorders never have a chance to make an impact because they are never made known to the practitioners, educators, administrators, and policy makers who would use them. A coordinated plan for dissemination of the fruits of prevention research is needed, whether it be through existing institutions or newly created brokering or linkage centers.

• In order for communities to learn how to obtain and make the best possible use of the research knowledge, they will need the help of a new breed of prevention program facilitator who can bridge research and practice.

REFERENCES

Battista, R. N.; Fletcher, S. W. (1988) Making recommendations on preventive practices: Methodological issues. In: R. N. Battista and R. S. Lawrence, Eds. Implementing Preventive Services. Suppl. to the American Journal of Preventive Medicine; 4(4). New York, NY: Oxford University Press; 53–67.

Buckner, J. C.; Trickett, E. J.; Corse, S. J. (1985) Primary Prevention in Mental Health: An Annotated Bibliography. Rockville, MD: DHHS Pub. No. (ADM) 85–1405.

GAO (Government Accounting Office). (1990) Home Visiting: A promising early intervention strategy for at-risk families. Report to the Chairman, Subcommittee on Labor, Health and Human Services, Education, and Related Agencies, Committee on Appropriations, U.S. Senate. GAO/HRD-90-93.

Goldston, S. E. (1991) A survey of prevention activities in state mental health authorities. Professional Psychology: Research and Practice; 22(4): 315–321.

Kuehnel, T. G.; Flanagan, S. G. (1984) Training the professionals: Guidelines for effective continuing education workshops. The Behavior Therapist; 7: 85–87.

Liberman, R. P.; Phipps, C. C. (1987) Innovative treatment and rehabilitation techniques for the chronic mentally ill. In: W. W. Merringer and G. Hannah, Eds. The Chronic Mental Patient—II. Washington, DC: American Psychiatric Press; 93–130.

Price, R. H.; Lorion, R. P. (1989) Prevention programming as organizational reinvention: From research to implementation. In: D. Shaffer, I. Philips, and N.B. Enzer, Eds. Prevention of Mental Disorders, Alcohol and other Drug Use in Children and Adolescents. Rockville, MD: Department of Health and Human Services.

Spitzer, W. O. (1979) Report of the Task Force on the Periodic Health Examination. Canadian Medical Association Journal; 121: 1193–1254.

Trickett, E. J.; Dahiyat, C.; Selby, P. (in press) Primary Prevention in Mental Health: An Annotated Bibliography. Rockville, MD: Department of Health and Human Services.

Yeaton, W. H.; Sechrest, L. (1981) Critical dimensions in the choice and maintenance of successful treatments: Strengths, integrity, effectiveness. Journal of Consulting and Clinical Psychology; 49: 156–167.

12

Infrastructure for Prevention: Funding, Personnel, and Coordination

Like any other field, preventive intervention research cannot thrive without providing for its infrastructure. What levels of funding and personnel are necessary to implement the prevention research activities outlined in the earlier chapters? How can the entire enterprise best be coordinated? To begin to answer these questions, the committee first reviewed the existing federal presence in the prevention of mental disorders. It determined which agencies have relevant research and service programs and reviewed the funding, personnel, and training resources supporting these programs. The committee then reviewed current coordination efforts among federal agencies.

FUNDING

Estimates of funding levels for research on prevention of mental disorders were difficult for the committee to obtain for several reasons. First, the definitions of prevention and prevention research vary immensely across and within agencies. Basic research, risk identification studies, preventive interventions, treatment, and maintenance are all included in the U.S. Public Health Service's definition of "prevention research." Some agencies use this inclusive definition, and others do not. (See Chapter 2 for more discussion of this issue.)

Second, the definition of mental disorder varies. Although many agencies are doing work in this area, some of them do not see their activities as having anything to do with "mental disorders" because they use a narrow definition of that term. A broader definition, for example, would include substance abuse and dependence. Other agencies use legal terminology such as "delinquency" rather than mental disorder diagnoses such as conduct disorder, although the terms often apply to the same people. Once it is generally acknowledged that precursors to mental disorders include behavioral dysfunction and clusters of serious psychological symptoms that do not yet meet full criteria for diagnosis, it is expected that more agencies will acknowledge their role in preventing these mental health problems. Moreover, agencies actively involved in prevention of physical illnesses, such as the National Institutes of Health (NIH) and the Centers for Disease Control and Prevention (CDC), often do not appreciate that an important outcome of their work is reduction of psychiatric morbidity. Thus the psychiatric consequences of preventive interventions for physical disorders need to be emphasized. With more consensus on these definitional issues, estimates of actual funding levels will be more easily obtained.

Third, data retrieval systems for information on research funding are difficult to access, inadequate, and sometimes misleading.*

Data from an NIH Retrieval System

The committee reviewed data from the Research Documentation Section, Information Systems Branch of the Division of Research Grants at NIH. The division supplied Computer Retrieval of Information on Scientific Projects (CRISP) files of funded prevention research across NIH and the former Alcohol, Drug Abuse, and Mental Health Administration (ADAMHA; which contained the three research institutes, the National Institute of Mental Health (NIMH), the National Institute on Drug Abuse (NIDA), and the National Institute on Alcohol Abuse and Alcoholism (NIAAA)). In the CRISP files, prevention research is classified by type: mental disorder prevention, alcoholism prevention, and drug abuse prevention. It is also classified by emphasis level, that is, the relevance of the indexing terms to the aims and objectives of the project. The emphasis codes are P = primary, S = secondary, T = tertiary, and M = main. (These codes should not be confused with terms used to describe types of intervention within the public health classification

---

*The Prevention Research Branches (PRBs) of NIMH, NIDA, and NIAAA initially found it difficult to comply with the committee's requests for lists of funded research grants back to 1988. The emphasis in the branches is on the current funding year, and hard-copy archives are not kept officially for more than a couple of years. (If they are, it is often by an efficient long-time support staff person.) Computers in the agency budget offices have eased these storage problems, and computerized lists are available.

system discussed in Chapter 2.) Main (M) emphasis codes are used only for parent projects of multiproject awards and are equivalent to the primary (P) emphasis level. Therefore, in the committee's review, main and primary levels were combined.

All items that appear in a CRISP printout are peer reviewed when they are proposals. However, the type of peer review required varies according to whether the monies are intended for a grant or a contract. A contract proposal is not reviewed by the same standards or mechanisms as a grant proposal. The contract proposals are reviewed through a process called a secondary review, in which the review committee is composed of a certain percentage of NIH personnel and a certain percentage of outside experts.

The difficulty in assessing the funding commitments by federal agencies to prevention research is dramatized by the CRISP recording system at NIH. The CRISP system has a number of serious problems when used to evaluate research programs. First, when funded projects come into the system, they are classified by a staff person. Classifications are not consistent, in part because a written definition of prevention has not been available for guidance. Second, the data are not complete. For example, the CRISP lists of research projects did not match the portfolios of funded grants supplied by the relevant program officers at NIMH and NIDA. Only 24 of 80 grants funded from 1988 to 1992 by the NIMH Prevention Research Branch (PRB) were even listed by CRISP as having a main/primary area of emphasis on prevention. Third, the same project can be classified in more than one prevention area, for example, alcoholism prevention and mental disorder prevention. Fourth, there is no limitation on how many times a particular project can be classified by emphasis code. For example, in fiscal year (FY) 1991, 41 research projects (which were funded by NIMH, NIDA, NIAAA, the National Institute of Child Health and Human Development (NICHD), and the National Center for Research Resources (NCRR)) were identified as having a main/primary emphasis in mental disorder prevention. The projects totaled $13,675,607. The numbers of other primary, secondary, and tertiary areas of emphasis that each particular grant was classified as having were counted. These included areas as diverse as "psychometrics" to "social control" to "immunopathology." The 41 projects had 264 primary areas of emphasis in addition to mental disorder prevention, 312 secondary areas, and 114 tertiary areas.

The committee concluded that the CRISP system can miss directly relevant projects, on the one hand, and also can produce extensive multiple counting of projects on the other, which can result in misleadingly large estimates of efforts in a particular area. However, CRISP is one of the few available sources of data on prevention research projects. Table 12.1 shows the dollars awarded and the number of research projects and subprojects for mental disorder prevention, alcoholism prevention, and drug addiction prevention by NIH and ADAMHA. All of these data were compiled from CRISP printouts.

A few of the agencies identified by CRISP as having scientific projects in mental disorder prevention, drug addiction prevention, or alcoholism prevention have received only contracts, not grants. For example, see the column on drug addiction prevention in Table 12.1 for FY 1992. The Office of Substance Abuse Prevention (OSAP; now the Center for Substance Abuse Prevention (CSAP)) had 22 projects or subprojects totaling $102,112,353. Upon examination, all of these projects were contracts. The Office for Treatment Improvement (OTI) also had only contracts. NIAAA and NIMH, on the other hand, had only grants. NIDA had 53 grants and 11 contracts. In total, 43 percent of the FY 1992 drug addiction prevention projects were contracts, not subject to the same standard of review as grants. They totaled $135,247,179. In contrast, the grant monies totaled $20,807,047.

From the CRISP data, the following points are clear:

• Research on prevention of mental disorders, alcoholism, or drug addiction is not the domain of any one agency; rather, many agencies are involved.

• Expenditures for research on prevention of alcoholism and drug addiction have been far more than for research on prevention of other types of mental disorders.

• OSAP was created in 1990. The following year, NIMH's role in research on the prevention of drug addiction and alcoholism was drastically decreased.

• OSAP is not listed as having had any role in research on the prevention of mental disorders, but it has received far more money for research on alcoholism prevention and drug addiction prevention than any other office or institute within the former ADAMHA or NIH.

• The type of peer review and the number of grants versus contracts vary enormously across the agencies.

Data from an ADAMHA Draft Report and from the PRBs

The ADAMHA Reorganization Act of 1992 transferred the three ADAMHA research institutes (NIMH, NIDA, and NIAAA) to NIH and established the Substance Abuse and Mental Health Services Adminis-

TABLE 12.1 Prevention Research Projects Funded by Agencies of NIH and the Former ADAMHA According to CRISP Definitions and Files

	Mental Disorder Prevention (1838 8404*)		Alcoholism Prevention (0080 8999*)		Drug Addiction Prevention (0962 7764*)	
	Dollars Awarded	Number of Projects and Subprojects	Dollars Awarded	Number of Projects and Subprojects	Dollars Awarded	Number of Projects and Subprojects
FY 1988						
NCRR	71,361	2	—	—	—	—
NIAAA	269,977	1	7,444,876	38	1,204,549	6
NIDA	245,143	1	955,839	5	12,868,727	44
NIDR	77,370	1	—	—	—	—
NIMH	4,596,638	18	5,467,078	2	5,983,948	3
NINDS	186,137	1	—	—	—	—
Totals	5,446,626	24	13,867,793	45	20,057,224	53
FY 1989						
DM-BHP	74,457	1	—	—	—	—
NCNR	271,759	1	—	—	—	—
NCRR	112,927	3	—	—	—	—
NIAAA	238,459	1	8,561,792	43	1,208,791	6
NICHD	121,729	1	—	—	—	—
NIDA	339,425	1	1,124,714	6	19,784,468	52
NIMH	5,253,651	22	7,015,665	17	7,532,535	18
Totals	6,412,407	30	16,702,171	66	28,525,794	76
FY 1990						
NCNR	151,814	1	—	—	—	—
NIAAA	343,634	1	12,711,923	51	1,790,248	8
NICHD	380,392	2	—	—	—	—
NIDA	381,426	1	3,664,251	9	31,894,783	73
NIMH	9,073,690	28	7,015,665	17	7,532,535	18
OSAP	—	—	37,802,237	6	44,001,150	10
Totals	10,330,956	33	61,194,076	83	85,218,716	109
FY 1991						
NCNR	—	—	25,000	1	—	—
NCRR	18,089	1	—	—	—	—
NIAAA	237,431	1	13,090,473	44	1,753,583	6
NICHD	1,654,804	4	—	—	—	—
NIDA	394,493	1	1,773,918	5	30,498,900	64
NIMH	11,370,790	34	487,432	5	487,432	5
OSAP	—	—	66,139,480	11	71,849,809	14
OTI	—	—	—	—	564,542	2
Totals	13,675,607	41	81,516,303	66	105,154,266	91

(continued)

TABLE 12.1 *(Continued)*

	Mental Disorder Prevention (1838 8404[a])		Alcoholism Prevention (0080 8999[a])		Drug Addiction Prevention (0962 7764[a])	
	Dollars Awarded	Number of Projects and Subprojects	Dollars Awarded	Number of Projects and Subprojects	Dollars Awarded	Number of Projects and Subprojects
FY 1992						
NCNR	194,672	1	25,000	1	—	—
NCRR	—	—	49,866	1	—	—
NIAAA	—	—	13,915,829	47	1,540,862	5
NICHD	1,773,029	3	—	—	—	—
NIDA	373,728	1	2,793,995	6	32,396,908	64
NIMH	13,444,251	40	487,432	5	487,432	5
OSAP	—	—	93,548,289	19	102,112,353	22
OTI	—	—	18,952,129	14	19,516,671	16
Totals	15,785,680	45	129,772,540	93	156,054,226	112

Abbreviations used are as follows:
  DM-BHP - Division of Medicine - Bureau of Health Professions
  NCNR - National Center for Nursing Research
  NCRR - National Center for Research Resources
  NIAAA - National Institute on Alcohol Abuse and Alcoholism
  NICHD - National Institute of Child Health and Human Development
  NIDA - National Institute on Drug Abuse
  NIDR - National Institute of Dental Research
  NIMH - National Institute of Mental Health
  NINDS - National Institute of Neurological Disorders and Stroke
  OSAP - Office of Substance Abuse Prevention
  OTI - Office for Treatment Improvement
[a]Codes used by CRISP to identify areas of emphasis.

NOTE: See text for problems related to definitions and classification in the NIH Computer Retrieval of Information on Scientific Projects (CRISP) system.

tration (SAMHSA) with the following three agencies: the Center for Substance Abuse Treatment (CSAT), CSAP (formerly OSAP), and the Center for Mental Health Services (CMHS) (see Table 1.1 in Chapter 1).* This division between research and services entailed intense debate, and the advantages and disadvantages created by the reorganization are likely to be reviewed for many years to come.

The original ADAMHA legislation required ADAMHA to prepare a report on its prevention activities every three years and submit this to

---

*This reorganization occurred in the middle of the committee's review of the status of prevention research.

TABLE 12.2   Prevention Activities Funded by NIMH, NIDA, and NIAAA (dollars)

	NIMH		NIDA		NIAAA	
	Total Institute	PRB[a]	Total Institute	PRB[a]	Total Institute	PRB[a]
1989	57,758,000	7,849,953	132,866,000	7,484,255	14,852,000	9,641,271
1990	77,945,000	15,153,315	168,853,000	16,612,418	21,337,000	16,521,839
1991	93,062,000	18,866,198	166,460,000	19,961,232	27,220,000	19,254,403
1992	—[b]	21,262,514	—[b]	19,731,873	—[b]	23,166,210

[a]Prevention Research Branch.

[b]No ADAMHA report was prepared for Congress.

NOTE: Figures for 1989–1991 totals are from the draft ADAMHA "Report to Congress on Prevention Activities 1989–1991." Figures for the NIMH and NIDA PRBs were compiled from the lists of grantees provided by the PRBs. Figures for the NIAAA PRB came from the NIAAA Budget Office. See text for problems related to definitions of prevention.

Congress. In 1992 a draft report was prepared by the ADAMHA director and submitted to the Secretary of the Department of Health and Human Services (DHHS). The committee used the figures from this draft report in its review of prevention. However, in 1993 the report was withdrawn; it was not submitted to Congress or released to the public.* This was because the legislative requirement for the report had been repealed by section 101 of the ADAMHA Reorganization Act of 1992.

The draft report included ADAMHA prevention activities and expenditures during fiscal years 1989, 1990, and 1991, including extramural and intramural research, service demonstrations, professional training and education, block grants, and miscellaneous activities, but excluding HIV/AIDS prevention. Prevention expenditures were reported as $382,529,000 in 1989, $643,792,000 in 1990, and $749,093,000 in 1991.

Table 12.2 shows the prevention expenditures reported by ADAMHA for each of the research institutes in 1989, 1990, and 1991. It also shows the grants funded by the Prevention Research Branches within those institutes during those years and 1992. These data came from the PRBs directly, not from the ADAMHA report. The differences in the expenditures are substantial. If the figures are accurate, most prevention activities took place outside the PRBs. However, this difference in reported expenditures dramatizes the problem of definition of prevention of mental disorders and the immense discrepancy in

---

*The committee acquired the report through the use of the Freedom of Information Act.

expenditures between service and research and between different types of research.

The ADAMHA report stated that during 1991 OSAP expenditures for prevention were $271,465,000, yet CRISP reported OSAP as having spent $71,849,809 on drug abuse prevention research and $66,139,480 on alcoholism prevention research during the same year. This difference reflects the amounts spent on services versus research, with the CRISP data reporting on research.

The Prevention Research Branches within the three research institutes—NIDA, NIAAA, and NIMH—vary in their research emphasis. Within the NIAAA PRB, there is both risk identification research and preventive intervention research. The branch increasingly has focused on youth and young adults, women, the elderly, and minorities. It has examined the effects of regulatory policies within the community and is interested in doing research on alcohol-related violence. The NIDA PRB is within the Division of Epidemiology and Prevention Research. The division has conducted several large, well-known epidemiological studies, but several of those have now been moved to SAMHSA; the division continues to sponsor risk identification research, and preventive intervention research at the individual, social environment, and community levels. A new initiative within this PRB is an effort to create prevention centers focused on testing culturally and ethnically sensitive preventive interventions. NIMH conducts prevention-related activities throughout its branches, but most of its preventive intervention research is within its PRB.

Only two of the three PRBs—those at NIDA and NIMH—have their own centers for prevention research. These centers are specialized, focusing on topics across the life span. NIAAA also has one, but it is not part of the branch. NIAAA's Prevention Research Center, in Berkeley, California, conducts basic research on identification of risk factors that contribute to alcoholism, including factors in the individual, family, peer group, work site, and community. It has initiated community preventive intervention trials to assess the effects of changes in availability of alcohol, such as minimum age of purchase and service interventions at restaurants and bars. Table 12.3 provides the history of funding levels for the NIMH prevention centers, called Preventive Intervention Research Centers (PIRCs), which were begun in 1983. Table 12.4 provides a similar history for the NIDA prevention centers, called Prevention Research Centers, which were begun in 1987. Overall, these centers in both institutes started with relatively modest support, and their current annual budgets average about $1 million per year per center. A major difference in the centers is that those at NIMH all focus on preventive

TABLE 12.3 Support Received for the NIMH PRB Preventive Intervention Research Centers (PIRCs) (dollars)

Fiscal Year	Hahnemann University (P50MH38425[a,b])	University of Michigan (P50MH39246[a])	Albert Einstein College of Medicine (P50MH38280[a])	Johns Hopkins University (P50MH38725[a])	Arizona State University (P50MH39246[a])	Oregon Social Learning Center (P50MH46690[a])
1983	289,000	245,814	461,124	—	—	—
1984	367,121	330,578	339,263	407,788	307,350	—
1985	295,750	263,007	506,829	439,761	282,361	—
1986	—	434,330	418,295	398,475	260,088	—
1987	—	497,988	497,948	427,810	312,207	—
1988	—	486,791	—	—	272,405	—
1989	—	130,000	806,500	—	130,000	—
1990	—	1,158,135	853,838	825,296	982,157	742,298
1991	—	807,757	925,456	1,102,418	765,815	1,099,980
1992	—	527,603	836,481	1,490,000	1,115,035	1,296,270
1993	—	722,947	672,145	1,637,851	1,282,436	1,348,120
Totals	951,871	5,604,950	6,317,879	6,729,399	5,709,854	4,486,668

[a]Research grant numbers.
[b]Discontinued.

NOTE: Figures are from the NIMH Budget Office.

TABLE 12.4 Support Received for the NIDA Epidemiology and Prevention Research Centers (dollars)

Fiscal Year	University of Colorado[a] (P50DA05131[b])	Western Psychiatric Institute, Pittsburgh, Pennsylvania[a] (P50DA05605[b])	Center for Prevention Research, Lexington, Kentucky (P50DA05312[b])	Columbia University (P50DA05321[b])	Colorado State University (P50DA07074[b])	Cornell University Medical College (P50DA07656[b])
1987	—	—	526,091	—	—	—
1988	399,500	—	527,965	658,451	—	—
1989	397,873	933,040	564,275	714,948	—	—
1990	414,671	952,960	431,299	676,427	779,485	—
1991	—	1,139,478	425,593	628,645	1,074,900	747,912
1992	844,653	1,200,835	1,003,734	844,820	1,072,500	1,003,626
1993	832,478	1,280,931	1,133,323	—	1,063,250	1,218,000
Totals	2,889,175	5,507,244	4,612,280	3,523,291	3,990,135	2,969,538

[a]Focused on epidemiology and risk research, not on preventive intervention research.
[b]Research grant numbers.

NOTE: Figures are from the NIDA Budget Office.

TABLE 12.5 Breakdown of NIMH Prevention Research Branch
Budget for FY 1992

	Number of Grants	Grant Amount (dollars)
Prevention of socioemotional problems among high-risk infants and toddlers	8	2,231,974
Prevention of conduct disorder in school-age children (including two PIRCs)	11	6,004,495
Prevention of anxiety and depression resulting from stressful life conditions (including three PIRCs)	15	4,498,796
Enhancement of coping mechanisms	2	202,664
Methodology	3	282,839
Research Scientist Award	2	197,618
Research training	3	206,136
Clinical training	19	1,112,993
Research demonstrations		
Prevention of conduct disorder	3	5,461,425*
Prevention of youth suicide	3	1,063,574
Suicide research conference	1	0
Totals	70	21,262,514

*This total includes a RO1 research grant of $1,102,000.

NOTE: Figures are from the NIMH Prevention Research Branch.

intervention research, whereas at NIDA two focus on risk research and four focus on preventive intervention research. These latter four are within the PRB.

The breakdown of the NIMH PRB budget for FY 1992 is shown in Table 12.5. Most of the research grants are in three important areas: socioemotional problems among high-risk infants and toddlers, conduct disorder in school-age children, and anxiety and depression resulting from stressful life conditions. Half of the budget supports RO1 research and research demonstrations in the area of conduct disorder. (The research demonstrations are not to be confused with large-scale field trials as described in Chapter 10.) Very few grants are awarded to research on enhancement of coping mechanisms or on the development of methodology, although some methods development does occur within the PIRCs. Five times more is spent on clinical training than on research training. A review of the clinical training grants showed them to be part of the Depression Awareness, Recognition and Treatment Program, which is clearly treatment rather than prevention by the committee's definition.

Overview of Government Involvement in Preventive Intervention Research

Research and services related to the prevention of mental disorders occur across a diverse array of federal and state agencies. Often this is not recognized or acknowledged by the agencies. Table 12.6 lists the federal agencies that are involved, though to varying degrees, in

TABLE 12.6   Federal Agencies Involved in Preventive Intervention Research and/or Preventive Intervention Services Related to Mental Disorders

Department of Agriculture

Department of Defense

Department of Education

Department of Health and Human Services
  Administration for Children and Families
    Administration on Children, Youth and Families
    Head Start Bureau
    National Center on Child Abuse and Neglect
  Public Health Service
    Centers for Disease Control and Prevention
    Health Resources and Services Administration
      Maternal and Child Health Bureau
    Indian Health Service
    National Institutes of Health
      National Center for Nursing Research
      National Institute on Aging
      National Institute on Alcohol Abuse and Alcoholism[a]
      National Institute of Child Health and Human Development
      National Institute on Drug Abuse[a]
      National Institute of Mental Health[a]
      Office of Disease Prevention
    Office of Health Promotion and Disease Prevention
    Substance Abuse and Mental Health Services Administration
      Center for Mental Health Services
      Center for Substance Abuse Prevention[a,b]

Department of Housing and Urban Development

Department of Justice
  Office of Juvenile Justice and Delinquency Prevention

Department of Transportation

Department of Veterans Affairs

[a]Formerly under the Alcohol, Drug Abuse, and Mental Health Administration (ADAMHA).
[b]Formerly the Office for Substance Abuse Prevention (OSAP).

preventive intervention research and/or services related to mental disorders. This compilation is based on direct contacts with agencies and reviews of agency program plans and annual reports and is arranged in alphabetical order.

The overall DHHS support for all types of prevention activities related to both physical and mental disorders in FY 1991 was $14,753,933,000 (DHHS, 1992). In Table 12.7 the funding levels for 3 of 23 priority areas—alcohol and other drugs, mental health and mental disorders, and violence and abusive behaviors—are given for DHHS agencies (DHHS, 1992). Unfortunately, these do not separate services and research.

The Maternal and Child Health Bureau within DHHS is an agency well-known for its services to women and their children. It is presented here as an example of an agency that is not well recognized as contributing to prevention of mental disorders. A careful review of its grants revealed otherwise (see Box 12.1).

Private Foundations

Many private foundations also support prevention services and research related to mental disorders. Some of the better-known examples include American Express Foundation, Ford Foundation, William T. Grant Foundation, Conrad N. Hilton, The J.M. Foundation, Henry Kaiser Family Foundation, Lilly Endowment, Inc., Meyer Memorial Trust, Annie E. Casey Foundation, The Robert Wood Johnson Foundation, the Carnegie Corporation, the W.K. Kellogg Foundation, The Pew Charitable Trusts, and the Colorado Trust.

Conclusions

Rational planning for the nation's prevention research agenda requires much more accurate monitoring and reporting of prevention activities related to mental disorders. The Computer Retrieval of Information on Scientific Projects (CRISP) system has resulted in incomplete and inaccurate data with extensive multiple counting of research projects. In 1991 DHHS reported expenditures of approximately $2 billion for prevention activities related to mental disorders and abuse of alcohol and other drugs. According to the draft ADAMHA report, the funding of prevention activities was substantial in 1991—$749,093,000. ADAMHA's $749 million is likely to be incorporated into DHHS's $2 billion, but it is not clear that they were using identical definitions of prevention activities. In contrast to both of these large figures, the total 1992 budget of the three Prevention Research Branches at NIMH, NIAAA,

TABLE 12.7 Department of Health and Human Services Agencies Reporting Prevention Activities in Priority Areas, 1991 (dollars)

	Alcohol and Other Drugs	Mental Health and Mental Disorders	Violent and Abusive Behavior	Overall Prevention Budget[a]
Public Health Service				
Food and Drug Administration	6,500,000	0	0	669,100,000
Health Resources and Services Administration	2,331,000	690,000	319,000	1,113,211,000
Indian Health Service	69,747,000	25,462,000	0	706,000,000
Centers for Disease Control	2,600,000	0	5,600,000	1,134,116,000
National Institutes of Health	2,840,000	6,112,000	1,652,000	1,927,963,000
Alcohol, Drug Abuse, and Mental Health Administration	426,703,000	43,134,000	5,364,000	753,907,000
Agency for Health Care Policy and Research	382,000	1,455,000	63,000	45,195,000
Office of the Assistant Secretary for Health	0	0	0	46,148,000
Total Public Health Service	511,103,000	76,853,000	12,998,000	6,395,640,000
Health Care Financing Administration	190,000,000	1,216,000,000	0	7,546,600,000
Administration for Children and Families	49,372,000	1,235,000	29,250,000	811,693,000
Total resources reported in 1991 for prevention (DHHS)[b]	750,475,000	1,294,088,000	42,248,000	14,753,933,000

[a]The overall prevention budget includes the three priority areas listed plus an additional 20 priority areas.
[b]Estimated.

SOURCE: Figures obtained from *Prevention '91/'92: Federal Programs and Progress* (DHHS, 1992).

BOX 12.1
Maternal and Child Health Bureau

The Maternal and Child Health Bureau (MCHB) is part of the Health Resources and Services Administration (HRSA) within the Public Health Service of the Department of Health and Human Services. In FY 1991, MCHB had a budget of approximately $637 million. Of this, $500 million was allocated for block grants to the states. The Maternal and Child Health Services Block Grant under Title V of the Social Security Act supports activities, through state block grants and project grants, to improve the health status of mothers and children.

Funds are used for the purpose of enabling states: (a) to assure mothers and children (particularly those with low income or with limited availability of health services) access to quality maternal and child health services; (b) to reduce infant mortality and the incidence of preventable diseases and handicapping conditions among children, to reduce the need for inpatient and long-term care services, to increase the number of children appropriately immunized and the number of low income children receiving health assessments and follow-up diagnostic and treatment services, and otherwise to promote the health of mothers and children (especially by providing preventive and primary care services for low income children, and prenatal, delivery, and postpartum care for low income mothers); (c) to provide rehabilitation services for blind and disabled individuals under age 16 receiving benefits under Title XVI of the Social Security Act; and (d) to provide services for locating, and for medical, surgical, corrective, and other services, and care for, and facilities for diagnosis, hospitalization, and aftercare for children with special health care needs or who are suffering from conditions leading to such status.

During the 1980s the MCHB state block grants were largely unregulated by the federal government. However, as a result of new legislation in 1989, the directing of the states' monies was shifted and placed under more federal control. This shift was made "to improve states' planning, accountability, and targeting of federal funds to priority populations" (OBRA, 1989). Previously, the states only had to submit a report of intended expenditures to receive the block grant monies. Now, obtaining this money entails an application process, state and federal reporting requirements, and submission of annual reports for review, as well as several other provisions as outlined in the Omnibus Budget Reconciliation Act of 1989.

The remaining 1991 budget monies constitute the MCHB discretionary fund. The formula for this, which is set by Congress, is 15 percent of all appropriated state block grant funds plus an extra 12.75 percent of state block grant funds over $600 million. The discretionary monies are used for service demonstration programs, research, implementation programs, and training. Included within these monies are programs of special projects of regional and national significance (SPRANS), as well as Community Integrated Services Systems (CISS). Additionally, support is provided for emergency medical services for children, pediatrics AIDS health care demonstration projects, and Healthy Start (not the Hawaii Healthy Start program described in Chapter 7).

Every year, MCHB publishes the abstracts of the active projects supported with discretionary funding. A review of the 1991 book, which included 591

continued

abstracts and an index, provided an overview of the breadth of the work done through MCHB. In 1991, $8 to $10 million was used for research.

Much of the discretionary work of MCHB is highly relevant to the issues of promotion of mental health and prevention of mental disorders. However, the agency does not conceptualize these issues in this way. The index of the 1991 book of abstracts does not include some of the main terms and definitions used in this report. For example, there is no mention of mental disorders, mental health, risk, risk reduction, mental health promotion, or universal/selective/indicated preventive interventions. On the other hand, listings in the index do include substance abuse (101), alcohol (18), injury prevention (21), preventive health care (21), mother-child interaction (10), health promotion (9), child abuse (4), child neglect (12), behavioral disorders (3), behavioral problems (1), violence (7), and low birthweight (32). All of these issues are related to mental health and mental disorders, especially within a conceptual framework of risk reduction.

Many of the service demonstration projects, implementation projects, and research projects of MCHB are preventive in orientation, whereas others are more treatment oriented. However, the grants are not categorized according to this distinction. Using this committee's definitions, some grants were selective preventive interventions, and others were indicated preventive interventions.

Research grants clearly had been required to meet standards of methodological rigor, but the service demonstrations and implementation projects varied along a continuum of evaluation rigor. Although some approached high standards of design and evaluation, others provided "process evaluations" of questionable value.

MCHB has collaborated with other federal agencies and private foundations in its use of discretionary funds, including the former ADAMHA, the Centers for Disease Control and Prevention, the National Institutes of Health, and the Administration for Children, Youth and Families. Two research projects that MCHB has co-funded with private foundations stand out as exemplary preventive interventions that demonstrate how preventive interventions can have effects on both physical and mental health. These are the Infant Health and Development Program, which was conducted at eight sites, and the Study of Home Visitation for Mothers and Children, in Memphis, Tennessee, which is a replication study to validate the findings of the previously completed Prenatal/Early Infancy Project, in Elmira, New York, which also received MCHB support. (These programs are reviewed in more depth in Chapters 7 and 11.)

The ADAMHA Reorganization Act authorized the Health Resources and Services Administration under Title IV to make grants to provide services to children of substance abusers and families in which a member is a substance abuser. The services to children are to include periodic evaluation for developmental, psychological, and medical problems as well as preventive counseling services and counseling related to the witnessing of chronic violence. Evaluation of the effectiveness of these programs is to include assessment of the prevention of adverse health conditions in children of substance abusers. HRSA was also authorized under Title V to make grants for home visiting services for at-risk families. Services are to be targeted to pregnant women at risk of delivering infants with a health or developmental condition. Services are also to be provided to children under age 3 who are experiencing or are at risk of (1) health or developmental complications or (2) child abuse or neglect. Again, evaluation to determine effectiveness was stipulated in the act. Although support for these services has not been appropriated, the act clearly has recognized the importance of HRSA's role in prevention of problems that are both physical and psychological. It would be beneficial—and not difficult—to employ rigorous methodological standards in these evaluations.

In light of the findings from this review, the committee makes the following suggestions:

- MCHB should be recognized for the critical role it has had and should continue to have in the prevention of mental disorders. More research needs to be done on the effects of risk reduction during gestation, infancy, and early childhood, and on the possible long-term effects on the reduction of new cases of mental illness. MCHB has access to and acceptance from high-risk populations because of its programs to provide physical health care.
- Efforts should be made to identify those projects that are related to a broad definition of mental health and mental disorders, using the conceptual framework of risk reduction.
- Preventive interventions within the mental health/mental disorder spectrum should be differentiated from treatment and from maintenance. Preventive interventions should be categorized according to the universal/selective/indicated classification scheme recommended in this report.
- Research of the quality of the two illustrative preventive interventions, the Infant Health and Development Program and the Study of Home Visitation for Mothers and Children (formerly the Prenatal/Early Infancy Project), should be encouraged.
- Evaluation of new projects should employ rigorous methodological standards.

and NIDA (all at that time part of ADAMHA) was $64,160,597. Expenditures at the PRBs included support for risk identification research, development of statistical methodology, training for identification and treatment of depression, alcohol treatment research, and other activities that, while worthy in their own right, are not preventive intervention research. Large preventive intervention demonstration projects were also included. While rigorous in their methodology, these have not been scaled up in size based on significant findings in prior pilot, confirmatory, and replication studies as recommended in Chapter 10.

In contrast to these findings, and using the definitions and guidelines developed in Chapters 2, 7, and 10 of this report, the committee's best estimate is that *the federal government's expenditure for rigorous preventive intervention research specifically targeted toward the prevention of mental disorders is approximately $20 million per year.*

For the reasons discussed in this chapter, it is difficult to precisely describe the current levels of expenditure by federal agencies. Nevertheless, this is the committee's best estimate of rigorous prevention research. Recommendations for increases in support (discussed in

Chapter 13) are derived from this estimate and the committee's analysis of the investment needed to enable the field of preventive intervention research on mental disorders to proceed.

PERSONNEL

Using multiple sources of information, the committee tried to determine the number of researchers working in the field of mental disorder preventive interventions. One source of data that the committee examined was the CRISP lists of grantees (1988 to 1992) for all three types of prevention (mental disorders, alcoholism, and drug addiction). The total number of grantees was 202. As discussed previously, there are many problems with CRISP information.

In late 1992 the Society for Prevention Research had 125 members. The aim of the society is to foster the scientific investigation of prevention issues. Because the initial issue that brought the society's organizers together was substance use prevention, the members are mostly from the substance abuse field, including alcoholism. In mid-1993 the National Association of Prevention Professionals and Advocates (NAPPA) had 524 members. The early focus of NAPPA was on alcohol and other drug abuse prevention, but it now includes social and health problems. Most of the membership is professional, but relatively few are researchers. The National Mental Health Association (NMHA) has a prevention constituency of 144, but how many of these are researchers is not known. Researchers who belong to NMHA are likely to have research grants and to belong to other research societies. Therefore they are likely to be identified through other sources. From FY 1985 through FY 1991, 112 researchers were funded by the NIMH PRB. Not all of them, however, were preventive intervention researchers, and some of them are no longer active in the prevention field.

Allowing for other researchers who may be funded by state agencies, universities, private foundations, and federal agencies not listed in CRISP, it is likely that there are no more than 500 researchers in the field of preventive interventions for mental disorders. The number who are fully trained to do the rigorous research described in Chapter 10 is much smaller than 500.

Probable Demand for Trained Prevention Researchers

Current and future budget constraints require that the proposed size of the training enterprise be congruent with the likely size of the research enterprise. Any proposal for training should be grounded in projections of demand for personnel. The committee's projection of demand is based not only on its judgment that the conventional university-based research effort focused on preventive intervention trials should increase in size, but also on its expectation that high-quality evaluations will be required for prevention service programs that are carried out in community organizations. Evaluation is critical when programs developed in research settings are adopted for the community. It is also essential when programs are developed in the community and have not been tested in research trials. This need for evaluation substantially increases the need for trained experts; the stakes are very high in terms of the national resources to be invested in these broad-based programs, whether they are universal, selective, or indicated. Thus the committee proposes that professionals trained in preventive intervention research are needed in federal, state, and local departments of education, social service, and public health. Although it is difficult to be precise, the steady-state national requirement of trained personnel, from various disciplines, is certainly at least 1,000 people.

Educational Background of Current Researchers

Few, if any, current researchers in preventive intervention research have completed a formal training program designed to produce researchers in the prevention of mental disorders. The committee obtained data on the type of degree for 97 of the 223 CRISP grantees funded from 1988 through 1992. This information came from agencies and professional membership listings. Of the 97, 81 are Ph.D.s (most in psychology), 12 are M.D.s, and 4 are Ed.D.s. Other data provided by NIMH further confirmed that the field of preventive intervention research is composed mainly of psychologists. There are some physicians and sociologists and almost no nurses or social workers. The scarcity of researchers in these other disciplines is in part due to the lack of emphasis on research and on prevention in their training programs.

Prevention is not a discipline but an interdisciplinary field of research. Most current researchers were trained in their primary discipline and then learned their research skills as apprentices on a research team. Moreover, a substantial proportion of the current researchers in the field migrated to prevention research after working in other related areas of inquiry. Many prevention researchers only do prevention research part time. As with some other fields, such as health services research, prevention of mental disorder research is impeded by traditional academic departments within universities that do not reward applied interdisciplinary studies, especially when the payoff is some time in the future. All of these observations are what one would expect in a new and developing field, still defining and organizing itself.

The Current Research Training Picture

The current preventive intervention research training effort is organized in such a fashion and funded at such a low level that an outside observer could reasonably conclude that policymakers wish to phase out investment in this field. Current institutional training programs are small and typically involve a 2-year training period. There may be five such programs in the entire United States, and the current output of trained (by the committee's standard) preventive intervention researchers from these institutional programs may be about 10 persons per year (assuming continuing funding and program viability). Additionally, there may be about 12 persons being trained on individual awards during any 1 year, with about half of them finishing their training each year.

The principal federal agencies that currently support research and training on prevention of mental disorders are NIMH, NIDA, and NIAAA. In FY 1992, NIMH supported three institutional training programs: Arizona State University at $117,237; Johns Hopkins University at $63,899; and Yale University at $25,000. The latter grant was terminated in FY 1993 because the principal investigator moved to another institution. During the last 6 years, these three programs have had a total of 23 postdoctoral students and 10 predoctoral students. Of the 23 postdoctoral students, 2 were physicians, 1 was a nurse, and 20 were psychologists. In 1992, the NIDA PRB had one institutional research training grant for 3 predoctoral and 3 postdoctoral trainees, all from nursing, and the NIAAA PRB awarded two institutional training grants, one for postdoctoral psychology training in alcohol research at the University of Washington and the other at the University of Georgia for research training on employee alcoholism. The program at the University of Washington, which has been in existence for 10 years, trains postdoctoral psychology students at a rate of 3 to 4 per year and some predoctoral students. The focus is on risk identification research as well as intervention research that is not restricted to prevention. The program at the University of Georgia, in existence for 5 years, has trained 9 postdoctoral students (5 sociologists, 3 psychologists, and 1 anthropologist; 6 women, 3 men; no minorities). The research focus of the center is on alcohol and the work site. Approximately half of the 9 students were interested in prevention, the other half in treatment. In 1993 the program had only 1 postdoctoral student and 7 predoctoral students.

TABLE 12.8   NIMH Grant Mechanisms That Can Be Used for
Research Training or Related Activities

F30	National Research Service Award for Individual Predoctoral Fellows (M.D./Ph.D. Fellowships)
F31	Predoctoral National Research Service Award Individual Fellowship
F32	Postdoctoral National Research Service Award Individual Fellowship
F34	Minority Access to Research Careers Faculty Fellowship
K02	Research Scientist Development Award
K05	Research Scientist Award
K21	Scientist Development Award
K20	Scientist Development Award for Clinicians
R24*	Minority Institutions Research Development Program
R24*	Research Infrastructure Support Program
T14 and R13	Research Conference Grant
T32	National Research Service Award for Institutional Grants
T34	Minority Access to Research Careers: Honors Undergraduate Research Training Grants
T35	Short-term Institutional National Research Service Award

*Minority Supplement Award as well as Disability Supplement Award can be applied.

In addition to the institutional training programs, the research institutes have awarded some individual traineeships. In 1992 the NIMH PRB had 2 Research Scientist Awards; the NIDA PRB had 2 postdoctoral individual fellowships, 1 Research Scientist Development Award, and 6 Minority Supplement Awards; and the NIAAA PRB awarded 2 individual fellowships. Other federal agencies such as MCHB, CDC, and the Department of Defense (DOD) have the potential for developing research training programs with a clear focus on preventive interventions for mental disorders.

The crisis in prevention research training reflects a larger crisis in training in the entire mental health area. Although there are many grant mechanisms available at NIMH for research training (see Table 12.8), the levels of support are inadequate. Stipends from NIH are $8,800 per year for a predoctoral student, in comparison with $15,000 at the Department of Defense, $15,500 at the National Science Foundation, and $15,000 at the Department of Education. Postdoctoral stipends at NIH are $18,600 to $33,300. These stipends are taxable and do not include health insurance. Training-related expenses that are covered for predoctoral students amount to $1,500 and $2,500 for postdoctoral students, and there are no funds for research support. Such small training grants have an especially adverse effect on minorities, who may be unable to supplement the stipends with personal or family funds.

The current demand for prevention research training can be estimated by the number of applicants for training positions. Because the numbers are small and fluctuate from year to year, the committee again must make rough estimates, but these numbers suggest that for now demand and supply are roughly in balance. There may be a slight surplus of applicants for training, but this may be desirable because it permits training institutions to make selections on the basis of quality. Until more high-quality research projects are funded, the supply of applicants for training positions is likely to remain small because many potential candidates will not see prevention as a viable and growing field.

The directors of training whom the committee has queried report that most graduates of their programs are employed, mostly at academic institutions and many in positions with responsibility for prevention research in funded projects.

A Model for Training Prevention Researchers

It is important to begin to identify optimal training models and to develop mechanisms for sustaining financial support. One way of looking at the training of preventive intervention researchers is to ask what should such researchers (or research teams) know? By its nature, research in the prevention of mental disorders requires the ability to

- assess evidence regarding risk and protective factors—both biological and psychosocial—for onset of the various mental disorders;
- transform this knowledge, if sufficient, into preventive interventions;
- design, conduct, and analyze preventive interventions in the real world; and
- incorporate sound decisions regarding cultural, ethical, and economic issues into preventive intervention research.

As is clear from the description of the preventive intervention research cycle in Chapter 10, this research is inherently interdisciplinary, requiring knowledge of several core sciences (including genetics, epidemiology, and psychology) as well as postdoctoral experience in the specific methods of preventive intervention research. It requires familiarity with all of the disciplines normally associated with mental health, as well as other disciplines that are relevant to innovations in various social and mental health services, school systems, and communities.

The committee believes that conventional disciplinary training in any one of the fields ordinarily concerned with the diagnosis, assessment, and treatment of mental illness is not sufficient to prepare individuals for a research career in prevention, although it is necessary. In other words, training in preventive intervention research should start with individuals who have already acquired knowledge and skills in such areas as nursing, social ecology, sociology, social work, public health, epidemiology, medicine (especially pediatrics, child psychiatry, and psychiatry), and clinical, developmental, social, and community psychology.

In addition to exposure to one or more of these basic approaches to a broad understanding of human behavior, training in preventive intervention research requires two other kinds of education or experience: (1) the design of interventions to prevent mental illness and (2) the analysis of the efficacy and effectiveness of an intervention. The intellectual orientations and methodological skills required for program design do not ordinarily receive much attention in the predoctoral programs of the behavioral sciences, and only slightly more in the practice-oriented fields of psychiatry and social work. Analysis demands still different orientations and skills, such as population perspective, that are almost entirely omitted from the "practice" disciplines and are only partially covered by other behavioral sciences. A program to train prevention researchers will require not only careful crafting of flexible and wide-ranging programs, but also close attention to each trainee's skills and knowledge deficiencies, careful mentoring and monitoring of progress, and suitable practicum experiences as well as didactic instruction.

Training in research design must be concerned with understanding the phenomena at issue: the nature and epidemiological distribution of the risk or protective factor that is to be reduced or enhanced. Knowledge of the particular mental disorder necessarily precedes and underlies an effective prevention strategy. Prevention programs should be based on sound research into the causes of mental disorders and also must go beyond that to understand how the disorders are manifest in everyday life. Further, training in design must invoke the know-how of implementing in practice an innovative idea that may have emerged from basic research.

Training in research focuses on learning how to obtain a dependable and unequivocal answer to the question of whether a particular intervention was indeed efficacious and effective in preventing mental disorder. Training also concentrates on learning about the processes by which the outcomes occurred, especially if the outcomes were not good. The questions are deceptively simple. The complications that make them difficult arise from the variability in human behavior, chance events in individual lives, errors in measurement, a tendency to overemphasize a few outstanding successes while ignoring a larger number of indifferent outcomes, and a myriad of other factors. Dependable answers almost always require comparing a group that did receive a particular preventive intervention with a group that did not, and that feature brings into question not only how the experimental group was selected, but also the ethical propriety of intervening with some individuals and not others. These are the generic issues that training in research must confront.

Training in preventive intervention research requires direct experience in established institutions or centers carrying out prevention studies. A central feature of this model training program is the incorporation of practicum or internship-like training, as well as classroom or other didactic instruction. The trainee's experience should include participation in all phases of an actual preventive intervention research program that is being conducted by the faculty of the training institution. The trainee's mentors need to have had actual experience in one or more phases of design and analysis, and at least some of them should be actively engaged in such tasks during a trainee's participation. A clear implication is that the training institution itself must be actively engaged in a continuing program of preventive intervention research, perhaps with shifting emphases and different types of intervention, but steadily engaged.

Although this kind of training is available in medical or relevant doctoral programs, it is not common in the education of human resources professionals. First, it is labor-intensive and expensive. Second, it is not easy to identify and bring together the range of talents needed for the training faculty. The model program depends, in most instances, on interdisciplinary collaboration, which can be disrupted by academic mobility. It is hard to see how such training could be provided without external support, for the costs of faculty as well as trainees. Fellowships for individual trainees alone will not suffice. As discussed earlier, current federal training grants cover only a small fraction of such training and are subsidized heavily by the training institution and by research grants from NIH.

The committee concludes that a long-term strategy for preventive intervention research training should be developed at the postdoctoral level. There is a significant demographic change that may have an impact on this strategy. In the last decade or so, the number of faculty positions at research universities has been limited, and many graduates of doctoral programs in the social and behavioral sciences, public health, and other fields have been willing to accept postdoctoral traineeships while they waited for openings to occur. In the next decade, a substantial number of retirements from the faculty are expected among those who were appointed during the expansion years of the 1960s. For other demographic reasons, there is likely to be, simultaneously, a smaller number of entrants into doctoral programs in fields related to prevention research. These two trends are likely to increase the demand for new Ph.D.s on faculties, thus making the traineeship less attractive, even with the prospect of an additional two years of training. Two possible solutions suggest themselves: one is to begin prevention research training earlier, say just before completion of disciplinary training. The other is to recognize the real costs of mid-career training for mature scientists with family obligations. The committee believes that support for both is necessary.

Postdoctoral training is a long-term strategy for increasing the number and quality of prevention researchers. What is needed immediately is a short-term strategy to "jump-start" the field. Mid-career scientists from related fields—risk identification research, epidemiology, treatment effectiveness research, and research on prevention of physical disorders—need to be recruited, trained, and adequately supported through increased stipends and increased availability of research grants.

It is possible that this presentation of a model training program may be misunderstood as being unduly narrow and rigid. The description should be taken as an indication of what the committee believes to be both desirable and feasible, without ruling out other possible approaches to the same goal. The field of prevention research should be open to additional training models as experience accumulates; a narrow prescription for training would be inappropriate at this time.

Conclusions

The committee concludes that the national interest in the prevention of mental disorders requires the following general strategies for building training capacity:

- A gradual increase in the number of investigators trained and experienced in preventive intervention research.
- An increase in the number of physicians, nurses, and social workers trained in preventive intervention research.
- To "jump-start" the field, fellowships as well as intensive short-term training for mid-career scientists who wish to change fields and spend all or part of their time collaborating with an interdisciplinary preventive intervention research team.
- The development of more postdoctoral training programs.
- An increase in funding for both training and research. A large part of the training the committee recommends occurs during participation

in research projects under the supervision of mentors. As indicated earlier, the training and research enterprises need to be coordinated so that the trainees are available to fill the need for researchers, both the need for researchers in an expanding research enterprise and the replacement of those who retire or leave the field.

- The creation of a career line that makes prevention research a rewarding profession, attracts high-quality talent, and sustains persistent attention to the difficult problems related to prevention of mental disorders. Such a career line includes forums for professional exchange, opportunities for continuing professional growth, and academic recognition of professional contributions, as well as mechanisms by which research, and researchers, can actually influence prevention programs and policy.

This capacity-building process will be a long-range effort, because the base from which it starts is small, and the start-up of new training programs is bound to be slower than the rate at which well-trained investigators can be effectively used. High-quality training is essential, and it will take time for potential new training institutions to assemble the required mix of professional talent. Leadership will have to be found within federal and state governments, universities, and foundations. Research training projects will require the cooperation of treatment and prevention agencies willing to try out new interventions and allow their efforts to be evaluated. Some training models may not be successful. The first 5 years will build capacity slowly, and it is important to have realistic goals for these years.

After a few years, with successful models for training programs, with developing career lines and the assurance of funding for prevention research, it is hoped that the curve of output growth will accelerate sharply—to the point where more ambitious long-range goals can be realistic. Accordingly, the committee suggests both 5-year and 10-year targets for the size of the training enterprise.

The committee's 5-year goal is to produce enough trained investigators in prevention research to provide staff for the larger number of training programs it envisions, for additional specialized prevention research centers in organizations that support research generally, and for research positions in some education and social service departments that now are, or soon will be, able to use their talents as these departments increase their standards for rigorous evaluation of program effectiveness. The committee's 10-year goal is to provide preventive intervention researchers in high-quality programs in major academic settings, in many departments of education and other social service agencies at the state level, and in all of the training programs and specialized prevention research centers that are expected to be in place at that time. To achieve such a goal will require support from federal, state, and private sources.

Finally, mechanisms must be created that make it feasible and even attractive for talented mid-career scientists to switch into preventive intervention research. Mechanisms to accomplish this include research scientist awards and awards to establish chairs for distinguished scientists in prevention research. Both of these mechanisms have precedents within NIH. As with the institutional training grants, it is essential that these programs cover the full costs. If policymakers decide that the national interest requires the development of this field, then barriers to that development must be completely removed.

COORDINATION

Federal agencies doing preventive intervention research and providing prevention services are decentralized and uncoordinated and have minimal awareness of each other's efforts. Few projects directly assess or attempt to intervene in the common phenomenon of co-morbidity among mental disorders, including drug and alcohol abuse. Even though NIMH is clearly the lead agency in research regarding the etiology and treatment of mental disorders, it has not taken a lead role in regard to the exchange of knowledge about preventive interventions with other federal agencies or with state agencies. In part, this lack of leadership regarding prevention knowledge exchange reflects the biomedical emphasis of NIMH, but it also is a result of NIMH's inability to coordinate its prevention programs with NIDA and NIAAA and other federal programs. Because many other DHHS agencies, such as SAMHSA, the Administration on Children, Youth and Families (ACYF), CDC, and HRSA; other departments, such as Education and Defense; and state agencies conduct their own preventive intervention research and provide prevention services, it is essential that coordination efforts include them as well as the NIH research institutes.

There is no central clearinghouse within the government on prevention of mental disorders. There have been few prevention conferences outside of a single institute or agency. There is no organized system for the exchange of knowledge regarding prevention research, including effective intervention programs, with state public health departments, advocacy groups, or universities (see Chapter 11).

Many problems that exist within the federal government also exist in the network of private foundations mentioned earlier in this chapter.

For many years, these foundations and many others have provided substantial research and service funds for prevention, including the reduction of various risk factors associated with the onset of mental disorders. The network for information sharing and joint funding of projects among federal agencies and private foundations is an informal one, relying heavily on the individuals involved, much as it is within the federal agencies.

The extent to which the private and public funding sources overlap to provide for the career development of prevention researchers and for joint sponsorship of research projects could not be determined because there is no mechanism for recording this type of information. However, it appears that the overlap, at least sequentially, for a particular project or researcher may be considerable.

To coordinate these diverse participants in prevention, a lead agency would require several attributes. The ability of the lead agency to bring together all the interested federal, state, and private parties to facilitate an open sharing of ideas and information, a commitment to the investigations of multiple, co-existing risk conditions for mental disorders and the co-morbidity of dysfunctions and disorders, and a willingness to participate in joint projects are all essential. A commitment to prevention, as distinguished from treatment and maintenance, is equally important in the lead agency.

To place such a leading role outside the federal government does not seem possible, because the bulk of funds for preventive intervention research and service will continue to come from the federal government.

The reorganization of ADAMHA complicates the picture. With the split between research and services, none of the remaining agencies covers all the bases. SAMHSA has a clear role in the delivery of preventive services regarding drug abuse, but its role in prevention of other mental disorders is less clear. Although prevention is part of the mandate to SAMHSA's Center on Mental Health Services, there is no mandate establishing an Office of Prevention, and no support for prevention coordination was authorized. Each of the three research institutes at NIH (NIMH, NIDA, and NIAAA) has an Office of Prevention. The new law does not, however, establish any overarching authority to coordinate their activities, and categorical funding has contributed to competitiveness and isolation of the institutes from each other. It remains to be seen how these three research institutes will dovetail with the already established Health and Behavior Committee and Prevention Coordinating Committee at NIH. The links between the research institutes and the service programs at ADAMHA were already tenuous; coordination may now be even more difficult.

Furthermore, the research grant review process is fraught with difficulties across the institutes. These include lack of high-quality proposals, lack of proposals from minority investigators, lack of expertise in preventive intervention research on review committees that sometimes consider epidemiology, treatment, and prevention grants, vested interests on review committees that are dominated by "inside" prevention scientists (partly because prevention is still a small and young field), and reluctance of some review committees to allow investigators to combine funding streams from different institutes or agencies or to cross from one institute to another.

Even though other agencies, such as the Maternal and Child Health Bureau and the Administration on Children and Families within DHHS, as well as the Department of Defense, the Department of Education, and the Department of Justice, are valuable contributors and should be included in any coalition-building effort, none has enough current expertise on mental disorders to become the lead agency. The Office of Health Promotion and Disease Prevention has had an important role in coordinating information about prevention services and research within DHHS, but it too lacks expertise on mental disorders. Some of these agencies also lack expertise in research methodology.

The Centers for Disease Control and Prevention clearly has the best delineated mandate for prevention among federal agencies, and it has excellent outreach capabilities through public health departments. Recently, it has taken a more active role in prevention of violence and the prevention of problems associated with low birthweight. However, its current expertise in mental disorders is quite limited.

Conclusions

There is little coordination of prevention research or prevention services across federal agencies, or among federal agencies, universities, and private foundations. In addition, research institutes and agencies frequently ignore issues of co-morbidity of mental disorders and of mental and physical disorders, as well as the co-existence of mental disorders and social and legal problems, such as delinquency. A less categorical approach to interventions may be productive to individuals as well as society, but there is no clear lead agency to provide such an approach. No agency has both the expertise in mental disorder preventive intervention research and an established track record in working collaboratively with other agencies and departments on prevention. Therefore the committee concludes that an alternative mechanism is needed so that research and services on prevention of mental disorders can be coordinated across the federal departments.

REFERENCES

ADAMHA (Alcohol, Drug Abuse, and Mental Health Administration). (1993) Prevention Activities of the Alcohol, Drug Abuse, and Mental Health Administration: Report to Congress FY 1989 to 1991; Draft received in 1993 through the Freedom of Information Act.

DHHS (Department of Health and Human Services). (1992) Public Health Service. Office of Disease Prevention and Health Promotion. Prevention '91/'92 Federal Programs and Progress. Washington, DC: Government Printing Office; 332–838.

OBRA (Omnibus Reconcilitation Act). (1989) Maternal and Child Health Block Grant Program. P.L. 101–239, Title VI, Subtitle C; Enacted December 19, 1989.

13

Conclusions and Recommendations: An Agenda for the Next Decade

When President Roosevelt announced in 1937 that "one third of our nation are ill housed, ill clad, ill nourished," our country was galvanized into action. Yet today, when careful population studies tell us that as many as one third of American adults will suffer a diagnosable mental disorder sometime in their life and that 20 percent have a mental disorder at any given time, there is little alarm. The Institute of Medicine's Committee on Prevention of Mental Disorders believes that strong action is warranted, and with this report it calls on the nation to mount a significant program to prevent mental disorders. Although research on the causes and treatment of mental disorders remains vitally important—and indeed major advances are leading to better lives for increasing numbers of people—much greater effort than ever before needs to be directed to prevention.

Public health experience has shown that when a critical mass of knowledge regarding a specific health problem accumulates and a core group of expert researchers have been identified, the time is ripe for launching a larger, coordinated research and training endeavor. The committee believes that such a moment has arrived for the field of mental health. Opportunities now exist to effectively exploit existing knowledge to launch a promising research agenda on the prevention of mental disorders. *Therefore the committee strongly recommends that an enhanced research agenda to prevent mental disorders be initiated and supported across all relevant federal agencies, including, but not limited to, the Departments of Health and Human Services, Education, Justice, Labor, Defense, and*

Housing and Urban Development, as well as state governments, universities, and private foundations. This agenda should facilitate development in three major areas:

- *Building the infrastructure to coordinate research and service programs and to train and support new investigators.*
- *Expanding the knowledge base for preventive interventions.*
- *Conducting well-evaluated preventive interventions.*

As previously stated, the committee's recommendations for funding of rigorous preventive intervention research are based on its best estimates of current efforts and its judgment of needed resources to create a robust federal research agenda.

The committee finds the need for prevention of mental disorders so great and the current opportunities for success so abundant that it recommends an increased investment across all federal agencies over the next five years (1995 through 1999) to facilitate the development of these three major areas of the research agenda. It recommends increased support of $50.5 million per year for the next two years, $53 million in year three, and $61 million per year in years four and five. These are modest increases considering the magnitude of the problem of mental illness in this country, and Congress may decide that an even greater investment is warranted.

Funding for the second five years should be recommended by a new coordinating body, such as a national scientific council on the prevention of mental disorders. The amount appropriated in year six should be no less than the amount of support in FY 1999. On the basis of positive results in the first five years, a considerably larger investment could be warranted during the second five years.

The three major areas to be developed are recommended in conjunction with use of the definitions of interventions for mental disorders and of prevention research developed in this report. The term prevention *is reserved for only those interventions that occur before the initial onset of a disorder. These preventive interventions can be further classified into universal, selective, and indicated types. The term* prevention research *refers only to preventive intervention research and is distinct from research that builds a broad scientific base for preventive interventions.*

BUILDING AN ENHANCED INFRASTRUCTURE FOR PREVENTIVE INTERVENTION RESEARCH

Preventive intervention research for mental disorders cannot thrive without providing for its infrastructure. Two areas are particularly important for moving ahead—coordination and research training.

The Coordination Role and Structure

Coordination among federal agencies is needed for four reasons: (1) variation in the application of definitions has made it virtually impossible to assess the current activities and expenditures in preventive intervention research; (2) duplication of research activities and the lack of piggybacking of smaller projects onto larger ones contribute to waste of dollars and time, and, at the same time, gaps in research go undetected; (3) agencies conduct research or provide interventions for mental disorders (including addictions), educational disabilities, criminal behavior, and physical disorders as though these were separate conditions, whereas, more often than not, coexisting disorders or problems occur; and (4) agencies have different strengths; for example, some are better at applying rigorous research methodologies to intervention programs, whereas others are better at reaching out into communities and forging alliances.

In arriving at its recommendations about coordination, the committee reviewed various alternatives. The decisions to be made include (1) how best to coordinate the various relevant activities, (2) where the coordination function should reside within the federal government, and (3) staffing and funding issues. The structure and function of the coordination mechanism are inextricably intertwined, so decisions 1 and 2 above cannot be readily separated. Staff and funding should be attached to the coordination mechanism wherever it is located. Four alternatives were considered regarding where the coordination function should reside. Although the committee does express a preference for coordination at the highest possible level, it believes that establishing a successful coordination mechanism across federal departments is more important than the details of where it is housed.

Initially, the committee considered the model of putting a coordination role in one agency, such as the National Institute of Mental Health (NIMH) or the National Institutes of Health's (NIH) Office of Disease Prevention. Locating the coordination role in a single agency is a natural way to keep coordination close to the science, because the personnel in NIMH or the director's office at NIH are likely to be more closely connected to the scientific network than those higher in the government. Although single agencies have mediated coordination among other parts of the same department and even among branches of different executive departments in the past, the breadth and extent of the need for multiagency collaboration in this case make a single agency lead seem unrealistic. One possible exception is the Centers for Disease Control and Prevention (CDC), which has a public health mandate for prevention activities and considerable experience in working collaboratively with federal, state, and local agencies.

Coordination from an office within one department that serves as an umbrella over several relevant agencies is a second alternative. The Office of the Assistant Secretary for Health within the Department of Health and Human Services (DHHS) already contains an Office for Disease Prevention and Health Promotion. This office could be charged with forming a subcommittee or task group to focus specifically on the coordination of research aimed at preventing mental disorders and substance abuse. These preventive efforts share many features with other disorders already subject to coordination within this office, but the involvement of the criminal justice system, the educational system, child and spousal protective services, civilian and military family support services, and other nonmedical services necessarily encompasses activities in an even broader array of federal agencies. Many of these services are housed in entirely separate cabinet departments. The committee thus believes that coordination at the departmental level is preferable to coordination by a single agency (with the possible exception of CDC), but the nature of the problem may well necessitate a higher-level coordination mechanism.

As a third alternative, the committee considered models developed within Congress, such as the Physician Payment Review Commission (PPRC) and the Prospective Payment Assessment Commission (PRO-PAC), for which appointments are made by an independent body—the Office of Technology Assessment. The question regarding these models is how well they would work in the prevention field, where many of the activities center on coordination of ongoing programs conducted within the executive branch.

As a fourth alternative, the committee considered other successful models—the ongoing White House Conferences, various presidential commissions, and the Office of Science and Technology Policy (OSTP)—within the White House. OSTP was originally created by President Eisenhower to focus national attention on science; after being disbanded, it was reestablished by President Ford upon the recommendation of the National Academy of Sciences (1974). This model has three components: (1) an office having coordinating responsibility regarding national science policy, (2) an individual who serves as the President's science advisor, and (3) a council with expertise in a broad range of scientific matters. The advantages of having a coordination structure under the White House are that it is at a natural level for coordinating activities of different cabinet departments and that it places a premium on interagency cooperation, which the committee believes is an essential element.

The committee thus leans toward the establishment of an overarching federal council, operated out of the White House Office of Science and Technology Policy or another coordinating office within the Executive Office of the President, to coordinate preventive intervention research. It recognizes that research and services related to the prevention of mental disorders have high relevance to the many other agendas and priorities of Congress and the President. These include the lack of high-quality education, deteriorating cities, drug problems, the lack of housing, poverty, and the lack of universal health care. Mental disorders contribute to these problems and vice versa; therefore the ultimate solutions must be broad in scope.

Adequate staffing and resources are essential to successful coordination of prevention research regardless of where it is located in the federal government. Moreover, the quality of leadership and extent of commitment among agencies are often far more important than the precise location of a coordination office. Leadership and commitment cannot be fully controlled, no matter how careful the plans may be. The competence of the particular individuals chosen to lead the effort and the politics of the day often determine whether interagency coordination is truly successful or merely an effort that consumes staff time and wastes increasingly scarce federal dollars. Despite these caveats, the committee nonetheless believes that a coordinating committee at the highest possible level with adequate staffing is necessary to weave together disparate federal activities in many different departments.

• *The committee strongly recommends that a mechanism be created to coordinate research and services on prevention of mental disorders across the federal departments. One model for accomplishing this would be the establishment of a national scientific council on the prevention of mental disorders by Congress and/or the President. Such an overarching federal council could be operated out of the White House Office of Science and Technology Policy or another coordinating office within the Executive Office of the President.* This council should formulate policies regarding preventive intervention research, evaluation of prevention services, knowledge exchange, coordination of interagency research efforts, and training. Because prevention activities span different departments, the members of the council should be appointed after soliciting nominations from a wide constituency who are willing to use the definitions and rigorous methodological criteria developed in this report to foster policies that will reduce the onset of mental disorders and related problems. Members should include—as equal partners—ex-officio high-level representatives of relevant federal agencies, including but not limited to the Departments of

Health and Human Services, Justice, Labor, Education, Defense, and Housing and Urban Development, as well as representatives from state agencies, private foundations, universities, and the public at large. A broad range of disciplines, including medicine (pediatrics, child psychiatry, psychiatry, primary care), psychology, nursing, social work, public health, sociology, and epidemiology, should be represented. The council should meet regularly to coordinate collaborative research across public and private agencies and should monitor the standards for rigorous methodological approaches to preventive intervention research. Terms on the council for nonfederal representatives should be limited. To provide ongoing executive leadership, the chair of the council should be appointed by the President. Other leadership positions could be selected from the nonfederal representatives. The council should have its own paid staff, including a coordinator with staff, who operates out of an office of prevention of mental disorders. The office should oversee and coordinate the daily operations of preventive intervention activities in all areas that are related to mental health across the federal government. The staff of the office should be responsible to the council. The council should report regularly, at least once a year, to the Congress and the President.

• *The committee also strongly recommends that Congress encourage the establishment of offices for prevention of mental disorders at the state level.* The current number of such offices is small even though the states have resources for prevention available to them through the state block grants. A mechanism to encourage the development of state offices would be a requirement attached to the block grants, and as health care reform is developed other possibilities may occur. The functions of these offices should be similar to those of the proposed national scientific council on the prevention of mental disorders. States that do establish such offices should, as a group, elect representatives to the national scientific council.

• *Agencies must be required to identify their funded programs for the prevention of mental disorders, separately accounting for universal, selective, and indicated preventive interventions, using the definitions developed in this report.* Congress should ask for separate accounting of these different kinds of preventive interventions when agencies report on the activities they support.

• *The National Institute of Mental Health (NIMH), the National Institute on Alcohol Abuse and Alcoholism (NIAAA), and the National Institute on Drug Abuse (NIDA) should consider including prevention researchers with broad mental health perspectives on their national advisory councils.* The prevention research field must produce more researchers of international stature who can serve on such advisory councils.

• *Mental health reimbursement from existing health insurance should be provided for preventive interventions that have proved effective under rigorous research standards such as those described in this report.*

• *Dissemination activities should receive much higher priority than they have in the past.* Agencies should disseminate results of research trials as well as evaluations of preventive intervention service programs. Funding of research trials should be continued only when investigators demonstrate a good publication record (including theoretical formulations and data from research trials). Interagency research conferences should be encouraged. A federal clearinghouse on preventive interventions in the mental health field should be considered, either as part of the council's function or as a separately funded initiative.

Research Training

• Training is an immediate and critical need in preventive intervention research. *Congress and federal agencies should immediately take steps to develop and support the training of additional researchers who can develop new preventive intervention research trials as well as evaluate the effectiveness of current service projects.* This training effort should include consortiums, seminars, fellowships, and research grants to attract existing researchers into prevention research, training programs for new investigators, and expansion of the training component of the specialized prevention research centers.

• *Research training should be focused on two groups—mid-career scientists and postdoctoral students.* Training for these groups should be developed simultaneously, but the expectation is that the training efforts for these groups will produce two waves of personnel. As an immediate strategy, training opportunities with adequate stipends should be developed to attract talented mid-career scientists from related fields, such as risk research, epidemiology, treatment effectiveness research, and research on prevention of physical illnesses, who seek to make the transition to research on prevention of mental disorders. This could be done through existing fellowships and career development awards and through the development of creative consortiums, seminars, and mentoring. All training should be tailored to the needs and schedules of these scientists. Such training could have a substantial impact on the number of personnel within three years if there is a simultaneous increase in the funds available for peer-reviewed research projects (RO1s).

As a second strategy, training opportunities with sufficient stipends should be developed to attract talented postdoctoral-level trainees to preventive intervention research. Much more effort should be made to attract trainees from a wide range of disciplines, including psychiatry, pediatrics, social work, nursing, public health, epidemiology, neuroscience, anthropology, and sociology, as well as psychology, which dominates the field today. If efforts to boost doctoral training begin concurrently with mid-career training, we might expect to see the benefits of an increased pool of researchers capable of securing their own research grants by year five of a 10-year plan.

● *The number of institutional training programs focusing on preventive intervention research should be increased from 5 to 12 over the next five years, including one at every specialized prevention research center, known at NIMH as Preventive Intervention Research Centers (PIRCs), that is productive.* Training of mid-career scientists and postdoctoral students should occur within every specialized prevention research center. To ensure that this happens, funding of specialized prevention research centers should be continued only when they demonstrate good track records in the production of published research and in the training of researchers capable of procuring their own research grants. In addition to the specialized prevention research centers, research training should be supported by federal agencies, schools of public health, and schools traditionally linked to service, such as social work, education, nursing, and medicine.

● *Support for faculty within institutional training programs should be increased.* Such support should increase the capacity of the faculty, program, and university to train preventive intervention researchers.

● *A major effort should be made to encourage the prevention research training of minorities.* Support should be offered to minority mental health research centers and other centers that focus on specific populations, such as low-income groups, the elderly, and minority groups. This would add more researchers to the field, but even more importantly, they would be researchers who specialize in populations with special needs.

● *The proposed national scientific council on the prevention of mental disorders should reevaluate the training needs for preventive intervention research after the first five years.* At that point the emphasis on mid-career scientists might be able to be decreased. If so, support for predoctoral training could be increased. An emphasis on postdoctoral training should be consistently high throughout the decade.

Funding

Coordination and training are the two most immediate and important needs in preventive intervention research on mental disorders (see

TABLE 13.1   Recommendations for Federal Government Support
Above 1993 Level of Support (dollars in millions)

	1995	1996	1997	1998	1999
Infrastructure					
Council/office/dissemination	2.0	2.0	2.0	2.0	2.0
Training	12.0	12.0	12.0	12.0	12.0
Knowledge Base Research					
Risk and protective factor research (biological/psychosocial interaction)	6.5	6.5	6.5	6.5	6.5
Child epidemiological study	2.5	2.5	2.5	2.5	2.5
Population studies	5.0	5.0	5.0	5.0	5.0
Mental health promotion study	0.5	0.5	0	0	0
Prevention Research					
Preventive intervention research projects	20.0	20.0	20.0	25.0	25.0
Preventive intervention research centers	2.0	2.0	5.0	8.0	8.0
Total Budget	50.5	50.5	53.0	61.0	61.0

NOTE: Figures are based on 1993 dollar amounts and are not adjusted for inflation. These recommendations for support are based on the committee's best estimates of current efforts and its judgment of needed resources to create a robust preventive intervention research agenda for mental disorders across the federal government.

Table 13.1). The national scientific council on the prevention of mental disorders and the office of prevention of mental disorders should have a combined budget of $1 million per year for five years. Dissemination activities should be budgeted at $1 million per year for five years. Support for training should be budgeted at $12 million above the current level for year one, and this level of funding should be maintained for each of the next four years. In the first few years, these researchers are needed for evaluating current prevention service projects; gradually, they also will be conducting original preventive intervention research projects. Stipends for mid-career scientists should be in the $60,000 to $120,000 range, plus travel expenses. Stipends for postdoctoral trainees should be in the $30,000 to $60,000 range, plus travel expenses.

EXPANDING THE KNOWLEDGE BASE

The committee believes, based on the review of literature for this report, that a viable research agenda for prevention of mental disorders rests on a firm stratum of health research in other fields. This knowledge base includes basic and applied research in the core sciences that is aimed at the causes and prevention of mental disorders. Included in this knowledge base are neurosciences, genetics, epidemiology, psychiatry, behavioral sciences (including developmental psychopathology), and risk research. It also includes evidence and lessons from other fields of research, such as prevention of physical illness and treatment of mental disorders.

- *Research to expand the knowledge base for preventive interventions should be continued.* Knowledge base research should continue to be supported for all five disorders reviewed in this report, in addition to other mental disorders. Basic research is essential to the understanding of mental disorders. New funds for the development of other knowledge base areas and for preventive intervention research should not be taken from funds currently used to support basic science. The committee also recommends that support be increased for the three specific knowledge base areas outlined below. Support of basic research will ensure the quality and continuity of the existing research effort and attract new investigators to those fields.
- *Support for research on potentially modifiable biological and psychosocial risk and protective factors for the onset of mental disorders should be increased. Priority should be given to research, regardless of the type of mental disorder, that illuminates the interaction of potentially modifiable biological and psychosocial risk and protective factors, rather than restricting the research to either biological or psychosocial factors.*
- *NIMH should support a series of prospective studies on well-defined general populations under the age of 18 to provide initial benchmark estimates of the prevalence and incidence of mental disorders and problem behaviors in this age group.* These epidemiological investigations should be oriented toward diagnosis but also should record a range of symptomatology, so that future changes in the diagnostic system, or developmental changes in individuals, do not preclude understanding of the development of psychopathology throughout this age range and into adult life. These prospective studies also should be oriented toward identification of modifiable risk factors in this age group with the explicit goal of recommending modifiable targets for preventive interventions in the future.
- *A population laboratory should be established with the capacity for conducting longitudinal studies over the entire life span in order to generate understanding as to how risk factors and developmental transitions combine to influence the development of psychopathology.* The primary goal of this laboratory should be the enhancement of knowledge for prevention and the development of new knowledge for the implementation of preventive intervention trials. Special attention should be paid to developmental transitions, such as childhood to adolescence, adolescence to adult-

hood, entry into marriage, and loss of a spouse; precursor signs and symptoms, prodromal periods, age periods just prior to when a specific mental disorder is most likely to occur; and the effects of race, ethnicity, and gender. Well-designed preventive intervention research trials might be conducted with these populations during the follow-up, as long as the goal of obtaining benchmark estimates of epidemiological data, especially in regard to developmental transitions, is not threatened. The population laboratory could be established as a branch in the intramural program of NIMH, although there are advantages to making it a multiagency project funded through agreements among DHHS agencies such as the Centers for Disease Control and Prevention (CDC), Substance Abuse and Mental Health Administration (SAMHSA), National Institute on Drug Abuse (NIDA), National Institute on Alcohol Abuse and Alcoholism (NIAAA), National Institute of Mental Health (NIMH), National Institute of Child Health and Human Development (NICHD), and Maternal and Child Health Bureau (MCHB), and departments such as the Departments of Justice, Education, and Defense. It could also be established as a unit outside the federal government funded through a special mechanism. An extragovernmental advisory panel, including experts in epidemiology, psychopathology, and prevention, should be formed to provide continuing scientific oversight to the population laboratory. Data from investigations of the population laboratory should be made available in anonymous form in a regular and timely fashion.

• *Whenever possible, research proposals relevant to the knowledge base for preventive interventions should explicitly state this connection, such as identification of potentially modifiable risk factors and possible avenues for preventive interventions.* This requirement should be applied across all federal agencies, and especially to research proposals funded from the additional support recommended by this committee. This clarification of relevance to prevention will help decrease confusion regarding definitions of prevention research and lead to findings relevant to preventive interventions.

• *Treatment intervention research conducted under rigorous methodological standards that is directly relevant to preventive intervention research should continue to be supported—but not from the prevention research budget.* The criteria for "direct relevance" should be reviewed by prevention researchers. Collaboration between treatment researchers and prevention researchers should be fostered. Principles from treatment research can and should be borrowed for use in prevention. Specialty areas in treatment research that are likely to yield payoffs for preventive intervention research include clinical psychopharmacology, cognitive-behavior therapy, and applied behavior analysis.

● *Research should continue to be supported to determine which risk and protective factors are similar and which ones are different for treatment and prevention of a variety of mental disorders.* Identifying potentially modifiable factors that are unique to first onset of a disorder increases possibilities for prevention.

● *Research should be supported to study the effects of social environments, such as families, peers, neighborhoods, and communities, on the individual and the effects of context on the onset of various mental disorders.*

● *Researchers working on relevant research in the core sciences should be encouraged to participate in activities such as forums and colloquia with preventive intervention researchers.*

● *A comprehensive, descriptive inventory of the activities in which the public engages to promote psychological well-being and mental health should be developed and supported.* This catalog of mental health promotion activities is expected to be substantial. Preliminary efforts should also be made to craft outcome criteria for these activities that could be used in rigorous evaluations down the road.

Funding

The committee recommends that $6.5 million be budgeted each year for the next five years for risk research on the complex interaction between biological and psychosocial risk and protective factors. This would augment the research base for those mental disorders furthest along the continuum in the understanding of etiology, emphasizing the identification of malleable risk factors that would augur well for further preventive intervention research. A child epidemiological study should be budgeted at a minimum of $2.5 million per year over the next five years, and a population laboratory should be budgeted at $5 million per year over the next five years. Over a two-year period, $1 million should be allocated to catalog mental health promotion activities and to craft outcome criteria.

CONDUCTING WELL-EVALUATED INTERVENTIONS

The knowledge base for some mental disorders is now advanced enough that preventive intervention research programs, targeted at risk factors for these disorders, can rest on sound conceptual and empirical foundations.

● *Increased methodological rigor in all research trials, demonstration projects, and service program evaluations should be required.* Wherever possible, the standards developed in this report, including hypothesis-driven randomized controlled trials and assessment of multiple outcome measures over time, should be instituted.

- *The concept of risk reduction, including the strengthening of protective factors, should be used as the best available theoretical model for guiding interventions to prevent the onset of mental disorders.* Other models for preventive interventions should continue to be explored; for example, as more becomes known about the mechanisms that link the presence of causal risk factors and absence of protective factors to the initial onset of symptoms, the possibilities for intervention may be increased.

- *Universal preventive interventions should continue to be supported in the areas of prenatal care, immunization, safety standards such as the use of seat belts and helmets, and control of the availability of alcohol.* These programs decrease brain injury and mental retardation, which are conditions associated with mental disorders. Although the main benefit of these interventions is the prevention of physical illness or injury, they may reduce the incidence of mental disorders as well. More evaluation is needed to assess their impact on mental disorders.

- *Research on selective and indicated interventions targeting high-risk groups and individuals should be given high priority.* Many of the programs described in this report are selective preventive intervention research programs, targeting multiple risk factors including poverty, job loss, caregiver burden, bereavement, medical problems, divorce, peer rejection, academic failure, and family conflict. These programs provide an impressive base for more rigorous research trials with larger samples.

- *Priority should be given to preventive intervention research proposals that address well-validated clusters of biological and psychosocial risk and protective factors within a developmental life-span framework.* Trials should measure short- and long-term outcomes for targeted disorders and should continue past the average age of onset. Sample size should be adequate for determining the validity of outcome measures.

- *Increased attention should be given to preventive intervention research that addresses the overlap between physical and mental illness.* For example, prevention trials with primary care populations should include examination of effects on physical well-being, use of health care (which at times may mean increased use), and social functioning.

- *Research support should be developed in two waves over the next decade, initially focusing primarily on increasing research grant support for individual investigators and later on increasing support for specialized prevention research centers throughout the appropriate federal agencies.* This strategy is based on the principle of building a prevention science from the ground up, rather than the top down. Individual investigators should compete for research grant support. As their academic track record becomes established, they should be encouraged to increase the size and scope of their trials and join with other solid investigators to form preventive intervention research centers. In the first wave, lasting five years, there should be a substantial increase in the funds available for peer-reviewed research projects. Preventive intervention research programs should be supported for any mental disorder for which there is well-validated evidence of risk factors that appear to be modifiable. After five years, with the impact of new mid-career researchers joining the field and evidence from five years of research programs, a review should be made of the evidence. It is highly likely that several other preventive intervention research centers could be warranted at that time. Research grant support should not decrease at this time.

- *Research on sequential preventive interventions aimed at multiple risks in infancy, early childhood, and elementary school age to prevent onset of multiple behavioral problems and mental disorders should be increased immediately and substantially.* This should include a large number of new research grants and at least one new specialized prevention research center. The knowledge base regarding multiple risk factors in infancy and childhood interacting in complex causal chains and resulting in multiple disorders is extensive. Data on the direct linkage to specific disorders that emerge in adolescence and adulthood are becoming available. Many rigorously designed preventive intervention programs document impacts on risk and protective factors that are likely to reduce incidence rates of mental disorders. Addressing clusters of risk and protective factors increases the chances of preventing multiple disorders, especially major depressive disorder and conduct disorder. A number of separate randomized controlled trials have demonstrated the efficacy, and in some studies the effectiveness, of specific preventive interventions across development from the prenatal period through adolescence in reducing risk factors and enhancing protective factors. These should now be combined and delivered in sequence to high-risk populations. The interventions should include high-quality prenatal care, childhood immunizations, home visiting and high-quality day care (such as the Prenatal/Early Infancy Project and the Infant Health and Development Program), high-quality preschool (such as the Perry Preschool Program), parenting training, and enhancement of social competence and academic performance. High priority should be given to interagency sponsorship of this research, including the specialized prevention research centers. The Department of Health and Human Services (including the Maternal and Child Health Bureau (MCHB), National Institute of Child Health and Human Development

(NICHD), Administration on Children, Youth, and Families (ACYF), Substance Abuse and Mental Health Services Administration (SAMHSA), and the National Institute of Mental Health (NIMH)) and the Departments of Education, Justice, and Defense might be interested in sponsoring such research.

● *Research on preventive interventions aimed at major depressive disorder should be increased immediately and substantially.* This should include a large number of new research grants and at least one new specialized prevention research center. The knowledge base in this area is extensive, and promising preventive interventions have been empirically tested across the life span. Research to prevent depressive disorders should be more focused on preventing co-morbid mental disorders than it has been in the past. Also, outcomes often extend beyond traditional boundaries of mental disorders. For example, prevention of depression has strong implications for reducing suicides, lost work productivity, and physical disorders. High priority should be given to interagency agreements for research projects and specialized prevention research centers. Gradually over the next five years, other new specialized prevention research centers should be initiated to focus on depression and co-occurring conditions. Links between these new centers and other research sites are essential, and monies should be set aside to provide for ongoing collaboration.

● *Research on preventive interventions aimed at alcohol abuse should be increased immediately.* The knowledge base is extensive, and promising preventive interventions have been empirically tested. A less categorical approach to alcohol abuse preventive intervention research is needed. Coexisting illnesses, such as depressive disorders and physical disorders, must be carefully studied. Prevention of alcohol abuse has strong implications for reducing drug abuse, spouse and child maltreatment, and physical injury. The outcomes of preventive interventions on these problems also should be considered. For alcohol abuse, it may be best to target children and young adolescents to delay the initiation of alcohol use.

● *Support for pilot and confirmatory preventive intervention trials should be increased for conduct disorder.* Priority should be given to research that addresses multiple risk factors for young children with early onset of aggressiveness, including parental psychopathology, poverty, and neurodevelopmental deficits in the child.

● *Research should be supported on alternative forms of intervention for the caregivers and family members of individuals with mental disorders, especially Alzheimer's disease and schizophrenia, to prevent the onset of stress-induced disorders among these caregivers.*

• *Over the next decade, as new specialized prevention research centers are initiated, priority should be given to those that are sponsored through interagency agreement.* In addition to the National Institute of Mental Health (NIMH), National Institute on Alcohol Abuse and Alcoholism (NIAAA), and National Institute on Drug Abuse (NIDA), other federal agencies, such as those in the Departments of Justice, Education, and Defense should be encouraged to become involved. Over the next 10 years, in addition to the new centers focusing on multiple childhood risks and depressive disorders, specialized prevention research centers could be developed for other risk factors or disorders if a review of the evidence suggests that such action is warranted.

• *Knowledge base research at the specialized prevention research centers should be supported by new research grants (RO1s) that do not use preventive intervention research dollars.* Specialized prevention research centers provide the structure, the personnel, and the study populations that could be used to increase the knowledge base for prevention through risk research and epidemiological studies as well as for increasing knowledge about preventive intervention research programs. When these two areas of research are combined in the same center, the definition of prevention research will be especially important.

• *Dissemination mechanisms, including publication in peer-reviewed journals, and knowledge exchange opportunities with other researchers and with representatives from the community should be mandated as part of the mission of each specialized prevention research center.*

• *The preventive intervention research cycle as described in this report should be used as a conceptual model for designing, conducting, and analyzing research programs.* Preventive intervention research should proceed from pilot studies to confirmatory and replication trials to large-scale field trials and finally be transferred into the community as service programs with rigorous evaluation.

• *Increased attention to cultural diversity, ethical considerations, and benefit-cost and cost-effectiveness analyses should be an essential component of preventive intervention research.*

• *Community involvement should be increased to help identify disorders and problems that merit research and to support preventive intervention research programs.* The committee believes strongly that the long-term interests of communities throughout the nation are best served if prevention services are based on well-crafted and thoroughly evaluated trial programs. Community groups that hope for the best long-term outcomes need to express an increased willingness to have service projects more rigorously evaluated and to bring promising prevention programs into the research cycle for a more complete analysis of efficacy and effectiveness.

Funding

Preventive intervention research (excluding the specialized prevention research centers) should be budgeted at $20 million above the FY 1993 level of support in years one, two, and three, with an additional $5 million (from $20 million to $25 million) in year four and year five. Support for new specialized prevention research centers is budgeted at $2 million per year in years one and two, $5 million in year three, and $8 million per year in years four and five. (The NIMH PIRCs receive, on average, $500,000 for core support per year.) Some of this support could come from reallocation and more prudent use of federal resources that currently are available for prevention in a broad sense. For example, huge demonstration projects are rarely warranted; scaling up from confirmatory and replication trials to large-scale field trials is a more cautious and constructive use of resources. Finding out the effectiveness of programs before they are widely disseminated is likely to save money in the long term. The support that is requested in this report is not necessarily new money, but it is new for the field of preventive intervention research for mental disorders. Much of the support should come from a wide array of federal agencies already supporting prevention services that currently lack rigorous evaluation.

A FINAL WORD

There could be no wiser investment in our country than a commitment to foster the prevention of mental disorders and the promotion of mental health through rigorous research with the highest of methodological standards. Such a commitment would yield the potential for healthier lives for countless individuals and the general advancement of the nation's well-being.

Even with the support of the federal government, the effort will not be easy. There will be no "magic bullet." No single prevention strategy or method of changing people's life-style, behavior, or environment will work across the broad range of risk factors and mental disorders that will be encountered. A program designed to prevent one public health problem will not exactly fit the needs and goals of another. Dedication to prevention service programs will not necessarily bring success without a corresponding commitment to rigorous evaluation to determine the effectiveness of these services. No single agency can accomplish the task outlined above. Overall, the effort will require the cooperation of numerous federal, state, and local agencies, universities, foundations, researchers, and communities.

Hardly a family in America has been untouched by mental illness. The need for effective preventive intervention programs is clear. It is equally clear that to obtain such programs we need to make a national commitment to rigorous research and increased support for the infrastructure to make that research possible.

REFERENCES

NAS (National Academy of Sciences). (1974) Science and Technology in Presidential Policymaking. Report of the *ad hoc* Committee on Science and Technology. Washington, DC: National Academy of Sciences.

Roosevelt, F. D. (1937) Second Inaugural Address, January 20.

APPENDIXES

A

Summary

Committee on Prevention of Mental Disorders

When President Roosevelt announced in 1937 that "one third of our nation are ill housed, ill clad, ill nourished," our country was galvanized into action. Yet today, when careful population studies tell us that as many as one third of American adults will suffer a diagnosable mental disorder sometime in their life and that 20 percent have a mental disorder at any given time, there is little alarm. The Institute of Medicine's Committee on Prevention of Mental Disorders believes that strong action is warranted, and with this report it calls on the nation to mount a significant program to prevent mental disorders. Although research on the causes and treatment of mental disorders remains vitally important—and indeed major advances are leading to better lives for increasing numbers of people—much greater effort than ever before needs to be directed to prevention.

Hardly a family in America has been untouched by mental illness. According to estimates from the National Institute of Mental Health, 20 percent of adults in our country suffer from an active mental disorder in a given year, and 32 percent can be expected to have such an illness sometime during their life (Robins and Regier, 1991).

The type and nature of mental disorders vary with age. At least 12 percent of the nation's 63 million children and adolescents suffer from one or more mental disorders—including autism, attention deficit hyperactivity disorder, severe conduct disorder, depression, and alcohol and psychoactive substance abuse and dependence (DHHS, 1991; IOM, 1989; OTA, 1986). The American Academy of Child and Adolescent

---

This summary of the report by the Institute of Medicine's Committee on Prevention of Mental Disorders was prepared for members of Congress as a stand-alone document.

Psychiatry (1990) reported that growing numbers of children and adolescents are at exceptionally high risk for developing a mental disorder: for example, 1.5 million children are reported abused or neglected each year. Toward the other end of the life span are the 4 million older Americans who, according to a National Institute on Aging estimate, are likely to be suffering from Alzheimer's disease (Evans, Scherr, Cook, Albert, Funkenstein, Smith et al., 1990) and the 15 to 25 percent of the elderly in nursing homes who are clinically depressed (NIH Consensus Panel on Depression in Late Life, 1992).

In addition to the cost in human suffering and lost opportunity, mental illness of this magnitude places an extraordinary burden on the financial and social resources of this country. According to one estimate, the economic costs for 1990 were $98 billion for alcohol abuse, $66 billion for drug abuse, and $147 billion for other mental illness (D. Rice, personal communication, April 1993). Mental and physical health are closely linked, and beyond the costs just described, the contribution of mental health to physical well-being has to be considered. Despite these enormous expenditures, it is estimated that only 10 to 30 percent of those in need receive appropriate treatment (DHHS, 1991; IOM, 1989; NMHA, 1986).

Problems on this scale require attacks on many fronts. Major advances in the prevention of health-related problems in several areas of physical health have led the way to an increased awareness of the promise of prevention in enhancing mental health (DHHS, 1991). Childhood immunization programs have prevented numerous physical diseases and large-scale prevention programs have demonstrated notable success in reducing the risk of onset of cardiovascular disease (Flora, Maccoby, and Farquhar, 1989). Could advances of the same magnitude occur in mental health? Could similar successes be achieved in the prevention of disorders such as depression and schizophrenia?

Over the years, there have been many efforts to address mental health problems from a prevention perspective (see Table 1). At the same time, Americans have begun to recognize that their physical health and mental health are intertwined. Many people are striving to improve their physical and mental well-being, not just to avoid illness but to achieve what they consider greater personal rewards, including a more active life and a generally more positive disposition (Breslow, 1990). In the report summarized herein, the Institute of Medicine's Committee on Prevention of Mental Disorders examines what is currently known about the prevention of mental disorders and promotion of mental health and outlines the prospects for advances in that knowledge and its application over the next decade.

TABLE 1 Time Line of Events Related to Prevention of Mental Disorders

1909 The Mental Health Association was founded; subsequently it became the National Association for Mental Health and then the National Mental Health Association (NMHA). Since its inception, it has advocated for prevention of mental illness and promotion of mental health.

1910 Public meeting on "Prevention of Insanity" organized by the New York Committee on Mental Hygiene. Topics included alcoholism, syphilis, drug addiction, head injuries, infectious diseases such as meningitis, and influences of fatigue and stress.

1915 *The Proceedings of the National Conference of Charities and Correction* contained papers on prevention of mental illness and mental retardation. The ideas included sterilization, reduced immigration, and more institutions to lower the numbers of "feeble-minded" in the community.

1920s The child guidance movement and the mental hygiene movement (fostered by the National Committee for Mental Hygiene that was organized by Clifford Beers) were begun. Both movements were committed to prevention as well as treatment of mental illness and highly valued the role of local communities in solving problems, including prevention of juvenile delinquency.

1930 The White House Conference on Child Health and Protection issued a report with an expanded focus that included social and environmental factors that affect the physical and mental health of children.

1930s The national commitment to prevention decreased, and the treatment-oriented approach began to dominate. Insurance plans created at this time reinforced the illness/treatment approach.

1946 Passage of the National Mental Health Act (P.L. 487) authorized the creation of the National Institute of Mental Health (NIMH).

1948 The World Federation for Mental Health, an independent organization with close ties to the United Nations, was created and included prevention within its purview.

1948 The Mental Health Study Center, a small NIMH community laboratory, was established in Prince Georges County, Maryland, to apply public health principles to the practice of mental health at the community level. For the next 34 years, research was done and treatment and prevention services were provided.

1954 The first organized training program in mental health consultation, which included a prevention component, began at the Harvard School of Public Health, Laboratory of Community Psychiatry.

1955 The Mental Health Study Act directed the Joint Commission on Mental Illness and Health to analyze and evaluate the needs and resources of the mentally ill and make recommendations for a national mental health program.

1961 The Joint Commission on Mental Illness and Health released *Action for Mental Health* to the Senate and House of Representatives.

1963 President John F. Kennedy, in a message to Congress, championed prevention as an approach to the problem of mental illness.

(continued)

TABLE 1   (Continued)

1963 The Community Mental Health Centers Act listed mental health consultation and education, which included prevention, as one of the five essential services necessary for such centers to qualify for federal funds. This was the first time in any federal health statute that a preventive service was declared mandatory.

1969 The Joint Commission on Mental Health of Children produced a report saying that millions of children were in need of services, and millions were at risk.

1973 NMHA formed a Prevention Task Force.

1975 The first Vermont Conference on the Primary Prevention of Psychopathology was sponsored by the World Federation for Mental Health, NIMH, and the John D. and Catherine T. MacArthur Foundation.

1976 The Conference on Primary Prevention sponsored by NIMH resulted in *Primary Prevention: An Idea Whose Time Has Come.*

1978 The President's Commission on Mental Health reported that (1) efforts to prevent mental illness and promote mental health were unstructured, unfocused, and uncoordinated and (2) preventive efforts received insufficient attention at the federal, state, and local levels. The commission recommended establishing a Center for Prevention in NIMH.

1978 The position of Coordinator for Disease Prevention and Health Promotion was established at the National Institutes of Health (NIH).

1979 The first annual Alcohol, Drug Abuse, and Mental Health Administration (ADAMHA) Conference on Prevention was held.

1980 The NIH Prevention Coordinating Committee was formed, with the NIH Coordinator for Disease Prevention and Health Promotion as the designated prevention coordinator.

1980 The Public Health Service Act (in response to the presidential endorsement of the 1978 President's Commission on Mental Health) was amended to give special attention to efforts to prevent mental disability. Among other requirements, this act and a 1983 amendment (1) established the Office of the Deputy Director for Prevention and Special Projects in NIMH, and (2) designated an Associate Administrator for Prevention within ADAMHA to promote and coordinate prevention programs, including those run by NIMH, the National Institute on Drug Abuse (NIDA), and the National Institute on Alcohol Abuse and Alcoholism (NIAAA). The Associate Administrator was made responsible for an annual report to Congress describing the prevention activities undertaken by ADAMHA and its agencies.

1980 NIDA established its Prevention Research Branch.

1981 The Select Panel for Promotion of Child Health (established by Public Law 95–626) presented its findings to the U.S. Congress and the Secretary of Health and Human Services. The panel reported a need for better coordination of mental health and health services due to the frequent concomitance of health and mental health problems in children.

1981 The Omnibus Budget Reconciliation Act folded the community mental health centers into alcohol, drug abuse, and mental health block grants to the states and introduced large cuts in all human service appropriations.

TABLE 1 (Continued)

1982 The Center for Prevention Research (CPR) was established at NIMH. This was a step toward consolidation of preventive intervention research throughout NIMH into one unit.

1983 NIMH Center for Prevention Research established its first Prevention Intervention Research Center (PIRC).

1983 ADAMHA Associate Administrator for Prevention was appointed, as mandated by an amendment to the Public Health Service Act, to promote and coordinate the research programs of its component agencies—NIAAA, NIDA, and NIMH.

1984 NMHA established the Commission on the Prevention of Mental-Emotional Disabilities.

1985 NIMH appointed its first Deputy Director for Prevention, mandated by the 1980 Public Health Service Act.

1985 The Office of Substance Abuse Prevention (OSAP) was established.

1985 NIDA published the first of several monographs dealing with preventing drug abuse.

1985 The Center for Prevention Research reorganized into the Prevention Research Branch within the newly created Division of Clinical Research in NIMH.

1986 A prevention initiative was undertaken by the American Academy of Child and Adolescent Psychiatry, and a Project Prevention Steering Committee was formed. The initiative resulted in a series of prevention monographs published by OSAP.

1986 NIAAA established the Prevention Research Branch within the Clinical and Prevention Research Division, created at the same time.

1986 The position of Assistant Director for Disease Prevention at the Office of Director level was established within NIH.

1986 The Office of Technology Assessment (OTA) issued a report entitled *Children's Mental Health: Problems and Services.* The report concluded that there was a substantial theoretical and research base to show that mental health interventions were effective for children.

1986 NMHA released a report by the Commission on the Prevention of Mental-Emotional Disabilities, *The Prevention of Mental-Emotional Disabilities.*

1987 NIMH published *Preventing Mental Disorders: A Research Perspective.*

1987 The National Prevention Coalition was established within NMHA.

1989 The U.S. General Accounting Office issued a report to Senator Inouye, *Mental Health: Prevention of Mental Disorders and Research on Stress-Related Disorders,* a critique of the implementation of prior recommendations in the prevention field.

1989 The Institute of Medicine (IOM) issued *Research on Children and Adolescents with Mental, Behavioral, and Developmental Disorders: Mobilizing a National Initiative.* Prevention was not emphasized.

1990 Because of a congressional mandate, NIMH entered into an agreement with IOM so that IOM could prepare an integrated report of current prevention research, with policy-oriented and detailed long-term recommendations for a prevention research agenda.

(continued)

TABLE 1   (Continued)

1990	The American Psychiatric Association published a report prepared by the Task Force on Prevention Research of the Council on Research with a review of research on the prevention of psychiatric disorders.
1990	The American Academy of Child and Adolescent Psychiatry published *Prevention in Child and Adolescent Psychiatry: The Reduction of Risk for Mental Disorders.*
1990	*A National Plan for Research on Child and Adolescent Mental Disorders* (National Advisory Mental Health Council) emphasized scientific research concerning biomedical risk factors and capacity building for scientific researchers.
1990	NIMH held its first National Conference on Prevention Research, and a NIMH Steering Committee on Prevention was established to write a report on the current status of prevention research within NIMH.
1992	The ADAMHA Reorganization Act abolished ADAMHA, organized the three research institutes (NIAAA, NIDA, and NIMH) under NIH, and provided for an Associate Director for Prevention in each research institute. The service components from ADAMHA were reorganized into the Substance Abuse and Mental Health Services Administration (SAMHSA) as the Center for Substance Abuse Treatment, the Center for Substance Abuse Prevention, and the Center for Mental Health Services.
1992	The IOM Committee on Prevention of Mental Disorders was formed in accordance with the NIMH agreement.
1993	NIMH Steering Committee on Prevention released *The Prevention of Mental Disorders: A National Research Agenda* at the third NIMH National Conference on Prevention Research.

OPPORTUNITIES AND OBSTACLES

The committee undertook its broad review of the status of prevention research at the request of Congress and the National Institute of Mental Health and co-funding agencies.* It found encouraging opportunities and strengths and a number of obstacles. To date, progress in prevention has been limited because efforts have been sporadic and often have lacked focus. Problems have included difficulties in identifying, defining, and classifying mental disorders; a perception that the knowledge base—including an understanding of etiologies and risk mechanisms—is too small to support preventive interventions; and confusion regarding the terms *prevention* and *prevention research*. But the knowledge base has undergone remarkable expansion within the past decade.

---

*The co-funding agencies were the National Institute of Mental Health (NIMH), the Administration on Children, Youth, and Families, the Maternal and Child Health Bureau, the Center for Substance Abuse Prevention, the Office of the Assistant Secretary for Planning and Evaluation, the Office of the Assistant Secretary for Health, and the Office of Disease Prevention and Health Promotion.

Fundamental advances in our understanding of the biological substrates and genetics underlying numerous mental disorders and the role of environmental factors in the onset of specific disorders have been made. There are a number of promising new preventive interventions. The committee believes that it is time to take a fresh look at prevention to see if it can be made to function as a full partner with new treatment approaches in addressing our nation's mental health care crisis.

NEW DIRECTIONS IN DEFINITIONS

An essential first step in a renewed prevention effort is to arrive at commonly agreed upon definitions for key terms. Two systems for classifying types of interventions for mental disorders are currently in use. But both the public health classification system of primary, secondary, and tertiary prevention (Commission on Chronic Illness, 1957) and Gordon's (1987, 1983) system of universal, selective, and indicated prevention are focused on prevention of disorders traditionally identified as medical disorders, and the application of these terms to a mental health framework is problematic.

"To prevent" literally means "to keep something from happening." But within the field of mental health, there are different notions about what that something is—first incidence, relapse, disability associated with a disorder, or the risk condition itself. Therefore, for application to mental disorders, the term *prevention* needs to be more carefully circumscribed than it is in either of these systems. In Chapter 2 of this report, the committee presents a classification system that is tailored for mental disorders and in which the term *prevention* is reserved for those interventions that occur before the initial onset of disorder. Treatment (for individuals who meet or are close to meeting diagnostic criteria) and maintenance (for diagnosed individuals whose illness continues) complete the committee's vision of the spectrum of interventions for mental disorders (see Figure 1).

The change in terminology that is used throughout this report, although perhaps not particularly useful to clinicians, who may find themselves providing elements of prevention, treatment, and maintenance to the same patient, is critical to a review of prevention research. Without a system for classifying specific interventions, there is no way to obtain accurate information on the type or extent of current activities, either public or private, and no way to ensure that prevention researchers, practitioners, and policymakers are speaking the same language.

To further classify interventions within prevention, the committee has adapted the terms used by Gordon. *Universal preventive interventions* for

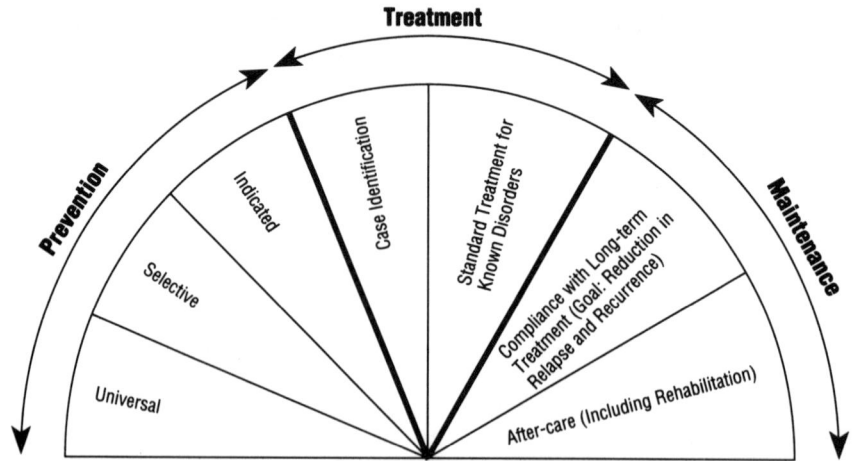

FIGURE 1   The mental health intervention spectrum for mental disorders.

mental disorders are targeted to the general public or a whole population group that has not been identified on the basis of individual risk. Such interventions have advantages when their cost per individual is low, the intervention is effective and acceptable to the population, and there is a low risk from the intervention. However, it is crucial to be realistic about costs. An intervention provided to every prospective marital couple, although low in cost per couple, would be very expensive overall because of the size of the target group.

Selective preventive interventions are targeted to individuals or a subgroup of the population whose risk of developing mental disorders is significantly higher than average. The risk may be imminent, or it may be a lifetime risk. Risk groups may be identified on the basis of biological, psychological, or social risk factors that are known to be associated with the onset of a mental disorder. Selective interventions are most appropriate if the interventions do not exceed a moderate level of cost and if negative effects are minimal or nonexistent.

Indicated preventive interventions are targeted to high-risk individuals who are identified as having minimal but detectable signs or symptoms foreshadowing mental disorder, or biological markers indicating predisposition for the mental disorder, but who do not meet DSM-III-R diagnostic levels at the current time. The term *indicated* is used differently here from how Gordon used it. Whereas he meant it to apply only to asymptomatic individuals, within this mental health classification system it can be applied to asymptomatic individuals with markers as well as to symptomatic individuals whose symptoms are still early and are not sufficiently severe to merit a diagnosis. Indicated interventions may be reasonable even if intervention costs are high and even if the intervention entails some risk.

The committee does not include mental health promotion within the spectrum of interventions focused on mental disorders because health promotion is not driven by an emphasis on illness, but rather by a focus on the enhancement of well-being. It is provided to individuals, groups, or large populations to enhance competence and self-esteem rather than to intervene to prevent psychological or social problems or mental disorders. Nevertheless, promotion is an important approach to mental health, and therefore Chapter 9 presents a capsulized look at its status.

THE RISK REDUCTION MODEL

The long-term goal of all three types of preventive intervention—universal, selective, and indicated—is the reduction of the occurrence of new cases of mental disorder. Usually, this is attempted through a risk reduction model, wherein the short-term goal is the reduction of the risk factors and the enhancement of the protective factors that have been shown to be associated with the onset of the disorder. Risk factors are those characteristics, variables, or hazards that, if present for a given individual, make it more likely that this individual, rather than someone selected from the general population, will develop a disorder (Werner and Smith, 1992; Garmezy, 1983). Many at-risk individuals also have variables in their background or life that serve as protective factors.

A well-documented description of the interplay between risk and protective factors is a critical scientific first step in establishing successful preventive intervention programs. Such a description is now available for some disorders, and research is under way to identify such factors for a number of others. The next step is to identify causal risk factors that may be malleable, that is, that can be altered through interventions. Then the effects of these interventions are tested in systematic, empirical, and rigorous ways, most often in preventive intervention trials. If risk factors can be decreased or in some way altered, and/or if protective factors can be enhanced, the likelihood that at-risk individuals would eventually develop the mental disorder would decrease.

As described in Chapter 3, this risk reduction model is widely used for prevention of physical illness. To prevent physical disorders due to complex multiple causes, the strategy is to determine risk factors and then to target interventions to such risk factors or to people with these risk factors. Progress has been notable in many areas, including the three used in this chapter as illustrations: cardiovascular disease, smoking cessation and prevention, and injury prevention. The universal preventive strategies mounted in these areas have demonstrated that effective interventions are possible even when knowledge about the mechanisms causing illness is incomplete.

THE KNOWLEDGE BASE

In order to formulate effective interventions, prevention researchers harvest methodologies, data, theories, and principles from a bounty of disciplines. The core sciences, including neuroscience, genetics, epidemiology, and developmental psychopathology; research on risk and protective factors for the onset of mental disorders; previous preventive intervention research programs; and research on treatment interventions for mental disorders all contribute to the knowledge base for research on preventive interventions for mental disorders. *For some mental disorders, the knowledge base is now at a stage comparable to that available for many physical disorders before successful large-scale prevention trials for those disorders were mounted.*

The Core Sciences

Two broad areas of science contribute to research on the prevention of mental disorders—the behavioral sciences, in which the study of mental disorders has its historical roots, and the biological sciences, which have begun to provide insights into these disorders more recently. The boundaries between these sciences should not be viewed as rigid and distinct. Interdisciplinary investigations that incorporate principles and findings from both the behavioral and the biological perspectives have vital implications for research on the prevention of mental disorders. The frontiers for the field of prevention can be moved forward through appropriate theoretical integration. Chapter 4 presents four of these integrative core sciences as illustrations—neuroscience, genetics, epidemiology, and developmental psychopathology—to highlight how they contribute to preventive intervention research.

Neuroscience research encompasses the acquisition of knowledge about fundamental biological processes of the brain and nervous system and about the pathophysiology of neurological disease processes, including cellular mechanisms underlying etiology, course, and outcome. The more that is known about etiology, the more possible it becomes to target preventive interventions to intervene in causal chains. In addition, recent advances in molecular biology have led to an increase in our understanding of the scope and complexity of neuronal function. The practical outcome so far has been the discovery of new classes of drugs, such as the calcium channel blockers. One goal of current research is to provide even greater effectiveness of drug therapy by increasing the number of cellular targets for drug action. The potential implications of this research for prevention, especially indicated interventions, may be considerable.

Research into the genetic causes of disease is among the most active and exciting areas of biomedical investigation and promises to make substantial contributions to our understanding of mental disorders. Genetic studies can tell us much about developmental processes and psychopathological mechanisms (Rutter, Simonoff, and Silberg, in press; Rutter, Silberg, and Simonoff, 1993). Eventually, it may become possible to determine the precise mechanisms by which environmental risk factors operate. In the absence of sound knowledge on these processes, there is some danger that prevention measures may be either wrongly targeted or so diffuse that they do not bring the expected benefits. Current and potential contributions to prevention center on the following areas of inquiry: causal processes, normal distributions, and co-morbidity of disorders; mechanisms of genetic risk; testing for environmental effects and individual differences in those effects; individual differences in exposure to risk factors; misleading environmental assumptions; genetic counseling; and gene therapy.

Another discipline that takes a developmental and integrative perspective on the etiology and course of psychopathology is epidemiology, which is the study of the distribution of disorders in populations. *Incidence* refers to the rate at which new cases of the disorder arise. *Prevalence* is the proportion of the population with the disorder. Preventive interventions are directed toward reducing incidence, whereas treatment interventions seek to reduce prevalence.

Epidemiological studies have yielded valuable data on the origins, life course, and risk factors for mental disorders. In studying the origins of a mental disorder, a prospective longitudinal design is particularly powerful. Two refinements of the concept of risk allow comparisons of various factors as they influence the development of disorder. *Relative risk* is the ratio of incidence for a given disorder in an exposed population to the incidence in an unexposed population. *Attributable risk* is the maximum proportion of cases that would be prevented if an intervention were 100 percent effective in eliminating the risk factor.

Data on prevalence and on attributable risk are especially germane to research on the prevention of mental disorders. To acquire these data, diverse strategies of research are needed. The prevalence of the disorder is required in order to assess its impact on the population. Prevalence is obtained efficiently from a cross-sectional survey. The attributable risk for a range of risk factors is required in order to select interventions that will have the most powerful effect. Attributable risk is probably most efficiently obtained via the case-control strategy.

An even more recent frontier is the conceptualization of the age of onset for specific disorders. Determination of age of onset is required in order to time the intervention appropriately, that is, before the first incidence of a disorder or problem. Recognizing the importance of such data, the committee commissioned new analyses of data from the National Institute of Mental Health's Epidemiologic Catchment Area study (Robins and Regier, 1991). The conceptualizations and methods used in these analyses, and the resulting fresh perspectives they permit, are presented in Chapter 5.

Many scientific areas of study with links to prevention research have their origins in the behavioral and social sciences. Contributions from these areas that offer substantial leads for research on the prevention of mental disorders include the impact of psychological stress on health; the role of social support mechanisms in decreasing risk factors and enhancing protective factors; usage of health care delivery systems; the relationship between theoretical concepts such as attachment, self-esteem, and self-efficacy and later social relationships and health behaviors; the importance of social frames of reference, including race, culture, gender, and community context; and the relevance of developmental psychopathology in understanding individual patterns of adaptation over time.

There is an increasing tendency within the biological and behavioral sciences to appreciate the complexity and interplay of genetic and environmental interactions. There is also an increased recognition of the utility of a developmental focus. From this developmental focus has arisen the concept of sensitive periods, which is especially relevant to the timing of preventive interventions.

Description of Illustrative Disorders

Whether a particular mental disorder and the risk factors associated with its onset warrant a major preventive research effort depends on a number of factors. In addition to information on incidence, prevalence, prodromal period, and age of onset, an understanding of the symptomatology, natural course, co-morbidity, and treatment effectiveness of the disorder is needed. For example, the incidence of a disorder will help determine the necessary size of the sample so that statistical analyses are meaningful; the demographics of a disorder will help determine who is at highest risk and what population groups should be targeted; and if a specific treatment is known to be effective, it could be considered for use before onset of the disorder.

In Chapter 5 the discussion of this knowledge is organized around five major mental disorders: conduct disorder, depressive disorders, alcohol abuse and dependence, schizophrenia, and Alzheimer's disease. These five disorders were chosen as illustrations for use throughout the report because they are all serious disorders that have enormous emotional and financial costs associated with them. They represent the great diversity of mental illness, have their onset at varying stages in the life cycle, and reflect a spectrum of causation, arising from primarily psychosocial factors in conduct disorder to clear biological contributions in Alzheimer's disease. The choice of these five disorders is by no means meant to imply that these are the only disorders that should be targeted for preventive intervention research programs. Anxiety disorders, post-traumatic stress disorder, obsessive-compulsive disorder, and other adult and childhood mental disorders may also be appropriate targets. These five disorders are simply illustrative of the range of factors and approaches that must be considered in designing preventive intervention research programs, and the brief descriptions given in Chapter 5 are examples of how the available information should be reviewed.

A disorder may be preventable up to the point of onset of first episode. Although onset can rarely be accurately pinpointed, the time at which an individual meets full criteria for diagnosis can be used as an approximation. As more becomes known about precursors and prodromes, the age of onset will become more accurately known. The *prodrome* is the period prior to onset of a disorder, when some early signs or symptoms are nevertheless present. But individuals with early signs and symptoms of disorder often do not go on to develop the full criteria for diagnosis. In this situation the signs and symptoms are not prodromal, in the strict sense of the word. Therefore, for a particular individual a prodrome can be known only in retrospect, after he or she has developed the disorder. If he or she never develops it, the early signs were not part of a prodrome. Signs and symptoms from a diagnostic cluster that precede disorder, but do not predict the onset of disorder with certainty, are referred to here as *precursor signs and symptoms*. Currently, there are few or no signs and symptoms that predict onset with certainty. Nevertheless, prospective epidemiological studies could identify precursor signs and symptoms, as well as the age of the first occurrence of these precursors. Thus it may be possible to identify individuals at heightened risk for developing the full-blown disorder, who would then become candidates for indicated preventive interventions.

Ideally, prevention efforts ought to be directed to specific age periods during which the causal events underlying the disorder are taking place: if the preventive intervention occurs too early, its positive effects may be washed out before onset; if it occurs too late, the disorder may already have had its onset. More research regarding the sensitive periods of risk factors, that is, when they contribute most to etiology, could lead to more strategic timing of preventive interventions. In addition, prospective epidemiological studies that estimate incidence of specific risk factors and disorders in childhood, adolescence, and during the age period of the transition to adulthood, from age 15 to 25, are greatly needed. Such studies could help clarify the mechanisms linking risk factors to the first occurrence of disorders. The epidemiological research on children and adults should gather and retain data on a wide range of signs and symptoms, as well as disorders, to help ensure that maturational changes and changes in the diagnostic classification system do not interfere with the study of the development of psychopathology over time.

Risk and Protective Factors for Onset

During the past 30 years a growing body of research has elucidated some of the risk factors that predispose children and adults to mental disorder. To qualify as a risk factor, a variable must be associated with an increased probability of disorder and must antedate the onset of disorder. Variables that are risk factors at one life stage might not be at another. Risk factors can reside with the individual or within the family, community, or institutions that surround the individual. They can be biological or psychosocial in nature. Some risk factors play a causal role, although this may not be known prior to an intervention study. If causal risk factors targeted in an intervention are malleable, the risk of onset of the disorder can be reduced. Other risk factors—for example, the unusual eye movement that is often associated with and predates schizophrenia—are identifying in nature rather than causal, and for these, therefore, malleability is not an issue. The committee uses the term *marker* for both biological and psychosocial risk factors of the latter sort. Incorporated into the definition of risk factor is the concept of vulnerability, which is a predisposition to a specific disease process. Having vulnerability traits may increase an individual's risk for developing a disorder, but other risk factors also may be necessary for the illness to be expressed.

Recently, researchers have been trying to understand why some children appear to be resilient, and why they come to maturity relatively unscathed by the organic and psychosocial risk insults that prevent so many of their peers from achieving optimal intellectual, social, and emotional functioning (Werner and Smith, 1992). Theoretical explanations for the phenomenon of resilience (Rutter, 1985; Garmezy, 1983) involve the interaction of risk factors, including individual vulnerability, and protective factors. Rutter (1985) defined protective factors as "those factors that modify, ameliorate or alter a person's response to some environmental hazard that predisposes to a maladaptive outcome." Protective factors also can reside with the individual or the family, community, or institutions and can be biological or psychosocial in nature.

Each mental disorder is likely to have multiple risk factors. Chapter 6 examines these factors for the five illustrative disorders. Over the past decade, evidence that genetic factors play a major role in vulnerability to Alzheimer's disease (AD) has accumulated. There is a suggestion that environmental factors may influence when symptoms begin, suggesting that prevention might work by delaying onset. The research base is not currently sufficient, however, to mount a preventive intervention campaign with potential AD victims. The best hope for prevention in the near future lies in the research focused on delaying the onset of AD, either through education early in life or through the prophylactic use of drugs to improve cognitive function or to impede amyloid deposition in high-risk individuals.

Although genetic vulnerability may predispose to schizophrenia, and may even be necessary, genetic factors by themselves cannot account for the illness. Many of the data are consistent with a developmental disorder that is set in place via genetic and biological factors early in life. This developmental pattern may be susceptible to psychosocial stress, which may trigger the symptomatic expression of the disorder or which may cross a threshold for disease expression. Universal and selective interventions to prevent the onset of schizophrenia are not warranted at this time. The best hope now for prevention of schizophrenia lies with indicated preventive interventions targeted at individuals manifesting precursor signs and symptoms who have not yet met full criteria for diagnosis. The children of schizophrenic parents are at increased risk for emotional problems of many types, including schizophrenia, and preventive intervention research should continue to study this high-risk group.

Alcohol abuse and dependence are genetically influenced disorders, and quantification of genetic risk has begun. Studies examining psychosocial risk factors for onset have often failed to control for family history of alcoholism or other mental disorders, especially antisocial personality disorder and depression. It appears likely that it is the accumulation of both genetic and psychosocial risk factors that increases the risk for alcohol abuse and dependence. Six risk factors are strongly associated with the onset of alcohol problems: (1) having a parent or other close biological relative with alcohol abuse or dependence; (2) having a biological marker that is highly associated with later onset of alcohol dependence, including decreased sensitivity to alcohol; (3) demonstrating antisocial behaviors or a combination of aggressiveness and shyness during childhood; (4) having low adaptability; (5) being exposed to group norms that foster alcohol use and abuse; and (6) having easy access to alcohol. Control of availability obviously continues to be a powerful prevention tool.

Five risk factors are likely to be associated with the onset of depression: (1) having a parent or other close biological relative with a mood disorder; (2) having a severe stressor such as a loss, divorce, marital separation, unemployment, job dissatisfaction, a physical disorder such as a chronic medical condition, a traumatic experience, or, in children, a learning disorder; (3) having low self-esteem, a sense of low self-efficacy, and a sense of helplessness and hopelessness; (4) being female; and (5) living in poverty. Approaches that have targeted either the prevention of clinical depression in high-risk adults or the prevention of depressive symptoms for those at high risk because of a major loss have all shown some promise. Definitive evidence of the prevention of the initial episode of major depressive disorder is not available at this time, but this area is one of the most promising for continued preventive intervention research.

Conduct disorder has the earliest average age of onset of the five illustrative disorders. Much remains to be learned about its risk and protective factors, but it is clear that the accumulation of risk factors as the child develops is more important than any specific risk factor. The lack of twin and adoption studies in conduct disorder is a major research gap. Such studies have provided tantalizing clues toward understanding the roles of genetic and environmental influences for the other illustrative disorders.

It has become evident that even though some risk factors, primarily genetic ones, may be specific to a particular disorder, others are common to many disorders. For a child, such factors as low birthweight, low IQ, and even gender can lead to a state of vulnerability in which other risk factors may have more effect (McGauhey, Starfield, Alexander, and Ensminger, 1991; Rutter, 1979). Factors that can contribute to resilience include positive temperament, above-average intelligence, and social competence (Rutter, 1985; Rutter, Tizard, and Whitmore,

1970), as well as good sibling relationships and adequate rule setting by parents (Werner and Smith, 1982). In general, protective factors in adulthood fall into two broad groupings—those that arise from the buffering effects of social support available to the individual and personality factors or personal characteristics that affect the individual's ability to cope with stress (O'Grady and Metz, 1987).

Understanding that risk and protective factors are common to many disorders is only a first step. It is also essential to understand that these factors do not function in isolation; instead, there exists a dynamic interaction among them that undergoes modification and change throughout an individual's life span. The concept of causal or etiological chains, in which one event calls forth another, is helpful in understanding risk and protective factor interaction. More likely, the patterns of interaction between the child's personal attributes and risk and protective factors in the family, school, and community are not linear but are woven like the threads in a Jacquard tapestry in patterns of increasing complexity. Research on child maltreatment has provided illustrations of this more complex conceptualization.

Because it appears that most risk and protective factors are not specific to a single disorder, the most fruitful approach for preventive interventions at this time may be to use a risk reduction model that includes the enhancement of protective factors and to aim at clusters or constellations of risk and protective factors. Markers can be used to identify high-risk populations, but the interventions will be aimed at those causal and malleable risk factors that appear to have a role in the expression of several mental disorders. Identification of relative and attributable risks associated with various clusters could greatly facilitate preventive intervention research.

Illustrative Preventive Intervention Research Programs

Although preventive intervention research is still a relatively young field and formidable tasks lie ahead, the past decade has brought encouraging progress. At present, there are many intervention programs that rest on sound conceptual and empirical foundations, and a substantial number are rigorously designed and evaluated. These research programs have been supported by a wide range of public agencies, including the specialized prevention centers at the research institutes, as well as private foundations.

Chapter 7 presents a limited number of these interventions to illustrate a range of promising program approaches to achieving diverse prevention goals. Most of the programs selected for inclusion have met rigorous criteria formulated by the committee for examining such programs, including the use of randomized controlled trials. The criteria pertain to (1) the risk and protective factors addressed, (2) the targeted population group, (3) the intervention itself, (4) the research design, (5) evidence concerning the implementation, and (6) evidence concerning the outcomes. Chapter 7 gives a full description of the criteria to serve as a guide for researchers, practitioners, and policymakers as they make critical decisions for this field. A framework for examinations using these criteria is presented in Figure 2. (See Table 2 for a summary of the research programs.)

The committee's examination of these programs brought several points to light. As yet, there is no evidence that preventive interventions reduce the incidence of mental disorders. However, although their numbers are relatively small, some excellent illustrations are available of preventive interventions that can reduce risk factors associated with the onset of mental disorders. Such programs can be mined for successful methodologies and strategies for future programs. Successful service programs also can provide good leads regarding intervention, community context, and exchange of ideas, but their effectiveness in reducing psychological symptoms and mental disorders needs to be tested experimentally.

Most prevention research programs are targeted to the needs of infants, preschoolers, elementary-age children, and adolescents. There is a nationwide and unfortunate lack of prevention research programs targeted to the needs of adults, especially the elderly. It has been shown that positive outcomes can be secured for both infants and their mothers from a single comprehensive intervention (Olds, Henderson, Tatelbaum, and Chamberlin, 1988, 1986), and it is possible that interventions that have been highly successful at certain developmental stages, such as home visiting with families with infants and preschoolers, might also be useful at other stages, such as with the elderly, who may be homebound. At the same time, it is clear that there is usually no single intervention at a single point in time that accomplishes comprehensive goals of prevention for a lifetime. The ultimate goal to achieve optimal prevention should be to build the principles of prevention into the ordinary activities of everyday life and into community structures to enhance development over the entire life span.

Risk factors that occur in multiple domains—home, school, peer group, neighborhood, or work site—require interventions in all of them. Preventive intervention programs from infancy to adolescence have shown the feasibility of multidomain interventions. Many prevention programs clearly demonstrate that education, physical health care, employment, and mental health care are not separable. Improvements

Program Name _____ Investigator(s): _____
Reference(s): _____

1. Description of the Risk and Protective Factors Addressed	2. Description of the Targeted Population Group	3. Description of the Intervention Program	4. Description of the Research Methodologies	5. Description of the Evidence Concerning Implementation	6. Description of the Evidence Concerning Outcomes
Documentation	Universal, selective, or indicated	Goals and Content	Methods of recruitment	Exposure of target group to intervention	Changes in status of risk and/or protective factors
Relationship to developmental task	Evidence that group is at risk for disorder or problem	Protocols	Sample size	Fidelity of delivery in accordance with design	Evidence of reduction of new cases
Causal status	Sociodemographic variables	Personnel delivering the intervention	Randomization		Evidence of delay of onset
Status in malleability		Site	Baseline measures		Side effects
Correlation with incidence and prevalence		Institutional or cultural content	Statistical analysis		Benefit-cost and cost-effectiveness analyses
		Ethical considerations	Attrition of subjects		
		Equipment or instrumentation			
		Method of delivery and techniques			
		Duration and extent			
		Multiple components			

FIGURE 2 A framework for examining preventive interventions. This format might be used as a worksheet in determining the methodological rigor of a specific program.

TABLE 2   Illustrative Preventive Intervention Programs Using Randomized Controlled Trial Design

	Targeted Population Group/Sample Size When Project Began	Risk Factors Addressed	Outcomes (for total intervention group or subgroups)	Principal Investigator(s) and Year(s)
Infants				
Prenatal/Early Infancy Project	Selective/ N=394	Economic deprivation, maternal prenatal health and damaging behaviors, poor family management practices	Improved maternal diet and reduced smoking during pregnancy, fewer preterm deliveries, higher-birthweight babies, less child abuse	Olds, 1988, 1986
Tactile/Kinesthetic Stimulation	Selective/ N=40	Preterm delivery, low birthweight	Better physical and mental development of infants	Field, 1986
Early Intervention for Preterm Infants	Selective/ N=60	Teenage parenthood, low socioeconomic status, preterm delivery	Better parenting behaviors and attitudes of mothers, better cognitive competence, better physical development, better temperament of infants	Field, 1980
Infant Health and Development Program	Selective/ N=985	Low birthweight, poor family management practices, academic failure, early behavior problems	Better cognitive competence, fewer behavior problems	Ramey, 1990
Carolina Abecedarian Project	Selective/ N=107	Academic failure, lack of readiness for school, economic deprivation, low commitment to school	Better cognitive competence, lower rates of retention in grade in school	Horacek and Ramey, 1987

Program	Type/N	Risk Factors	Outcomes	Citation
Young Children				
Houston Parent-Child Development Center	Selective/ N=~700	Economic deprivation, academic failure, early behavior problems, poor family management practices	Better family management practices, fewer behavior problems	Johnson, 1991, 1990
Mother-Child Home Program of Verbal Interaction Project	Selective/ N=156	Academic failure, economic deprivation, poor family management practices, early behavior problems	Better family management practices, better cognitive competence	Levenstein, 1992, 1984
Parent-Child Interaction Training	Indicated/ N=105	Economic deprivation, early behavior problems, poor family management practices, maternal depressive symptoms	Lower rates of attention deficits and conduct problems	Strayhorn, 1991
High/Scope Preschool Curriculum Comparison Study (including Distar)	Selective/ N=68	Academic failure, early behavior problems, economic deprivation	Better cognitive competence	Weikart and Schweinhart, 1992, 1986
Perry Preschool Program (using High/ Scope curriculum)	Selective/ N=123	Academic failure, economic deprivation, early behavior problems, low commitment to school	Better cognitive competence, greater achievement and school completion, better vocational outcomes, fewer conduct problems and arrests	Weikart and Schweinhart, 1987, 1984
I Can Problem Solve: Interpersonal Cognitive Problem-Solving Program	Selective/ N=219 (N=60 in pilot study)	Economic deprivation, poor impulse control, early behavior problems	Better cognitive problem-solving skills, fewer behavior problems	Shure and Spivack, 1982, 1979
Elementary-Age Children				
Assertiveness Training Program (program 1)	Universal/ N=343	Early behavior problems, academic failure	Improved social assertiveness, improved academic performance	Rotheram, 1982

(continued)

TABLE 2 (*Continued*)

	Targeted Population Group/Sample Size When Project Began	Risk Factors Addressed	Outcomes (for total intervention group or subgroups)	Principal Investigator(s) and Year(s)
Assertiveness Training Program (program 2)	Indicated/ N=101	Early behavior problems, academic failure	More assertive behavior, better school achievement, fewer behavior problems	Rotheram, 1982
Children of Divorce Intervention Program	Selective/ N=75	Marital conflict and separation, early conduct problems	Lower anxiety, fewer learning problems, better adjustment	Pedro-Carroll and Cowen, 1989, 1986, 1985
Family Bereavement Program	Selective/ N=72	Child bereavement, poor family management practices, early behavior problems	Lower levels of symptoms of depression and conduct disorder	Sandler, 1992
Social Skills Training	Selective/ N=28	Peer rejection, early conduct problems	Less peer rejection, better interpersonal skills	Bierman, 1986
Social Relations Intervention Program	Indicated/ N=86	Early behavior problems (aggression), peer rejection, impulsivity	Less aggression, less peer rejection, more prosocial behavior	Lochman, in press
Montreal Longitudinal-Experimental	Indicated/ N=172	Poor family management practices, peer rejection, academic failure, early behavior problems, violence on television	Less aggressive behavior, less delinquent behavior, better school achievement	Tremblay, 1992, 1991
Community Epidemiological Preventive Intervention: Mastery Learning and Good Behavior Game	Universal/ N=2314	Academic failure, aggressive and antisocial behavior, concentration problems, depressive symptoms, shy behavior	Less aggressive and shy behavior, better cognitive competence—especially among those with early depressive symptoms	Kellam and Rebock, 1992

Program	Type/N	Risk factors targeted	Outcomes	Citation
Academic Tutoring and Social Skills Training	Selective/N=40	Academic failure, peer rejection, early behavior problems, early depressive symptoms	Better cognitive competence, less peer rejection	Coie and Krehbiel, 1984
Seattle Social Development Project	Universal/N=908	Poor family management practices, early behavior problems, low commitment to school, academic failure	Better family management practices and family bonding, greater attachment to school, lower rates of delinquency and drug use initiation	Hawkins and Catalano, 1988
Adolescents				
Changing Teaching Practices	Selective/N=1166	Low commitment to education, academic failure, behavior problems	Greater attachment and commitment to school, lower rates of school suspension for misbehavior	Hawkins, 1988
Positive Youth Development Program	Universal/N=282	Early drug use onset, favorable attitudes toward drugs, social influences to use	Better coping skills, better stress management strategies, better conflict resolution and impulse control, less excessive alcohol use	Caplan and Weissberg, 1992
Adolescent Alcohol Prevention Trial	Universal/N=3011	Attitudes favorable to the use of drugs, social influences to use, early onset of drug use	Lower rates of tobacco, alcohol, and marijuana use, lower prevalence of problem alcohol use and drunkenness	Hansen and Graham, 1991
ALERT Drug Prevention	Universal/N=6527	Social influences to use, early onset of drug use, attitudes favorable to the use of drugs	Lower rates of tobacco, alcohol, and marijuana use	Ellickson and Bell, 1990
Alcohol Education Project	Universal/N=2536	Favorable attitudes toward alcohol consumption, early onset of alcohol use, association with alcohol-consuming friends, community norms favorable toward alcohol use	Less initiation of alcohol use, increased knowledge about alcohol, decreased use among those drinking prior to study	Perry et al., 1989

(continued)

TABLE 2 (Continued)

	Targeted Population Group/Sample Size When Project Began	Risk Factors Addressed	Outcomes (for total intervention group or subgroups)	Principal Investigator(s) and Year(s)
Midwestern Prevention Project	Universal/ N=5065	Social influences to use, early onset of drug use, attitudes favorable to the use of drugs	Lower rates of tobacco, alcohol, and marijuana use	Pentz, 1989
Behaviorally Based Preventive Intervention	Indicated/ N=80	Academic failure, early behavior problems, alienation from family, low commitment to school	Less conduct problems and delinquency	Bry, 1992
Intervention Campaign Against Bully-Victim Problems	Universal/ N=2400	Aggressive behavior, poor family management practices, favorable attitudes toward bullying/aggression	Less bullying, less delinquent behavior, more attachment to school	Olweus, 1991
Adults				
Prevention and Relationship Enhancement Program (PREP):An Empirically Based Preventive Intervention Program for Couples	Universal/ N=135	Couple relationship problems	Better marital adjustment, less divorce, less physical violence	Markman, 1992
University of Colorado Separation and Divorce Program	Selective/ N=153	Marital separation/divorce, anxiety, depression, childrearing problems, economic problems	Fewer symptoms of anxiety and depression, better vocational outcomes	Bloom and Hodges, 1985, 1982

Program	Selective/N	Problem/Risk Factors	Outcomes	Reference
Perceived Personal Control Preventive Intervention for a Caesarean Birth Population	Selective/N=70	Caesarean delivery, depressive symptoms	Lower levels of postpartum depression, more rapid physical and psychological recovery	Tadmor and Brandes, 1988, 1984
Prenatal/Early Infancy Project	Selective/N=394	Single parent status, school dropout, economic hardships, joblessness, subsequent pregnancy	Better vocational adjustment, fewer second pregnancies, better educational achievement	Olds, 1988
Caregiver Support Program for Coping with Occupational Stress	Selective/N=247	Occupational stress, distress, anxiety, depression	Lower psychological distress, better job satisfaction	Heaney, 1992
JOBS Project for the Unemployed: Michigan Prevention Research Center	Selective/N=928	Involuntary job loss, anxiety, depression, alcohol abuse, marital stress	Fewer depressive symptoms, higher pay, cost-effective outcomes	Vinokur, Price, Caplan, and van Ryn, 1992, 1991
San Francisco Depression Prevention Research Project: A Randomized Trial with Medical Outpatients	Selective/N=150	Depressive symptoms, medical problems, low income, minority status in public primary care setting	Lower levels of depressive symptoms	Muñoz, 1993, 1990, 1987
Projecto Bienestar: An Intervention for Preventing Depression in Hispanic Immigrant Women in the Community	Selective/N=399	Low income, immigrant minority status, distress, depressive symptoms	Fewer depressive symptoms	Vega, 1990, 1987
Peer- and Professionally-Led Groups to Support Family Caregivers	Selective/N=56	Caregiver burden, anxiety, depression	Lower levels of psychiatric symptoms, including anxiety and depression, better coping skills	Toseland, 1990, 1989
Elderly				
Widow-to-Widow: A Mutual Help Program for the Widowed	Selective/N=162	Widowhood, bereavement, depression, anxiety, social isolation	Fewer depressive symptoms, less social withdrawal	Vachon, 1982, 1980, 1979

in one area can affect other areas. A logical extension of this finding is support for collaboration among the agencies and institutions in these domains.

A number of interventions show promise for the prevention of behavior problems. Social competence enhancement has been shown to be successful with young children and should probably be included in risk reduction interventions seeking to strengthen resilience in populations at risk for early behavior problems. Prevention research suggests the importance of using interventions beginning in preschool and elementary school to create normative consensual behavior regarding substance use and bullying. Those at risk might then be more committed to the normative standards of the larger community. In addition, some proportion of conduct disorder may be preventable. Developmentally adjusted interventions throughout childhood and adolescence have, in isolated experiments and with some confirmatory data from quasi-experimental studies, shown modest but statistically significant effects in preventing later delinquent behaviors and related indicators of conduct disorder during adolescence. Successful components include early childhood education, parent training, enhancement of social and academic competence, and school curricula promoting consensual norms antithetical to risk behavior for disorder, such as substance use. As yet, there are no communitywide prevention research programs that target multiple age groups and attempt to change community norms.

A number of programs have successfully focused on prevention of depressive symptoms in adults and the elderly, and preventive trials with adequate sample sizes are now needed to determine whether the first episode of a major depressive disorder can also be prevented. Changes in laws and pricing have affected the availability of alcohol and appear to be successful in the prevention of alcohol use.

Even though biological risk factors have a significant role in the onset of mental disorders, few prevention programs other than prenatal care and childhood immunizations address these factors. As knowledge grows in this area over the next decade, growth in the number of programs addressing these factors is expected.

Much remains to be learned about tailoring interventions to groups in which they will have the most impact. Consideration will need to be given to benefit-cost issues as well as the potential harmful effects of screening and labeling individuals as being at risk.

In the committee's examination of prevention research programs, certain methodological complications recurred, among them difficulty in adhering to a strict randomized controlled trial design; high attrition of participants; lack of documentation of fidelity in delivering the intervention; lack of multiple measures of outcomes from multiple sources; and insufficient long-term follow-up, which can prevent the collection of outcome data on incidence of multiple disorders. Perhaps the best chance to deal effectively with these sorts of problems lies in the application of a comprehensive set of rigorous standards for preventive intervention research.

Treatment Intervention Research

Effective psychosocial and pharmacological treatments are now available for many mental disorders (Kaplan and Sadock, 1989; Karasu, 1989; Dobson and Shaw, 1988). When these treatment interventions are used, they can substantially reduce the morbidity, chronicity, and disability of mental disorders. One justification for mining the principles grounded in treatment intervention research for use in preventive intervention research programs is that preventive interventions and treatment interventions are often based on similar multifactorial causal models. Therefore it is possible that if a particular treatment intervention is effective for treating an already developed mental disorder, the same or similar intervention may be effective in preventing the disorder in individuals who are at high risk.

For example, many treatment studies have shown that when language, communication, and social skills are improved—giving individuals more functional control in their environments—disruptive, aggressive, self-injurious, and stigmatizing behaviors can be greatly reduced (Liberman, 1988). In addition, identification of prodromal phases for disorders such as depression, schizophrenia, and agoraphobia, combined with educational campaigns designed to promote early identification, could facilitate use of interventions, such as cognitive-behavioral approaches for the individual and his or her family, to push the boundaries from treatment into indicated preventive interventions for individuals at high risk for developing a disorder.

In addition to lessons on risk and protective factors and causal chains, Chapter 8 lists a number of other possible applications to prevention from treatment. All are presented with cautious optimism and the realization that only a growing body of empirical trials of preventive interventions can validate their applicability. For example, evidence from treatment research has shown that there is a high rate of co-morbidity in mental disorders. Half of persons with mental disorders have more than one diagnosis (Wolf, Schubert, Patterson, Grande, Brocco, and Pendleton, 1988). This evidence on co-morbidity suggests several rationales for preventive intervention research (Kessler and

Price, in press), among them the approach that when one disorder causes or leads to a second, prevention of the first disorder is a plausible preventive strategy for the second. Other applications include the importance of recognizing the progressive course of maladaptive behavior and the enormous range of individual differences, the benefits of modular and multimodal approaches, and lessons regarding the timing, duration, and environment of interventions. Lessons applicable to research methodology, ethical and cultural concerns, and dissemination can also be drawn from the treatment perspective. Over the next decade, progress is expected in the development of mutual respect, equal opportunity, and pragmatic collaboration among the scientists and advocates in the prevention and treatment fields.

MENTAL HEALTH PROMOTION

Chapter 9 shifts the focus from mental disorder and the attendant risk-oriented approaches for preventive intervention to mental health and the research and intervention specific to its promotion. As explained in Chapter 2, mental health promotion activities are offered to people to enhance competence, self-esteem, and a sense of well-being rather than to prevent a disorder.

In many respects, the goals of decreasing risk and increasing protection in the disease-oriented model and the goals of promoting mental health are not mutually exclusive, either in practice or in outcome. There is also overlap in the techniques used to achieve these goals. Consequently, it sometimes may be difficult to distinguish the pursuit of prevention from the pursuit of promotion; moreover, achieving one can result in the other. However, there are enormous differences, conceptually and philosophically, between these two goal orientations that must be recognized. Such differences have far-reaching implications for how people talk about these endeavors, why they participate in them, what they expect to gain, and the manner and extent to which they are willing to support them.

Substantial, but largely incalculable, resources—public as well as private—are currently being expended in the attempt to promote mental health. Examples are readily apparent in schools, health service organizations, businesses, industries, and municipal governments. Other, perhaps not so apparent, examples can be found in religion, recreation, and physical exercise, all of which can be used to enhance mental well-being. The enthusiasm of commitment to such activities is infectious; personal testimony in regard to success abounds. Yet careful, rigorous examination of the effectiveness of these activities and of their associated costs and benefits has not been conducted.

Although a useful body of theory exists, the current level of understanding is basic and elemental, and no body of applied knowledge comparable to that presented in Chapter 7 for prevention is available with respect to mental health promotion. The gaps in knowledge are considerable. What is the motivation for psychological well-being, and what are the conditions under which it emerges? Do the different forms of alternative mental health promotion reflect significant needs that have not been met by other mental health interventions? Has the multicultural nature of our society been a significant factor in the emergence of diverse modes of mental health promotion? How many people participate in mental health promotion activities? Of what kind? Where are mental health promotion activities occurring, and where else could they be implemented? What criteria are to be used in evaluating the outcomes of these activities? Are particular forms of mental health promotion likely to cause harm?

In the quest to understand and ultimately attempt to prevent suffering, it is important to not lose sight of another, equally powerful imperative, that is, the need to nurture positive regard for one's self and the world around us. There appear to be many ways of accomplishing this goal of promotion of mental health; clearly, each entails more than seeking freedom from disease or ailment. People in our society are deeply committed to such pursuits, expending enormous resources to attain happiness and dignity. Because little is known about the outcomes of health promotion activities, it would be useful to assess them scientifically. A research agenda could begin by cataloging mental health promotion activities across the life course and crafting outcome criteria that could be used in rigorous evaluations down the road.

DESIGNING, CONDUCTING, AND ANALYZING PROGRAMS WITHIN THE PREVENTIVE INTERVENTION RESEARCH CYCLE

Successful science benefits from cumulative progress, and the field of prevention of mental disorders is no exception. The task over the next decade will be to enlarge the body of work represented in Chapter 7 into a prevention science by instituting rigorous standards for designing, conducting, and analyzing future preventive intervention research programs, as described in Chapter 10. By adhering to such standards, prevention can achieve the credibility and validity necessary for its interventions to reduce the incidence of mental disorders.

Rigorous standards can also lead to an enrichment of the knowledge base undergirding prevention. Outcomes from trials built on such standards can serve to refine hypotheses and concepts related to risk and protective factors. The model building and hypothesis testing inherent in prevention research can elucidate pathways taken by individuals as they move toward or away from the onset of a mental disorder, as well as intervening mechanisms and brain-behavior-environment interactions that result in mental disorders or avert their occurrence, even in individuals at very high risk. In addition, empirical validation of preventive interventions can usefully inform and broaden clinical practice.

The Preventive Intervention Research Cycle

Just as the development of prevention into a science requires a series of rigorously designed research programs for its collective progress, so an individual research program requires a series of carefully planned and implemented steps for its success. Figure 3 presents the committee's concept of how these steps build upon one another in the preventive intervention research cycle.

The first step is to identify and operationally and reliably define the mental disorder(s) or problem. The second step is to consider relevant information from the core biological and behavioral sciences and from research on the treatment of mental disorders, and to review risk and protective factors associated with the onset of the disorder(s) or problem, as well as prior physical and mental disorder prevention intervention research. The investigator then embarks on designing and testing the preventive intervention, by conducting rigorous pilot studies and confirmatory and replication trials (the third step) and extending the initial positive findings in large-scale field trials (the fourth step). If the trials are successful, the researcher facilitates the dissemination, adoption, and ongoing evaluation of the program into community service settings (the fifth step). Most of the research programs presented as illustrations in Chapter 7 are at the third step.

Although the review processes that constitute the first and second steps in Figure 3 are considered to be part of the preventive intervention research cycle, the original studies in these areas, with the exception of the previous studies on the prevention of mental disorders or problems, are not. For the individual researcher, it is the activities in the third and fourth steps that constitute preventive intervention research per se. Likewise, it is not the community service program and its evaluation but the facilitation by the investigator of the program's widespread dissemination and adoption (the fifth step) that is part of the cycle. The knowledge exchange processes that operate between the researcher and the community at this step are discussed in more detail in Chapter 11. The final steps in the cycle, represented by the feedback loop, are to review the results of any subsequent epidemiological studies to determine if the prevention program actually resulted in reductions in incidence of the targeted problem or disorder and to respond to community representatives regarding their research interests and suggestions for further work.

In this discussion the terms *preventive intervention program* and *preventive intervention trial* are carefully delineated. The preventive intervention program is the activity or activities that are provided to the target population (e.g., home visitation with mothers and their infants or a substance use resistance training curriculum delivered to school children by their teacher). The preventive intervention trial is the research component designed with experimental protocols to evaluate and validate the success of the intervention program. *Preventive intervention research program* is the inclusive term for the program plus the trials.

Researchers involved in activities in steps three and four of the cycle face a host of issues. These include methodological issues pertaining to experimental design, sampling, measurement, and statistics and analysis, as well as documentation issues. Cultural, ethical, and economic issues require attention throughout the cycle.

Methodological Issues

It is essential to delineate the goals of the research program at the outset. Is the goal to reduce an occupational, social, educational, family, or personal risk factor? Is it also to enhance protective factors? Is the goal to intervene with mechanisms, triggers, and processes related to the onset of disorder? The ultimate goal of preventing or delaying the development of a full-blown mental disorder(s) should be explicitly stated even though at this stage that may not be the goal of the preventive intervention itself. These goals will influence the choice of research methodology.

The randomized controlled trial, in which members of a population are randomly allocated into experimental and control groups, usually is the preferred experimental design in research studies. It provides the most rigorous means for hypothesis testing available for preventive intervention trials. Randomized control groups are particularly important in selective and indicated prevention trials. The interventions in these trials are working against the probabilities associated with the "natural" course of the pathological process. If this course is increas-

518

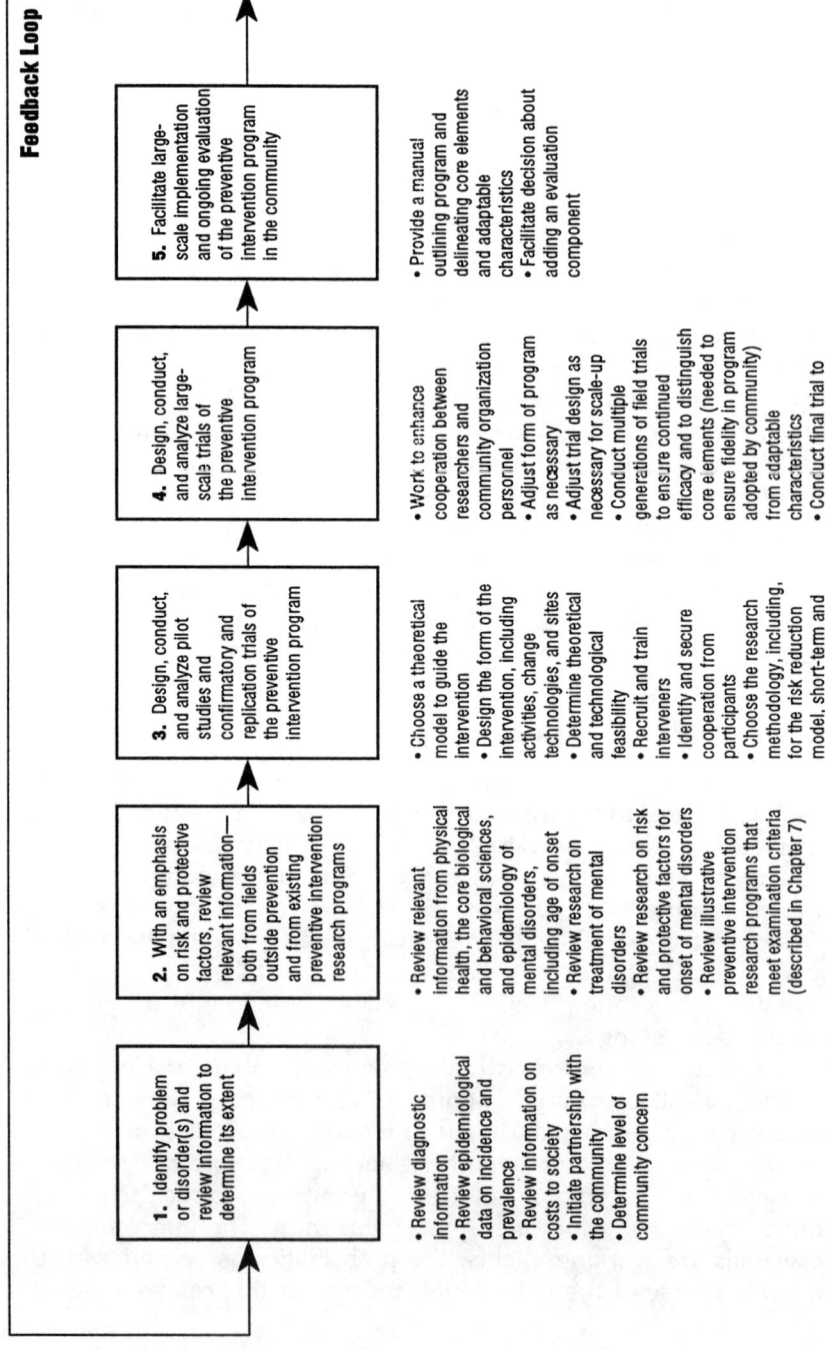

Feedback Loop

1. Identify problem or disorder(s) and review information to determine its extent

- Review diagnostic information
- Review epidemiological data on incidence and prevalence
- Review information on costs to society
- Initiate partnership with the community
- Determine level of community concern

2. With an emphasis on risk and protective factors, review relevant information—both from fields outside prevention and from existing preventive intervention research programs

- Review relevant information from physical health, the core biological and behavioral sciences, and epidemiology of mental disorders, including age of onset
- Review research on treatment of mental disorders
- Review research on risk and protective factors for onset of mental disorders
- Review illustrative preventive intervention research programs that meet examination criteria (described in Chapter 7)

3. Design, conduct, and analyze pilot studies and confirmatory and replication trials of the preventive intervention program

- Choose a theoretical model to guide the intervention
- Design the form of the intervention, including activities, change technologies, and sites
- Determine theoretical and technological feasibility
- Recruit and train interveners
- Identify and secure cooperation from participants
- Choose the research methodology, including, for the risk reduction model, short-term and intermediate outcome measures to determine

4. Design, conduct, and analyze large-scale trials of the preventive intervention program

- Work to enhance cooperation between researchers and community organization personnel
- Adjust form of program as necessary
- Adjust trial design as necessary for scale-up
- Conduct multiple generations of field trials to ensure continued efficacy and to distinguish core elements (needed to ensure fidelity in program adopted by community) from adaptable characteristics
- Conduct final trial to determine effectiveness
- Document thoroughly

5. Facilitate large-scale implementation and ongoing evaluation of the preventive intervention program in the community

- Provide a manual outlining program and delineating core elements and adaptable characteristics
- Facilitate decision about adding an evaluation component

malleability of theorized
risk and protective factors
and long-term outcome
measures to determine
effects on incidence of
problem or disorder(s)
• Determine efficacy in
pilot studies and
confirmatory and
replication trials
• Document thoroughly

FIGURE 3   The preventive intervention research cycle. Preventive intervention research is represented in boxes three and four. Note that although information from many different fields in health research, represented in the first and second boxes, is necessary to the cycle depicted here, it is the review of this information, rather than the original studies, that is considered to be part of the preventive intervention research cycle. Likewise, for the fifth box, it is the facilitation by the investigator of the shift from research project to community service program with ongoing evaluation, rather than the service program itself, that is part of the preventive intervention research cycle. Although only one feedback loop is represented here, the exchange of knowledge among researchers and between researchers and community practitioners occurs throughout the cycle. The feedback loop demonstrates both the continuity of the cycle and the necessity to incorporate many different types of feedback into each step, including community responses, additions to the knowledge base, and ultimate effects of programs on incidence and prevalence of disorders. Cross-cutting issues regarding methodology, documentation, and cultural, ethical, and economic concerns are treated in the text.

ingly negative, the results can appear to be an increase in problems that did not exist before the intervention. On the other hand, some problems are self-limiting, and positive results may be due to the passage of time rather than the intervention. A finding of lower incidence of disorder in the experimental group as compared to a higher incidence in the control group is the best way of documenting the effect of the intervention.

The length of the intervention—short enough to be practical and yet long enough to be effective—governs the length of the trial. In addition, because a decrease in the incidence of the disorder is the major long-term goal, participants should be followed longitudinally in pro- spective designs. Follow-up periods can be quite lengthy. The longer the duration of follow-up, the greater the power—that is, the statistical capacity to be able to demonstrate a significant result—may be to detect the efficacy of the program in showing short-term as well as long-term positive effects. Long time frames also may be necessary in order to get beyond the age of risk of onset. Lengthy follow-up periods, however, do have complications. The longer the trial and follow-up, the greater the cost and difficulty, and the longer the delay in obtaining answers to the research questions. Also, if multiple factors are involved in the onset of a disorder, lengthy follow-up provides more opportunity for uncon- trolled factors to influence outcome. Therefore a balance must be found between the gain in power and precision resulting from long-term follow-up and the loss in relevance and quality of content or substance that may be incurred. The practical limitations placed on the duration of a preventive intervention trial and follow-up in part can be dealt with by timing the implementation carefully. Selecting participants who are moving into their period of highest risk for the onset of the disorder, a period of critical developmental challenge and maturation, or a period of high responsiveness to protective effects permits detection of effects that are sufficiently large and immediate.

The choice of the sample from the targeted population also has methodological repercussions. The major problem in using selective and indicated preventive interventions is the identification of the high-risk group. Obviously, it is critical that the definition of high risk be a valid one. Also, if any group is excluded from a trial, the results may not generalize to that group.

The use of a universal population presents methodological problems of a different sort. Such a population is typically diverse and may include participants who are not receptive to the program. The hetero- geneity, combined with the likely low incidence rates, creates a situation in which very large sample sizes are necessary to detect any indication of efficacy or effectiveness. Because the effects may seem quite small, the clinical or policy significance of the prevention program may be under-estimated. One solution is to plan secondary analyses to focus on those subgroups likely to be most receptive to the intervention, in order to generate results comparable to those that would be obtained with selective or indicated populations.

Although the processes of focusing attention on the questions that require answers, selecting the appropriate measures (and thus exclud-ing the rest), deciding when and how often to measure, choosing the best measurement techniques or instruments, and taking steps to ensure the reliability and validity of the selected measures are perhaps the most tedious and difficult parts of a trial, these are also among the most essential procedures in determining its success or failure.

Careful selection of primary outcome measures, that is, the measures used most often to document the results of the trial, is essential. These are usually the measures of changes in the theorized mediating vari-ables, including risk and protective factors, that are assumed to be responsible for the reduction in risk. It is particularly desirable for prevention research programs to include measures of the incidence of mental disorders. Measures of process—which reflect certain character-istics of the participants, program, activities, change technologies, and so on, and of the interaction of these, that might help to generate hypotheses as to why and how the program might work—are also appropriate, as are measures of compliance. Finally, because random assignment does not yield groups that are identical on all baseline variables, an extensive collection of baseline information, including targeting variables, is also necessary.

Whether the chosen measures are continuous (that is, a scaled or dimensional response) or categorical (that is, a number of nonhierarchial responses), they should display high internal consistency and construct validity (an expression of the degree to which a measurement measures what it purports to measure) as well as high reliability (replicability) with different assessors. They should also be relatively independent and limited to a carefully chosen few. To ensure validity, outcome measures ideally should be assessed "blind" to the group to which the partici-pants have been assigned. For many randomized controlled trials, however, it is simply not possible to blind all assessors (or, for self-reporting, all participants) to the group membership of the partici-pants. This situation places a premium on measures that are objective.

Randomized controlled trials in which participants are followed longitudinally inevitably entail collection of a great deal of data, no matter how careful the investigator has been in choosing the type and frequency of measures and instruments. Many statistical methods for analyzing these data exist. As more data regarding age of onset are gathered, the preferred analytic strategy for comparing incidence rates across groups is likely to be survival analysis. Survival analysis is a flexible and powerful statistical method for analyzing incidence of illness when time to onset is known. An interesting aspect of survival analysis is the hazard function, which is the probability of becoming ill at each point in time. Analyses of changes in risk over time may be particularly sensitive indicators of a program's efficacy and effectiveness. The hope is that the intervention program might begin to exert an effect at its inception and gradually build to its full effect as it is fully implemented with desired impacts on the participants' risk and protective factors. The hazard function curve quantifies the probability per unit time that a participant who has survived up to a particular time will have the onset of the disorder in the very short ensuing time interval. For an insidiously developing disorder, such as schizophrenia, the time to onset may be difficult to ascertain, however, and, at least from the point of view of analyzing a prevention research program, relatively unimportant. Therefore, if survival methods cannot be used, random effects regression models permit the best use of incomplete follow-up data for participants and help avoid some of the problems of sample bias associated with low retention rates during a trial. However, such problems do not disappear; every missing data point or dropout from the study costs some degree of power.

Power calculations should precede the initiation of a preventive intervention trial to determine the requisite sample size. For example, for a universal trial targeting the general population with a short follow-up period to measure the onset of a disorder that has a low baseline frequency and unreliable diagnosis, having one million participants may not yield adequate power to detect statistically significant effects. On the other hand, for a trial of a potent selective preventive intervention sampling a relatively high risk population and using frequent, repeated measurements that are valid and reliable, with a long follow-up period and good retention of subjects, a sample size of 50 per group might be adequate.

Documentation Issues

When the research program has been completed, the design, sampling, measurement, and analytic decisions should be specified in the peer-reviewed literature and manuals in sufficient detail that they can be replicated by others. The background and rationale are also relevant. When the results have been analyzed, the statistical methods used should be reported in such a way that the proper inferences can be made about the effectiveness of the program. Details should also be provided about recruitment, randomization, dropout rate, and compliance so that readers can judge how convincing the results are. Documentation of the quality of measurement (reliability or validity) is also always valuable.

Issues of Culture, Ethnicity, and Race

Given the cultural diversity that characterizes this country, no discussion of the current and future status of preventive intervention research could possibly be complete without systematic attention to issues of culture, ethnicity, and race. Throughout the preventive intervention research cycle, investigators must be sensitive to the attitudes, values, beliefs, and practices of the cultural groups with whom they are working, as matters of good science and therapeutic leverage, as well as professional ethics (Kavanagh and Kennedy, 1992; Locke, 1992; Vega, 1992; Galanti, 1991). However, they must strive for more, namely, a set of skills and a perspective that have become commonly known as *cultural competence* (Isaacs and Benjamin, 1991; Cross, Bazron, Dennis, and Isaacs, 1989; Lefley, 1982). Competence is achieved through personal experience, either closely supervised practice or actual immersion in the field, which leads to the acquisition and mastery of the skills needed to fit intervention to context.

The committee has identified a number of activities throughout the cycle in which issues of cultural competence become especially salient: (1) Forging relationships between researchers and community. Mutual respect, appropriate responsibility, equity in decision-making, and shared commitment to negotiating differences are central. (2) Identifying risks, mechanisms, triggers, and processes. Attempts to understand these should allow for the possibility of alternative explanation and circumstances among cultural groups (Neighbors, 1990). (3) Employing relevant theoretical frameworks. Choosing theory to guide the intervention entails more than attending to the presumed links between cause and effect. It also must accommodate the relationship between what participants will (or are expected to) learn and those things valued by them. (4) Preparing the content, format, and delivery of preventive interventions. Attending to the historical and evolving nature of the ethnocultural niches—defined in familial, social, political, and economic terms—of the targeted individuals and groups can help avoid unintended negative effects. (5) Adopting appropriate narrative structures and discourse. How individuals refer to and discuss a given disorder or problem, for example, can differ markedly by ethnicity and culture.

"Down in the dumps," "feeling blue," and "feeling low"—expressions commonly used in white, middle-class America to refer to depression—do not have the same currency among Asian-Americans (Kinzie, Manson, Do, Nguyen, Bui, and Than, 1982) or Native Americans (Manson, 1993; Manson, Shore, and Bloom, 1985). (6) Tapping critical decision-making processes. These processes and those who engage in them can be quite different from one ethnic or cultural group to another. For example, though their role has been slightly eroded, family councils among Hmong refugees from Vietnam remain central to conflict resolution and mediation of domestic disputes (Norton and Manson, 1993; Bloom, Kinzie, and Manson, 1985). Imagine the probability of success of preventive interventions that ignore, or even run counter to, such decision-making processes. (7) Determining points of intervention leverage. Social structure influences access to people. For example, a home visiting model for prevention would need, among the Navajo, to take into account seasonal household migration (Dinges, 1982). Other activities that can be enhanced through cultural competence include (8) recognizing social networks and natural helpers, (9) seeking fidelity of implementation, and (10) replicating interventions across diverse populations.

Ethical Issues

Three factors combine to complicate the ethical issues involved in research on the prevention of mental disorders. First, the various disciplines and techniques that are being integrated into prevention research programs each carry their own complex ethical issues. Second, prevention research programs conducted in communities often require commitments, promises, and risks not encountered in basic research. Third, in many cultures mental disorders carry a special stigma.

The development of a specific ethical code for prevention research is premature and perhaps not even desirable. What is needed is not only a sensitivity on the part of the individual investigator, and within the research community in general, regarding the importance of ethical issues throughout the preventive intervention research cycle, but also the ability to recognize these issues in changing circumstances and respond responsibly—with appropriate questions, skills, and decisions—to them. The development of this competence begins with formal training in basic principles but then requires a continuing process of self-education to instill the habit of ethical accountability.

In addition to being bound by the values and standards that guard scientific integrity and by policies of the Institutional Review Board at the home institution, researchers must address numerous specific ethical issues regarding participants. Pope (1990) has suggested several general guidelines for investigators to consider. Briefly, these are do no harm, practice with competence, do not exploit, treat participants with respect and dignity, protect confidentiality, obtain informed consent, and promote equity and justice.

Although there is consensus about the importance of ethics in prevention research on mental disorders, ethical accountability in this area has not yet received the emphasis it deserves. This remains a developing field, in need of increasing numbers of individuals and organizations possessing heightened sensitivity to ethical concerns and new skills for designing and conducting ethically appropriate intervention programs.

Economic Issues

The allocation of available resources to activities aimed at reducing the burden of mental health problems in our society requires some capacity to estimate the benefits and costs of our efforts. There are two main methods for doing this analysis. In cost-benefit analysis, costs and benefits are expressed in dollars. Assigning dollar amounts is difficult or nearly impossible for measures such as life and health, however. Cost-effectiveness analysis, on the other hand, uses two categories of outcome measures—dollars and health outcomes, presented, for example, as "years of healthy life gained."

The assumption is often made that preventive efforts are cost-effective. Some programs provide evidence that this may be true, but much more confirmation is desirable. In a useful framework for analyzing the cost-effectiveness of potential preventive efforts (adapted from work by Russell, 1986), the following factors must be taken into account: (1) population and risk—the more specific the definition of risk groups, the more likely the intervention will be cost-effective, other factors being equal; (2) cost and frequency of administration of the intervention; (3) potency of the intervention; (4) uncertainty of risk—when risk is low and uncertain, thought must be given to the costs associated with exposing large populations to interventions that offer no advantages to most and possible adverse effects to some; and (5) time, that is, the temporal proximity of the result of the intervention to its administration.

Cost-benefit and cost-effectiveness analyses appear only infrequently in the treatment literature (Cardin, McGill, and Falloon, 1985; Weisbrod, Test, and Stein, 1980; Paul and Lentz, 1977) and are almost nonexistent in the prevention literature. As requests for these analyses increase over the next decade, there are several important points that policymakers and prevention researchers should consider (Gramlich, 1984). For example, benefits from prevention programs may increase over time. Short-term evaluations may show small or nonexistent benefits, but benefits may accrue as children are engaged over time in less crime, depend less on welfare, or begin to reap the benefits of higher levels of educational achievement. In addition, a well-designed and sensitive benefit-cost analysis can identify gainers and losers in society. Net social benefits may be received by participants in the program themselves, taxpayers, and potential victims of crime. One example of a pioneering benefit-cost analysis of a prevention program is that done for the Perry Preschool Program, a selective preventive intervention described in Chapter 7 (Berrueta-Clement, Schweinhart, Barnett, Epstein, and Weickert, 1984). The investigators documented the costs of high-quality preschool education and the benefits resulting from positive program outcomes. The total net benefit to preschool participants themselves was approximately $5,000. On the other hand, the total net benefit to taxpayers and potential crime victims was estimated at around $23,000 for one year of preschool by the time the program recipients reached age 19.

THE KNOWLEDGE EXCHANGE PROCESS: FROM RESEARCH INTO PRACTICE

The success of the preventive intervention research cycle for a given research program lies only partly in how well it works to expand the knowledge base for prevention. The cycle's ultimate merit—and the justification for the expenditure of large amounts of research monies—lies in how effectively that knowledge can be exchanged among researchers, community practitioners, and policymakers to successfully implement the program in real-life settings and ultimately, with widespread societal application, to reduce the incidence of mental disorders.

Chapter 11 focuses on the process of exchanging knowledge. Researchers and community practitioners come to the knowledge exchange table with very different perspectives and value systems. Most researchers, by nature, are cautious. They have high standards for the quality of the evidence they believe is needed before practice recommendations can be made. But community practitioners are faced on a daily basis with the need for preventive services, and they cannot wait for the results of completed field trials within the research cycle.

The Role of the Community

The role of the community—defined here as policymakers, community practitioners, and representatives of host organizations—in the knowledge exchange process includes the following steps: defining the problem and assessing the needs, ensuring the readiness of the host organization, selecting a model program, balancing fidelity and adaptability while implementing the program, evaluating the program's effectiveness, and providing feedback to the researchers.

For a community searching for a model program, practicality is paramount. An ideal model that has proved its efficacy and effectiveness through confirmatory, replication, and large-scale field trials is as yet, owing to the status of current prevention research, unlikely to be available. Nevertheless, communities can measure the evidence that is available against a hierarchial scale, such as that adapted from work by the Canadian Task Force on the Periodic Health Examination and the U.S. Preventive Service Task Force (Battista and Fletcher, 1988; Spitzer, 1979) to determine its quality.

Information Sources

Throughout the cycle, there can be information and data ready to be exchanged with community practitioners and policymakers for general use. There are five main routes by which research findings are commonly disseminated: academic journals and books, manuals, clearinghouses, professional conferences, and direct working relationships between researchers and communities to facilitate implementation of the prevention programs. When a research program is being reviewed by a community, published papers and manuals should be obtained from libraries, clearinghouses, or the researchers themselves. The criteria listed in Chapter 7 can then be used to assess the quality of the research.

The committee reviewed the amount of knowledge dissemination currently available. There were exceptionally few articles in professional journals that reported the results from randomized controlled trial designs. For example, many NIMH Prevention Research Branch researchers, including those whose projects are completed, have never published their findings in peer-reviewed academic journals. The publication rates generated from the NIMH Preventive Intervention Research Centers (PIRCs) have been uneven. It is recognized that many preventive interventions require a long follow-up period to assess the effects of the programs and investigators are reluctant to publish findings prematurely. However, if the theory, methods, and results are not published in a timely fashion, communities and practitioners have little access to this information and cannot use it in designing their local programs. It is likely that as increased methodological rigor is applied to the design of preventive intervention research programs over the next decade, more articles will be published in high-quality journals. Published manuals, important vehicles for disseminating information about which elements in an intervention are adaptable and which are "core," are also in short supply. In addition, there is no federal clearinghouse, little in the way of crossover between agencies in each other's meetings, and no federally funded mechanism for researchers to work directly with communities to develop programs.

Finally, evaluation of the program during and after implementation is needed, not only to critique the program but also to provide feedback about its effects on the needs and problems originally identified by the community, feedback that is then in turn provided to the original researchers.

Strategies for Overcoming Barriers to the Knowledge Exchange Process

Barriers to the adoption of innovative prevention programs include those related to the prevention programs themselves; to the practitioners, clinicians, educators, and administrators; and to the host organizations. Techniques to overcome these barriers include making program packages more "user-friendly"; working to reshape attitudes toward prevention by providing relevant training to equip practitioners, educators, and other human service workers with new knowledge and competences; and engaging the active support of the host organization—from top management to local unit chiefs and team leaders.

Improving Community Access to Research Knowledge

Many research findings relevant to the prevention of mental disorders never have a chance to make an impact because they are never made known to the practitioners, educators, administrators, and policymakers who would use them. Any national research agenda for prevention of mental disorders will have to include the development of mechanisms for promoting the proper application of prevention technologies that have been validated in confirmatory, replication, and large-scale field trials. In order for communities to learn how to obtain and make the best possible use of the research knowledge, they will need the help of a new breed of prevention program facilitator who can bridge research and practice. Also, a coordinated plan for dissemination of the fruits of prevention research is needed, whether it be through existing institutions or newly created centers. One model that could be considered is the regional or national research knowledge exchange center, adapted from work by Liberman and Phipps (1987), which could serve as the broker, linkage center, or central agent between prevention researchers and scientists on the one hand, and practitioners, educators, administrators, and policymakers on the other.

INFRASTRUCTURE FOR PREVENTION: FUNDING, PERSONNEL, AND COORDINATION

Preventive intervention research cannot thrive without providing for its infrastructure. What levels of funding and personnel are necessary to implement the prevention research activities outlined in this report? How can the entire enterprise best be coordinated? To begin to answer these questions, the committee first reviewed the existing federal presence in the prevention of mental disorders. It determined which agencies have relevant research and service programs and reviewed the funding, personnel, and training resources supporting these programs. The committee then reviewed current coordination efforts among federal agencies. Full results are presented in Chapter 12.

Funding

Estimates of funding levels for research on prevention of mental disorders were difficult for the committee to obtain for several reasons. First, the definitions of prevention and prevention research vary immensely across and within agencies. Second, although many agencies are doing work in this area, some of them do not see their activities as having anything to do with "mental disorders" because they use a narrow definition of that term. A broader definition, for example, would include substance abuse and dependence. Third, data retrieval systems for funding information are difficult to access, inadequate, and sometimes misleading. The Computer Retrieval of Information on Scientific Projects (CRISP) at the National Institutes of Health (NIH), for example, can miss directly relevant projects, on the one hand, and also can produce extensive multiple counting of projects on the other, which can result in misleadingly large estimates of efforts in a particular area.

On the basis of direct contacts with agencies and reviews of agency program plans and annual reports, the committee has determined that

TABLE 3   Federal Agencies Involved in Preventive Intervention
Research and/or Preventive Intervention Services Related to Mental
Disorders

Department of Agriculture

Department of Defense

Department of Education

Department of Health and Human Services
  Administration for Children and Families
    Administration on Children, Youth and Families
    Head Start Bureau
    National Center on Child Abuse and Neglect
  Public Health Service
    Centers for Disease Control and Prevention
    Health Resources and Services Administration
      Maternal and Child Health Bureau
    Indian Health Service
    National Institutes of Health
      National Center for Nursing Research
      National Institute on Aging
      National Institute on Alcohol Abuse and Alcoholism[a]
      National Institute of Child Health and Human Development
      National Institute on Drug Abuse[a]
      National Institute of Mental Health[a]
      Office of Disease Prevention
    Office of Health Promotion and Disease Prevention
    Substance Abuse and Mental Health Services Administration
      Center for Mental Health Services
      Center for Substance Abuse Prevention[a,b]

Department of Housing and Urban Development

Department of Justice
  Office of Juvenile Justice and Delinquency Prevention

Department of Transportation

Department of Veterans Affairs

[a]Formerly under the Alcohol, Drug Abuse, and Mental Health Administration (ADAMHA).
[b]Formerly the Office for Substance Abuse Prevention (OSAP).

many federal agencies are involved in prevention research and services related to mental disorders—though to varying degrees and
perhaps not recognized or acknowledged by the agencies themselves
(see Table 3).

Many private foundations also support prevention services and research related to mental disorders. Some of the better-known examples
include American Express Foundation, Ford Foundation, William T.

Grant Foundation, Conrad N. Hilton, The J.M. Foundation, Henry Kaiser Family Foundation, Lilly Endowment, Inc., Meyer Memorial Trust, Annie E. Casey Foundation, The Robert Wood Johnson Foundation, the Carnegie Corporation, the W.K. Kellogg Foundation, the Pew Charitable Trusts, and the Colorado Trust.

Rational planning for the nation's prevention research agenda requires much more accurate monitoring and reporting of prevention activities related to mental disorders. The CRISP system has resulted in incomplete and inaccurate data with extensive multiple counting of research projects. In 1991 the Department of Health and Human Services (DHHS) reported expenditures of approximately $2 billion for prevention activities related to mental disorders and abuse of alcohol and other drugs. According to the draft Alcohol, Drug Abuse, and Mental Health Administration (ADAMHA) report, the funding of prevention activities was substantial in 1991—$749,093,000. ADAMHA's $749 million is likely to be incorporated into DHHS's $2 billion, but it is not clear that they were using identical definitions of prevention activities. In contrast to both of these large figures, the total 1992 budget of the three Prevention Research Branches (PRBs) at NIMH, National Institute on Alcohol Abuse and Alcoholism (NIAAA), and National Institute on Drug Abuse (NIDA) (all at that time part of ADAMHA) was $64,160,597. Expenditures at the PRBs included support for risk identification research, development of statistical methodology, training for identification and treatment of depression, alcohol treatment research, and other activities that, while worthy in their own right, are not preventive intervention research. Large preventive intervention demonstration projects were also included. While rigorous in their methodology, these have not been scaled up in size based on significant findings in prior pilot, confirmatory, and replication studies as recommended in Chapter 10.

In contrast to these findings, and using the definitions and guidelines developed in Chapters 2, 7, and 10 of this report, the committee's best estimate is that *the federal government's expenditure for rigorous preventive intervention research specifically targeted toward the prevention of initial onset of mental disorders is approximately $20 million per year.*

For reasons discussed in this chapter, it is difficult to precisely describe the current levels of expenditure by federal agencies. Nevertheless, this is the committee's best estimate of rigorous prevention research. Recommendations for increases in support (discussed in Chapter 13) are derived from this estimate and the committee's analysis of the investment needed to enable the field of preventive intervention research on mental disorders to proceed.

Personnel

Using multiple sources of information, the committee tried to determine the number of researchers working in the field of mental disorder preventive interventions. One source of data that the committee examined was the CRISP lists of grantees (1988 to 1992) for all three types of prevention (mental disorders, alcoholism, and drug addiction). The total number of grantees was 202. Allowing for others who may be funded by state agencies, universities, private foundations, and other federal agencies not listed in CRISP, it is likely that there are no more than 500 researchers in the field. The number who are fully trained to do the rigorous research described in Chapter 10 is much smaller than 500.

Any proposal for training should be grounded in projections of demand for personnel, both for the research enterprise and for the performance of high-quality evaluations of service programs. Thus the committee proposes that professionals trained in preventive intervention research are needed in federal, state, and local departments of education, social service, and public health. Although it is difficult to be precise, the steady-state national requirement of trained personnel, from various disciplines, is certainly at least 1,000 people.

Few, if any, of the current researchers in preventive intervention research have completed a formal training program to produce researchers in the prevention of mental disorders. Most were trained in their primary discipline and then learned their research skills as apprentices on a research team.

The current preventive intervention research training effort is organized in such a fashion and funded at such a low level that an outside observer could reasonably conclude that policymakers wish to phase out investment in this field. Current institutional training programs are small and typically involve a 2-year training period. There may be 5 such programs in the entire United States, and the current output of trained (by the committee's standard) preventive intervention researchers from these institutional programs may be about 10 persons per year (assuming continuing funding and program viability). Additionally, there may be about 12 persons being trained on individual awards during any 1 year, with about half of them finishing their training each year. The principal federal agencies that currently support research and training on prevention of mental disorders are NIMH, NIDA, and NIAAA.

It is important to begin to identify optimal training models and to develop mechanisms for sustaining financial support. Training in preventive intervention research should start with individuals who have already acquired knowledge and skills in such areas as nursing, social ecology, sociology, social work, public health, epidemiology, medicine (especially pediatrics, child psychiatry, and psychiatry), and clinical, developmental, social, and community psychology. In addition, education or experience is required in two other areas: (1) the design of interventions to prevent mental illness and (2) the analysis of the efficacy and effectiveness of an intervention. One central feature of the model training program envisioned by the committee is the incorporation of practicum or internship-like training in established centers carrying out prevention studies, as well as classroom or other didactic instruction. It is hard to see how such training could be provided without external support, for the costs of faculty as well as trainees. Fellowships for individual trainees alone will not suffice. Current federal training grants cover only a small fraction of such training and are subsidized heavily by the training institution and by research grants from NIH.

The committee concludes that a long-term strategy for preventive intervention research training should be developed at the postdoctoral level. However, what is needed immediately is a short-term strategy to "jump-start" the field. Mid-career scientists from related fields—risk identification research, epidemiology, treatment effectiveness research, and research on prevention of physical disorders—need to be recruited, trained, and adequately supported through increased stipends and increased availability of research grants. A career line needs to be created that makes prevention research a rewarding profession and attracts high-quality talent.

Coordination

There is little coordination of prevention research or prevention services across federal agencies, or among federal agencies, universities, and private foundations. In addition, research institutes and agencies frequently ignore issues of co-morbidity of mental disorders and of mental and physical disorders, as well as the co-existence of mental disorders and social and legal problems, such as delinquency. A less categorical approach to interventions may be productive to individuals as well as society, but there is no clear lead agency to provide such an approach. No agency has both the expertise in mental disorder preventive intervention research and an established track record in working collaboratively with other agencies and departments on prevention.

To coordinate these diverse participants in prevention, a lead agency would require several attributes. Of first importance would be the ability of the lead agency to bring together all the interested federal, state, and private parties to facilitate an open sharing of ideas and information, a commitment to the investigation of multiple, co-existing risk conditions for mental disorders and the co-morbidity of dysfunctions and disorders, and a willingness to participate in joint projects. Of equal importance would be the commitment of the lead agency to prevention, as distinguished from treatment and maintenance. Because no single agency seems able to accomplish these tasks, the committee concludes that an alternative mechanism is needed so that research and services on prevention of mental disorders can be coordinated across the federal departments.

CONCLUSIONS AND RECOMMENDATIONS

When President Roosevelt announced in 1937 that "one third of our nation are ill housed, ill clad, ill nourished," our country was galvanized into action. Yet today, when careful population studies tell us that as many as one third of American adults will suffer a diagnosable mental disorder sometime in their life and that 20 percent have a mental disorder at any given time, there is little alarm. The Institute of Medicine's Committee on Prevention of Mental Disorders believes that strong action is warranted, and with this report it calls on the nation to mount a significant program to prevent mental disorders. Although research on the causes and treatment of mental disorders remains vitally important—and indeed major advances are leading to better lives for increasing numbers of people—much greater effort than ever before needs to be directed to prevention.

Public health experience has shown that when a critical mass of knowledge regarding a specific health problem accumulates and a core group of expert researchers have been identified, the time is ripe for launching a larger, coordinated research and training endeavor. The committee believes that such a moment has arrived for the field of mental health. Opportunities now exist to effectively exploit existing knowledge to launch a promising research agenda on the prevention of mental disorders. *Therefore the committee strongly recommends that an enhanced research agenda to prevent mental disorders be initiated and supported across all relevant federal agencies, including, but not limited to, the Departments of Health and Human Services, Education, Justice, Labor, Defense, and Housing and Urban Development, as well as state governments, universities, and private foundations. This agenda should facilitate development in three major areas:*

- *Building the infrastructure to coordinate research and service programs and to train and support new investigators.*

- *Expanding the knowledge base for preventive interventions.*
- *Conducting well-evaluated preventive interventions.*

As previously stated, the committee's recommendations for funding of rigorous preventive intervention research are based on its best estimates of current efforts and its judgment of needed resources to create a robust federal research agenda.

The committee finds the need for prevention of mental disorders so great and the current opportunities for success so abundant that it recommends an increased investment across all federal agencies over the next five years (1995 through 1999) to facilitate the development of these three major areas of the research agenda. It recommends increased support of $50.5 million per year for the next two years, $53 million in year three, and $61 million per year in years four and five. These are modest increases considering the magnitude of the problem of mental illness in this country, and Congress may decide that an even greater investment is warranted.

Funding for the second five years should be recommended by a new coordinating body, such as a national scientific council on the prevention of mental disorders. The amount appropriated in year six should be no less than the amount of support in FY 1999. On the basis of positive results in the first five years, a considerably larger investment could be warranted during the second five years.

The three major areas to be developed are recommended in conjunction with use of the definition of interventions for mental disorders and of prevention research developed in this report. The term prevention *is reserved for only those interventions that occur before the initial onset of a disorder. These preventive interventions can be further classified into universal, selective, and indicated types. The term* prevention research *refers only to preventive intervention research and is distinct from research that builds a broad scientific base for preventive interventions.*

Building an Enhanced Infrastructure for Preventive Intervention Research

Preventive intervention research for mental disorders cannot thrive without providing for its infrastructure. Two areas are particularly important for moving ahead—coordination and research training.

The Coordination Role and Structure

Coordination among federal agencies is needed for four reasons: (1) variation in the application of definitions has made it virtually impossible to assess the current activities and expenditures in preventive intervention research; (2) duplication of research activities and the lack of piggybacking of smaller projects onto larger ones contribute to waste of dollars and time, and, at the same time, gaps in research go undetected; (3) agencies conduct research or provide interventions for mental disorders (including addictions), educational disabilities, criminal behavior, and physical disorders as though these were separate conditions, whereas, more often than not, coexisting disorders or problems occur; and (4) agencies have different strengths; for example, some are better at applying rigorous research methodologies to intervention programs, whereas others are better at reaching out into communities and forging alliances.

In arriving at its recommendations about coordination, the committee reviewed various alternatives. The decisions to be made include (1) how best to coordinate the various relevant activities, (2) where the coordination function should reside within the federal government, and (3) staffing and funding issues. The structure and function of the coordination mechanism are inextricably intertwined, so decisions 1 and 2 above cannot be readily separated. Staff and funding should be attached to the coordination mechanism wherever it is located. Four alternatives were considered regarding where the coordination function should reside. Although the committee does express a preference for coordination at the highest possible level, it believes that establishing a successful coordination mechanism across federal departments is more important than the details of where it is housed.

Initially, the committee considered the model of putting a coordinating role in one agency, such as the National Institute of Mental Health (NIMH) or the National Institute of Health's (NIH) Office of Disease Prevention. Locating the coordination role in a single agency is a natural way to keep coordination close to the science, because the personnel in NIMH or the director's office at NIH are likely to be more closely connected to the scientific network than those higher in the government. Although single agencies have mediated coordination among other parts of the same department and even among branches of different executive departments in the past, the breadth and extent of the need for multiagency collaboration in this case make a single agency lead seem unrealistic. One possible exception is the Centers for Disease Control and Prevention (CDC), which has a public health mandate for prevention activities and considerable experience in working collaboratively with federal, state, and local agencies.

Coordination from an office within one department that serves as an umbrella over several relevant agencies is a second alternative. The Office of the Assistant Secretary for Health within the Department of

Health and Human Services (DHHS) already contains an Office for Disease Prevention and Health Promotion. This office could be charged with forming a subcommittee or task group to focus specifically on the coordination of research aimed at preventing mental disorders and substance abuse. These preventive efforts share many features with other disorders already subject to coordination within this office, but the involvement of the criminal justice system, the education system, child and spousal protective services, civilian and military family support services, and other nonmedical services necessarily encompasses activities in an even broader array of federal agencies. Many of these services are housed in entirely separate cabinet departments. The committee thus believes coordination at the departmental level is preferable to coordination by a single agency (with the possible exception of CDC), but the nature of the problem may well necessitate a higher-level coordination mechanism.

As a third alternative, the committee considered models developed within Congress, such as the Physician Payment Review Commission (PPRC) and the Prospective Payment Assessment Commission (PRO-PAC), for which appointments are made by an independent body—the Office of Technology Assessment. The question regarding these models is how well they would work in the prevention field, where many of the activities center on coordination of ongoing programs conducted within the executive branch.

As a fourth alternative, the committee considered other successful models—the ongoing White House Conferences, various Presidential commissions, and the Office of Science and Technology Policy (OSTP)—within the White House. OSTP was originally created by President Eisenhower to focus national attention on science; after being disbanded, it was reestablished by President Ford upon the recommendation of the National Academy of Sciences (NAS, 1974). This model has three components: (1) an office having coordinating responsibility regarding national science policy, (2) an individual who serves as the President's science advisor, and (3) a council with expertise in a broad range of scientific matters. The advantages of having a coordination structure under the White House are that it is a natural level for coordinating activities of different cabinet departments and that it places a premium on interagency cooperation, which the committee believes is an essential element.

The committee leans toward the establishment of an overarching federal council, operated out of the White House Office of Science and Technology Policy or another coordinating office within the Executive Office of the President, to coordinate preventive intervention research.

It recognizes that research and services related to prevention of mental disorders have high relevance to the many other agendas and priorities of Congress and the President. These include the lack of high-quality education, deteriorating cities, drug problems, the lack of housing, poverty, and the lack of universal health care. Mental disorders contribute to these problems and vice versa; therefore, ultimate solutions must be broad in scope.

Adequate staffing and resources are essential to successful coordination of prevention research regardless of where it is located in the federal government. Moreover, the quality of leadership and extent of commitment among agencies are often far more important than the precise location of a coordination office. Leadership and commitment cannot be fully controlled, no matter how careful the plans may be. The competence of the particular individuals chosen to lead the effort and the politics of the day often determine whether interagency coordination is truly successful or merely an effort that consumes staff time and wastes increasingly scarce federal dollars. Despite these caveats, the committee nonetheless believes that a coordinating committee at the highest possible level with adequate staffing is necessary to weave together disparate federal activities in many different departments.

- *The committee strongly recommends that a mechanism be created to coordinate research and services on prevention of mental disorders across the federal departments. One model for accomplishing this would be the establishment of a national scientific council on the prevention of mental disorders by Congress and/or the President. Such an overarching federal council could be operated out of the White House Office of Science and Technology Policy or another coordinating office within the Executive Office of the President.* This council should formulate policies regarding preventive intervention research, evaluation of prevention services, knowledge exchange, coordination of interagency research efforts, and training. Because prevention activities span different departments, the members of the council should be appointed after soliciting nominations from a wide constituency who are willing to use the definitions and rigorous methodological criteria developed in this report to foster policies that will reduce the onset of mental disorders and related problems. Members should include—as equal partners—ex-officio high-level representatives of relevant federal agencies, including but not limited to the Departments of Health and Human Services, Justice, Labor, Education, Defense, and Housing and Urban Development, as well as representatives from state agencies, private foundations, universities, and the public at large. A broad range of disciplines, including medicine (pediatrics, child psychiatry, psychiatry, primary care), psychology, nursing, social work, public health, sociology, and epidemiology should be represented. The council should meet regularly to coordinate collaborative research across public and private agencies and should monitor the standards for rigorous methodological approaches to preventive intervention research. Terms on the council for nonfederal representatives should be limited. To provide ongoing executive leadership, the chair of the council should be appointed by the President. Other leadership positions could be selected from the nonfederal representatives. The council should have its own paid staff, including a coordinator with staff, who operates out of an office of prevention of mental disorders. The office should oversee and coordinate the daily operations of preventive intervention activities in all areas that are related to mental health across the federal government. The staff of the office should be responsible to the council. The council should report regularly, at least every year, to the Congress and the President.

• *The committee also strongly recommends that Congress encourage the establishment of offices for prevention of mental disorders at the state level.* The current number of such offices is small even though the states have resources for prevention available to them through the state block grants. A mechanism to encourage the development of state offices would be a requirement attached to the block grants, and as health care reform is developed other possibilities may occur. The functions of these offices should be similar to those of the proposed national scientific council of the prevention of mental disorders. States that do establish such offices should, as a group, elect representatives to the national scientific council.

• *Agencies must be required to identify their funded programs for the prevention of mental disorders, separately accounting for universal, selective, and indicated preventive interventions, using the definitions developed in this report.* Congress should ask for separate accounting of these different kinds of preventive interventions when agencies report on the activities they support.

• *The National Institute of Mental Health (NIMH), the National Institute on Alcohol Abuse and Alcoholism (NIAAA), and the National Institute on Drug Abuse (NIDA) should consider including prevention researchers with broad mental health perspectives on their national advisory councils.* The prevention research field must produce more researchers of international stature who can serve on such advisory councils.

• *Mental health reimbursement from existing health insurance should be provided for preventive interventions that have proven effective under rigorous research standards such as those described in this report.*

- *Dissemination activities should receive much higher priority than they have in the past.* Agencies should disseminate results of research trials as well as evaluations of preventive intervention service programs. Funding of research trials should be continued only when investigators demonstrate a good publication record (including theoretical formulations and data from research trials). Interagency research conferences should be encouraged. A federal clearinghouse on preventive interventions in the mental health field should be considered, either as part of the council's function or as a separately funded initiative.

Research Training

- Training is an immediate and critical need in preventive intervention research. *Congress and federal agencies should immediately take steps to develop and support the training of additional researchers who can develop new preventive intervention research trials as well as evaluate the effectiveness of current service projects.* This training effort should include consortiums, seminars, fellowships, and research grants to attract existing researchers into prevention research, training programs for new investigators, and expansion of the training component of the specialized prevention research centers.
- *Research training should be focused on two groups—mid-career scientists and postdoctoral students.* Training for these groups should be developed simultaneously, but the expectation is that the training efforts for these groups will produce two waves of personnel. As an immediate strategy, training opportunities with adequate stipends should be developed to attract talented mid-career scientists from related fields, such as risk research, epidemiology, treatment effectiveness research, and research on prevention of physical illnesses, who seek to make the transition to research on prevention of mental disorders. This could be done through existing fellowships and career development awards and through the development of creative consortiums, seminars, and mentoring. All training should be tailored to the needs and schedules of these scientists. Such training could have a substantial impact on the number of personnel within three years if there is a simultaneous increase in the funds available for peer-reviewed research projects (RO1s).

As a second strategy, training opportunities with sufficient stipends should be developed to attract talented post-doctoral level trainees to preventive intervention research. Much more effort should be made to attract trainees from a wide range of disciplines including psychiatry, pediatrics, social work, nursing, public health, epidemiology, neuroscience, anthropology, and sociology, as well as psychology, which dominates the field today. If efforts to boost doctoral training begin concurrently with mid-career training, we might expect to see the benefits of an increased pool of researchers capable of securing their own research grants by year five of a 10-year plan.

● *The number of institutional training programs focusing on preventive intervention research should be increased from 5 to 12 over the next five years, including one at every specialized prevention research center, known at NIMH as Preventive Intervention Research Centers (PIRCs), that is productive.* Training of mid-career scientists and postdoctoral students should occur within every specialized prevention research center. To ensure that this happens, funding of specialized prevention research centers should be continued only when they demonstrate good track records in the production of published research and in the training of researchers capable of procuring their own research grants. In addition to the specialized prevention research centers, research training should be supported by federal agencies, schools of public health, and schools traditionally linked to service, such as social work, education, nursing, and medicine.

● *Support for faculty within institutional training programs should be increased.* Such support should increase the capacity of the faculty, program, and university to train preventive intervention researchers.

● *A major effort should be made to encourage the prevention research training of minorities.* Support should be offered to minority mental health research centers and other centers that focus on specific populations, such as low-income groups, the elderly, and minority groups. This would add more researchers to the field, but even more importantly, they would be researchers who specialize in populations with special needs.

● *The proposed national scientific council on the prevention of mental disorders should reevaluate the training needs for preventive intervention research after the first five years.* At that point the emphasis on mid-career scientists might be able to be decreased. If so, support for predoctoral training could be increased. An emphasis on postdoctoral training should be consistently high throughout the decade.

Funding

Coordination and training are the two most immediate and important needs in preventive intervention research on mental disorders (see Table 4). The national scientific council on the prevention of mental disorders and the office of prevention of mental disorders should have a combined budget of $1 million per year for five years. Dissemination

TABLE 4   Recommendations for Federal Government Support Above 1993 Level of Support (dollars in millions)

	1995	1996	1997	1998	1999
Infrastructure					
Council/office/dissemination	2.0	2.0	2.0	2.0	2.0
Training	12.0	12.0	12.0	12.0	12.0
Knowledge Base Research					
Risk and protective factor research (biological/psychosocial interaction)	6.5	6.5	6.5	6.5	6.5
Child epidemiological study	2.5	2.5	2.5	2.5	2.5
Population studies	5.0	5.0	5.0	5.0	5.0
Mental health promotion study	0.5	0.5	0	0	0
Prevention Research					
Preventive intervention research projects	20.0	20.0	20.0	25.0	25.0
Preventive intervention research centers	2.0	2.0	5.0	8.0	8.0
Total Budget	50.5	50.5	53.0	61.0	61.0

NOTE: Figures are based on 1993 dollar amounts and are not adjusted for inflation. These recommendations for support are based on the committee's best estimates of current efforts and its judgment of needed resources to create a robust preventive intervention research agenda for mental disorders across the federal government.

activities should be budgeted at $1 million per year for five years. Support for training should be budgeted at $12 million above the current level for year one, and this level of funding should be maintained for each of the next four years. In the first few years, these researchers are needed for evaluating current prevention service projects; gradually, they also will be conducting original preventive intervention research projects. Stipends for mid-career scientists should be in the $60,000 to $120,000 range, plus travel expenses. Stipends for postdoctoral trainees should be in the $30,000 to $60,000 range, plus travel expenses.

Expanding the Knowledge Base

The committee believes, based on the review of literature for this report, that a viable research agenda for prevention of mental disorders rests on a firm stratum of health research in other fields. This knowledge base includes basic and applied research in the core sciences that is aimed at the causes and prevention of mental disorders. Included in this knowledge base are neurosciences, genetics, epidemiology, psychiatry, behavioral sciences (including developmental psychopathology), and risk research. It also includes evidence and lessons from other fields of research, such as prevention of physical illness and treatment of mental disorders.

- *Research to expand the knowledge base for preventive interventions should be continued.* Knowledge base research should continue to be supported for all five disorders reviewed in this report, in addition to other mental disorders. Basic research is essential to the understanding of mental disorders. New funds for the development of other knowledge base areas and for preventive intervention research should not be taken from funds currently used to support basic science. The committee also recommends that support be increased for three specific knowledge base areas outlined below. Support of basic research will ensure the quality and continuity of the existing research effort and attract new investigators to those fields.
- *Support for research on potentially modifiable biological and psychosocial risk and protective factors for the onset of mental disorders should be increased. Priority should be given to research, regardless of the type of mental disorder, that illuminates the interaction of potentially modifiable biological and psychosocial risk and protective factors, rather than restricting the research to either biological or psychosocial factors.*
- *NIMH should support a series of prospective studies on well-defined general populations under the age of 18 to provide initial benchmark estimates of the prevalence and incidence of mental disorders and problem behaviors in this age group.* These epidemiological investigations should be oriented toward diagnosis but also should record a range of symptomatology, so that future changes in the diagnostic system, or developmental changes in individuals, do not preclude understanding of the development of psychopathology throughout this age range and into adult life. These prospective studies also should be oriented toward identification of modifiable risk factors in this age group with the explicit goal of recommending modifiable targets for preventive interventions in the future.
- *A population laboratory should be established with the capacity for conducting longitudinal studies over the entire life span in order to generate understanding as to how risk factors and developmental transitions combine to influence the development of psychopathology.* The primary goal of this laboratory should be the enhancement of knowledge for prevention and the development of new knowledge for the implementation of preventive intervention trials. Special attention should be paid to developmental transitions, such as childhood to adolescence, adolescence to adulthood, entry into marriage, and loss of a spouse; precursor signs and symptoms, prodromal periods, age periods just prior to when a specific mental disorder is most likely to occur; and the effects of race, ethnicity,

and gender. Well-designed preventive intervention research trials might be conducted with these populations during the follow-up, as long as the goal of obtaining benchmark estimates of epidemiological data, especially in regard to developmental transitions, is not threatened. The population laboratory could be established as a branch in the intramural program of NIMH, although there are advantages to making it a multiagency project funded through agreements among DHHS agencies such as the Centers for Disease Control and Prevention (CDC), Substance Abuse and Mental Health Services Administration (SAMHSA), National Institute on Drug Abuse (NIDA), National Institute on Alcohol Abuse and Alcoholism (NIAAA), National Institute of Mental Health (NIMH), National Institute of Child Health and Human Development (NICHD), and Maternal and Child Health Bureau (MCHB), and departments such as the Departments of Justice, Education, and Defense. It could also be established as a unit outside the federal government funded through a special mechanism. An extragovernmental advisory panel, including experts in epidemiology, psychopathology, and prevention, should be formed to provide continuing scientific oversight to the population laboratory. Data from investigations of the population laboratory should be made available in anonymous form in a regular and timely fashion.

● *Whenever possible, research proposals relevant to the knowledge base for preventive interventions should explicitly state this connection, such as identification of potentially modifiable risk factors and possible avenues for preventive interventions.* This requirement should be applied across all federal agencies, and especially to research proposals funded from the additional support recommended by this committee. This clarification of relevance to prevention will help decrease confusion regarding definitions of prevention research and lead to findings relevant to preventive interventions.

● *Treatment intervention research conducted under rigorous methodological standards that is directly relevant to preventive intervention research should continue to be supported—but not from the prevention research budget.* The criteria for "direct relevance" should be reviewed by prevention researchers. Collaboration between treatment researchers and prevention researchers should be fostered. Principles from treatment research can and should be borrowed for use in prevention. Specialty areas in treatment research that are likely to yield payoffs for preventive intervention research include clinical psychopharmacology, cognitive-behavior therapy, and applied behavior analysis.

● *Research should continue to be supported to determine which risk and protective factors are similar and which ones are different for treatment and prevention of a variety of mental disorders.* Identifying potentially modifiable factors that are unique to first onset of a disorder increases possibilities for prevention.

- *Research should be supported to study the effects of social environments, such as families, peers, neighborhoods, and communities, on the individual and the effects of context on the onset of various mental disorders.*
- *Researchers working on relevant research in the core sciences should be encouraged to participate in activities such as forums and colloquia with preventive intervention researchers.*
- *A comprehensive, descriptive inventory of the activities in which the public engages to promote psychological well-being and mental health should be developed and supported.* This catalog of mental health promotion activities is expected to be substantial. Preliminary efforts should also be made to craft outcome criteria for these activities that could be used in rigorous evaluations down the road.

Funding

The committee recommends that $6.5 million be budgeted each year for the next five years for risk research on the complex interaction between biological and psychosocial risk and protective factors. This would augment the research base for those mental disorders furthest along the continuum in the understanding of etiology, emphasizing the identification of malleable risk factors that would augur well for further preventive intervention research. A child epidemiological study should be budgeted at a minimum of $2.5 million per year over the next five years, and a population laboratory should be budgeted at $5 million per year over the next five years. Over a two-year period, $1 million should be allocated to catalog mental health promotion activities and to craft outcome criteria.

Conducting Well-evaluated Interventions

The knowledge base for some mental disorders is now advanced enough that preventive intervention research programs, targeted at risk factors for these disorders, can rest on sound conceptual and empirical foundations.

- *Increased methodological rigor in all research trials, demonstration projects, and service program evaluations should be required.* Wherever possible, the standards developed in this report, including hypothesis-driven randomized controlled trials and assessment of multiple outcome measures over time, should be instituted.

- *The concept of risk reduction, including the strengthening of protective factors, should be used as the best available theoretical model for guiding interventions to prevent the onset of mental disorders.* Other models for preventive interventions should continue to be explored; for example, as more becomes known about the mechanisms that link the presence of causal risk factors and absence of protective factors to the initial onset of symptoms, the possibilities for intervention may be increased.

- *Universal preventive interventions should continue to be supported in the areas of prenatal care, immunization, safety standards such as use of seat belts and helmets, and control of the availability of alcohol.* These programs decrease brain injury and mental retardation which are conditions associated with mental disorders. Although the main benefit of these interventions is the prevention of physical illness or injury, they may reduce the incidence of mental disorders as well. More evaluation is needed to assess their impact on mental disorders.

- *Research on selective and indicated interventions targeting high-risk groups and individuals should be given high priority.* Many of the programs described in this report are selective preventive intervention research programs, targeting multiple risk factors including poverty, job loss, caregiver burden, bereavement, medical problems, divorce, peer rejection, academic failure, and family conflict. These programs provide an impressive base for more rigorous research trials with larger samples.

- *Priority should be given to preventive intervention research proposals that address well-validated clusters of biological and psychosocial risk and protective factors within a developmental life-span framework.* Trials should measure short- and long-term outcomes for targeted disorders and should continue past the average age of onset. Sample size should be adequate for determining the validity of outcome measures.

- *Increased attention should be given to preventive intervention research that addresses the overlap between physical and mental illness.* For example, prevention trials with primary care populations should include examination of effects on physical well-being, use of health care (which at times may mean increased use), and social functioning.

- *Research support should be developed in two waves over the next decade, initially focusing primarily on increasing research grant support for individual investigators and later on increasing support for specialized prevention research centers throughout the appropriate federal agencies.* This strategy is based on the principle of building a prevention science from the ground up, rather than the top down. Individual investigators should compete for research grant support. As their academic track record becomes established, they should be encouraged to increase the size and scope of their trials and join with other solid investigators to form preventive intervention research centers. In the first wave, lasting five years, there should be a substantial increase in the funds available for peer-reviewed research projects. Preventive intervention research programs should be supported for any mental disorder where there is well-validated evidence of risk factors that appear to be modifiable. After five years, with the impact of new mid-career researchers joining the field and evidence from five years of research programs, a review should be made of the evidence. It is highly likely that several other preventive intervention research centers could be warranted at that time. Research grant support should not decrease at this time.

- *Research on sequential preventive interventions aimed at multiple risks in infancy, early childhood, and elementary school age to prevent onset of multiple behavioral problems and mental disorders should be increased immediately and substantially.* This should include a large number of new research grants and at least one new specialized prevention research center. The knowledge base regarding multiple risk factors in infancy and childhood interacting in complex causal chains and resulting in multiple disorders is extensive. Data on the direct linkage to specific disorders that emerge in adolescence and adulthood are becoming available. Many rigorously designed preventive intervention programs document impacts on risk and protective factors that are likely to reduce incidence rates of mental disorders. Addressing clusters of risk and protective factors increases the chances of preventing multiple disorders, especially major depressive disorder and conduct disorder. A number of separate randomized controlled trials have demonstrated the efficacy, and in some studies the effectiveness, of specific preventive interventions across development from the prenatal period through adolescence in reducing risk factors and enhancing protective factors. These should now be combined and delivered in sequence to high-risk populations. The intervention should include high quality prenatal care, childhood immunizations, home visiting and high-quality day care (such as the Prenatal/Early Infancy Project and the Infant Health and Development Program), high quality preschool (such as the Perry Preschool Program), parenting training, and enhancement of social competence and academic performance. High priority should be given to interagency sponsorship of this research, including the specialized prevention research centers. The Department of Health and Human Services (including the Maternal and Child Health Bureau (MCHB), National Institute of Child Health and Human Development (NICHD), Administration on Children, Youth, and Families (ACYF), Substance Abuse and Mental Health Services Administration (SAMHSA), and the National Institute of Mental Health (NIMH)) and the

Departments of Education, Justice, and Defense might be interested in sponsoring such research.

● *Research on preventive interventions aimed at major depressive disorder should be increased immediately and substantially.* This should include a large number of new research grants and at least one new specialized prevention research center. The knowledge base in this area is quite extensive, and promising preventive interventions have been empirically tested across the life span. Research to prevent depressive disorders should be more focused on preventing co-morbid mental disorders than it has been in the past. Also, outcomes often extend beyond traditional boundaries of mental disorders. For example, prevention of depression has strong implications for reducing suicides, lost work productivity, and physical disorders. High priority should be given to interagency agreements for research projects and specialized prevention research centers. Gradually over the next five years, other new specialized prevention research centers should be initiated to focus on depression and co-occurring conditions. Links between these new centers and other research sites are essential, and monies should be set aside to provide for ongoing collaboration.

● *Research on preventive interventions aimed at alcohol abuse should be increased immediately.* The knowledge base is extensive, and promising preventive interventions have been empirically tested. A less categorical approach to alcohol abuse preventive intervention research is needed. Co-existing illnesses, such as depressive disorders and physical disorders, must be carefully studied. Prevention of alcohol abuse has strong implications for reducing drug abuse, spouse and child maltreatment, and physical injury. The outcomes of preventive interventions on these problems also should be considered. For alcohol abuse, it may be best to target children and young adolescents to delay the initiation of alcohol use.

● *Support for pilot and confirmatory preventive intervention trials should be increased for conduct disorder.* Priority should be given to research that addresses multiple risk factors for young children with early onset of aggressiveness, including parental psychopathology, poverty, and neurodevelopmental deficits in the child.

● *Research should be supported on alternative forms of intervention for the caregivers and family members of individuals with mental disorders, especially Alzheimer's disease and schizophrenia, to prevent the onset of stress-induced disorders among these caregivers.*

● *Over the next decade, as new specialized prevention research centers are initiated, priority should be given to those that are sponsored through interagency agreement.* In addition to the National Institute of Mental Health (NIMH), National Institute on Alcohol Abuse and Alcoholism (NIAAA), and National Institute on Drug Abuse (NIDA), other federal agencies, such as those in the Departments of Justice, Education, and Defense, should be encouraged to become involved. Over the next 10 years, in addition to the new centers focusing on multiple childhood risks and depressive disorders, specialized prevention research centers could be developed for other risk factors or disorders if a review of the evidence suggests that such action is warranted.

• *Knowledge base research at the specialized prevention research centers should be supported by new research grants (RO1s) that do not use preventive intervention research dollars.* Specialized prevention research centers provide the structure, the personnel, and the study populations that could be used to increase the knowledge base for prevention through risk research and epidemiological studies as well as for increasing knowledge about preventive intervention research programs. When these two areas of research are combined in the same center, the definition of prevention research will be especially important.

• *Dissemination mechanisms, including publication in peer-reviewed journals, and knowledge exchange opportunities with other researchers and with representatives from the community should be mandated as part of the mission of each specialized prevention research center.*

• *The preventive intervention research cycle as described in this report should be used as a conceptual model for designing, conducting, and analyzing research programs.* Preventive intervention research should proceed from pilot studies to confirmatory and replication trials to large scale field trials and finally be transferred into the community as service programs with rigorous evaluation.

• *Increased attention to cultural diversity, ethical considerations, and benefit-cost and cost effectiveness analyses should be an essential component of preventive intervention research.*

• *Community involvement should be increased to help identify disorders and problems that merit research and to support preventive intervention research programs.* The committee believes strongly that the long-term interests of communities throughout the nation are best served if prevention services are based on well-crafted and thoroughly evaluated trial programs. Community groups that hope for the best long-term outcomes need to express an increased willingness to have service projects more rigorously evaluated and to bring promising prevention programs into the research cycle for a more complete analysis of efficacy and effectiveness.

Funding

Preventive intervention research (excluding the specialized prevention research centers) should be budgeted at $20 million above the FY

1993 level of support in years one, two, and three, with an additional $5 million (from $20 million to $25 million) in year four and year five. Support for new specialized prevention research centers is budgeted at $2 million per year in years one and two, $5 million in year three, and $8 million per year in years four and five. (The NIMH PIRCs receive, on average, $500,000 for core support per year.) Some of this support could come from reallocation and more prudent use of federal resources that currently are available for prevention in a broad sense. For example, huge demonstration projects are rarely warranted; scaling up from confirmatory and replication trials to large-scale field trials is a more cautious and constructive use of resources. Finding out the effectiveness of programs before they are widely disseminated is likely to save money in the long term. The support that is requested in this report is not necessarily new money, but it is new for the field of preventive intervention research for mental disorders. Much of the support should come from a wide array of federal agencies already supporting prevention services that currently lack rigorous evaluation.

A Final Word

There could be no wiser investment in our country than a commitment to foster the prevention of mental disorders and the promotion of mental health through rigorous research with the highest of methodological standards. Such a commitment would yield the potential for healthier lives for countless individuals and the general advancement of the nation's well-being.

Even with the support of the federal government, the effort will not be easy. There will be no "magic bullet." No single prevention strategy or method of changing people's life-style, behavior, or environment will work across the broad range of risk factors and mental disorders that will be encountered. A program designed to prevent one public health problem will not exactly fit the needs and goals of another. Dedication to prevention service programs will not necessarily bring success without a corresponding commitment to rigorous evaluation to determine the effectiveness of these services. No single agency can accomplish the task outlined above. Overall, the effort will require the cooperation of numerous federal, state, and local agencies, universities, foundations, researchers, and communities. The need for effective preventive programs in clear. It is equally clear that to obtain such programs we need a national commitment to rigorous research and increased support for the infrastructure to make that research possible.

REFERENCES

American Academy of Child and Adolescent Psychiatry. (1990) Prevention in Child and Adolescent Psychiatry: The Reduction of Risk for Mental Disorders. Washington, DC: American Academy of Child and Adolescent Psychiatry.

Battista, R. N.; Fletcher, S. W. (1988) Making recommendations on preventive practices: Methodological issues. In: R. N. Battista and R. S. Lawrence, Eds. Implementing Preventive Services. Suppl. to the American Journal of Preventive Medicine 4(4). New York, NY: Oxford University Press; 53–67.

Berrueta-Clement, J. R.; Schweinhart, L. J.; Barnett, W. S.; Epstein, A. S.; Weikart, D. P. (1984) Changed Lives: The Effects of the Perry Preschool Program on Youths Through Age 19 (High/Scope Educational Research Foundation, Monograph 8). Ypsilanti, MI: High/Scope Press.

Bloom, J. D.; Kinzie, J. D.; Manson, S. M. (1985) Halfway around the world to prison: Vietnamese in Oregon's criminal justice system. International Journal of Medicine and Law; 4: 563–572.

Breslow, L. (1990) A health promotion primer for the 1990's. Health Affairs; 9: 7–21.

Cardin, V. A.; McGill, C. W.; Falloon, I. R. H. (1985) An economic analysis: Costs, benefits and effectiveness. In: I. R. H. Falloon, Ed. Family Management of Schizophrenia. Baltimore, MD: Johns Hopkins University Press; 115–123.

Commission on Chronic Illness. (1957) Chronic Illness in the United States. Vol. 1. Published for the Commonwealth Fund. Cambridge, MA: Harvard University Press.

Cross, T. L.; Bazron, B. J.; Dennis, K. W.; Isaacs, M. R. (1989) Toward a Cultural Competent System of Care: Vol. I. Washington, DC: Georgetown University Child Development Center.

DHHS (Department of Health and Human Services). (1991) Healthy People 2000. Washington, DC: Government Printing Office; DHHS Pub. No. (PHS) 91–50212.

Dinges, N. G. (1982) Mental health promotion with Navajo families. In: S. M. Manson, Ed. New Directions in Prevention Among American Indian and Alaska Native Communities. Portland, OR: Oregon Health Sciences University; 119–143.

Dobson, K. S.; Shaw, B. F. (1988) The use of treatment manuals in cognitive therapy: Experience and issues. Journal of Consulting and Clinical Psychology; 56(5): 673–680.

Evans, D. A.; Scherr, P. A.; Cook, N. R.; Albert, M. S.; Funkenstein, H. H.; Smith, L. A.; Hebert, L. E.; Wetle, T. T.; Branch, L. G.; Chown, M.; Hennekens, C. H.; Taylor, J. O. (1990) Estimated prevalence of Alzheimer's disease in the United States. Milbank Quarterly; 68: 267–289.

Flora, J. A.; Maccoby, N.; Farquhar, J. W. (1989) Communication campaigns to prevent cardiovascular disease: The Stanford Community Studies. In: R. Rice and C. Atkin, Eds. Public Communication Campaigns. Beverly Hills, CA: Sage Publications; 233–252.

Galanti, G. (1991) Caring for Patients from Different Cultures. Philadelphia, PA: University of Pennsylvania Press.

Garmezy, N. (1983) Stressors of childhood. In: N. Garmezy and M. Rutter, Eds. Stress, Coping and Development in Children. New York, NY: McGraw-Hill; 43–84.

Gordon, R. (1987) An operational classification of disease prevention. In: J. A. Steinberg and M. M. Silverman, Eds. Preventing Mental Disorders. Rockville, MD: DHHS; 20–26.

Gordon, R. (1983) An operational classification of disease prevention. Public Health Reports; 98: 107–109.

Gramlich, E. M. (1984) Commentary on changed lives. In: J. R Barreuta-Clement, L. J.

Schweinhart, W. S. Barnett, A. S. Epstein and D. P. Weikart, Eds. Changed Lives: The Effects of the Perry Preschool Program on Use through Age 19. Ypsilanti, MI: Monographs of the High Scope Educational Research Foundation; 8: 200–203.

IOM (Institute of Medicine). (1989) Research on Children and Adolescents with Mental, Behavioral, and Developmental Disorders. Washington, DC: National Academy Press.

Issacs, M. R.; Benjamin, M. P. (1991) Toward a Culturally Competent System of Care: Vol. II. Washington, DC: Georgetown University Child Development Center.

Kaplan, H.; Sadock, B. J., Eds. (1989) Comprehensive Textbook of Psychiatry. Baltimore, MD: Williams & Wilkins.

Karasu, T. B. (1989) New frontiers in psychotherapy. Journal of Clinical Psychiatry; 50(4): 148.

Kavanagh, K. H.; Kennedy, P. H. (1992) Promoting Cultural Diversity: Strategies for Health Care Professionals. Newbury Park, CA: Sage Publications.

Kessler, R. C.; Price, R. H. (in press) Primary prevention of secondary disorders: A proposal and an agenda. American Journal of Community Psychology.

Kinzie, J. D.; Manson, S. M.; Do, T. V.; Nguyen, T. T.; Bui, A.; Than, N. P. (1982) Development and validation of a Vietnamese-language depression rating scale. American Journal of Psychiatry; 139(10): 1276–1281.

Lefley, H. P. (1982) Cross-cultural training for mental health personnel. Final Report. Miami, FL: University of Miami School of Medicine; NIMH Training Grant Number 5-T24-MH15249.

Liberman, R. P. (1988) Psychiatric Rehabilitation of Chronic Mental Patients. Washington, DC: American Psychiatric Press.

Liberman, R. P.; Phipps, C. C. (1987) Innovative treatment and rehabilitation techniques for the chronic mentally ill. In: W. W. Merringer and G. Hannah, Eds. The Chronic Mental Patient—II. Washington, DC: American Psychiatric Press; 93–130.

Locke, D. C. (1992) Increasing Multicultural Understanding: A Comprehensive Model. Newbury Park, CA: Sage Publications.

Manson, S. M. (1993) Culture and depression: Discovering variations in the experience of illness. In: W. J. Lonner and R. S. Malpass, Eds. Psychology and Culture. Needham, MA: Allyn and Bacon.

Manson, S. M.; Shore, J. H.; Bloom, J. D. (1985) The depressive experience in American Indian communities: A challenge for psychiatric theory and diagnosis. In: A. Kleinman and B. Good, Eds. Culture and Depression. Berkeley, CA: University of California Press; 331–368.

McGauhey, P. J.; Starfield, B.; Alexander, C.; Ensminger, M. E. (1991) Social environment and vulnerability of low birth weight children: A social-epidemiological perspective. Pediatrics; 88(5): 943–953.

NAS (National Academy of Sciences). (1974) Science and Technology in Presidential Policymaking. Report of the *ad hoc* Committee on Science and Technology. Washington, DC: National Academy of Sciences.

NIH Consensus Development Panel on Depression in Late Life. (1992) NIH Consensus conference: Diagnosis and treatment of depression in late life. Journal of the American Medical Association; 268(8): 1018–1024.

NMHA (National Mental Health Association). (1986) The Prevention of Mental-Emotional Disabilities. Alexandria, VA: NMHA.

Neighbors, H. W. (1990) The prevention of psychopathology in African Americans: An epidemiologic perspective. Community Mental Health Journal; 26(2): 167–179.

Norton, I. M.; Manson, S. M. (1993) An association between domestic violence and depression among Southeast Asian refugee women. Journal of Nervous and Mental Disease; 180(11): 729–730.

OTA (Office of Technology Assessment). U.S. Congress. (1986) Children's Mental Health: Problems and Services—A Background Paper. Washington, DC: Government Printing Office.

O'Grady, D.; Metz, J. R. (1987) Resilience in children at high risk for psychological disorder. Journal of Pediatric Psychology; 12: 3–23.

Olds, D. L.; Henderson, C. R.; Tatelbaum, R.; Chamberlin, R. (1988) Improving the life-course development of socially disadvantaged mothers: A randomized trial of nurse home visitation. American Journal of Public Health; 78(11): 1436–1444.

Olds, D. L.; Henderson, C. R.; Tatelbaum, R.; Chamberlin, R. (1986) Preventing child abuse and neglect: A randomized trial of nurse home visitation. Pediatrics; 78(1): 65–78.

Paul, G. L.; Lentz, R. (1977) Psychosocial Treatment of Chronic Mental Patients. Cambridge, MA: Harvard University Press.

Pope, K. S. (1990) Identifying and implementing ethical standards for primary prevention. In: E. J. Trickett and G. B. Levin, Eds. Ethical Issues of Primary Prevention. New York, NY: The Haworth Press.

Robins, L. N.; Regier, D. A.; Eds. (1991) Psychiatric Disorders in America: The Epidemiologic Catchment Area Study. New York, NY: The Free Press.

Roosevelt, F. D. (1937) Second Inaugural Address, January 20.

Russell, L. B. (1986) Is Prevention Better Than Cure? Washington, DC: The Brookings Institution.

Rutter, M. (1985) Resilience in the face of adversity: Protective factors and resistance to psychiatric disorder. British Journal of Psychiatry; 147: 598–611.

Rutter, M. (1979) Protective factors in children's responses to stress and disadvantage. In: M. W. Kent and J. E. Rolf, Eds. Primary Prevention of Psychopathology, Vol. 3: Social Competence in Children. Hanover, NH: University Press of New England.

Rutter, M.; Silberg, J.; Simonoff, E. (1993) Whither behaviour genetics? A developmental psychopathology perspective. In: R. Plomin and G. E. McClearn, Eds. Nature, Nurture and Psychology. Washington, DC: American Psychiatric Association.

Rutter, M.; Simonoff, E.; Silberg, J. (in press) How informative are twin studies of child psychopathology? In: T. J. Bouchard and P. Propping, Eds. Twins as a Tool of Behaviour Genetics. Chichester, England: John Wiley and Sons.

Rutter, M.; Tizard, J.; Whitmore, K. (1970) Education, Health and Behaviour. London, England: Longman.

Spitzer, W. O. (1979) Report of the Task Force on the Periodic Health Examination. Canadian Medical Association Journal; 121: 1193–1254.

Vega, W. A. (1992) Theoretical and pragmatic implications of cultural diversity for community research. American Journal of Community Psychology; 20(3): 375–391.

Weisbrod, B. A.; Test, M. A.; Stein, L. I. (1980) Alternative to mental hospital treatment: III. Economic benefit-cost analysis. Archives of General Psychiatry; 37: 400–405.

Werner, E. E.; Smith, R. S. (1992) Overcoming the Odds: High Risk Children from Birth to Adulthood. New York, NY: Cornell University Press; 185.

Werner, E. E.; Smith, R. S. (1982) Vulnerable but Invincible: A Longitudinal Study of Resilient Children and Youth. New York, NY: McGraw-Hill.

Wolf, A. W.; Schubert, D. S. P.; Patterson, M. B.; Grande, T. P.; Brocco, K. J.; Pendleton, L. (1988) Associations among major psychiatric diagnosis. Journal of Consulting and Clinical Psychology; 56: 292–294.

B

Contributors

Biographical Sketches

ROBERT J. HAGGERTY (*Chair*) is Professor of Pediatrics Emeritus, at the University of Rochester School of Medicine and Dentistry and formerly the president of the William T. Grant Foundation. He is a pediatrician; a graduate of Cornell University and its Medical College; Editor of *Pediatrics in Review*, the continuing education journal of The American Academy of Pediatrics, as well as a past president of that organization; Editor-in-Chief of *The Bulletin of the New York Academy of Medicine: A Journal of Urban Health*; and Executive Director of the International Pediatrics Association. He is a member of numerous professional societies, including The American Pediatric Society, The Board of Overseers for the Social Sciences at Tufts University, Board of Visitors of the School of Public Health at Oklahoma University, and a Fellow of the American Association for the Advancement of Science. He has been Co-editor of *Pediatrics*, Associate Editor of *The New England Journal of Medicine*, and Chairman of the Health Services Research Study Section of the National Center for Health Services Research. He received the Martha Eliot Award in Maternal and Child Health from the American Public Health Association; the Clifford C. Grulee Award, the Dale Richmond Award, and the Andrew Aldrich Award from the American Academy of Pediatrics; the Joseph St. Geme Award for the Future of Pediatrics from the American Pediatric Society; and the Gustav Leinhard Award for contributions to health services from the Institute of Medicine. He chaired the Mayor's Committee on Maternal and Child Health

(New York City) and the Subcommittee on Adolescents and AIDS of the Governor's Commission on AIDS (New York). He has been a member of the New York State Council of Graduate Medical Education, the Carnegie Council on Children, the Board of Alliance for Health Care for All, and the MacArthur Foundation Committee on Successful Adolescence. His initial faculty experiences were at Harvard Medical School and Children's Hospital Medical Center of Boston, where he developed a training and research program in general family pediatrics. There his interest in the effects of psychosocial stress as a cause of many children's illnesses began. His next career position was at the University of Rochester's School of Medicine and Dentistry, where he was Professor and Chairman of the Department of Pediatrics. In Rochester, he and his colleagues developed community-based health services for children, and coined the phrase "the new morbidity" for the psychosocial problems of children. He then returned to Boston, where he was the Roger I. Lee Professor of Health Services at The Harvard School of Public Health and Chairman of the Department of Health Services (a department that included maternal and child health, behavioral sciences, and health services administration). He is author of more than 120 original papers, editor or author of three books, one of which is now in its fourth edition (*Ambulatory Pediatrics*), and author of nearly 200 book chapters, editorials, and abstracts. He has been Visiting Professor and/or named lecturer at over 50 institutions. He is a member of the Institute of Medicine and was formerly a member of its council.

BEATRIX A. HAMBURG (*Vice-Chair*) is the President of the William T. Grant Foundation and is Professor of Psychiatry and Pediatrics at the Mount Sinai School of Medicine, where she was formerly Director of the Division of Child and Adolescent Psychiatry. She received her A.B. from Vassar College and her M.D. from Yale University School of Medicine. Her prior professional appointments were at the Stanford University School of Medicine and Harvard Medical School in their respective Departments of Psychiatry. She is a member of the Institute of Medicine and is a member of the IOM Board on Biobehavioral Sciences and Mental Disorders. She was a member of the Commission on Behavioral and Social Sciences and Education (CBASSE) of the National Research Council. In New York State she is a member of The Public Health Council of the Department of Health; a member of the Governor's Task Force on Life and Law; and a member of the New York State Council on Graduate Medical Education. She is a Fellow of the American Association for the Advancement of Science (AAAS) and a former member of the Board of Directors of the AAAS. She has served on study sections and ad hoc review panels for NIMH and is currently a member of the National Advisory Mental Health Council. She is a member of numerous professional societies, including the American Academy of Child and Adolescent Psychiatry, the Society for Adolescent Research, the Society for Research in Child Development, The American Public Health Association, the Society for Adolescent Medicine, and the Royal Society of Medicine. Her research has been in normal adolescent development, adolescent psychopathology, and endocrine-behavior interactions. She is most noted for her studies of early adolescence, her pioneering work on peer counseling, and studies of diabetic children and adolescents. She is the author of many books and papers on these topics. She has received many honors and awards, including Phi Beta Kappa, the Brownell Prize, the T. Ross Gallagher Award, and the ADAMHA Administrators' Award for Outstanding Achievement. She currently serves on the boards of the Bush Foundation, the Revson Foundation, and the Greenwall Foundation. She is a member of the Committee on Successful Adolescence of the John D. and Catherine T. MacArthur Foundation, and a member of the Carnegie Council on Adolescence.

WILLIAM R. BEARDSLEE is the Clinical Director and Vice Chairman of the Department of Psychiatry at Children's Hospital in Boston, and Associate Professor of Psychiatry at Harvard Medical School. He received his B.A. from Haverford College and his M.D. from Case Western Reserve University. He trained in general psychiatry at Massachusetts General Hospital and in child psychiatry and psychiatric research at the Children's Hospital in Boston. He has a longstanding research interest in the development of children at risk because of severe parental mental illness. He has been especially interested in the protective effects of self-understanding in enabling youngsters and adults to cope with adversity and has studied self-understanding in civil rights workers, survivors of cancer, and children of parents with mood disorders. He has received the Blanche F. Ittleson Award of the American Psychiatric Association for outstanding published research contributing to the mental health of children and has been a faculty scholar of the William T. Grant Foundation. Currently, he directs the Preventive Intervention Project at Judge Baker Children's Center, an NIMH-funded study to explore the effects of a clinician-centered, family-based preventive intervention designed to enhance resiliency and family understanding for children of parents with mood disorder. He has served on the NIMH's Life Course and Prevention Research Committee, Subcommittee on Child and Family Prevention, and is active with numerous professional organizations, for both research and advocacy for children.

ROLAND D. CIARANELLO is Nancy Friend Pritzker Professor of Psychiatry and Behavioral Sciences at Stanford University Medical Center. He is Director of the Nancy Friend Pritzker Laboratory of Developmental and Molecular Neurobiology and Director of the Division of Child Psychiatry and Child Development. He received his B.S. from Union College and his M.D. from Stanford University. He has been the recipient of Research Scientist Development Awards and Research Scientist Awards since 1978 and the John Merck Fund Award for Research in Autism since 1982. He received the Daniel H. Efron Research Award from the American College of Neuropsychopharmacology and the Distinguished Mentor Award from the American Academy of Child and Adolescent Psychiatry. He has served on the editorial boards of the *American Journal of Medical Genetics, Journal of the American Academy of Child and Adolescent Psychiatry, Neuropsychopharmacology, Pediatric Psychopharmacology,* and *Psychiatric Genetics,* and he is Co-editor-in-Chief of *Neuropsychopharmacology.* He has also served on the Council of the American College of Neuropsychopharmacology as well as on NIMH's Extramural Science Advisory Board, Basic Psychopharmacology and Neuropsychology Research Review Committee, and Mental Health Special Projects Review Committee. He is author of over 140 scientific papers and book chapters.

JOSEPH T. COYLE is the Eben S. Draper Professor of Psychiatry and of Neuroscience and Chair of the Consolidated Department of Psychiatry at Harvard Medical School. He received his A.B. from the College of the Holy Cross and his M.D. from The Johns Hopkins University School of Medicine. After an internship in pediatrics at The Johns Hopkins University Hospital, he spent three years as a research fellow with Julius Axelrod at NIMH. He completed his residency training in psychiatry at The Johns Hopkins University Hospital, where he then served as Distinguished Service Professor and Director of the Division of Child Psychiatry until 1991. His research contributions have been recognized by the reception of the John Jacob Abel Award from the American Society for Pharmacology and Experimental Therapeutics, the Gold Medal Award from the Society for Biological Psychiatry, the Foundation Fund Research Award from the American Psychiatric Association, and the McAlpin Award from the National Mental Health Association. His research interests include developmental neurobiology, mechanisms of neuronal vulnerability, and psychopharmacology, and he has published over 400 scientific articles. He is currently a member of the Institute of Medicine and the Institute of Medicine's Board on Biobehavioral Sciences and Mental Disorders. He serves on the

Advisory Board for NIMH, and is past president of the Society for Neuroscience.

WILLIAM W. EATON is Professor in the Department of Mental Hygiene, School of Hygiene and Public Health at The Johns Hopkins University Hospital. He received his B.A. from Wesleyan University and his M.S. and Ph.D. in sociology from the University of Wisconsin-Madison. He was Staff Investigator at the Institute of Community and Family Psychiatry at Jewish General Hospital in Montreal and Assistant Chief of the Center for Epidemiologic Studies at NIMH. He has membership in various professional societies, including the American Sociological Association, the Society for Epidemiologic Research, the American Public Health Association, and the American Psychopathologic Association. His major research interests are in the epidemiology of schizophrenia, the sociology of mental disorders, and the quantitative approaches to understanding social life. His research and publications have also included studies of migration and ethnic relations, anxiety disorders, occupations and psychopathology, incidence of mental disorders, and analysis of longitudinal data on psychopathology.

J. DAVID HAWKINS is Professor of Social Work and Director of the Social Development Research Group at the School of Social Work, University of Washington in Seattle. He received his B.A. from Stanford University and his M.A. and his Ph.D. in sociology from Northwestern University. His research focuses on understanding and preventing child and adolescent health and behavior problems by seeking to identify risk and protective factors, discovering how these factors interact, and testing comprehensive prevention strategies which seek to reduce risk through the enhancement of protective factors in families, schools, peer groups, and communities. Since 1981, he has been conducting the Seattle Social Development Project, a longitudinal prevention study testing a risk reduction strategy based on his theoretical work. His prevention work has recently been published in the book *Communities That Care*. He has served as a member of the National Institute on Drug Abuse's Epidemiology, Prevention, and Services Research Review Committee and on the former Office for Substance Abuse Prevention's National Advisory Committee, and as a member of the National Education Goals Panel Resource Group. He is a member of the American Sociological Association, the American Society of Criminology, the Council on Social Work Education, and the National Association of Social Workers. He has authored over 70 publications.

FRITZ A. HENN is Professor and Chairman of the Department of Psychiatry and Behavioral Medicine at the State University of New York at Stony Brook and Director of the Institute for Mental Health Research. He is responsible for a network of mental health services covering eastern Long Island. Before his current position, Dr. Henn was Professor of the Department of Psychiatry at the University of Iowa College of Medicine. He received his B.A. from Wesleyn University, his Ph.D. from The Johns Hopkins University, was a visiting scientist at the Institute of Neurobiology at the University of Goteborg, Sweden, and received his M.D. from the University of Virginia. He has held several appointments to federal advisory committees and has membership in many professional societies, including the American College of Neuropsychopharmacology, the American Psychiatric Association, the Society for Neuroscience, and the Society for Biological Psychiatry. He is a past president of the Winter Conference on Brain Research. He is on the scientific board of the Anika Monica Foundation and Dalheim Workshops and has also served on the editorial boards of the *Journal of Neurochemistry*, the *Archives of General Psychiatry*, and the *Journal of Schizophrenia Research*. He has authored over 100 publications.

ROBERT P. LIBERMAN is Professor of Psychiatry at UCLA School of Medicine, where he directs the NIMH-funded Clinical Research Center for Schizophrenia and Psychiatric Rehabilitation. He developed the Social and Independent Living Skills Program at the West Los Angeles Veterans Affairs Medical Center, which has produced, validated, and disseminated modules for training and rehabilitating persons with serious and disabling mental disorders. The modules have been translated into Japanese, French, German, and seven other languages and have been recognized with Significant Achievement Awards from the American Psychiatric Association and the World Association of Psychosocial Rehabilitation. He has directed the Camarillo/UCLA Clinical Research Unit at Camarillo State Hospital since 1970, where biobehavioral treatments for refractory schizophrenia have been designed and experimentally evaluated. The Camarillo/UCLA Research Center received the Exemplary Award for State-University Collaboration by the American Psychiatric Association in 1991. He received his A.B. from Dartmouth College, where he also attended medical school. He received his M.D. from The Johns Hopkins University School of Medicine and his M.S. in pharmacology from the University of California School of Medicine, San Francisco. He is on the Executive Council of the Association for Clinical Psychosocial Research and has served on the Board of Directors of the Association for Advancement of Behavior Therapy and the American Association of Community Psychiatrists. He has been the recipient of the Silvano Arieti Award for Schizophrenia Research from the American Academy of Psychoanalysis, the Samuel Hibbs Award for innovations in treatment from the American Psychiatric Association, the Van Ameringen Award for Psychiatric Rehabilitation from the American Psychiatric Association, and the Howard Davis Award from the Society for Knowledge Utilization and Planned Change. His research team is guided by a heuristic conceptual framework based upon vulnerability, stress, and protective factors that determine the etiology, course, and treatment outcome of schizophrenia and other major mental disorders. Among his more than 300 publications are the books *Psychiatric Rehabilitation of Chronic Mental Patients* and *Social Skills Training for Psychiatric Patients*.

BEVERLY B. LONG is President-Elect of the World Federation for Mental Health, an international nongovernmental organization in consultative status to the United Nations and its specialized agencies. Previously, she has been president of the Atlanta, the Georgia, and the National Mental Health Associations. She received her B.S. and her M.S. in psychology from the University of Georgia and her M.S. in public health from the University of North Carolina. She served as a member of President Carter's Commission on Mental Health. From 1984 to 1986, she chaired a National Commission on the Prevention of Mental-Emotional Disabilities, and in 1987 she founded and chaired the National Prevention Coalition, both under the auspices of the National Mental Health Association. She is a member of the NIMH Prevention Research Steering Committee, and she chairs the World Federation's International Committee for Primary Prevention. Her interest is in attaining government policies and action that recognize the interface of health and mental health and that strive toward a balanced research and service agenda for mental health that includes prevention of disorder, promotion of health, and effective treatment for those who are disordered.

SPERO M. MANSON is Professor of Psychiatry at the University of Colorado Health Sciences Center and Director of the National Center for American Indian and Alaska Native Mental Health Research, also located at the University of Colorado. He received his Ph.D. in medical anthropology from the University of Minnesota in 1978. From 1978 to 1986, he was a member of the Department of Psychiatry, Oregon Health Sciences University in Portland. In 1986, he left Oregon to join the University of Colorado Health Sciences Center faculty, where he assumed his present position. He has served on numerous boards of directors, including those of the Denver Community Mental Health Commission and the State of Oregon Governor's Commission on Alcohol and Drugs. He spent four years as a member of the NIMH's Epidemiology Research Review Committee and is nearing the end of a four-year term on the NIMH's Services Research Review Committee. His professional interests encompass psychiatric epidemiology, mental health services research, and cross-cultural psychiatry, with special emphasis on depression, anxiety, suicide, and substance abuse/ dependence across the developmental life span. He has published extensively and has been supported by funds from federal research grants, contracts, state/tribal research grants, and private foundation grants. He is currently a member of the Institute of Medicine's Board on Biobehavioral Sciences and Mental Disorders.

DAVID MECHANIC is the Rene Dubos Professor of Behavioral Sciences and Director of the Institute for Health, Health Care Policy, and Aging Research at Rutgers University. He received his B.A. from City College of New York, and his M.A. and Ph.D. from Stanford University. He served on the National Committee on Vital and Health Statistics of the Department of Health and Human Services and is a member of the Health Advisory Board of the General Accounting Office. He chaired the NIMH's Advisory Group on Research Resources in Mental Health Services Research and has had numerous other government assignments. He is a member of the Institute of Medicine, the National Academy of Sciences, and the Commission on Behavioral and Social Sciences and Education. He has served on numerous committees for these National Research Council organizations. He is a fellow of the American Association for the Advancement of Science. He received the Distinguished Investigator Award from the Association for Health Services Research, and the first Carl Taube Award of the American Public Health Association. He has served as a consultant to numerous nonprofit organizations. He has written or edited 23 books and more than 250 research articles, chapters, and other publications in the fields of medical sociology, health policy, health services research, and social and behavioral sciences.

RICARDO F. MUÑOZ is Professor of Psychology in the Department of Psychiatry at the University of California, San Francisco (UCSF), where he serves as Director of the Clinical Psychology Training Program and Chief Psychologist at UCSF's San Francisco General Hospital (SFGH) campus. He earned his A.B. from Stanford and his Ph.D. from the University of Oregon. His research program is focused on the development and evaluation of linguistically and culturally appropriate screening, prevention, and treatment approaches to major depression, using a social learning orientation and cognitive-behavioral self-control approaches. He was founding Director of the SFGH Depression Clinic and the Depression Prevention Research Project, which has received an honorable mention for the Lela Rowland Prevention Award of the National Mental Health Association. He is a recipient of the Health Promotion Award from the National Coalition of Hispanic Mental Health and Human Services Organization and the Martin Luther King, Jr. Award from UCSF. He is a member of the National Hispanic Psychological Association, the American Association for Artificial Intelligence, the American Association of Applied and Preventive Psychology, the American Association for the Advancement of Science, and a Fellow of the American Psychological Association. He serves on the editorial boards of the *Journal of Consulting and Clinical Psychology, Community Mental Health Journal*, and the *Revista Interamericana de Psicologia*. He is a member of the Institute of Medicine's Board on Health Promotion and Disease Prevention. He has published many articles and chapters, and five books, including *Depression Prevention: Research Directions* and *The Prevention of Depression: Research and Practice* (with Y.W. Ying).

HERBERT W. NICKENS is the first Vice-President of Minority Health, Education, and Prevention at the Association of American Medical Colleges. He received his A.B. from Harvard College and an M.D. and M.A. (in sociology) from the University of Pennsylvania. He is board certified by the American Board of Psychiatry and Neurology. He has held positions as the first Director of the Office of Minority Health at the U.S. Department of Health and Human Services; Director of the Office of Policy, Planning, and Analysis at the National Institute on Aging; and Deputy Chief, Center on Aging at NIMH. He is a member of the National Medical Association, the American Public Health Association, Black Psychiatrists of America, the Board of Directors of the American Association for Geriatric Psychiatrists, the Task Force on Minority Aging of the Gerontological Society of America, and the Board of Trustees of the Scientists' Institute for Public Information. He also serves as a consultant to the Council on Aging of the American Psychiatric Association. He has written numerous articles, and has lectured frequently on geriatrics, minority health, and AIDS.

RICHARD H. PRICE is Professor of Psychology and Research Scientist in the Survey Research Center, Institute for Social Research, University of Michigan. He is also Director of the Michigan Prevention Research Center, which focuses on the impact of working life on mental health. He is also chair of the Organizational Psychology Program at the University of Michigan. He received his A.B. from Lawrence College, and his A.M. and Ph.D. from the University of Illinois, Urbana. He has served as an advisor to NIMH, National Institute on Drug Abuse, the former Alcohol, Drug Abuse, and Mental Health Administration, the Carnegie Corporation of New York, and serves as a member of the board of directors of the William T. Grant Foundation. He is chair of the NIMH Prevention Research Steering Committee. He is a recipient of the Lela Rowland Prevention Award from the National Mental Health Association, and the Distinguished Contribution Award from the American Psychological Association. He is a Fellow of the American Psychological Association, the American Psychological Society, and the American Orthopsychiatric Association. He is the author or editor of a number of books and articles on mental health and prevention, including *Fourteen Ounces of Prevention: A Casebook for Practitioners* and *Prevention in Mental Health: Research, Policy, & Practice.*

NAOMI RAE GRANT is Professor and Head of the Division of Child Psychiatry and Professor of Pediatrics at The University of Western Ontario. She is also the Director of Treatment, Training, and Research at Child and Parent Resource Institute (CPRI). She received her medical and psychiatric education at the University of London (England), and has had extensive clinical experience in Canada and the United States. She came to Canada to head the Children's Services Branch of the Mental Health Division of the Ministry of Health. She has held senior positions in child psychiatry in London and Hamilton, and she was Clinical Director of the Child and Family Centre at Chedoke-McMaster Hospitals in Hamilton. She has held academic appointments at Washington University, University of Maryland, University of Toronto, and McMaster University. From 1986 to 1987, she was Chairman of the Association of Agencies for Treatment and Development in Hamilton. She is past president of the London Coordination Council for Children and Youth. She was formerly a member of the Premier's Council on Health Strategies, and of the Board of the Canadian Academy of Child Psychiatry. She is currently a member of the Board of the Group for the Advancement of Psychiatry, for which she also serves as Chairman of the Committee on Preventive Psychiatry. Her areas of special interest and research are prevention and the promotion of mental health in children and adolescents.

PATRICIA J. MRAZEK is Senior Program Officer and Study Director in the Institute of Medicine's Division of Biobehavioral Sciences and Mental

Disorders. She obtained her M.S.W. in social work from Smith College and her Ph.D. in family development from Union Graduate School. She was a Sheldon Fellow in the Advanced Family Therapy Program at the Tavistock Clinic in London, England. For many years she worked with C. Henry Kempe as the Assistant Director of the National Center for the Prevention and Treatment of Child Abuse and Neglect at the University of Colorado Health Sciences Center. Her interests and publications have focused on child maltreatment and the prevention of asthma in young children. She recently became the Executive Director of the Institute for the Advancement of Social Work Research in Washington, D.C.

CAROLYN E. PETERS is Research Assistant for the Committee on Prevention of Mental Disorders. Her previous experience at the Institute of Medicine involved work in the Division of Biobehavioral Sciences and Mental Disorders and on the AIDS Roundtable. She received her B.A. in English from Dickinson College.

CAROL M. HOSPENTHAL serves as Project Assistant for the Committee on the Prevention of Mental Disorders. Before joining the Institute of Medicine, she received her B.A. from Davenport College of Business and worked as Administrative Assistant for the Lions Clubs of Michigan State Office.

ROSEANNE PRICE received her B.A. degree in American literature and experimental psychology from Rockford College, where she was elected to Phi Beta Kappa. She received her scientific editorial training at the American Geophysical Union in Washington, D.C. From 1978 to 1990, she served as Staff Editor for various units of the National Academy of Sciences, most recently as the Director of the Editorial Office of the Commission on Physical Sciences, Mathematics, and Resources of the National Research Council. Since 1990, she has worked independently as an editor and writer for a number of scientific organizations.

Acknowledgments

Ron Abeles, National Institute on Aging

Naleen Andrade, University of Hawaii

Virginia Anthony, American Academy of Child and Adolescent Psychiatry

Joan Asarnow, University of California, Los Angeles

Cheryl Austein, Office of the Assistant Secretary for Planning and Evaluation, DHHS

Mohamet Badawi, The Johns Hopkins University

Jack Barchas, Cornell University Medical College

Kathryn Barnard, University of Washington

Heather Barton, National Mental Health Association

Rhoda Baruch, The Institute for Mental Health Initiatives

Leila Beckwith, University of California, Los Angeles

Myron Belfer, Substance Abuse and Mental Health Services Administration

Richard Bonnie, University of Virginia

Gail Boyd, National Institute of Alcohol Abuse and Alcoholism

Lester Breslow, University of California, Los Angeles

William Bukoski, National Institute on Drug Abuse

William Bunney, University of California, Irvine

Thomas Burroughs, Consultant, Durham, NC

William Carpenter, Maryland Psychiatric Research Center

Wendy Chavkin, Columbia University

Dante Cicchetti, University of Rochester

John Coie, Duke University

James Cromwell, National Alliance for the Mentally Ill

Cal Crutchfield, National Association of Prevention Professionals and Advocates

Robert Czeh, National Institute of Mental Health

Patrick DeLeon, Senator Inouye's Office

Norman Dinges, University of Alaska, Fairbanks

Carl Dunst, Western Carolina Center, Morganton, NC

Felton Earls, Harvard Medical School

Byron Egeland, University of Minnesota

Leona Eggert, University of Washington

Leon Eisenberg, Harvard Medical School

John Farquhar, Stanford University

Stephen Fawcett, University of Kansas

Manning Feinleib, National Center for Health Statistics

Tiffany Field, University of Miami Medical School

Michael Fishman, Maternal and Child Health Bureau

Laurie Flynn, National Alliance for the Mentally Ill

L. Patt Franciosi, National Prevention Coalition

Vincent Francisco, University of Kansas

Loretta Fuddy, Hawaii State Department of Health

Ronald Gallimore, University of California, Los Angeles

Helen Gee, Consultant, Washington, DC

Miriam Gersfield, National Institutes of Health

Shirley Glynn, West Los Angeles VA Medical Center

Thomas Glynn, National Cancer Institute

Frederick Goodwin, National Institute of Mental Health

Irving Gottesman, University of Virginia

Mark Greenberg, University of Washington

Bernard Guyer, The Johns Hopkins University

Barbara Haight, Medical University of South Carolina

Laura Hall, Office of Technology Assessment

William Hansen, Bowman Gray School of Medicine

James Harrell, Office of Disease Prevention and Health Promotion, DHHS

Nancy Henkin, Temple University

James Herbert, Medical College of Pennsylvania at EPPI

Ralph Hingson, Boston University

Harold Holder, Prevention Research Center, Berkeley, CA

Wade Horn, Administration for Children, Youth and Families

Jan Howard, National Institute of Alcohol Abuse and Alcoholism

Mary Jansen, Substance Abuse and Mental Health Services Administration

Leonard Jason, DePaul University

Peter Jensen, National Institute of Mental Health

Dale Johnson, University of Houston

Marshall Jones, Milton S. Hershey Medical Center

John Kalberer, National Institutes of Health

Robert Katzman, University of California, San Diego

Sheppard Kellam, The Johns Hopkins University

Edward Kelty, National Institute of Mental Health

Zaven Khatchaturian, National Institute on Aging

Ruth Knee, American Orthopsychiatric Association

Robert Koegel, University of California, Santa Barbara

Doreen Spilton Koretz, National Institute of Mental Health

Helena Chmura Kraemer, Stanford University

Leonard Lash, National Institute of Mental Health

James Leckman, Yale University

Alan Leshner, National Institute of Mental Health

Vicki Levin, National Institute of Mental Health

Peter Lewinsohn, University of Oregon

Rhonda Lewis, University of Kansas

Alicia Lieberman, San Francisco General Hospital

Maurey Lieberman, Substance Abuse and Mental Health Services Administration

Marsha Liss, National Center on Child Abuse and Neglect

Kenneth Lutterman, National Institute of Mental Health

Harriet MacMillan, McMaster University

Beryce MacLennan, Private practice, Washington, DC

Wallace Mandell, The Johns Hopkins University

Ann Maney, National Institute of Mental Health

Katie Maslow, Office of Technology Assessment

Neil Mazer, Hawaii State Department of Health

Sandy McElhaney, National Mental Health Association

Dan McFerran, Department of Defense

Roger Meyer, University of Connecticut

Jim Mintz, University of California, Los Angeles

Leonard Mitnick, National Institute of Mental Health

Terrie Moffitt, University of Wisconsin, Madison

Bill Mollerstrom, Department of Defense

John Morgan, Chesterfield Community Services Board, Chesterfield, VA

Eve Moscicki, National Institute of Mental Health

Marilyn Moses, National Institute of Justice

Joseph Mottola, Administration for Children, Youth and Families

David Mrazek, Children's National Medical Center, Washington, DC

Peter Muehrer, National Institute of Mental Health

Kim Mueser, Medical College of Pennsylvania at EPPI

Holly Neckerman, Harborview Injury Prevention Research Center, Seattle, WA

Harold Neighbors, University of Michigan

Godfrey Oakley, Centers for Disease Control and Prevention

Dan Offord, Chedoke-McMaster Hospital, Hamilton, Ontario

Adrienne Paine, University of Kansas

Paula Panzer, Columbia University

Delores Parron, National Institute of Mental Health

David Pauls, Yale University

Roseanne Price, Consultant, Silver Spring, MD

Juan Ramos, National Institute of Mental Health

John Reid, Oregon Social Learning Center

David Reiss, George Washington University Medical Center

Dorothy Rice, University of California, San Francisco

Kimber Richter, University of Kansas

Henry Riecken, University of Pennsylvania

John Romano, University of Rochester

William Roper, Centers for Disease Control and Prevention

Mark Rosenberg, Centers for Disease Control and Prevention

Jack Rothman, University of California, Los Angeles

Michael Rutter, Institute of Psychiatry, London, England

Irwin Sandler, Arizona State University

James Schlie, Department of Defense

Marc Schuckitt, University of California, San Diego

Myrna Shure, Hahnemann University

Lonnie Snowden, University of California, Berkeley

Ruth Stein, Albert Einstein College of Medicine
Barbara Strane, Institute of Social Research
Joseph Strayhorn, Allegheny General Hospital, PA
Frank Sullivan, Substance Abuse and Mental Health Services Administration
Ruby Takinishi, Carnegie Council on Adolescent Development
Stephen Teret, The Johns Hopkins Injury Prevention Center
E. Fuller Torrey, St. Elizabeth's Hospital, Washington, DC
Edward Trickett, University of Maryland

William Vega, University of California, Berkeley
Alexander Wagenaar, University of Minnesota
Joseph Webb, Centers for Disease Control and Prevention
Roger Weissberg, University of Illinois at Chicago
Myrna Weissman, Columbia University
Valerie Welsh, Office of the Assistant Secretary for Health, DHHS
Peter Whitehouse, Case Western Reserve University
Susan Wolf, Harvard University
Stuart Youngner, University Hospitals of Cleveland

Institute of Medicine and National Research Council Staff:

Laura Baird	Michael Edington	Nina Spruill
Enriqueta Bond	Gary Ellis	Susanne Stoiber
Claudia Carl	Michael Lai	Mike Stoto
Rosemary Chalk	Constance Pechura	Betsy Turvene
Robert Cook-Deegan	Kenneth Shine	Audrey Ward
Molla Donaldson	Gail Spears	Karl Yordy

NOTE: Individuals are listed with the affiliations they had at the time they contributed to the report.

C

Workshops

WORKSHOP ON APPLICATION OF RISK FACTOR/PREVENTIVE MODEL FROM PHYSICAL HEALTH CARE TO MENTAL DISORDERS

July 20, 1992

Institute of Medicine
2101 Constitution Avenue, N.W.
Washington, D.C. 20418

Agenda

8:00 am   Continental Breakfast (available in meeting room)

8:30 am   Welcome and Introduction to the Work Group Objectives
             William Beardslee, M.D., Chair

8:45 am   Introduction of Members of Work Group and Guests

9:00 am   Topic I: Cardiovascular Risk Factors and Prevention
             Presenter
             John Farquhar, M.D.
             Professor of Health Research and Policy
             Stanford Center for Research in Disease Prevention
             Palo Alto, CA

9:40 am   Response from Mental Health Field: Depression
William Beardslee, M.D.
Associate Professor of Psychiatry
Harvard Medical School
Clinical Director, Department of Psychiatry
Judge Baker Children's Center, Boston

10:00 am   Discussion

10:30 am   BREAK

10:40 am   Topic II: Smoking Prevention and Cessation
Presenter
Thomas Glynn, Ph.D.
Chief, Prevention and Control Extramural Research Branch
Division of Cancer Prevention and Control
National Cancer Institute

11:20 am   Response from Mental Health Field: Substance Abuse
Roger Meyer, M.D.
Professor and Chair
Department of Psychiatry
Executive Dean
University of Connecticut School of Medicine

11:40 am   Discussion

12:10 pm   Comments and Discussion of Policy Implications of the
(20 min)   Morning Discussion
Leon Eisenberg, M.D.
Presley Professor
Department of Social Medicine
Harvard Medical School

                    Doreen Koretz, Ph.D.
Assistant Chief
Prevention Research Branch
National Institute of Mental Health

12:45 pm   LUNCH IN MEETING ROOM
Welcome from Committee Chair
Robert Haggerty, M.D., Chair and
Professor of Pediatrics Emeritus

University of Rochester School of Medicine and Dentistry, and
Former President
William T. Grant Foundation

1:30 pm   Topic III: Safety and Trauma Prevention
                Stephen Teret, J.D., M.P.H.
                Director
                Johns Hopkins Injury Prevention Center
                Baltimore, MD

2:10 pm   Respondent from Mental Health Field: Violence
                Mark Rosenberg, M.D., M.P.P.
                National Center for Injury Prevention and Control
                Centers for Disease Control

2:30 pm   BREAK

2:35 pm   Respondent from Mental Health Field: Violence
                Paula G. Panzer, M.D.
                Postdoctoral Clinical Fellow
                College of Physicians and Surgeons
                Columbia University
                Public Psychiatry Fellow
                NY State Psychiatric Institute

3:00 pm   Comments and Discussion of Policy Implications of the
(20 min)   Afternoon Discussion
                Leon Eisenberg, M.D.
                Presley Professor
                Department of Social Medicine
                Harvard Medical School

                Doreen Koretz, Ph.D.
                Assistant Chief
                Prevention Research Branch
                National Institute of Mental Health

3:20 pm   Comments on the Day and Round Table Discussion Led By
                Lester Breslow, M.D., M.P.H.
                Dean Emeritus and Professor of Public Health
                UCLA School of Public Health

4:30 pm   ADJOURN

Participants

WILLIAM BEARDSLEE, M.D. (Workshop Chair), Associate Professor of Psychiatry at Harvard Medical School, Clinical Director, Department of Psychiatry, Judge Baker Children's Center, Boston, Massachusetts

LESTER BRESLOW, M.D., M.P.H., Dean Emeritus and Professor of Public Health, UCLA School of Public Health, University of California, Los Angeles, Los Angeles, California

LEON EISENBERG, M.D., Presley Professor, Department of Social Medicine, Harvard Medical School, Boston, Massachusetts

JOHN W. FARQUHAR, M.D., Professor of Medicine, Professor of Health Research and Policy, Director, Stanford Center for Research in Disease Prevention, Palo Alto, California

THOMAS J. GLYNN, Ph.D., Chief, Prevention and Control, Extramural Research Branch, Division of Cancer Prevention and Control, National Cancer Institute, Bethesda, Maryland

ROBERT J. HAGGERTY, M.D., Professor of Pediatrics Emeritus, University of Rochester School of Medicine and Dentistry, Rochester, New York

DOREEN SPILTON KORETZ, Ph.D., Assistant Chief, Prevention Research Branch, National Institute of Mental Health, Rockville, Maryland

ROGER MEYER, M.D., Professor and Chair, Department of Psychiatry, Executive Dean, University of Connecticut School of Medicine, Farmington, Connecticut

PAULA PANZER, M.D., College of Physicians and Surgeons, Columbia University, New York, New York

MARK ROSENBERG, M.D., M.P.P., National Center for Injury Prevention and Control, Centers for Disease Control and Prevention, Atlanta, Georgia

STEPHEN TERET, J.D., M.P.H., Director, Johns Hopkins Injury Prevention Center, Baltimore, Maryland

Invited Guests

BERNARD GUYER, M.D., M.P.H., Professor and Chairman, Department of Maternal and Child Health, Johns Hopkins School of Hygiene and Public Health, Baltimore, Maryland

BEATRIX A. HAMBURG, M.D., President, William T. Grant Foundation, New York, New York

BEVERLY LONG, M.S., M.S.P.H., Chair, International Committee on Primary Prevention, World Federation for Mental Health, Atlanta, Georgia

ANN MANEY, Ph.D., Social Science Analyst, Office of Prevention and Special Projects, National Institute of Mental Health, Rockville, Maryland

JUAN RAMOS, Ph.D., Deputy Director, Office of Prevention and Special Projects, National Institute of Mental Health, Rockville, Maryland

Institute of Medicine and National Research Council Staff

JESSICA BACKER, Research Assistant, Panel on Research on Child Abuse and Commission on Behavioral and Social Sciences and Education (CBASSE)

ROSEMARY A. CHALK, Study Director, Panel on Research on Child Abuse and Neglect, CBASSE

ROBERT M. COOK-DEEGAN, M.D., Director, Division of Biobehavioral Sciences and Mental Disorders

MOLLA S. DONALDSON, M.S., Senior Staff Officer

GARY B. ELLIS, Ph.D., Director, Division of Health Promotion and Disease Prevention

CAROL M. HOSPENTHAL, Project Assistant, Study on Prevention of Mental Disorders

PATRICIA J. MRAZEK, M.S.W., Ph.D., Study Director, Committee on Prevention of Mental Disorders

CAROLYN E. PETERS, Research Assistant, Study on Prevention of Mental Disorders

SUSANNE A. STOIBER, Director, Division on Social and Economic Studies, CBASSE

MICHAEL A. STOTO, Ph.D., Deputy Director, Division of Health Promotion and Disease Prevention

SPECIAL POPULATIONS WORK GROUP

December 14, 1992

Hyatt Regency San Francisco Airport
Burlingame, California

Participants

NALEEN ANDRADE, M.D., Associate Professor, Department of Psychiatry, University of Hawaii, Honolulu, Hawaii

SPERO MANSON, Ph.D. (Work Group Chair), Professor and Director, National Center for American Indians and Alaska Natives Mental Health Research, University of Colorado Health Sciences Center, Denver, Colorado

RICARDO MUÑOZ, Ph.D., Professor of Psychology, Department of Psychiatry, University of California, San Francisco, San Francisco, California

HAROLD NEIGHBORS, Ph.D., Research Scientist, Research Center for Black Americans, Institute for Social Research, Ann Arbor, Michigan

JUAN RAMOS, Ph.D., Deputy Director, Office of Prevention and Special Projects, National Institute of Mental Health, Rockville, Maryland

LONNIE SNOWDEN, Ph.D., School of Social Welfare, University of California, Berkeley, California

RUBY TAKANISHI, Ph.D., Executive Director, Carnegie Council on Adolescent Development, Washington, D.C.

WILLIAM VEGA, Ph.D., Professor, School of Public Health, University of California, Berkeley, California

Institute of Medicine Staff

PATRICIA J. MRAZEK, M.S.W., Ph.D., Study Director, Committee on Prevention of Mental Disorders, Institute of Medicine, Washington, D.C.

WORKSHOP ON ETHICAL CONSIDERATIONS IN PREVENTIVE INTERVENTION RESEARCH

March 22, 1993

Institute of Medicine
The Foundry Building
1055 Thomas Jefferson Street, NW
Washington, DC 20007

Participants

ROSEMARY A. CHALK, Study Director, Panel on Research on Child Abuse and Neglect, CBASSE

WENDY CHAVKIN, M.D., Associate Professor of Clinical Public Health and Obstetrics-Gynecology, Columbia University School of Public Health and College of Physicians and Surgeons, New York, New York

SUSAN WOLF, J.D., Fellow, Program in Ethics and the Professions, Harvard University, Cambridge, Massachusetts

STUART YOUNGNER, M.D., Associate Professor of Medicine, Psychiatry and Biomedical Ethics, University Hospitals of Cleveland, Division of General Internal Medicine, Cleveland, Ohio

Committee Members

ROBERT J. HAGGERTY, M.D. (Committee Chair), Professor Emeritus, Department of Pediatrics, University of Rochester School of Medicine and Dentistry, Rochester, New York

BEATRIX HAMBURG, M.D. (Committee Vice-Chair), President, William T. Grant Foundation, New York, New York

Institute of Medicine Staff

PATRICIA MRAZEK, M.S.W., Ph.D., Study Director

CAROLYN PETERS, Research Assistant

CAROL HOSPENTHAL, Project Assistant

Consultant

TOM BURROUGHS, Science Writer

D

Background Materials

The background materials for this report consist of the following:

- 6 commissioned papers and 2 commentaries,
- 39 abstracts of illustrative preventive intervention programs using randomized controlled trial design (see Chapter 7), and
- a bibliography of over 2,000 background references in Pro-Cite and ASCII format.

These materials can be accessed in the following ways:

- The commissioned papers and abstracts are available on disk (in Wordperfect 5.0) from the Institute of Medicine only until June 1, 1994. The disk can be obtained by returning the card found inside this book or by calling (202) 334-2328.
- After June 1, 1994, the commissioned papers and abstracts will become available through the National Technical Information Service (NTIS) at (703) 487-4650 or 800-553-6847, or through the National Institute of Mental Health while supplies last. When calling NTIS, please have the following order number ready: PB94-121860.
- The bibliography and supporting documentation are available on the National Academy of Sciences' anonymous ftp server (ftp.nas.edu), in the directory /reports/reducing_risks.

The complete table of contents of *Reducing Risks for Mental Disorders: Frontiers for Preventive Intervention Research* appears in each of these data bases. The table of contents for the background materials is as follows:

Commissioned Papers and Commentaries

Prevention of Mental Disorders in Children .... Joan Asarnow
and Robert Koegel
Mental Health Promotion .... Norman G. Dinges
Conducting Preventive Interventions for
Community Mental Health .... Stephen B. Fawcett,
Adrienne L. Paine, Vincent T. Francisco,
Kimber P. Richter, and Rhonda K. Lewis
Commentary on Fawcett et al. paper .... Ronald Gallimore
Commentary on Fawcett et al. paper .... Jack Rothman
Treatment of Adult Psychiatric Disorders: Implications for
Prevention Efforts .... Shirley M. Glynn, Kim T. Mueser,
and James D. Herbert
Design and Analysis Issues for Trials of Prevention
Programs in Mental Health Research ...... Helena Chmura Kraemer
and Karen L. Kraemer
Genetic Knowledge and Prevention of
Mental Disorders .... Michael Rutter

Abstracts of Illustrative Preventive Intervention Research Programs

Infants
Prenatal/Early Infancy Project
Tactile/Kinesthetic Stimulation
Early Intervention for Preterm Infants
Infant Health and Development Program
Carolina Abecedarian Project

Young Children
Houston Parent-Child Development Center
Mother-Child Home Program of Verbal Interaction Project
Parent-Child Interaction Training
High/Scope Preschool Curriculum Comparison Study (including Distar)
Perry Preschool Program (using High/Scope curriculum)
I Can Problem Solve: Interpersonal Cognitive Problem-Solving Program

Elementary-Age Children
Assertiveness Training Program (program 1)
Assertiveness Training Program (program 2)
Children of Divorce Intervention Program
Family Bereavement Program

Social Skills Training
Social Relations Intervention Program
Montreal Longitudinal-Experimental Study
Community Epidemiological Preventive Intervention: Mastery Learning and Good Behavior Game
Academic Tutoring and Social Skills Training
Seattle Social Development Project

Adolescents

Changing Teaching Practices
Positive Youth Development Program
Adolescent Alcohol Prevention Trial
ALERT Drug Prevention
Alcohol Education Project
Midwestern Prevention Project
Behaviorally Based Preventive Intervention
Intervention Campaign Against Bully-Victim Problems

Adults

Prevention and Relationship Enhancement Program (PREP): An Empirically Based Preventive Intervention Program for Couples
University of Colorado Separation and Divorce Program
Perceived Personal Control Preventive Intervention for a Caesarean Birth Population
Prenatal/Early Infancy Project
Caregiver Support Program for Coping with Occupational Stress
JOBS Project for the Unemployed: Michigan Prevention Research Center
San Francisco Depression Prevention Research Project
Projecto Bienestar: An Intervention for Preventing Depression in Hispanic Immigrant Women in the Community
Peer- and Professionally-Led Groups to Support Family Caregivers

Elderly

Widow-to-Widow: A Mutual Help Program for the Widowed

Bibliography of Background References

E

Journals Publishing Prevention Articles Related to Mental Disorders

The following list contains the 224 journals that published prevention articles related to mental disorders, as compiled in the NIMH prevention bibliography, 1983 to 1991 (Trickett, E. J.; Dahiyat, C.; Selby, P. (in press) *Primary Prevention in Mental Health: An Annotated Bibliography.* Rockville, MD: Department of Health and Human Services). The bibliography has 1,326 entries, 109 of which were excluded from this analysis because they centered on AIDS, a topic outside the committee's purview. Of the remaining entries, 808 are journal articles. The number of articles in each journal is listed below.

Academic Medicine (1)
Acta Psychiatrica Scandinavica (6)
Addictive Behaviors (3)
Administration in Mental Health (2)
Adolescence (3)
Adolescent Psychiatry (1)
Advances in Adolescent Mental Health (1)
Advances in Developmental and Behavioral Pediatrics (1)
Advances in Learning and Behavioral Disabilities (1)
Aging and Prevention (3)
Alcohol and Alcoholism (2)

Alcoholism Treatment Quarterly (1)
American Educational Research Journal (1)
American Indian and Alaska Native Mental Health Research (1)
American Journal of Community Psychology (49)
American Journal of Diseases of Children (1)
American Journal of Drug and Alcohol Abuse (3)
American Journal of Family Therapy (1)

American Journal of Mental Deficiency (1)

American Journal of Mental Retardation (1)

American Journal of Orthopsychiatry (19)

American Journal of Preventive Medicine (2)

American Journal of Psychiatry (6)

American Journal of Public Health (4)

American Psychologist (18)

Analysis and Intervention in Developmental Disabilities (1)

Annual Progress in Child Psychiatry and Child Development (2)

Annual Review of Psychology (2)

Annual Review of Public Health (2)

Applied Psychology: An International Review (1)

Archives of General Psychiatry (1)

Archives of Physical Medicine and Rehabilitation (1)

Archives of Psychiatric Nursing (1)

Australasian Journal of Special Education (1)

Australia and New Zealand Journal of Psychiatry (1)

Australian Psychologist (1)

Behavior Genetics (1)

Behavior Therapy (2)

Behaviour Change (1)

Biological Psychiatry (1)

British Journal of Addiction (2)

British Journal of Psychiatry (1)

British Review of Bulimia and Anorexia Nervosa (1)

Bulletin of the Hong Kong Psychological Society (1)

Bulletin of the Society of Psychologists in Addictive Behaviors (1)

Canada's Mental Health (2)

Canadian Journal of Behavioral Science (1)

Canadian Journal of Community Mental Health (1)

Canadian Journal of Counselling (1)

Canadian Journal of Psychiatry (5)

Child Abuse and Neglect: The International Journal (18)

Child and Youth Services (1)

Child Development (5)

Child Psychiatry and Human Development (1)

Child Welfare (3)

Children and Youth Services Review (4)

Clinical Medicine in North America (1)

Clinical Nursing in North America (1)

The Clinical Psychologist (1)

Clinical Psychology Review (4)

College Student Journal (1)

Community Mental Health in New Zealand (1)

Community Mental Health Journal (10)

The Counseling Psychologist (2)

Criminal Justice and Behavior (2)

Critical Social Policy CSP (1)

Death Studies (1)

Developmental and Behavioral Pediatrics (1)

Developmental Psychology (2)

Deviant Behavior (1)

Early Child Development and Care (1)

Education and Treatment of Children (3)

Education and Urban Society (1)

Educational and Child Psychology (1)

Elementary School Guidance and Counseling (1)

Estudios de Psicologia (1)

Evaluaciaon Psicolaogica (1)

Evaluation Review (2)

Evaluation and the Health Professions (4)

Exceptional Children (3)

Family and Community Health (1)

Family Planning Perspectives (2)

Family Process (1)

Family Relations (2)

Family Relations Journal of Applied Family and Child Studies (1)

Family Systems Medicine (1)

Gerontologist (2)

Health and Social Work (1)

Health Education (1)

Health Education Quarterly (4)

Health Education Research (2)

Health Promotion (1)

Health Psychology (6)

High School Journal (1)

Hospice Journal (1)

Hospital and Community Psychiatry (3)

Human Organization (1)

Infant Mental Health Journal (10)

Integrative Psychiatry (1)

Interchange (1)

International Journal of Eating Disorders (1)

International Journal of Educational Development (1)

International Journal of Health Services (1)

International Journal of Offender Therapy and Comparative Criminology (1)

International Journal of Social Psychiatry (1)

International Journal of the Addictions (7)

International Nursing Review (2)

Issues in Mental Health Nursing (2)

Journal for Specialists in Group Work (2)

Journal of Abnormal Child Psychology (3)

Journal of Abnormal Psychology (1)

Journal of Adolescence (2)

Journal of Advanced Nursing (1)

Journal of Alcohol and Drug Education (4)

Journal of American College Health (3)

Journal of Applied Behavior Analysis (3)

Journal of Applied Developmental Psychology (1)

Journal of Applied Psychology (2)

Journal of Applied Social Psychology (5)

Journal of Behavioral Medicine (6)

Journal of Child and Adolescent Psychiatric and Mental Health Nursing (1)

Journal of Child Psychiatry (1)

Journal of Child Psychology and Psychiatry (2)

Journal of Children in Contemporary Society (3)

Journal of Clinical Child Psychology (4)

Journal of Clinical Psychiatry (1)

Journal of College Student Psychotherapy (1)

Journal of Community Psychology (13)

Journal of Counseling and Development (2)

Journal of Counseling Psychology (1)

Journal of Consulting and Clinical Psychology (18)

Journal of Developmental and Behavioral Pediatrics (1)

Journal of Divorce (3)

Journal of Drug Education (24)

Journal of Drug Issues (6)

Journal of Educational Psychology (1)

The Journal of Educational Research (1)

Journal of Health and Social Behavior (1)

Journal of Pediatric Psychology (1)

Journal of Personality (1)

Journal of Preventive Psychiatry and Allied Disciplines (25)

Journal of Primary Prevention (82)

Journal of Psychoactive Drugs (3)

Journal of Psychosocial Nursing and Mental Health Services (2)

Journal of Psychosocial Oncology (1)

Journal of Public Health Policy (2)

Journal of Reading, Writing and Learning Disabilities International (1)

Journal of Research in Crime and Delinquency (1)

Journal of School Health (15)

Journal of School Psychology (2)

Journal of Social Issues (1)

Journal of Social Service Research (1)

Journal of Sociology and Social Welfare (1)

Journal of Studies on Alcohol (6)

Journal of Youth and Adolescence (2)

Journal of the American Academy of Child and Adolescent Psychiatry (8)

Journal of the American Medical Association (4)

Journal of the Division for Early Childhood (2)

Journal of the Florida Medical Association (1)

Journal of the Multihandicapped Person (1)

Language, Speech and Hearing Services in Schools (1)

Medical Law (1)

Mental Retardation (1)

Military Medicine (1)

MOBIUS (1)

Narcotics Bulletin (2)

Neurologic Clinics (1)

New Directions for Child Development (1)

New Directions for Mental Health Services (3)

New Directions for Student Services (1)

Occupational Medicine (2)

Oxford Review of Education (1)

Patient Education and Counseling (1)

Pediatrics (2)

Personality and Social Psychology Bulletin (1)

Personnel and Guidance Journal (23)

Pointer (1)

Prevention in Human Services (92)

Preventive Medicine (2)

Professional Psychology (3)

Professional School Psychology (1)

Progress in Behavior Modification (1)

Psychiatric Annals (1)

Psychiatric Clinics of North America (1)

Psychiatric Quarterly (1)

Psychiatrie and Psychobiologie (1)

Psychiatry (3)

Psychological Bulletin (3)

Psychology and Aging (2)

Psychology and Health (1)

Psychology in the Schools (2)

Psychology of Addictive Behaviors (1)

Psychotherapy and Psychosomatics (3)

Psychotherapy Bulletin (1)

Public Health Nursing (1)

Public Health Reports (7)

Public Health Reviews (1)

Public Welfare (1)

Residential Treatment for Children and Youth (1)

Review of Educational Research (1)

Schizophrenia Bulletin (4)

The School Counselor (3)

School Psychologist (1)

School Psychology Review (10)

Schweizer Archiv fuer Neurologie, Neurchirurgie und Psychiatrie (1)

Science (1)

Seminars in Perinatology (1)

Social Policy (1)

Social Psychiatry and Psychiatric Epidemiology (1)

Social Science and Medicine (7)

Social Service Review (1)

Social Work (2)

Social Work in Education (1)

Social Work Research and Abstracts (1)

Southern Exposure (1)

Special Services in the Schools (3)

Suicide and Life-Threatening Behavior (2)

Teaching and Teacher Education (1)

Updating School Board Policies (1)

Violence and Victims (1)

White Cloud Journal of American Indian Mental Health (1)

Women and Health (1)

Youth and Society (1)

Zero to Three (2)

Index